BIOPSY INTERPRETATION SERIES

BIOPSY INTERPRETATION OF THE BONE MARROW

BIOPSY INTERPRETATION SERIES

BIOPSY INTERPRETATION OF THE BONE MARROW

Laura M. Wake, MD
Assistant Professor of Pathology
Program Director, Hematopathology Fellowship
Department of Pathology
Johns Hopkins
Baltimore, Maryland

Genevieve Crane, MD, PhD
Staff Hematopathologist
Medical Director Manual Hematology
Pathology and Lab Medicine Institute
Cleveland Clinic, Cleveland, OH

Michael J. Borowitz, MD, PhD
Professor of Pathology and Oncology
Johns Hopkins Medical Institutions
Baltimore, Maryland

Wolters Kluwer

Philadelphia • Baltimore • New York • London
Buenos Aires • Hong Kong • Sydney • Tokyo

Acquisitions Editor: Nicole Dernoski
Senior Development Editor: Ariel S. Winter
Editorial Coordinator: Sunmerrilika Baskar
Marketing Manager: Kirsten Watrud
Production Project Manager: Justin Wright
Design Coordinator: Stephen Druding
Manufacturing Coordinator: Beth Welsh
Prepress Vendor: S4Carlisle Publishing Services

First Edition

9 8 7 6 5 4 3 2 1

Printed in Mexico

Library of Congress Cataloging-in-Publication Data

ISBN-13: 978-1-4963-0059-1
ISBN-10: 1-4963-0059-9

Library of Congress Control Number: 2023908197

shop.lww.com

QUADM0623

DEDICATION

We are privileged to work alongside some of the most dedicated and hardworking pathology residents and fellows in the nation. We wrote this book with these learners in mind.

PREFACE

Producing a volume devoted to the bone marrow for the excellent "Biopsy Interpretation" series presented a unique challenge. More than virtually any other organ, histologic examination of a bone marrow represents only a small portion of what is needed to establish a patient diagnosis. Complete workup of hematologic diseases also requires examination of Wright-Giemsa-stained marrow aspirates and blood smears, and numerous ancillary tests, ranging from histochemical stains to flow cytometry to genetic sequencing. Clinical presentation and treatment history also impact interpretation of results. We wanted neither to write yet another textbook of hematopathology, nor to simply provide an atlas of morphologic curiosities, but rather to help guide readers through the sometimes complex morphologic and ancillary interpretations necessary for reaching a diagnosis. Although the bulk of the book takes the reader through myeloid and lymphoid diseases that involve the marrow, introductory chapters also cover the approach and basic tools needed to study marrow diseases. The book starts with a discussion of the peripheral blood and the abnormalities that may prompt an initial bone marrow examination. Also included is a separate chapter describing the important ancillary techniques needed for diagnosis with illustrations both in that chapter and, as appropriate, throughout the book.

Each of the major chapters also includes text about the entities illustrated, describing both their diagnostic and clinical characteristics to better contextualize the illustrations. This presented us with our second challenge. During the writing of this book, both the World Health Organization (WHO) and the International Consensus Classification (ICC) published new classifications of myeloid and lymphoid neoplasms. These updates incorporated new knowledge about the biology of hematopoietic neoplasms and created new categories not previously recognized. In addition, however, the updates also introduced new words for categories we previously knew, and sometimes the two efforts recognized the same entities but gave them different names. In writing this, we tried to be accurate in our use of the new terminology, but not to overwhelm the reader in the language nor with the complex and rapidly changing understanding of the disease biology. It may comfort the reader to know that we experts in this field are also striving for clarity throughout these changes. However, rather than focusing on names, or on the differences between the two classification schemes, our aim in this book is to focus on general principles, starting with morphology. Terminology and classifications change over time, but certain qualities remain constant; whatever one might call them, the pictures in this book represent real diseases that afflict real patients. We hope that our illustrations and the discussion of pertinent and relevant points of these diseases will help pathologists care for the patients they see throughout their careers.

CONTENTS

1

PERIPHERAL BLOOD FINDINGS AND THE INDICATIONS FOR A BONE MARROW EXAMINATION

The most common indications for a bone marrow (BM) examination are abnormalities of the complete blood count (CBC; Table 1.1), primarily cytopenias or cytoses. Cytopenias and cytoses can be hereditary or acquired and may reflect either reactive or neoplastic conditions.

Cytopenia: Decreased quantity of cells or platelets in the peripheral blood (PB), which may be symptomatic, causing a noticeable detriment to the patient, or may be asymptomatic, detected only with routine bloodwork

Anemia: decreased red blood cell (RBC) number and/or hemoglobin (Hgb) or hematocrit (Hct)
Leukopenia: decreased white blood cell (WBC) count
Thrombocytopenia: decreased platelet count

Cytosis: Increased quantity of cells or platelets in the PB, a finding that is less common than cytopenia

Erythrocytosis: increased RBC number and/or Hgb or Hct
Leukocytosis: elevated WBC count
Thrombocytosis: increased platelet count

In most cases, patients with abnormal blood counts will not need a BM examination as clinical assessment and other laboratory tests can

TABLE 1.1 **Normal CBC**

CBC indices	Adult females	Adult males
White blood cell count	3.4-9.6 K/μL	3.4-9.6 K/μL
Red blood cell count	3.92-5.13 M/μL	4.35-5.65 M/μL
Hemoglobin	11.6-15 g/dL	13.2-16.6 g/dL
Hematocrit	35.5%-44.9%	38.3%-48.6%
Platelet count	157-371 K/μL	135-317 K/μL

CBC, complete blood count; K, thousand; M, million.

be used to help establish a diagnosis. In addition, patients with only mild quantitative abnormalities will often be followed clinically. However, persistent or unexplained abnormalities in blood counts may necessitate a BM examination and an accompanying PB film review.

Conversely, patients with normal PB counts may need a biopsy in various circumstances, such as when staging a patient to assess for BM metastasis or when a radiographic abnormality is detected.

In this chapter, we will discuss the cells of the PB and how their morphologic changes can help to interpret the marrow abnormalities discussed in more detail in subsequent chapters.

ANALYSIS OF CELLULAR ELEMENTS IN THE PB

Today most blood films are produced by automatic slide makers and stainers. Evaluation of blood morphology requires that the RBCs in the smear do not touch, but also not so spread apart as to produce artifacts, including the inability to see the normal biconcave disk shape of an RBC. Although automated slide makers typically adjust for the Hct, they often have a relatively limited area of optimal spread. For this reason, direct smears (on a pair of coverslips made by touching a drop of blood and spreading it on both coverslips quickly but smoothly) provide a larger optimal area for viewing.

GOLDEN ZONE

The ideal area to microscopically evaluate the slide is in the "golden zone," between the feathered edge with the "zone of holes" and the dense area, or "zone of cells," where the cellular morphology is easiest to interpret (Figure 1.1; eFigure 1.1).

RED BLOOD CELLS

Several RBC parameters are assessed during PB review, including the cellular composition, cellular morphology, and other factors. Noting the RBC quantity, size, shape, color, and the presence of inclusions will direct further laboratory testing and/or help develop a differential diagnosis.[1]

RBC Quantity

A thorough morphologic assessment includes assessing the quantity of RBCs, best appreciated as either an increase or a decrease in the "spaces" between RBCs on a PB smear. This should be correlated with RBC parameters on the CBC, as well as reticulocyte quantitation,[2,3] which helps determine the proliferative capacity of the BM and is often necessary for subclassifying anemias.

Morphologic Assessment of RBCs

RBC Size and Shape

Normal RBCs are round, anucleate biconcave disk-shaped cells with central pallor (Figure 1.2), 7 to 8 μm in size, or approximately the same size

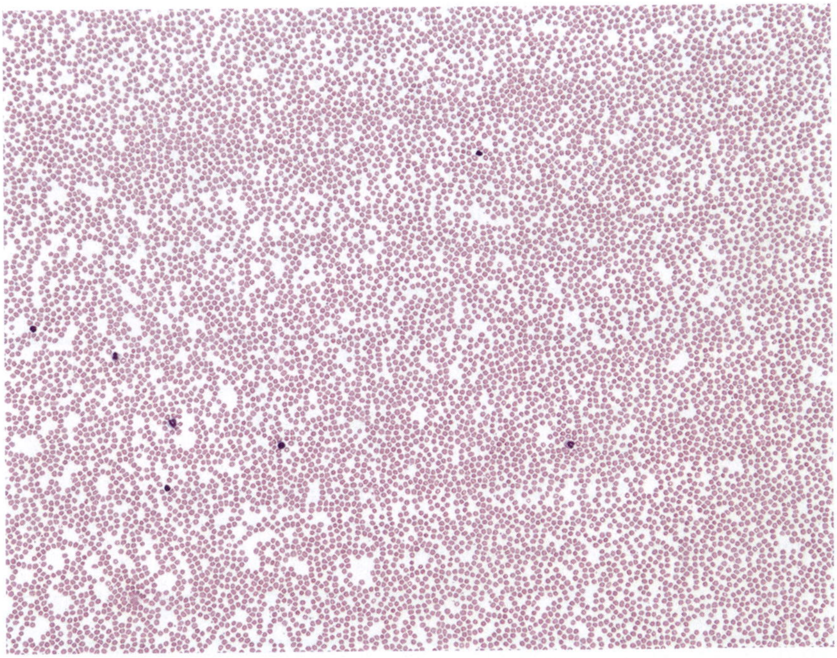

FIGURE 1.1 The "golden zone" in the peripheral blood smear is the optimal place to view cellular morphology.

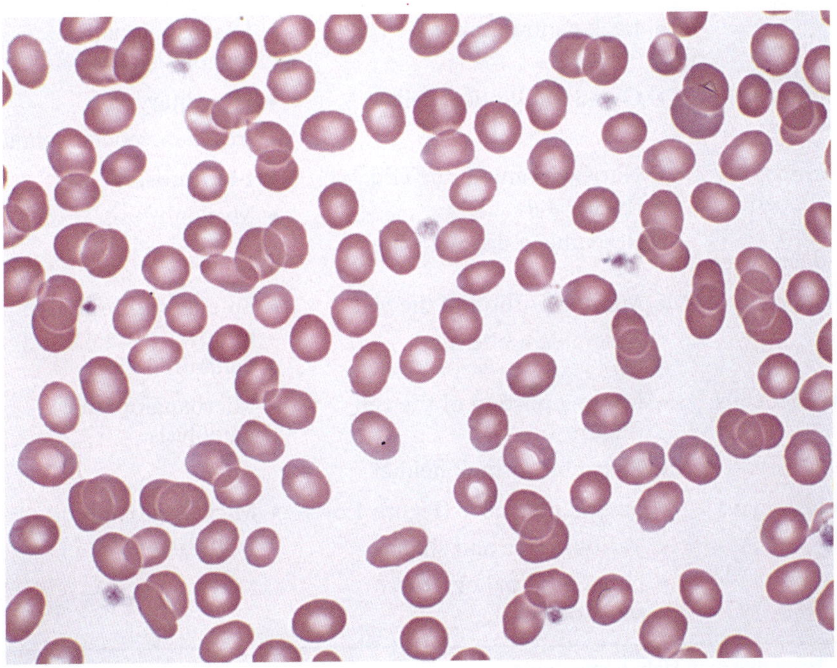

FIGURE 1.2 Normal red blood cells are round, anucleate biconcave disk-shaped cells with central pallor.

as a normal lymphocyte nucleus.[4] Abnormalities in RBC size (macrocytosis, microcytosis, or anisocytosis) or shape (poikilocytosis) may provide clues to the underlying pathology (Tables 1.2 and 1.3; Figures 1.3 to 1.6; eFigures 1.2 to 1.8). Although these are morphologic parameters, RBCs are objectively assessed in the CBC via the mean corpuscular volume (MCV) or, in the case of anisocytosis, the RBC distribution width (RDW). Marked anisopoikilocytosis can be seen in different reactive conditions and disease states, including myelodysplastic syndrome (MDS) (Figure 1.7).

TABLE 1.2 RBC Size

RBC size	Definition	Example of associated anemia
Microcytic	MCV <80 fL	Iron deficiency
Normocytic	MCV 80-100 fL	Blood loss
Macrocytic	MCV >100 fL	Vitamin B_{12} or folate deficiency

fL, femtoliters; MCV, mean corpuscular volume.

TABLE 1.3 RBC Shape

RBC shape	Description	Causes
Target cells	• Targetoid shape (Figure 1.3) • Abundant membrane	• Artifact • Thalassemia
Spherocytes	• Small, round • Lack central pallor	• Hereditary • Microangiopathic hemolysis
Elliptocytes	• Ovoid or elliptical cells	• Hereditary • Iron deficiency anemia
Teardrop-shaped cells/dacrocytes	• Narrow point at one end (Figure 1.4) • Resemble a drop of water	• BM fibrosis • Myelophthisis
Bite cells	• Missing portion of the cell • Resemble a bite mark	• Splenic macrophages remove RBCs with denatured Hgb
Helmet cells	• Missing portion of the cell (Figure 1.5) • Resemble a small helmet	• Microangiopathic hemolysis
Schistocytes	• Fragmented cells (Figure 1.6) • Various sizes and shapes • No central pallor (true schistocyte)	• Microangiopathic hemolysis

BM, bone marrow; Hgb, hemoglobin.

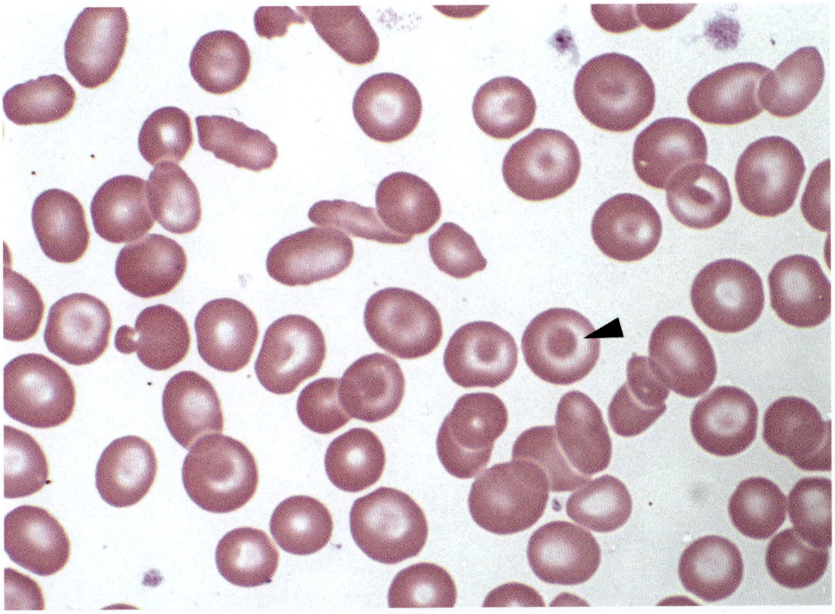

FIGURE 1.3 Target cells (arrowhead) represent red cells with excess membrane and may be seen in Thalassemia and liver disease, but may also be an artifact.

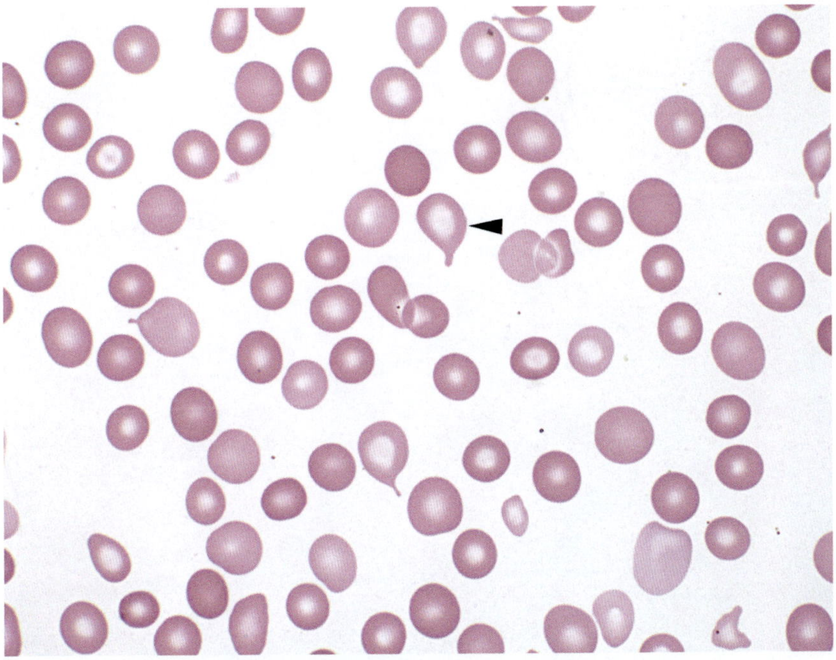

FIGURE 1.4 Dacrocytes (arrowhead) are teardrop-shaped red blood cells seen in the peripheral blood of patients with bone marrow fibrosis.

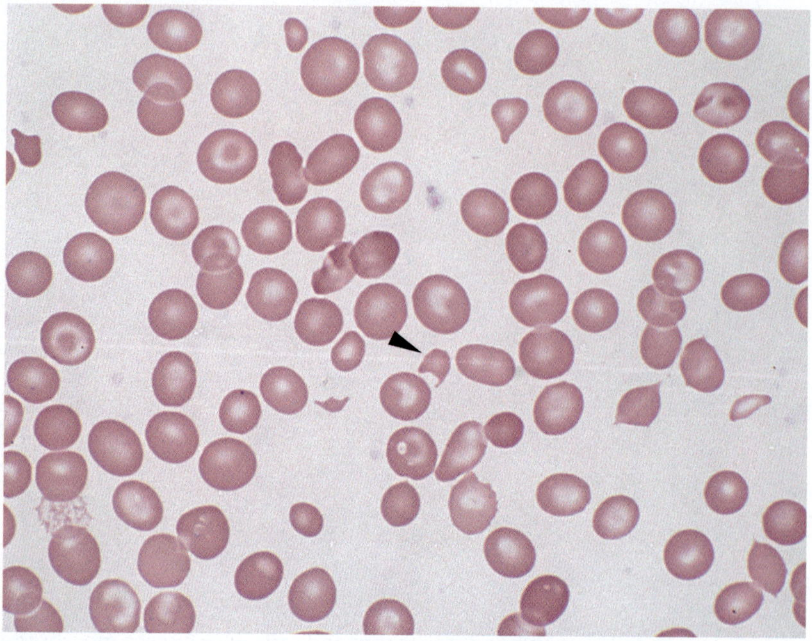

FIGURE 1.5 Helmet cells (arrowhead) are red blood cells with membrane defects due to mechanical destruction most often caused by microangiopathic hemolysis.

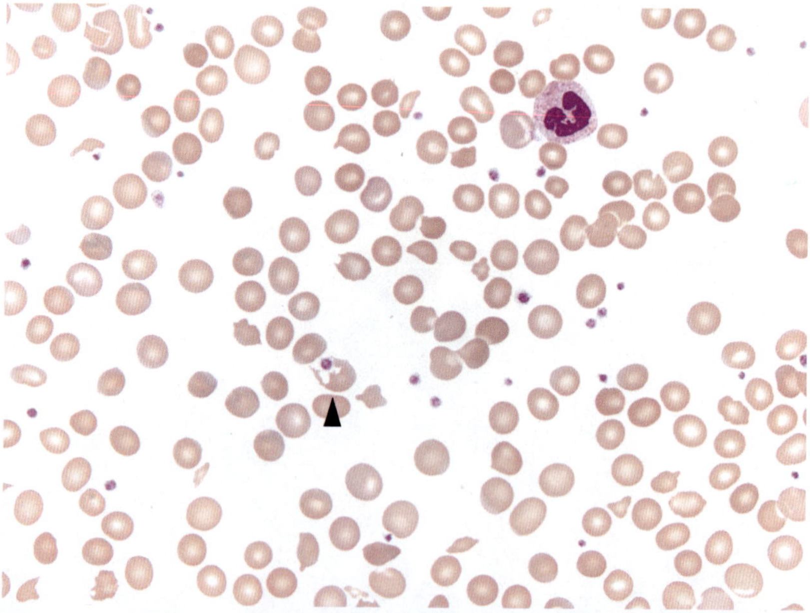

FIGURE 1.6 Schistocytes (arrowhead) are always pathologic and are typically a sign of intravascular mechanical red cell destruction as in microangiopathic hemolytic anemia.

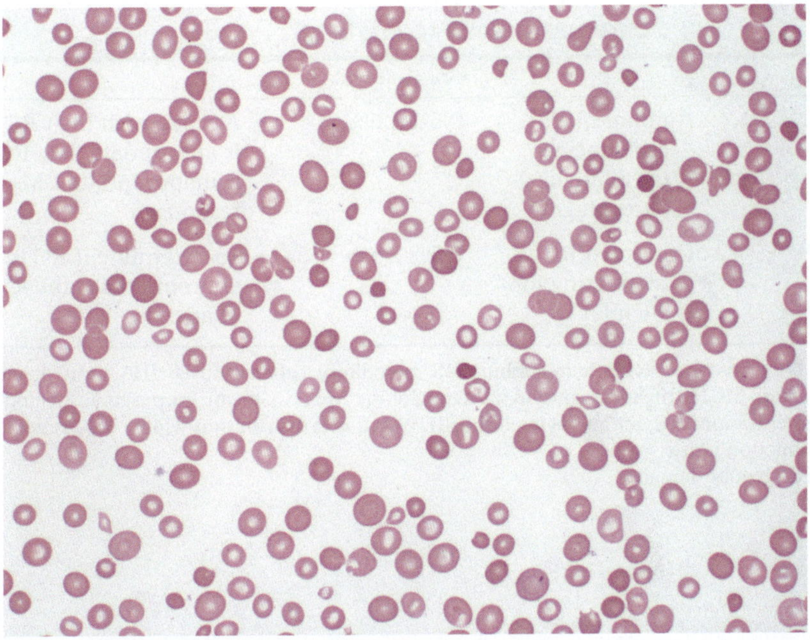

FIGURE 1.7 Marked anisopoikilocytosis is a common abnormality seen in different disease states but is not specific of any one diagnosis.

RBC Color

This reflects the Hgb content and is assessed by the mean corpuscular hemoglobin concentration (MCHC) (Table 1.4). Reticulocytes, as the youngest mature RBCs in the PB, have the highest iron content and appear larger and bluer than other RBCs on a Wright-Giemsa (WG) stain because of greater residual RNA content (Figure 1.8; eFigure 1.9). Reticulocyte count/index indicates the number of reticulocytes in circulation, an indicator of

TABLE 1.4 RBC Chromasia/Color

Parameter	Definition	Normal range[a]	Notes
MCH	Average Hgb per RBC	26.6-33.0 pg	• Hypochromia is associated with IDA • Hyperchromia is associated with HS
MCHC	Amount of Hgb per RBC unit volume	31.5-35.7 g/dL	• Similar to MCH, but takes into account RBC size
RDW	Measurement of RBC size variability	11.7%-15.4%	• High RDW may indicate anisocytosis or increased reticulocytes

(*continued*)

TABLE 1.4 RBC Chromasia/Color (*continued*)

Parameter	Definition	Normal range[a]	Notes
RC	Amount of reticulocytes (absolute or percentage)	0.6%-1.6%	• Anemia with high RC is appropriate; low RC is inappropriate BM response
RPI	Corrected RC (correcting for anemia)	0.5%-2.5%	• To determine if RC is appropriate for the level of anemia

BM, bone marrow; Hgb, hemoglobin; HS, hereditary spherocytosis; IDA, iron deficiency anemia; MCH, mean corpuscular hemoglobin; MCHC, mean corpuscular hemoglobin concentration; RC, reticulocyte count; RDW, red cell distribution width; RPI, reticulocyte production index.

[a]Based on adult female.

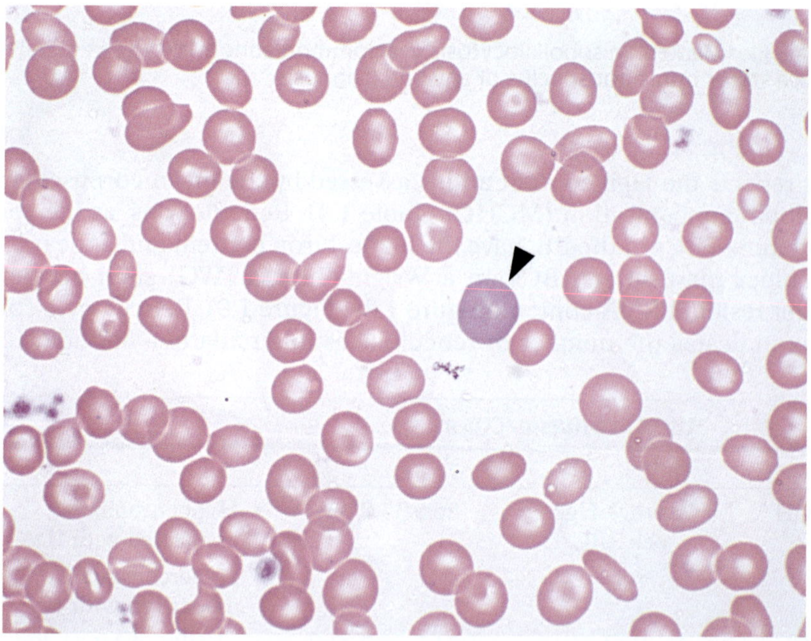

FIGURE 1.8 Reticulocytes (arrowhead) are the youngest mature red blood cells (RBCs) in the peripheral blood (PB), have the highest iron content, and appear larger and more amphophilic than other RBCs on a Wright-Giemsa (WG) stain because of their RNA content.

normal regeneration in the BM. Patients with iron deficiency anemia often have microcytic and hypochromic RBCs, whereas patients with spherocytosis may have microcytic and hyperchromic RBCs.

RBC Inclusions

Inclusions may or may not be seen on the WG stain, depending on the type of inclusion (eFigure 1.10). Some require special stains or supravital stains. The most common RBC inclusions are detailed in Table 1.5 and Figures 1.9 and 1.10.

Circulating Immature RBC Precursors

Outside of infancy, the presence of nucleated RBCs in blood usually indicates a pathologic process (Figure 1.11; eFigure 1.11). These may be seen in states of stressed erythropoiesis, splenic disorders, or may reflect a primary marrow disorder or an inflammatory or neoplastic space-occupying lesion in the marrow.

WHITE BLOOD CELLS

As the main defenders of the immune system, WBCs are constantly patrolling the body. This cadre of cells, including neutrophils, monocytes, eosinophils, basophils, and lymphocytes, circulate in the PB, travel through tissue, transverse lymph nodes via lymphatics, and home to the BM. The WBC

TABLE 1.5 RBC Inclusions

Inclusions	RBC appearance	Stain	Associated with
Pappenheimer bodies	Irregularly shaped intracellular iron granules	WG	• Iron overload
Basophilic stippling	Small blue dots (Figure 1.9) Clusters of ribosomes	WG	• Lead poisoning • Thalassemia • Megaloblastic anemia • Sideroblastic anemia
Howell-Jolly bodies	Round, regular inclusions (Figure 1.10)	WG	• Asplenia
Heinz bodies	Fragments of denatured hemoglobin	Supravital stain (identified as "bite cells" on WG)	• G6PD deficiency

G6PD, glucose-6-phosphate dehydrogenase; WG, Wright-Giemsa.

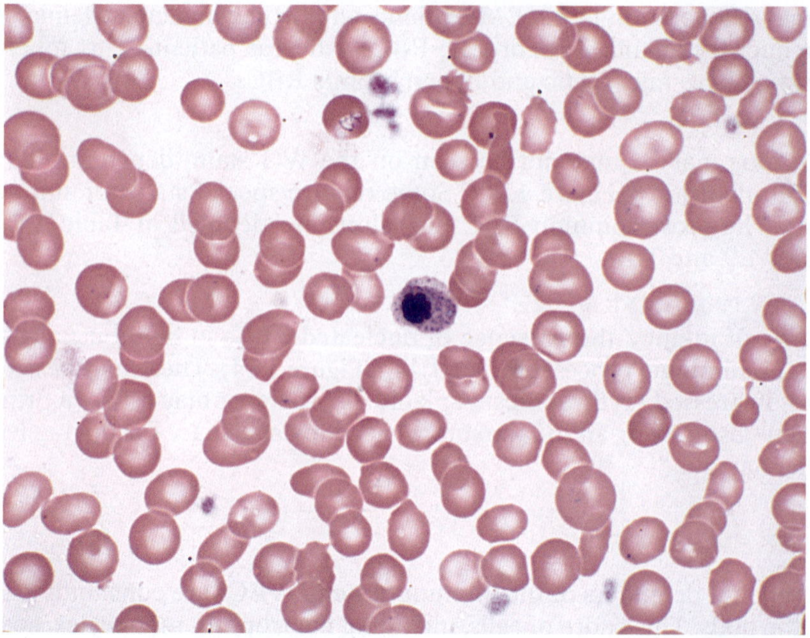

FIGURE 1.9 **Basophilic stippling is thought to represent residual fragments of RNA and appears as small blue dots in red cells.** Although abnormal, it may be seen in a wide variety of diseases.

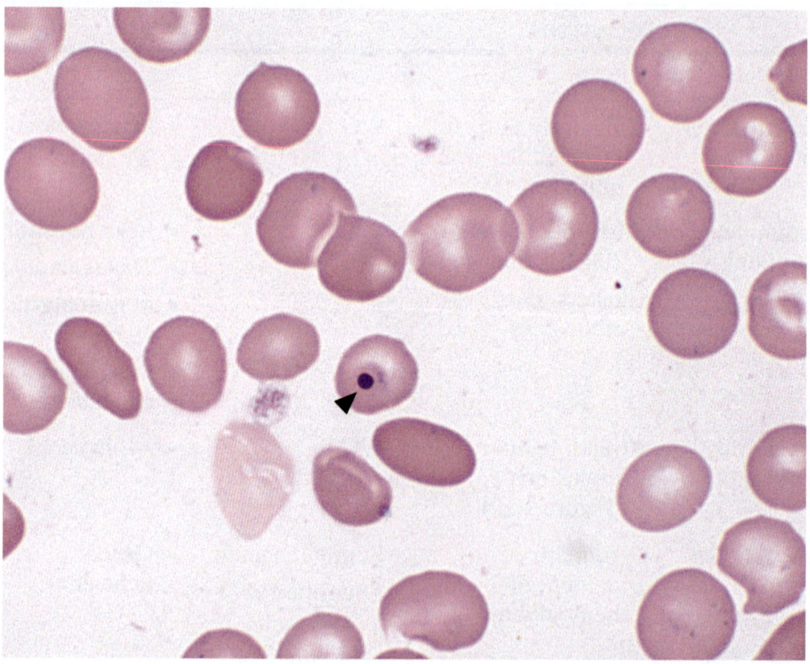

FIGURE 1.10 **Howell-Jolly bodies (arrowhead) are nuclear remnants that indicate asplenia.**

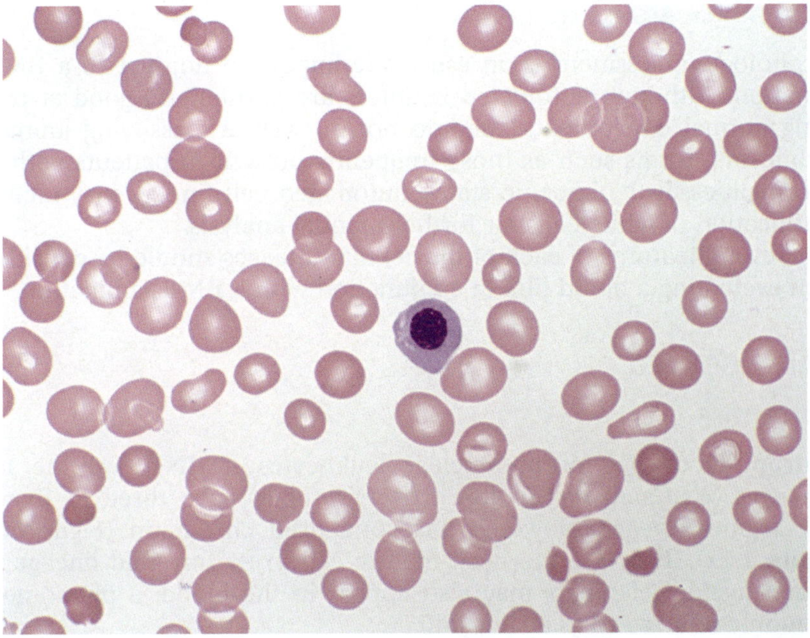

FIGURE 1.11 Nucleated red cells in the peripheral blood (PB) usually indicate a pathologic process.

count and the differential count are critically important pieces of information necessary for evaluation of a BM (Table 1.6).

WBC Quantity

Abnormalities in WBC counts, namely leukocytosis and leukopenia, arise because of a wide variety of situations, conditions, and/or disease states, and detailed discussion of these is outside the scope of this chapter. Consideration of cell types involved and whether the involved cells are mature, immature, or morphologically abnormal are all important considerations when forming a differential diagnosis and in planning further workup.

TABLE 1.6 WBC Differential Counts

Cell type	Absolute count (K/μL)	WBC count (%)
Neutrophils	2.5-8.0	55-70
Lymphocytes	1.0-4.0	20-40
Monocytes	0.1-0.7	2-8
Eosinophils	0.05-0.5	1-4
Basophils	0.025-0.1	0.5-1
Blasts	0	0

K, thousand.

Morphologic Assessment of WBCs

Morphologic assessment is an especially important adjunct to a BM examination. Although automated counters are particularly good at recognizing normal constituents, they do not do well at classifying immature or abnormal forms such as those frequently present in patients with BM abnormalities. In leukopenic states, automated cell finders may facilitate identification of white cells for further manual analysis.

Several features of each of the cellular lineages should be considered when evaluating a blood film in conjunction with a BM examination.

GRANULOCYTES

Neutrophils

Neutrophils or polymorphonuclear leukocytes (PMNs) are the most numerous WBCs in circulation. They normally have three to five nuclear segments, each of which has condensed chromatin (Figure 1.12; eFigure 1.12). They are the most mature cell in the myeloid lineage. Immature myeloid elements may also appear in the blood, a phenomenon commonly referred to as a "left shift."

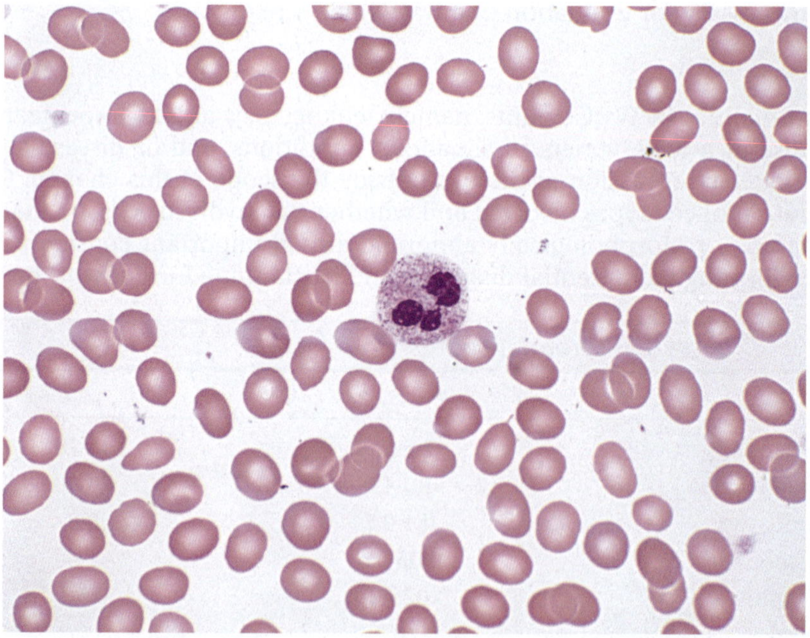

FIGURE 1.12 **Neutrophils are the most common blood leukocyte.** They have three to five nuclear segments and eosinophilic secondary granules.

Immature Granulocytes

Immature granulocytes, such as bands, myelocytes, and metamyelocytes, are commonly seen in low numbers in PB as a reaction to normal physiologic stress or infection (Figure 1.13; eFigure 1.13), but in many cases finding these significant numbers or finding these in association with promyelocytes and/or myeloblasts (Figure 1.14; eFigure 1.14) will prompt a BM examination.

Nuclear or cytoplasmic abnormalities in mature or immature neutrophilic granulocytes may provide important information. Hypersegmentation of neutrophils may indicate vitamin B_{12} or folate abnormalities, as these defects impair nuclear maturation (Figure 1.15; eFigure 1.15). Hyposegmented neutrophils (eFigure 1.16), often with abnormally clumped nuclear chromatin, may indicate dysplasia (see Chapter 5) or may be seen in rare hereditary conditions like Pelger-Huet anomaly (Figure 1.16).

The cytoplasm of mature neutrophils is evenly distributed with secondary pink cytotoxic granules.[5] Hypergranulation may indicate granulocyte colony–stimulating factor (GCSF) administration, infections, or sepsis (Figure 1.17; eFigure 1.17) and, less commonly, MDS. Döhle bodies, which

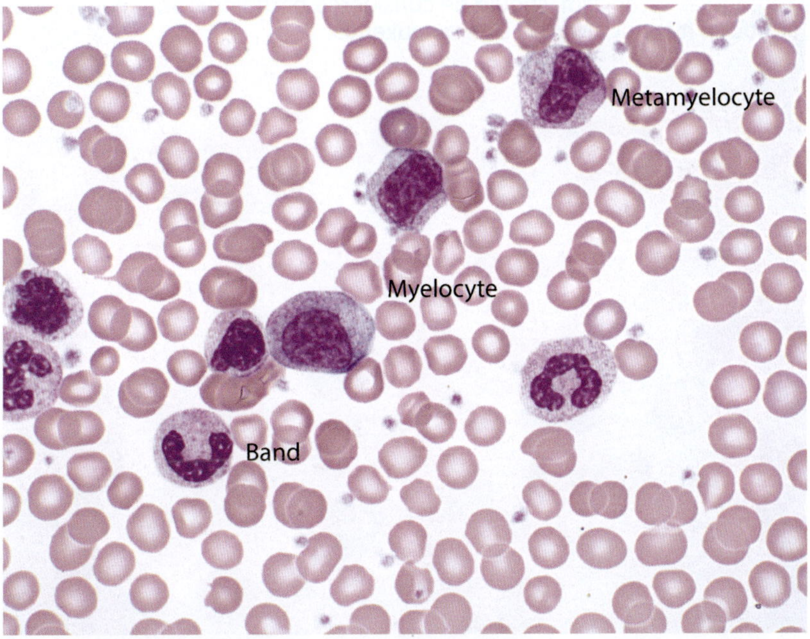

FIGURE 1.13 **Myeloid precursors may be seen in low numbers in the peripheral blood (PB) as a reaction to stress or in infection, although when as numerous as shown here, chronic myeloid leukemia should be excluded.** Bands have horseshoe-shaped nuclei without any significant constriction; metamyelocytes have a small indentation, and myelocytes have round-to-oval nuclei with a Golgi zone. Granules are present in all stages.

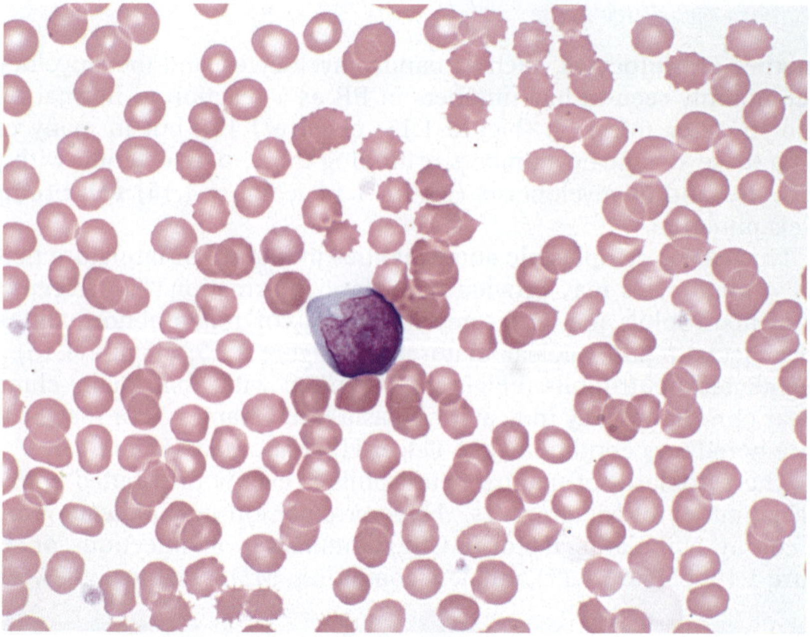

FIGURE 1.14 A circulating myeloblast, such as this cell with fine chromatin and a rim of agranular cytoplasm, should be considered pathologic and merits investigation, although it is not always a sign of leukemia.

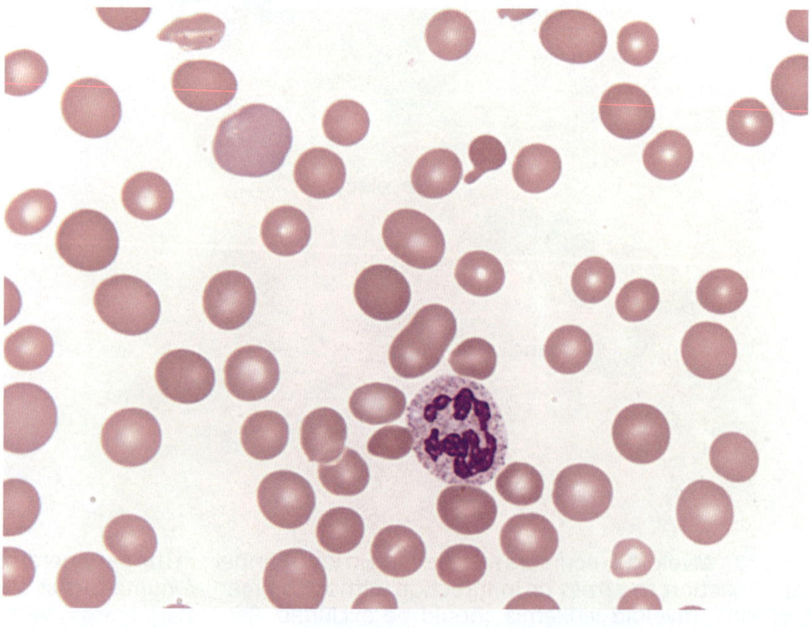

FIGURE 1.15 Neutrophil hypersegmentation (typically more than five nuclear segments) is characteristically seen in megaloblastic anemia.

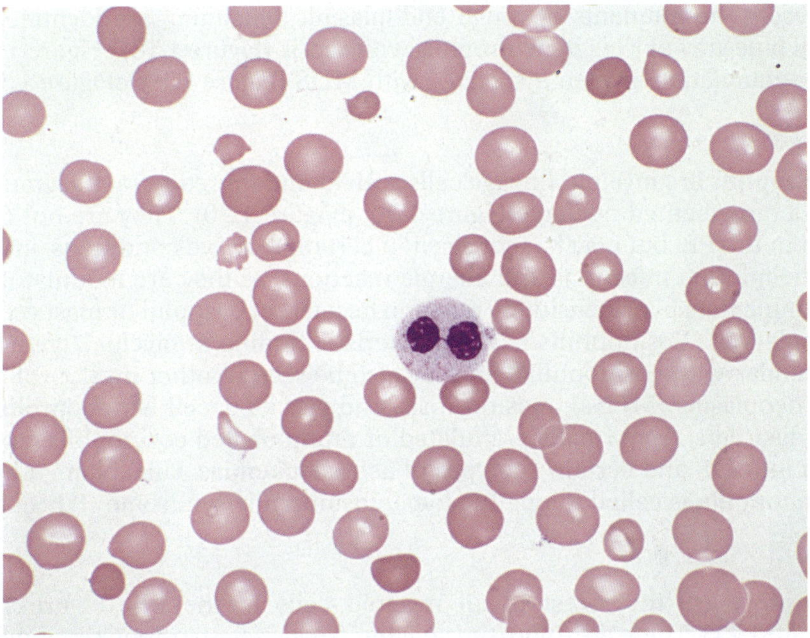

FIGURE 1.16 Hyposegmented neutrophils may be found in myelodysplastic syndromes or Pelger-Huet anomaly.

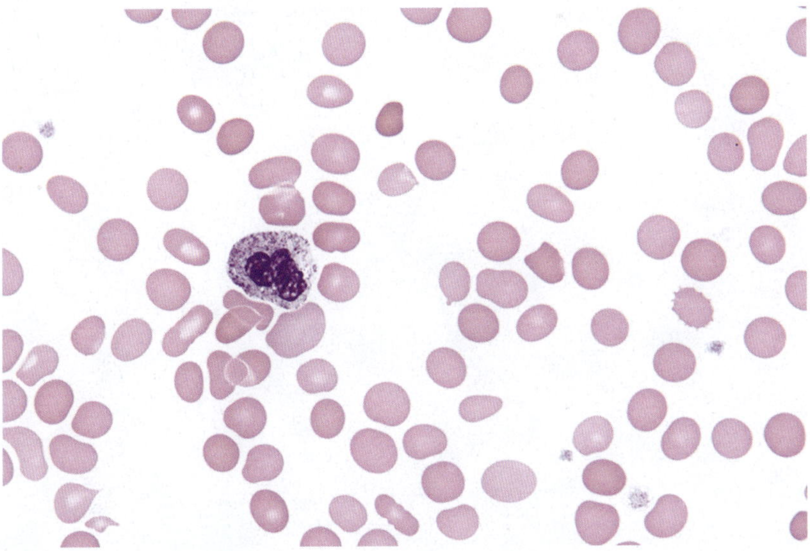

FIGURE 1.17 Hypergranulation may indicate growth factor/granulocyte colony-stimulating factor administration, infections, sepsis, or myelodysplastic syndrome (MDS).

represent the remnants of rough endoplasmic reticulum, are identified as small blue-gray objects in neutrophils with sepsis (Figure 1.18; eFigure 1.18). Hypogranulation is often associated with MDS (Figure 1.19; eFigure 1.19).

Eosinophils

Eosinophils are myeloid-lineage cells with abundant red refractile granules and a bisegmented nucleus (Figure 1.20; eFigure 1.20). They are not common in the PB, but may be increased in certain reactive conditions, including helminthic infections and allergic reactions, as they are modulators of the immediate hypersensitivity reaction because of basophil or mast cell degranulation.[6] Eosinophilia is a characteristic finding in myeloid/lymphoid leukemias with eosinophilia but may also be seen in other myeloproliferative neoplasms (MPNs), mastocytosis, and certain T cell lymphoproliferative disorders. Abnormally granulated or monolobated eosinophils may be seen in MDS and certain subtypes of acute leukemias. Unexplained hypereosinophilia is called idiopathic hypereosinophilic syndrome (HES).

Basophils

Basophils are the rarest of all myeloid cells in the PB (Figure 1.21; eFigure 1.21). These are approximately the same size as eosinophils and have coarse basophilic cytoplasmic granules that initiate allergic and hypersensitivity reactions.[6-8] Increased basophils are seen in MPNs and are invariably present in chronic myeloid leukemia.

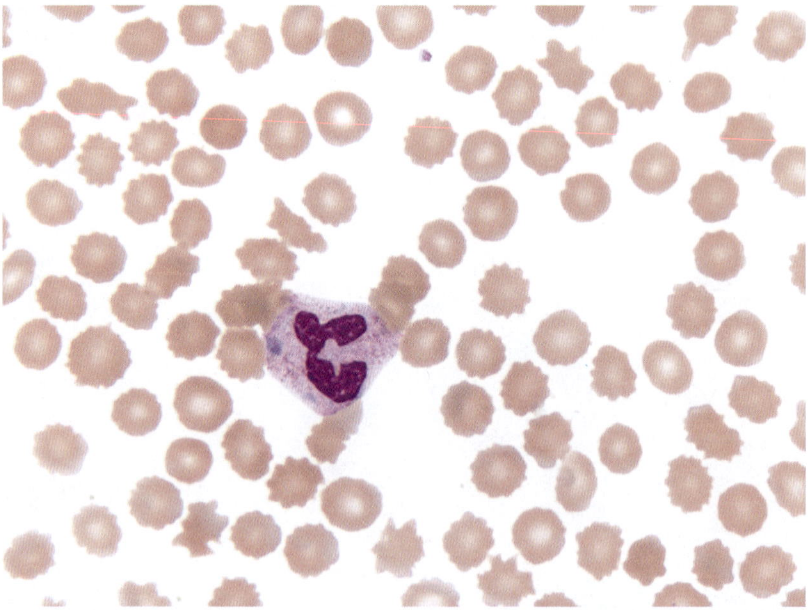

FIGURE 1.18 Döhle bodies, the small blue structures seen at the left edge of this neutrophil's cytoplasm, consist of ribosomes and endoplasmic reticulum and are seen in a wide variety of conditions.

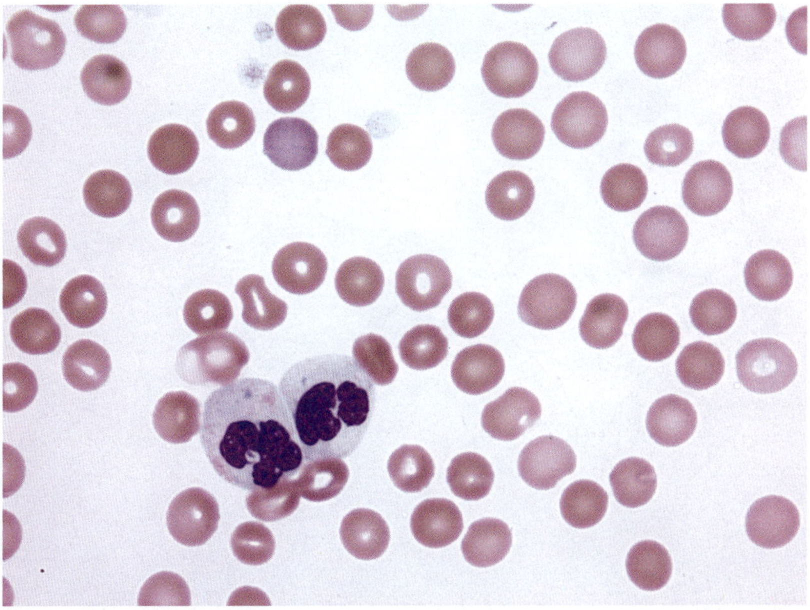

FIGURE 1.19 Hypogranular neutrophils have very pale-appearing cytoplasm and are a common finding in myelodysplastic syndrome (MDS).

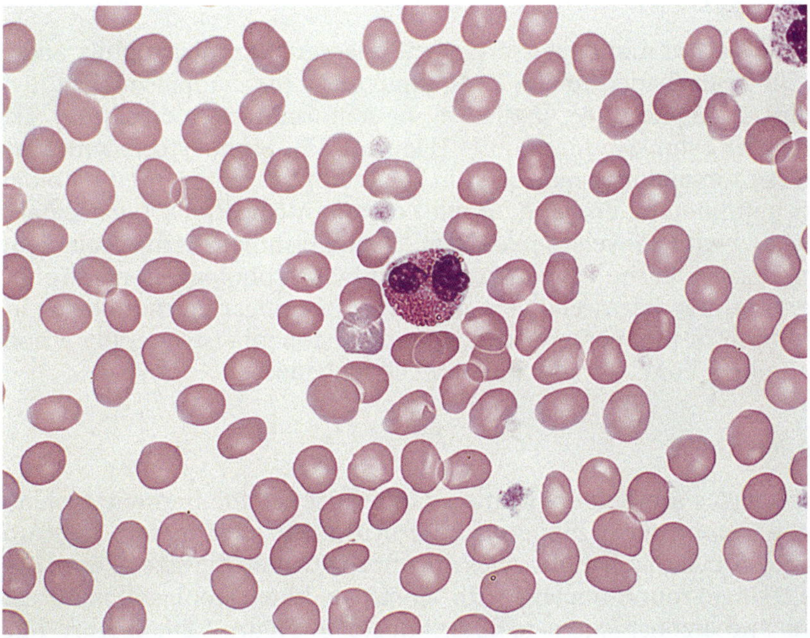

FIGURE 1.20 Eosinophils have abundant refractile red granules and a bisegmented nucleus.

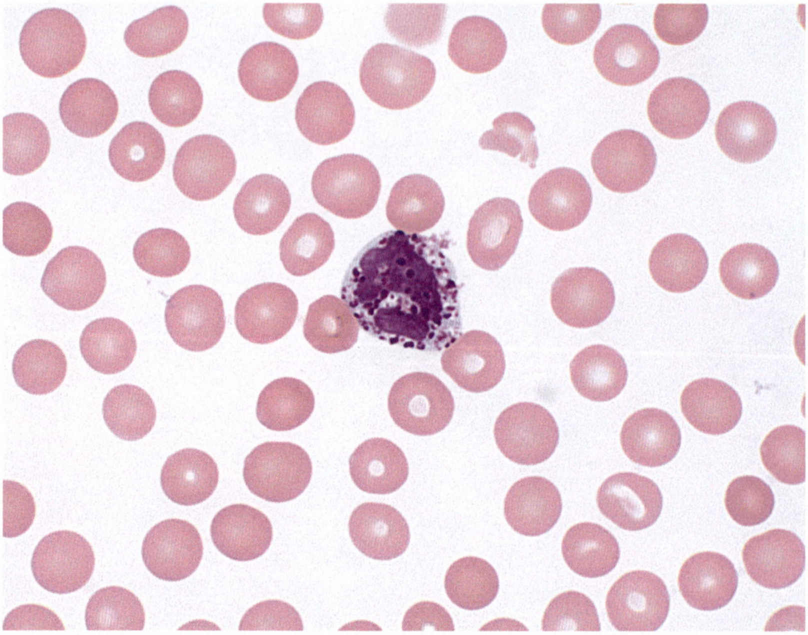

FIGURE 1.21 **Basophils are recognized by their coarse basophilic granules; the nucleus, when not obscured is often irregularly shaped, as in this case.**

MONOCYTES

Normal mature monocytes are slightly larger than neutrophils and have oval- or bean-shaped nuclei and ample gray-blue cytoplasm (Figure 1.22; eFigure 1.22). Reactive, immature, or abnormal monocytes may display nucleoli or cytoplasmic vacuoles (Figure 1.23). Monocytosis with variable degrees of immaturity may be seen in certain infections, rheumatologic or other autoimmune diseases, or with certain medications, but may also be associated with a myeloid neoplasm. Distinguishing reactive from neoplastic monocytes in the PB can be difficult by morphology alone. Monocytic leukemias may have relatively more mature-appearing monocytes in the blood than in the marrow. Relative monocytopenia is generally a nonspecific finding, but is notable in hairy cell leukemia.

LYMPHOCYTES

Lymphocytes are fighters in the adaptive arm of the immune system and are the second most numerous cell in the PB after mature neutrophils. Normal circulating lymphocytes are approximately the size of an RBC and have a single round nucleus with scant pale blue cytoplasm, mature chromatin, and inconspicuous-to-absent nucleoli (Figure 1.24; eFigure 1.23). It is not possible to identify the lymphocyte lineage (B cell vs T cell vs natural killer [NK] cell) by morphologic features alone. In most cases, patients with

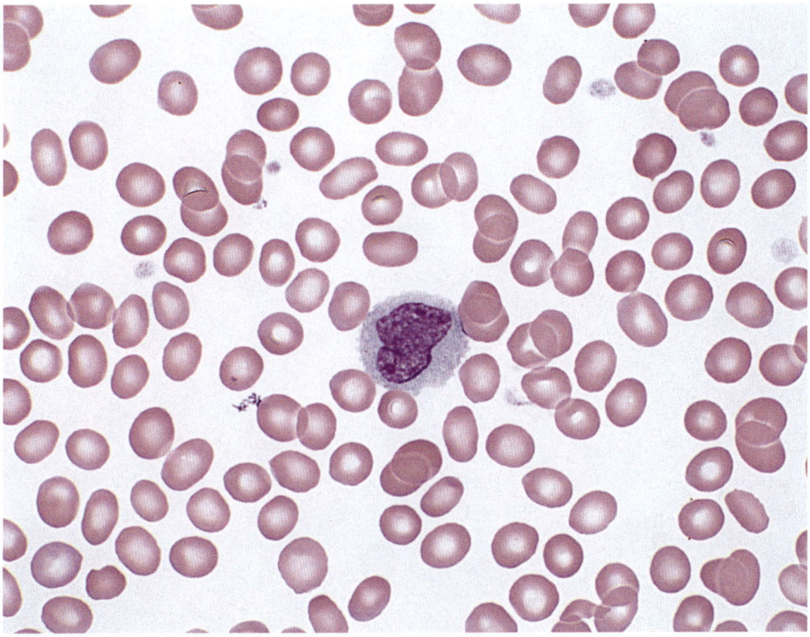

FIGURE 1.22 Normal mature monocytes have oval- or bean-shaped nuclei and ample gray-blue cytoplasm.

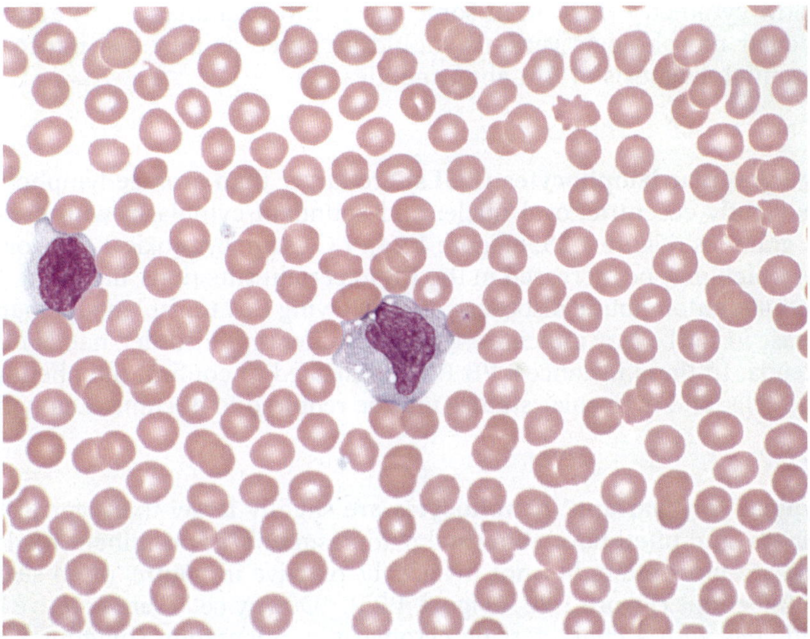

FIGURE 1.23 Reactive monocytes may display nucleoli or cytoplasmic vacuoles.

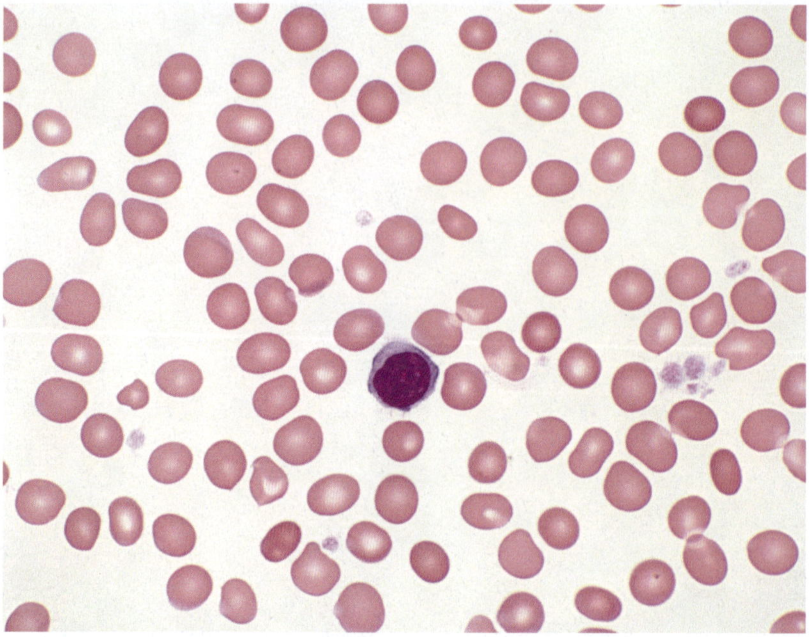

FIGURE 1.24 Normal circulating lymphocytes have mature chromatin and inconspicuous-to-absent nucleoli.

absolute lymphocytosis will require further workup, either in the form of PB flow cytometry (FC) or, in some cases, BM examination. In addition, particular morphologic variants should be noted as they can inform the differential diagnosis of BM abnormalities.

Large Granular Lymphocytes

Large granular lymphocytes (LGLs) are larger than average lymphocytes with slightly eccentric, oval nuclei and abundant cytoplasm with delicate pink granules (Figure 1.25; eFigure 1.24). LGLs are cytotoxic T cells or NK cells, which may be increased in the PB in certain situations, including viral infections, autoimmune disorders, and following BM transplants. A marked increase in LGLs may indicate a lymphoproliferative disorder, namely LGL leukemia. In these instances, PB FC is indicated to confirm the phenotype of the cells, and molecular studies may be required to document clonality.

"Atypical" or "Variant" Lymphocytes

"Atypical" or "variant" lymphocytes are slightly larger-than-typical lymphocytes, and often have abnormal cytoplasm and/or prominent nucleoli. These are most often, but not invariably, reactive in nature, often seen in viral infections (Figure 1.26; eFigure 1.25). "Downy cells" are reactive lymphoid cells with a characteristic cytoplasmic indentation sometimes seen in the PB of patients with infectious mononucleosis.

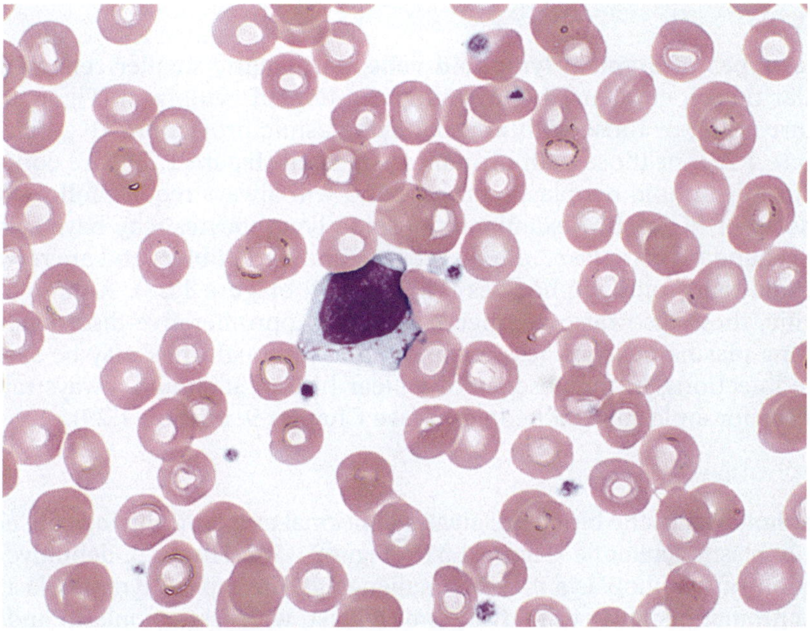

FIGURE 1.25 Large granular lymphocytes (LGLs) are larger-than-average lymphocytes with slightly eccentric, oval nuclei and abundant cytoplasm with delicate pink granules.

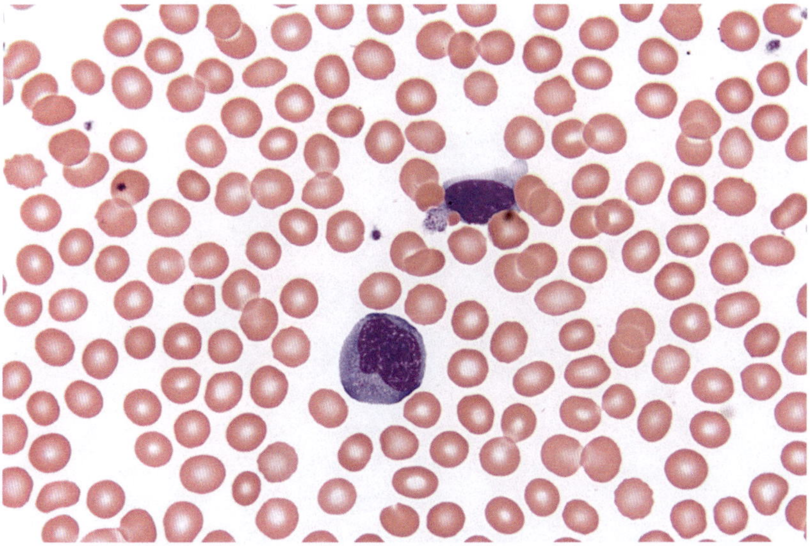

FIGURE 1.26 Lymphoid cells in cases of viral infection typically have more abundant cytoplasm than normal lymphocytes, ranging from pale to darker blue. Their cytoplasm may be compressed by red cells.

Other Types of Atypical Lymphoid Cells

Other types of atypical lymphoid cells, particularly smaller cells with irregular nuclei, condensed chromatin, and limited cytoplasm (Figure 1.27; eFigure 1.26); or those with unusual cytoplasmic projections (Figure 1.28; eFigure 1.27); or those with prominent nucleoli (Figure 1.29), are concerning for a lymphoid neoplastic process and will always require follow-up in the form of FC or BM examination. Some lymphocytes may have slightly more abundant cytoplasm, often eccentric and darker blue, and are referred to as plasmacytoid lymphocytes (Figure 1.30; eFigure 1.28). Although not specific, these also raise a concern for lymphoproliferative disorders. Circulating plasma cells are less common, and although they may be seen in some infections, in the absence of a clear history, it should always raise a concern for a plasma cell neoplasm (see Chapter 9; eFigure 1.29).

Lymphoblasts

Lymphoblasts in the blood are always abnormal and typically indicate acute lymphoblastic leukemia (Figure 1.31; eFigure 1.30). However, definitive recognition of lymphoblasts may be challenging. The typical lymphoblast has fine chromatin similar to that of a myeloblast, with less cytoplasm and less conspicuous nucleoli. The morphology can vary considerably, to include cells indistinguishable from myeloblasts to cells that look like mature lymphocytes, which is why FC is a critical tool when evaluating PB lymphocytosis.

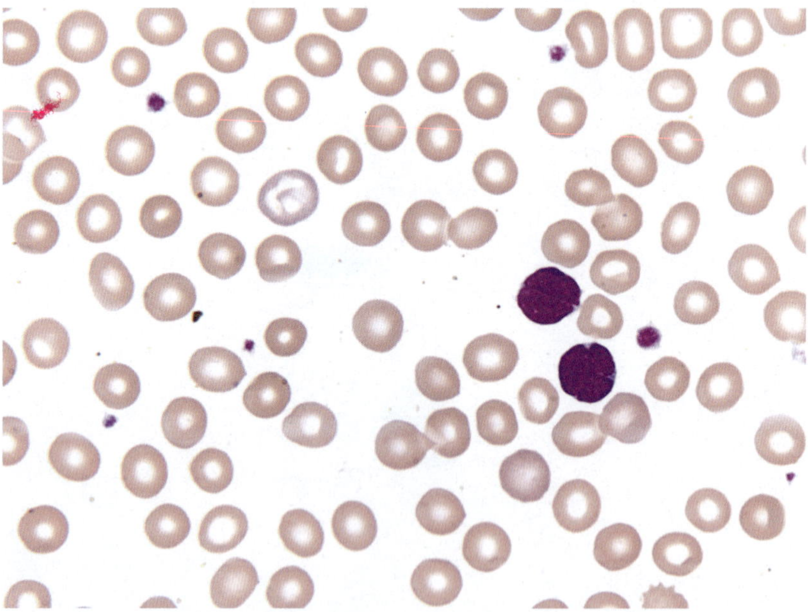

FIGURE 1.27 Lymphocytes with irregular nuclei or clefted shape, as seen here, are never normal and are most often associated with circulating low-grade lymphoma, particularly follicular lymphoma.

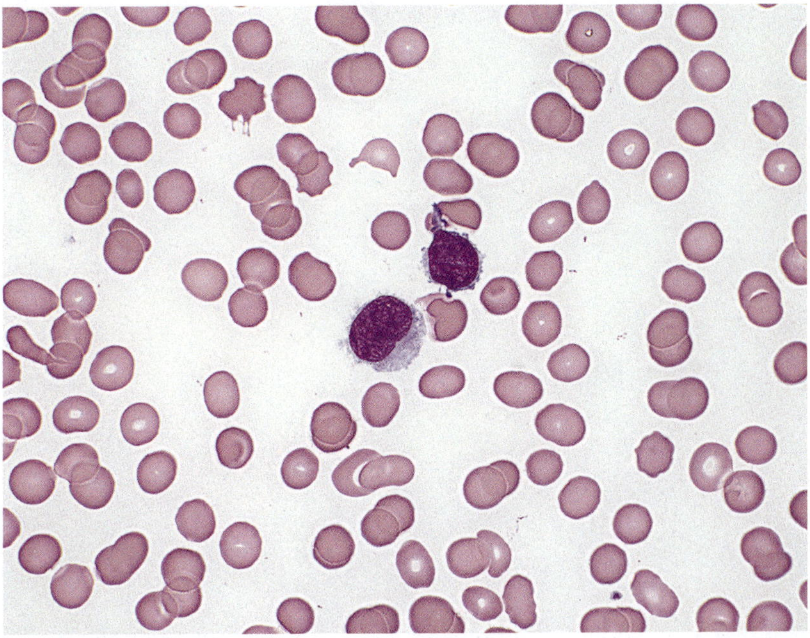

FIGURE 1.28 Hairy cell leukemia lymphocytes have characteristic projections and a nucleus with more open chromatin than a normal lymphocyte, but typically lack (or have very small) nucleoli.

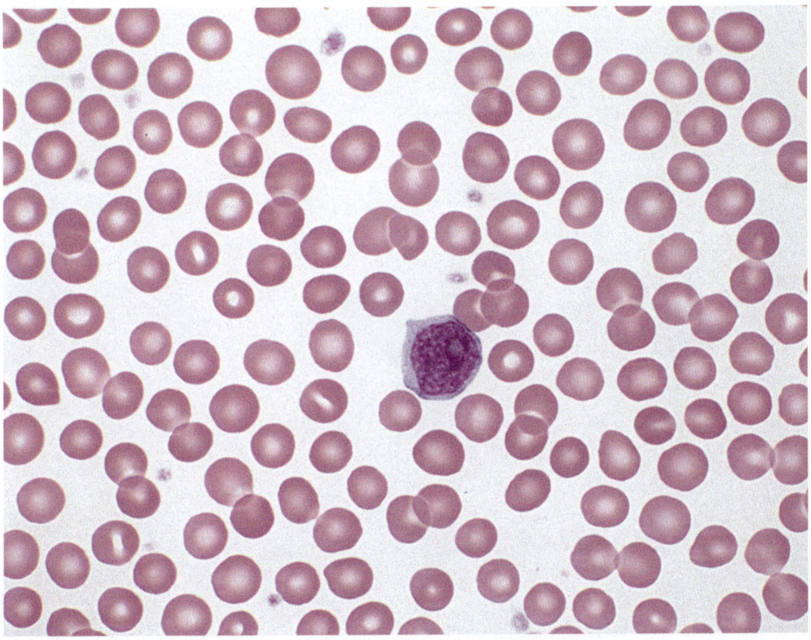

FIGURE 1.29 Prolymphocytes are larger than normal lymphocytes with abundant blueish cytoplasm and prominent nucleoli.

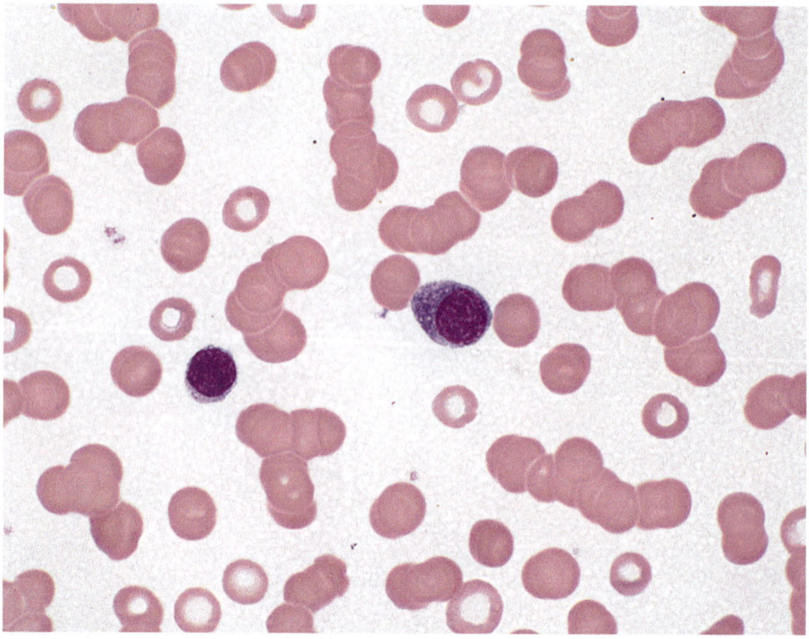

FIGURE 1.30 **Plasmacytoid lymphocytes or circulating plasma cells are uncommon in the blood.** They have eccentric, dark blue cytoplasm that varies in amount, and their nuclear chromatin is condensed. Although they often suggest a neoplastic process, they may also be seen in cases of polyclonal B cell activation.

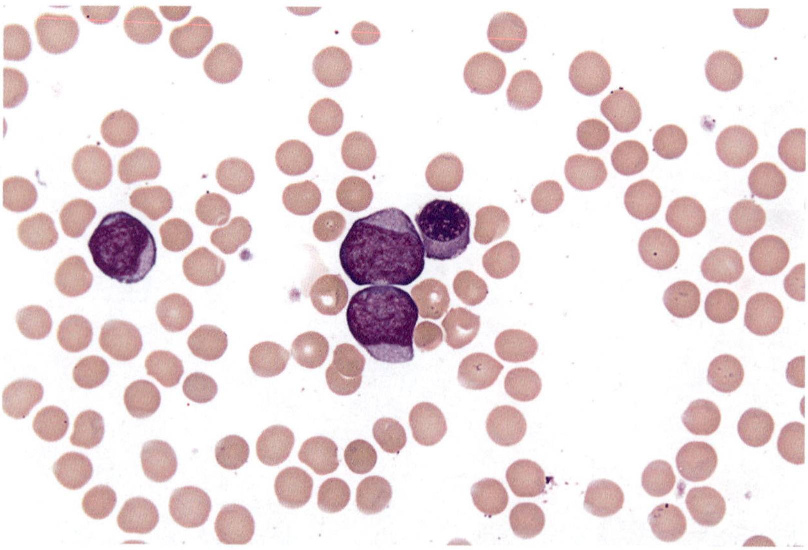

FIGURE 1.31 **Lymphoblasts have fine chromatin but, in contrast to that of a myeloblast, typically have less cytoplasm and less conspicuous nucleoli.**

PLATELETS

The smallest components in the PB are derived from megakaryocytes, the largest hematopoietic cells in the BM. Platelets are anucleate cell fragments, less than one-fourth the size of an RBC (Figure 1.32; eFigure 1.31). In a normal PB smear, there should be at least 8-10 platelets per high-power field.[9] A morphologic estimate of platelet counts can be important to help identify spurious thrombocytopenia, which may occur as a consequence of ethylenediaminetetraacetic acid (EDTA)–induced platelet clumping resulting in an abnormally low automated platelet count (Figure 1.33). In some cases, blood films made after clotting begins can result in platelet clumping on the film, making platelet estimation impossible.

In addition to assessing platelet number, platelet size and cytoplasmic granularity should also be assessed (Figure 1.34); this can provide clues to the diagnosis of certain congenital and acquired disorders. Many BM disorders, including MDS and MPN, are associated with abnormalities in circulating platelets, particularly larger than normal platelets (eFigure 1.32). Fragments of megakaryocytes may also rarely be seen (eFigure 1.33).

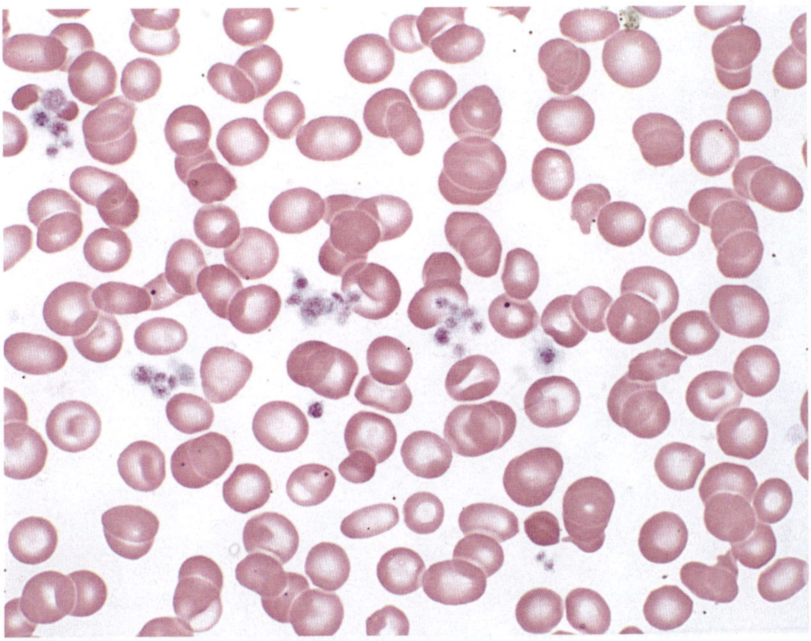

FIGURE 1.32 Normal platelets range in size from about a tenth to a fourth of the cross-sectional area of red cells and have a dark center with wispy blue periphery.

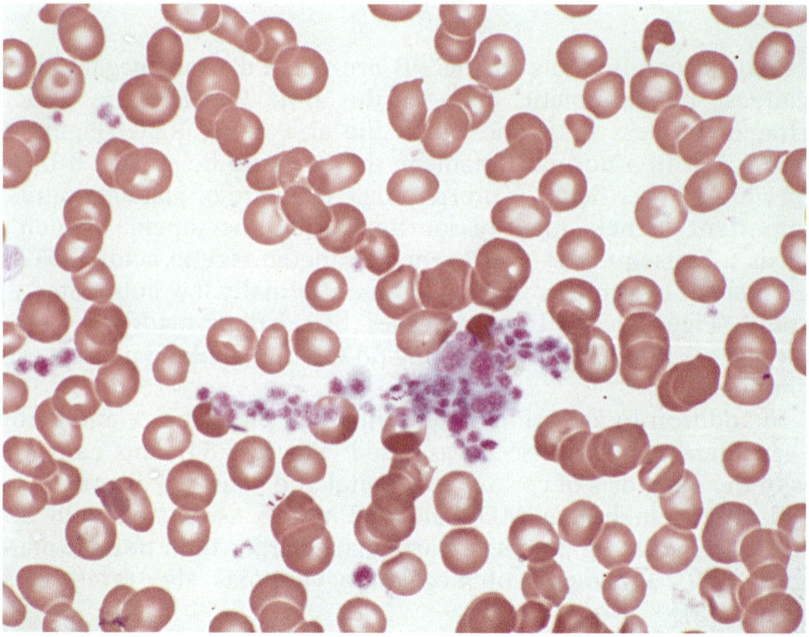

FIGURE 1.33 **Platelet clumping may lead to a spuriously low automated platelet count.**

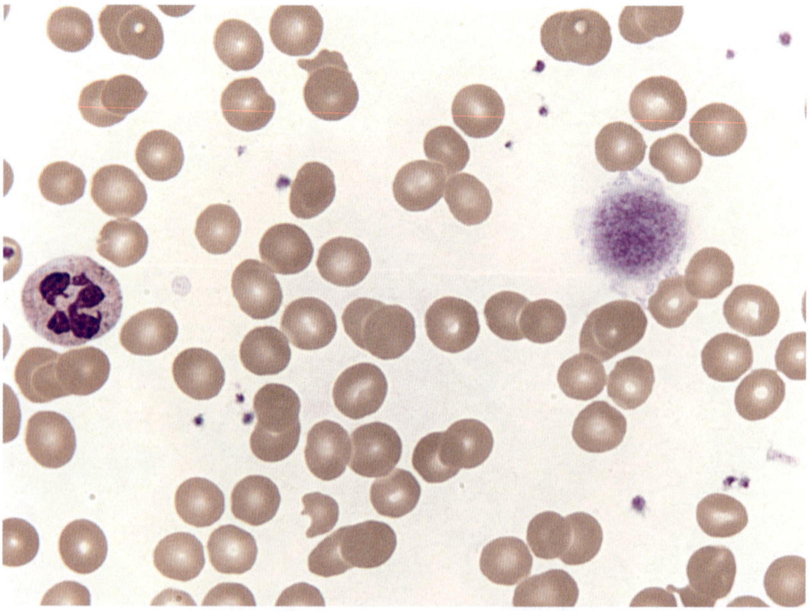

FIGURE 1.34 **Giant platelets (on the right) are always abnormal but not specific of any disease.** They can be large enough to be counted as lymphocytes on some blood counters.

OTHER CELLS AND OBJECTS IDENTIFIED IN THE PB

Smudge Cells

These are cells that are destroyed or "smudged" during the smearing process. Numerous smudge cells may be seen in conditions like chronic lymphocytic leukemia (CLL)/small lymphocytic lymphoma (SLL) or acute leukemia (Figure 1.35; eFigure 1.34). It is not possible to definitively categorize smudge cells. A smear preparation with albumin may improve morphologic evaluation.

Staining Artifacts

Bacterial colonies are sometimes identified in a PB smear; this usually indicates a contaminated WG stain that needs to be replaced. Rarely, a truly septic patient may have bacteria identified on the PB smear.

Organisms

Malaria, ehrlichiosis, and/or babesiosis organisms are identifiable in the PB (Figure 1.36; eFigure 1.35) and do not require a BM biopsy. A BM biopsy is only indicated if a patient has a fever of unknown origin or after a non-informative infectious disease workup. Occasionally, severe infections are accompanied by hemophagocytosis, which is discussed in Chapter 10.

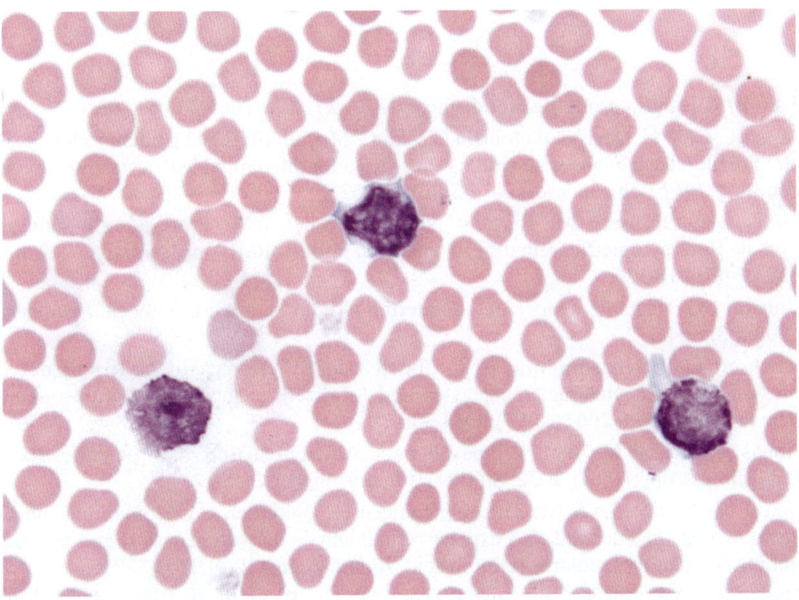

FIGURE 1.35 **Smudge cells, such as the one on the lower left, are cells that are destroyed during the process of making a blood film.** Although their original cell type can sometimes be recognized, they are typically skipped when performing a differential blood count.

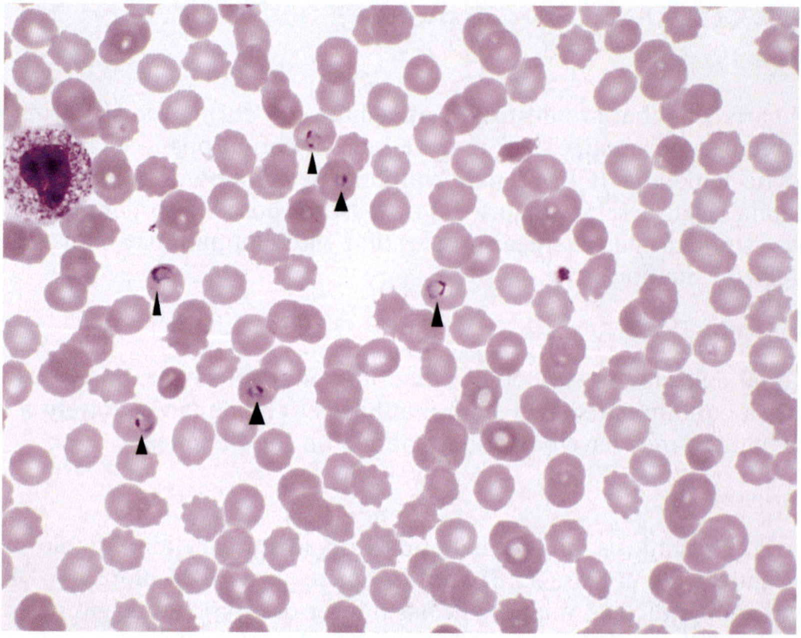

FIGURE 1.36 *Plasmodium* organisms (arrowheads) may occasionally be seen within RBCs on routine blood smears, although malaria detection is typically done on a special thick blood film.

REFERENCES

1. Bain BJ. Diagnosis from the blood smear. *N Engl J Med.* 2005;353(5):498-507.
2. Briggs C, Culp N, Davis B, d'Onofrio G, Zini G, Machin SJ. ICSH guidelines for the evaluation of blood cell analysers including those used for differential leucocyte and reticulocyte counting. *Int J Lab Hematol.* 2014;36(6):613-627.
3. Davis BH, DiCorato M, Bigelow NC, Langweiler MH. Proposal for standardization of flow cytometric reticulocyte maturity index (RMI) measurements. *Cytometry.* 1993;14(3):318-326.
4. Borovoi AG, Naats EI, Oppel UG. Scattering of light by a red blood cell. *J Biomed Opt.* 1998;3(3):364-372.
5. Jacobsen LC, Theilgaard-Mönch K, Christensen EI, Borregaard N. Arginase 1 is expressed in myelocytes/metamyelocytes and localized in gelatinase granules of human neutrophils. *Blood.* 2007;109(7):3084-3087.
6. Abbas M, Moussa M, Akel H. Type I hypersensitivity reaction. In: *StatPearls.* StatPearls Publishing. Copyright © 2022, StatPearls Publishing LLC; 2022.
7. Spiegl N, Didichenko S, McCaffery P, Langen H, Dahinden CA. Human basophils activated by mast cell-derived IL-3 express retinaldehyde dehydrogenase-II and produce the immunoregulatory mediator retinoic acid. *Blood.* 2008;112(9):3762-3771.
8. Didichenko SA, Spiegl N, Brunner T, Dahinden CA. IL-3 induces a Pim1-dependent antiapoptotic pathway in primary human basophils. *Blood.* 2008;112(10):3949-3958.
9. Stiff PJ. Platelets. In: Walker HK, Hall WD, Hurst JW, editors. Clinical Methods: The History, Physical, and Laboratory Examinations. Butterworths. Copyright © 1990, Butterworth Publishers, a division of Reed Publishing; 1990.

2

BONE MARROW BIOPSY PROCEDURE AND EVALUATION

BONE MARROW BIOPSY AND ASPIRATE PROCEDURE

An examination of a bone marrow (BM) biopsy and aspirate is the gold standard to evaluate hematopoiesis and diagnose certain disorders. The BM evaluation consists of several key components. The proper procedures and techniques are important not only to obtain the materials necessary for accurate diagnosis but also to ensure patient safety and health (Table 2.1).

Preparation: The biopsy may be performed by a surgeon in the operating room, by interventional radiology, or by a practitioner or pathologist in the outpatient clinical setting. Once the patient is laying prone and the operator is sterile, the patient's skin on the posterior hip is cleaned. Identifying and manually palpating the posterior iliac crest may be difficult on obese patients, but once found, the site is marked, and the skin is numbed using local anesthetic. A scalpel is used to make a small incision in the skin and subcutaneous tissue. The exterior surface of the bone (periosteum) is innervated and must also be anesthetized.

Aspirate: A trocar needle is inserted into the incision. Using pressure, the operator manually rotates the trocar into the bone using a corkscrew motion. The interior trocar advances with the turning and allows the operator to estimate the depth of the biopsy. At a depth of 1 to 2 cm, the inner trocar is removed and a syringe is attached. The syringe plunger is quickly retracted to extract the liquid BM aspirate; this typically causes significant patient discomfort. After obtaining 2 to 3 mL of aspirate, the syringe is replaced by another, and additional aspirate samples are removed as needed for indicated special studies, including flow cytometry (FC), cytogenetics, and molecular testing. The liquid in the syringe is expelled onto a slide to assess for the presence of particles, which indicates a good specimen. Several slides are made at the bedside and allowed to air-dry. These samples are later stained and reviewed morphologically.

Clot section: The remainder of the aspirate in the syringe is allowed to clot and is placed into formalin for fixation. It is then sectioned and processed normally. Unlike the core biopsy, which is decalcified and generally unsuitable for molecular studies, the clot section may be used after fixation if necessary.

TABLE 2.1 **Bone Marrow Biopsy Specimens**

Specimen	Description	Common stains	Adequacy
Core biopsy	• Tissue biopsy • Formalin fixed • Decalcified	• H&E • Special stains (reticulin, etc) • IHC stains	• 1-2 cm • Intact
Clot	• Clotted liquid aspirate • Formalin fixed • Not decalcified	• H&E • Special stains • IHC	• Several particles
Aspirate smear	• Liquid aspirate • Smeared at bedside (or preserved in EDTA)	• WG • Cytochemical stains • Iron stain	• Spicules and cells • Well-spread and stained
Peripheral blood smear	• Liquid sample • Finger stick • Smeared at bedside	• WG • Cytochemical stains	• Well-spread and stained

EDTA, ethylenediaminetetraacetic acid; H&E, Hematoxylin & Eosin; IHC, immunohistochemical; WG, Wright-Giemsa.

Core biopsy: After obtaining the aspirate, a core biopsy is obtained by repositioning the trocar about 2 mm away from the aspirate site; repositioning is important to avoid sampling marrow that has previously been aspirated. The core is obtained by rotating the trocar into the bone. At a depth of 1 to 2 cm, the trocar is removed. The core biopsy is removed from the needle by gently pushing the core out with the inner trocar. In cases in which the marrow is inaspirable, it is important to create a touch imprint by gently pressing the core biopsy onto a slide. Care should be taken not to rotate the biopsy, as this will result in shearing of cells. The BM core is placed into formalin and subsequently decalcified before processing or, in some cases, directly immersed in a decalcifying fixative.

ASSESSING ADEQUACY OF BM SAMPLES

Aspirate smear: The slide should be well-stained with Wright-Giemsa (WG) and coverslipped. An adequate BM aspirate should have intact cells and spicules (Figure 2.1; eFigure 2.1). Spicules are collections of stroma and cells found in the BM, and their presence is necessary to prove that the BM was accessed during the biopsy. By contrast, a hemodilute aspirate will not be representative of marrow and can result in spurious counts (Figure 2.2; eFigure 2.2). Smears without spicules ("aspiculate") may be a

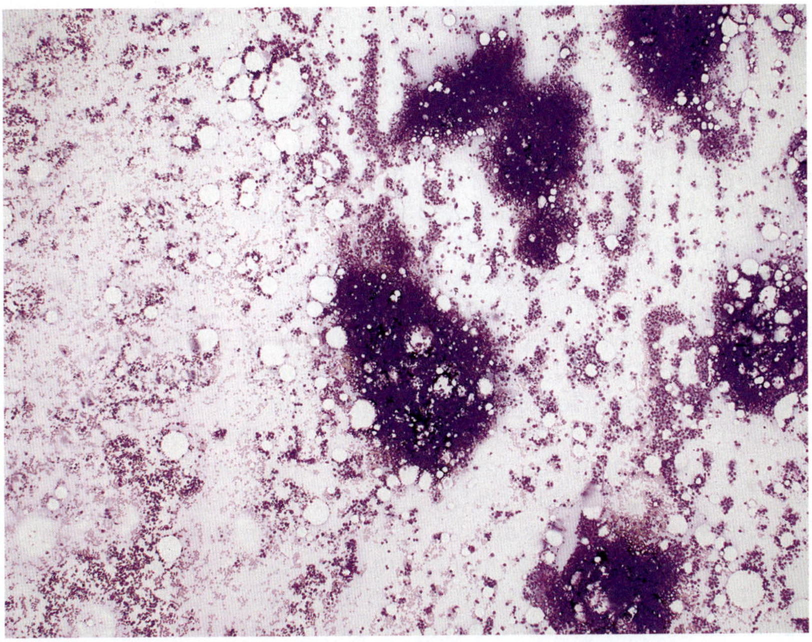

FIGURE 2.1 Low-power view of an adequate bone marrow aspirate with multiple dark spicules and well-spread intact marrow cells at the edges.

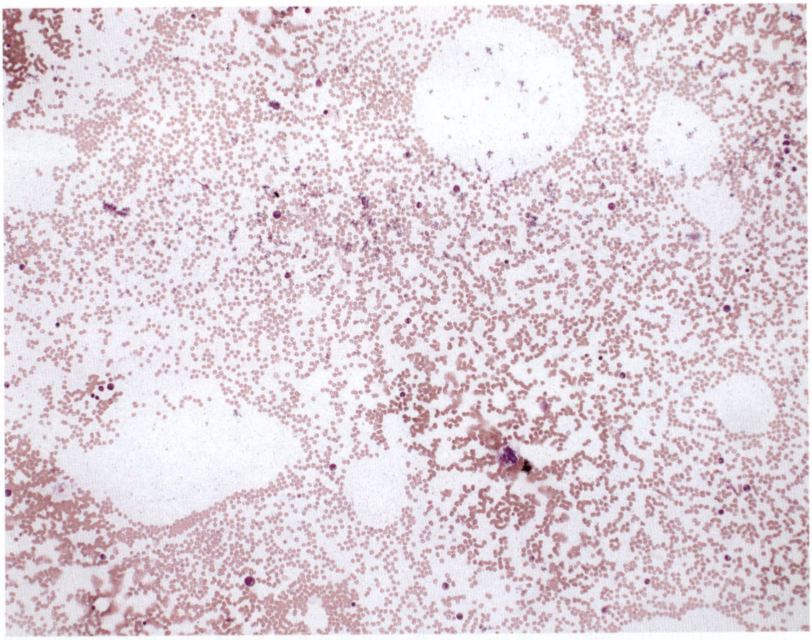

FIGURE 2.2 This aspiculate aspirate smear has mostly blood and scattered hematopoietic elements and is inadequate to evaluate the bone marrow.

result of a dry tap, and in these cases, a touch prep of the core is necessary (Figure 2.3; eFigure 2.3). In some cases, when it is not possible to make a direct smear at the bedside, the marrow aspirate may be placed into ethylenediaminetetraacetic acid (EDTA) and a smear may be made from this sample as if it were blood. Such samples may be fine for assessing cytomorphology, although estimates of cellularity and examination of the types of cells more likely to be associated with spicules (such as mast cells and megakaryocytes) may be compromised.

The best place to assess the aspirate is at the feathered edge, where the cells are not too crowded nor too hemodilute (Figure 2.4; eFigure 2.4). However, certain cell types, particularly clusters of metastatic tumor cells, are frequently pushed to the periphery of the aspirate so the entire slide should be scanned at low power. Multiple fields are morphologically assessed, and 500 nucleated cells are counted to obtain the differential cell count. The differential includes nucleated erythroid cells, lymphocytes, plasma cells, and myeloid cells of all maturation stages, including blasts (Table 2.2). Megakaryocytes are not included in the differential count. Aspirate artifacts include stripped nuclei and crush artifact (Figure 2.5).

Clot section: The clot section is an aggregate of cellular particles obtained from the clotted aspirate (Figure 2.6; eFigure 2.5), typically stained with hematoxylin and eosin (H&E), periodic acid-Schiff (PAS), or Giemsa. If there is no aspirate smear, no clot section will be available. The clot is usually similar in composition to the core biopsy, but occasionally, disease may be patchy in the BM and may be present in one specimen and not another.

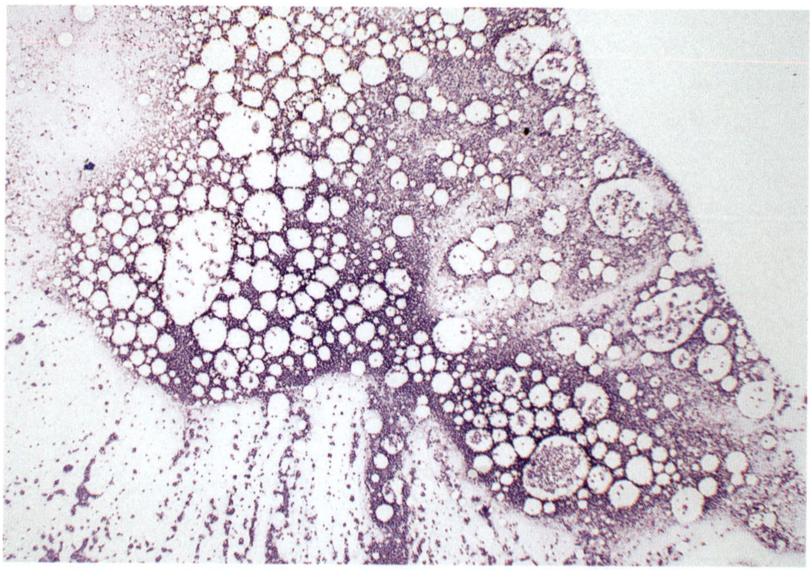

FIGURE 2.3 A good quality touch prep will have areas with intact cells that are not smudged or disrupted.

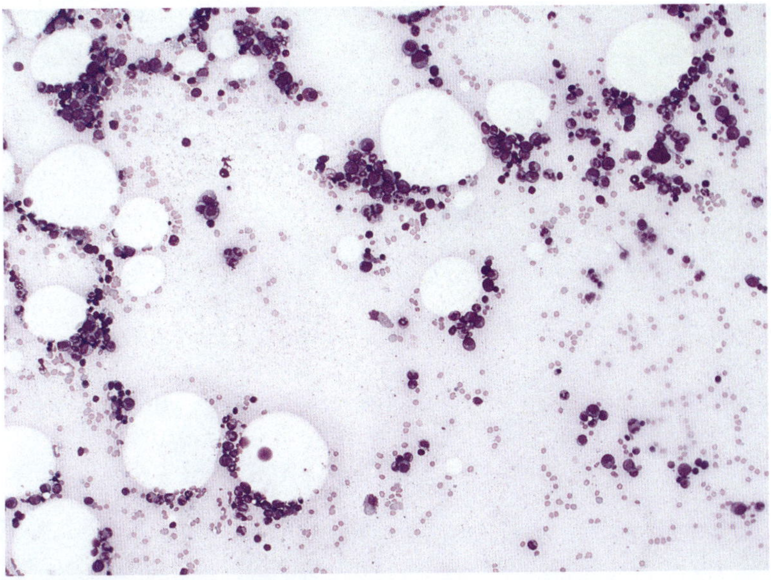

FIGURE 2.4 This area shows well-spread and well-stained cells at the feathered edge outside of a spicule.

TABLE 2.2 Bone Marrow Differential Count

Cell	Adult reference range (%)
Myeloid	
Blasts	0.2
Promyelocytes	2-4
Myelocytes	8-16
Metamyelocytes	10-25
Bands	9-18
Neutrophils	7-14
Eosinophils (myelo/meta)	1-4
Eosinophils (bands)	0-3
Eosinophils	1-2
Basophils	0-0.2
Monocytes	0-2
Pronormoblasts	0-1
Normoblasts	16-32
Lymphocytes	11-23
Plasma cells	0-3
Other cells	
Myeloid:erythroid (M:E) ratio	1.5-3.3

meta, metamyelocyte; myelo, myelocyte.

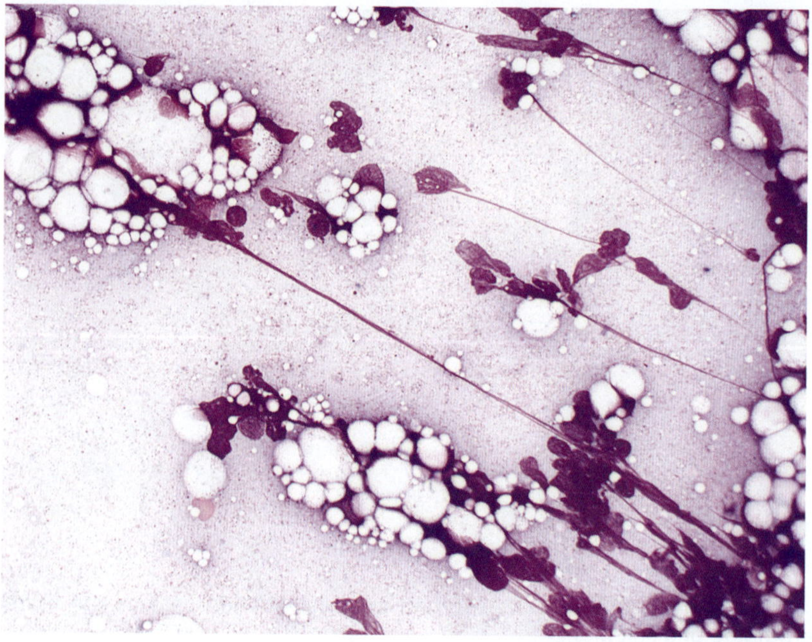

FIGURE 2.5 **A poor-quality aspirate with smeared nuclei, precluding identification of cell types.**

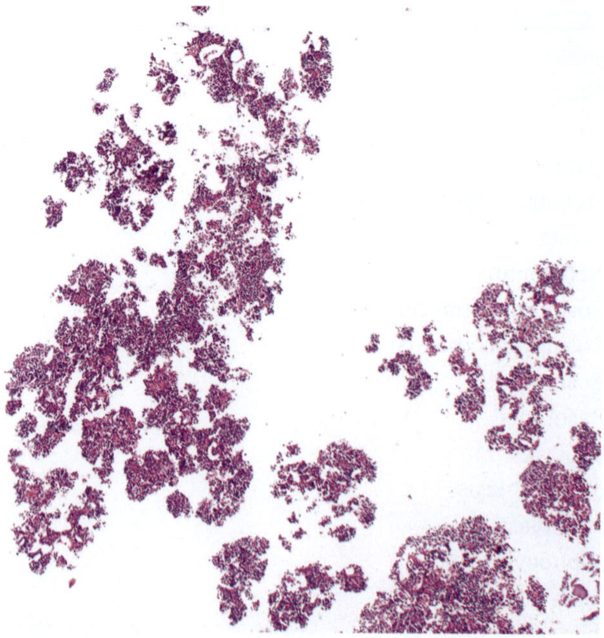

FIGURE 2.6 **Clot sections represent the aggregate of cellular particles, variably associated with clotted red cells.** In this case, spicules were separated from the remainder of the blood and fixed before clotting was complete.

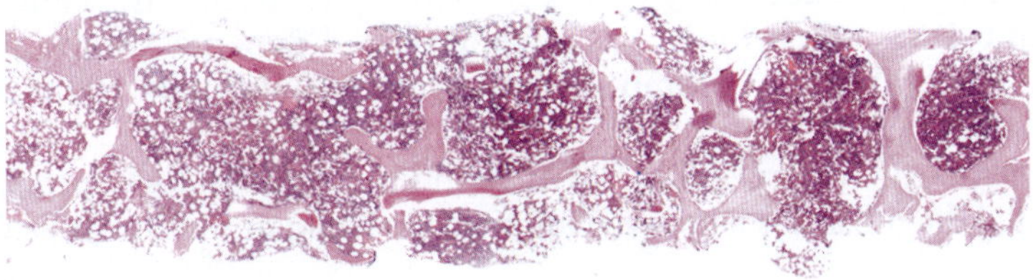

FIGURE 2.7 **A good quality core biopsy should be intact without areas of distortion by hemorrhage from aspiration artifact, and preferably at least 1 cm in length.**

Core biopsy: The core should be 1 to 2 cm or more in length, with minimal hemorrhage or fragmentation (Figure 2.7; eFigure 2.6). The most common cause of a disrupted biopsy is the inability to reposition the trocar after obtaining the aspirate, although it may be difficult to obtain an intact biopsy in some patients with significant osteoporosis or other causes of bone resorption, particularly myeloma. The core biopsy is the best specimen to assess cellularity and megakaryocyte morphology. The most encountered artifacts include aspiration artifact, hemorrhage, crush, and fragmentation. A cortical or subcortical biopsy may not be representative because the marrow is typically acellular or hypocellular in these areas (Figure 2.8; eFigure 2.7).

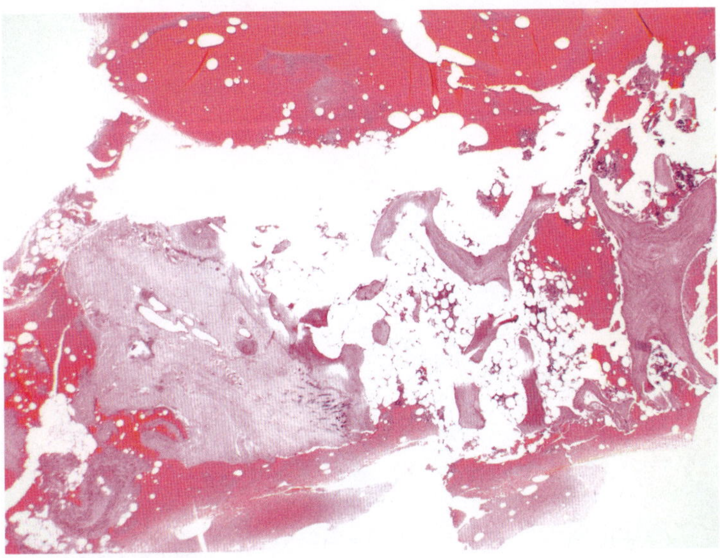

FIGURE 2.8 **A poor-quality biopsy.** Not only is there hemorrhage and clot distorting the specimen, but it is also subcortical, where marrow cellularity is normally markedly decreased and may not be representative.

CELLULARITY

After assessing the adequacy of a specimen, evaluation of the cellularity is important. BM cellularity is a relative term and depends on the patient's age. The general rule of thumb is that normal cellularity is 100 minus the patient's age ± 10%.

A hypo- or hypercellular BM may indicate a pathologic process. The differential diagnosis for a hypercellular or hypocellular marrow is listed next.

Hypocellular BM

Hypocellular BM is a hypoplastic marrow, with decreases in one or more cell lines (Figure 2.9; eFigure 2.8). Most commonly, a patient with a hypocellular BM also has peripheral blood (PB) cytopenias. The differential includes:

Toxin/drug: Following chemotherapy or after exposure to cytotoxic agents; mustard gas; agent orange; atomic bomb; pesticides; chronic alcoholism

Viral infection: Common colds, as well as other viral infections. Some viruses, including HIV, produce a hypercellular BM with a polytypic plasmacytosis.

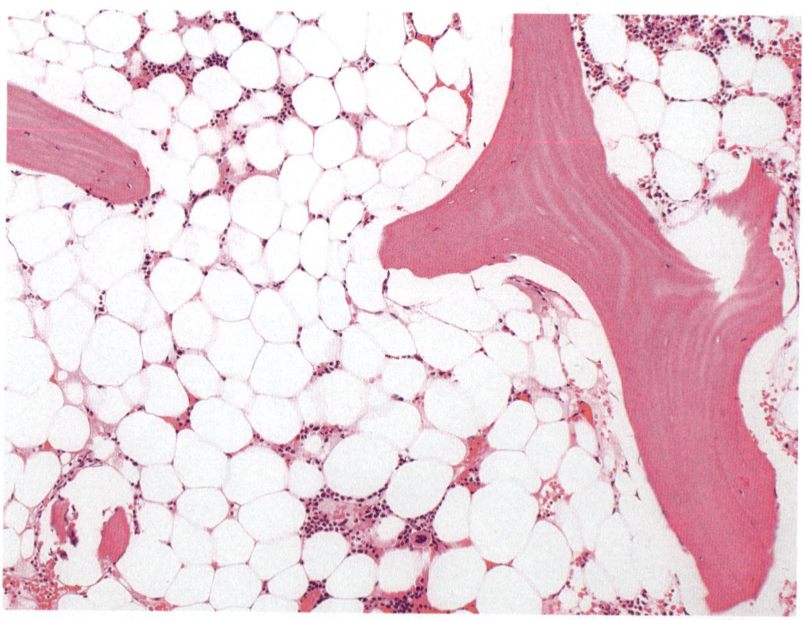

FIGURE 2.9 This marrow biopsy from a patient following chemotherapy shows mostly fat with just a few islands of hematopoietic cells, including a rare megakaryocyte.

Aplastic anemia (congenital or acquired): Aplastic anemia appears as a markedly hypocellular BM with trilineage hypoplasia and near-absent myeloblasts. All three lineages are affected, which results in anemia, leukopenia (specifically neutropenia), and thrombocytopenia. These may be congenital or acquired, after a toxin or viral infection or, most commonly, via immune-mediated destruction of marrow stem cells.

Hypocellular myelodysplastic syndrome (MDS): This is uncommon because MDS typically produces a hypercellular BM with ineffective hematopoiesis; hypocellular MDS can often be distinguished from other causes of hypocellular marrows because blasts are increased or megakaryocytes are atypical.

Hypercellular BM

Hypercellular BM: Different diagnostic considerations depend on which type of cell(s) is/are increased. These are discussed in detail in subsequent chapters.

Increased hematopoietic cells:

- Normal regeneration
- Following infection
- Hemolytic anemia (erythroid hyperplasia)
- Immune thrombocytopenia
- Clonal expansions: acute leukemia, myeloproliferative neoplasms (MPNs), MDS, MDS/MPN

Increased lymphocytes or plasma cells:

- Lymphoma or myeloma

Increased "other" cells:

- Metastatic tumor
- Histiocytic disorders

ORGANIZATION OF THE BM AND NORMAL HEMATOPOIESIS

Thorough evaluation of a BM is essential to assess all the scenarios described earlier. The core biopsy and aspirate smear are each utilized to assess certain aspects of the marrow.

BM architecture is best appreciated on the core biopsy. At first glance, the BM core biopsy appears as a chaotic mixture of cells, and discerning the cellular composition is a big undertaking, especially for beginners. However, with practice, it is evident that although the normal BM is heterogeneous, it has a characteristic organizational pattern.

The aspirate smear is the gold standard specimen for assessing blast count, cellular composition, and cellular cytology. Erythroid and myeloid

TABLE 2.3 Hematopoietic Morphologic Maturation

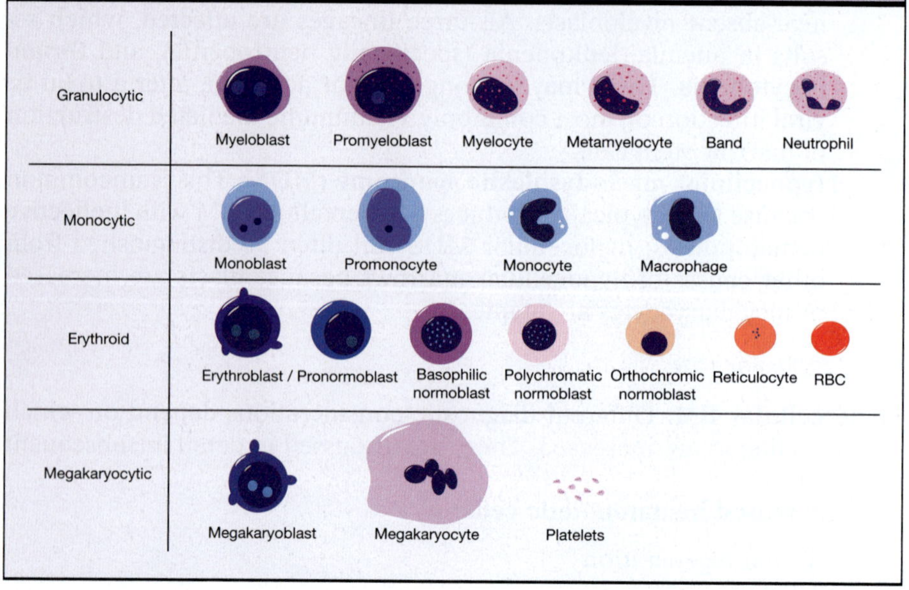

RBC, Red blood cell.

maturation are especially well-visualized on the aspirate smear, discussed further below, as are dyserythropoiesis and/or maturation asynchrony and dysmyelopoiesis, discussed at length in Chapter 5. Table 2.3 shows a schematic diagram outlining the morphologic changes associated with maturation of all the BM lineages.

MYELOID CELLS

Location—core biopsy: The least mature myeloid cells are found immediately adjacent to the bony trabecula, in layers of five to seven cells deep on average (Figure 2.10; eFigure 2.9). More mature forms, including bands and mature neutrophils, are located centrally in the interstitium; combined, the latter forms should equal about half of all myeloid cells in the marrow. Under normal circumstances, only bands and mature neutrophils pass into the PB. Rare myeloblasts are scattered throughout the core biopsy, as highlighted by CD34 (Figure 2.11).

Myelopoiesis—aspirate smear: Myeloid cells progress through several stages of maturation, each with characteristic morphology, best recognized on the aspirate smear (Figure 2.12; eFigure 2.10), and immunophenotype, as recognized by FC (Table 2.4). The common myeloid progenitor also gives rise to eosinophilic and basophilic cell lines. Although myelopoiesis is continuous, we typically recognize distinct morphologic differentiation stages.

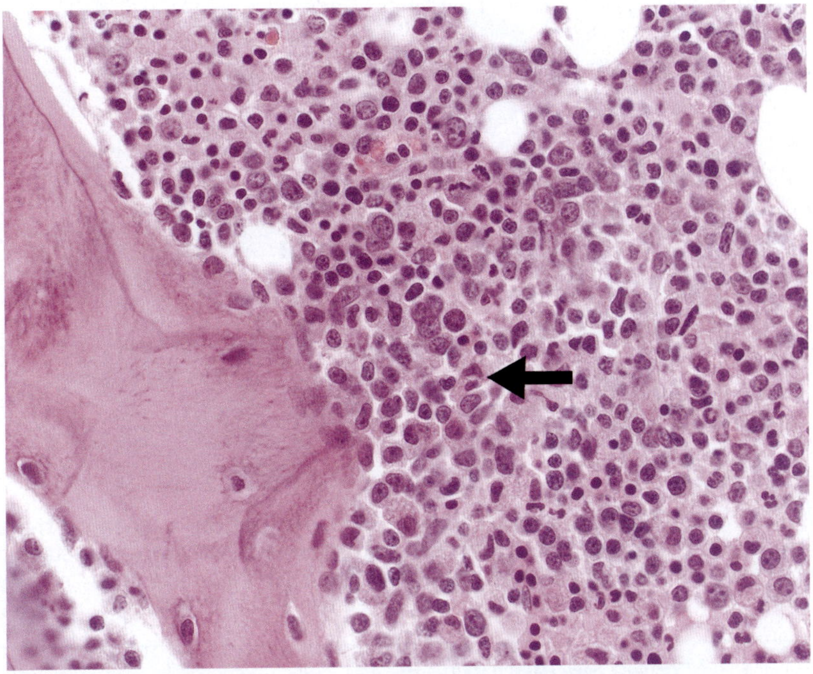

FIGURE 2.10 **Less mature myeloid cells (arrow) are found immediately adjacent to the bony trabeculae, in layers of five to seven cells deep on average.** Further away from the bone myeloid, cells mature to bands and neutrophils.

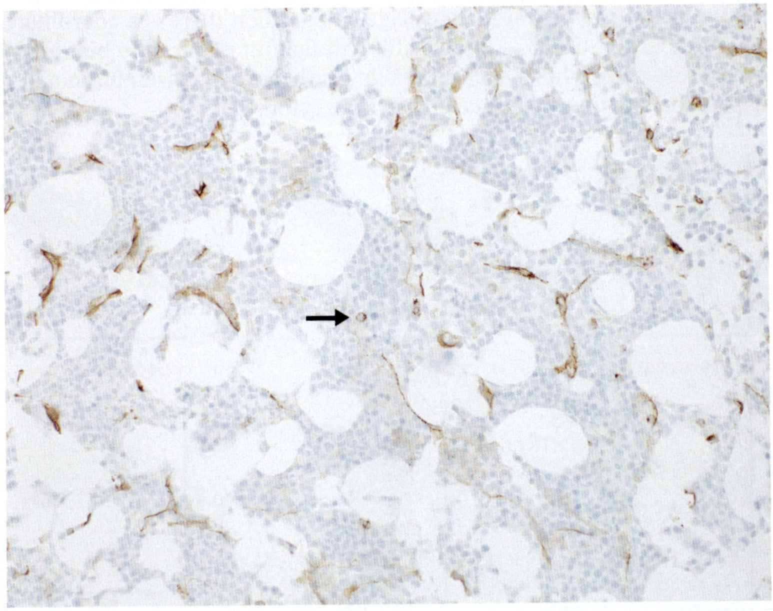

FIGURE 2.11 **Normal myeloblasts (arrow) can be identified on the core biopsy with a CD34 immunostain.**

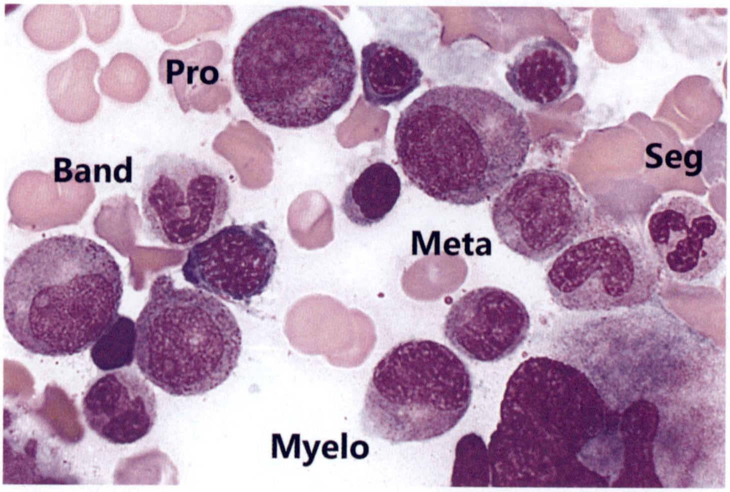

FIGURE 2.12 **Myeloid cells at different stages of maturation, as seen on the aspirate smear.** As the cells progress from the promyelocyte to the myelocyte stage, they become smaller, acquire secondary granules, and have lower N:C ratios. Meta, metamyelocyte; Myelo, myelocyte; Pro, promyelocyte; Seg, segmented neutrophil.

TABLE 2.4 **Myeloid Maturation by FC**

Myeloid cells gain CD10 and CD16 as they mature. Normal myeloid maturation shows characteristic changes by FC, shown here with deepening shades of green with maturation. Earliest promyelocytes have bright CD13, which decrease to a minimum at around the myelocyte stage, after which there is a coordinated increase with CD16. CD33 is more stable throughout maturation but decreases in most mature cells, whereas CD11b is low early and increases, but much more slowly past the late myelocyte stage. FC, flow cytometry.

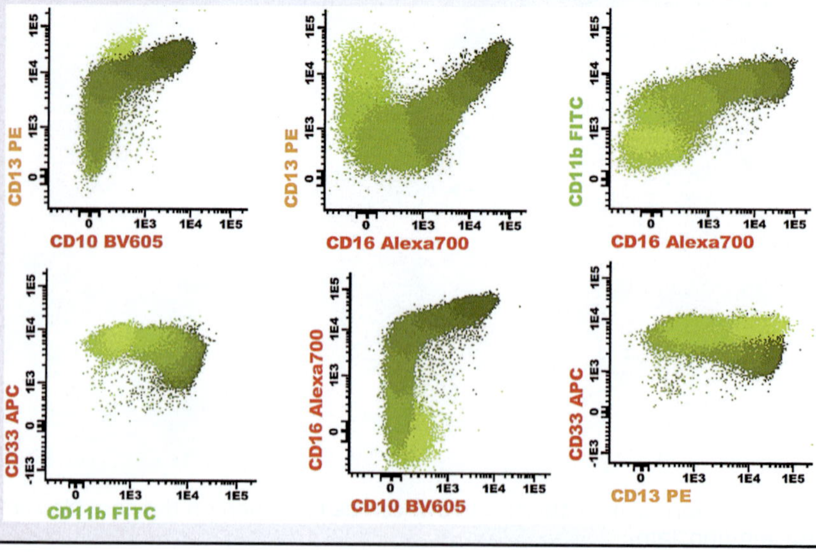

Myeloblasts comprise <5% of BM total cellularity. Although it is impossible to differentiate between a myeloid blast and a lymphoid blast in all cases, some clues include cytoplasmic granulation and cell size. Myeloid blasts are usually slightly larger than lymphoid blasts and may have more abundant cytoplasm and cytoplasmic granules (Figure 2.13; eFigure 2.11). However, the only definitive way to differentiate between them is by phenotyping with cytochemistry, immunohistochemistry (IHC), and/or FC.

Promyelocytes are typically larger than blasts, with a slightly eccentric round nucleus with prominent nucleoli. The cytoplasm is typically dark blue with basophilic primary granules and a perinuclear Hof (eFigure 2.12).

Myelocytes are recognizable as slightly smaller than blasts, with a round-to-oval nucleus, absent or inconspicuous nucleoli, and secondary granules, imparting a pinkish hue to the cytoplasm (eFigure 2.13).

Metamyelocyte nuclei have clumped chromatin and an indentation or fold, imparting a bean-shaped appearance (eFigure 2.14).

Band neutrophils and mature neutrophils (PMNs, or polymorphonuclear leukocytes) have clumped nuclear chromatin and pink secondary cytoplasmic granules. The former is distinguished by the lack of nuclear segmentations (eFigure 2.15). Bands and mature neutrophils are described in Chapter 1.

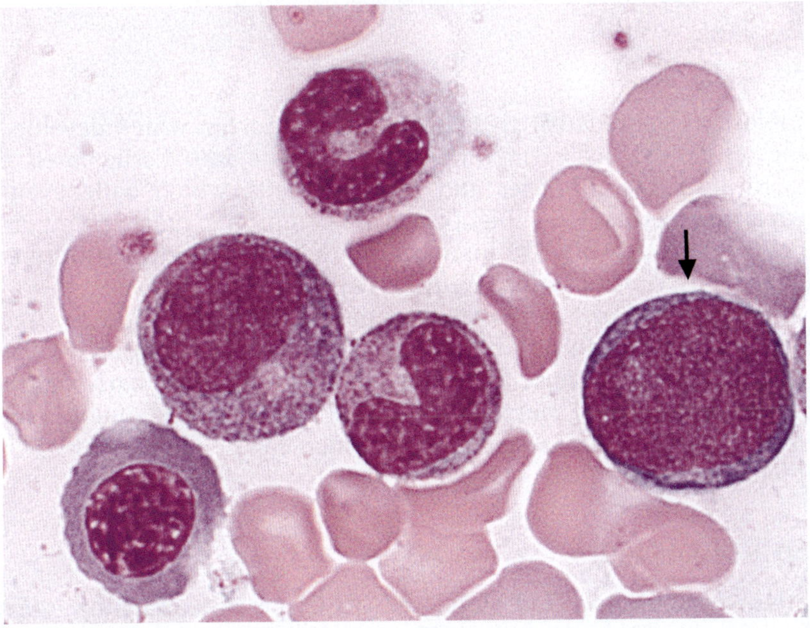

FIGURE 2.13 **Myeloblasts (arrow) have nuclei with fine smooth chromatin, pale nucleoli, and typically agranular pale blue cytoplasm, although rare granules may be seen.** Also in this field are a polychromatic normoblast and some differentiating myeloid cells.

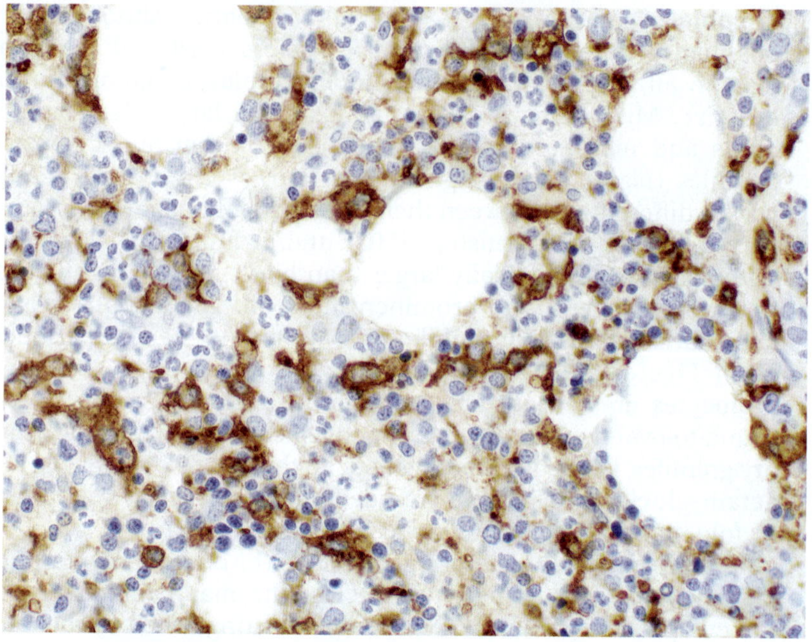

FIGURE 2.14 **This CD163 stain highlights bone marrow macrophages.** Individual cells with nuclei can be recognized but the processes of macrophages between and around other hematopoietic elements are also highlighted.

MONOCYTIC CELLS

Monoblasts (eFigure 2.16) give rise to promonocytes, which develop into monocytes. These cells can further differentiate into tissue-based cells, including both macrophages and dendritic cells, which collectively are known as histiocytes. These histiocytes are common in marrow and distributed evenly through the BM interstitium; they are sometimes more easily visualized with special stains (Figure 2.14; eFigure 2.17).

Like myeloid cells, the stages of monocytic maturation are accompanied by different morphology, which may be difficult to appreciate on the aspirate smear because there are typically not many early monocyte precursors in a normal marrow. They show characteristic changes in surface protein expression as they mature, which can be identified by FC (see Chapter 3 and Table 2.5).

ERYTHROID CELLS

Location–core biopsy: Red blood cell (RBC) precursors mature together in clusters in the BM interstitium (Figure 2.15; eFigure 2.18). Myeloid cells typically outnumber erythroid cells, with a ratio of (2-3):1. The myeloid to erythroid (M:E) ratio varies under many circumstances, reflecting a myeloid or erythroid hyperplasia or hypoplasia; distinguishing hyperplasia of one lineage from hypoplasia of the other is accomplished by assessing cellularity.

TABLE 2.5 Monocytic Maturation by FC

Monocyte maturation by FC is shown here as a deepening color as monocyte precursors mature. Earliest monocytes have bright CD33 and HLA-DR but dim CD64 and lack CD11b. As they mature, they acquire CD64 and lose HLA-DR as they begin to acquire CD14. CD11b and CD14 are both acquired relatively late in maturation, with CD11b before CD14. CD14, CD11b, and CD13 are brightest on the most mature cells. FC, flow cytometry; HLA-DR, human leukocyte antigen-D related.

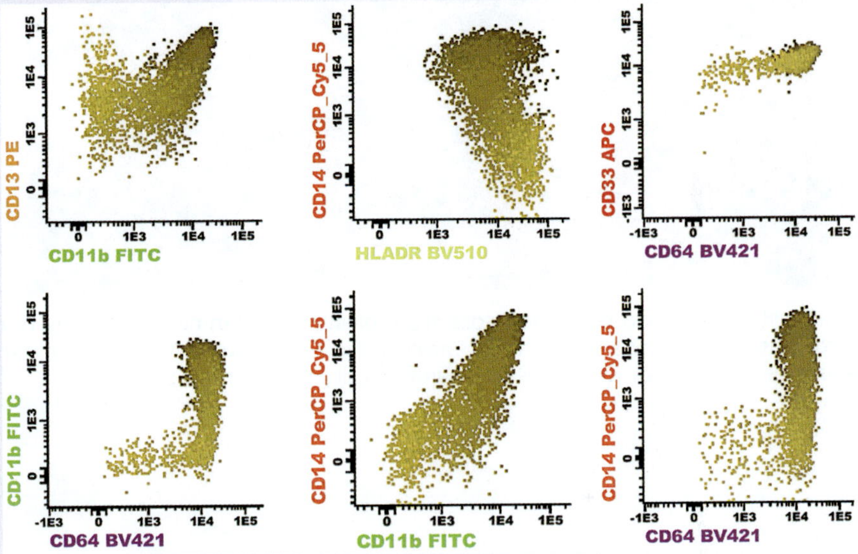

Erythropoiesis–aspirate smear (eFigure 2.19)**:** The common RBC/megakaryocyte progenitor differentiates into a large blast with basophilic cytoplasm and occasional cytoplasmic blebs (Figure 2.16); it can be difficult to distinguish megakaryoblasts from erythroblasts. Erythroid cells undergo a stepwise process of nuclear and cytoplasmic maturation, from pronormoblast to basophilic normoblast, then polychromatic normoblast, then orthochromic normoblast (Figure 2.17). Aggregates of immature and mature erythroid cells may be seen together in the aspirate, occasionally surrounding an iron-laden histiocyte,[1,2] sometimes referred to as a "nurse cell" (Figure 2.18; eFigure 2.20). The extrusion of the nucleus is the last step in maturation in the BM before RBCs are released into the PB. RBCs circulate for about 120 days in the periphery before they are removed by macrophages in the spleen. RBC maturation defects/asynchrony in the BM results in megaloblastic changes, seen in megaloblastic anemia, rare congenital abnormalities, and MDS.

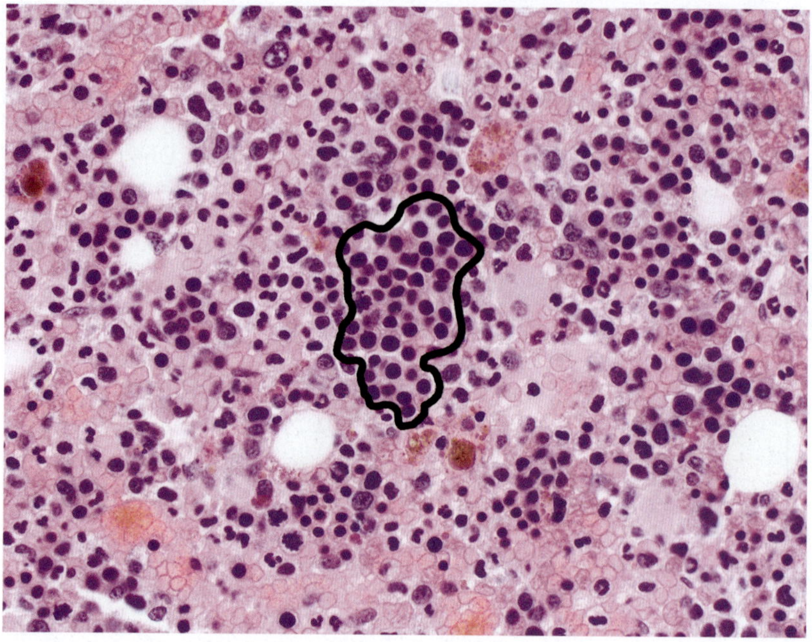

FIGURE 2.15 **Red blood cell precursors are typically found in clusters in the bone marrow interstitium away from bone.** The encircled area shows relatively mature forms characterized by dark homogeneous nuclei and a small amount of cytoplasm.

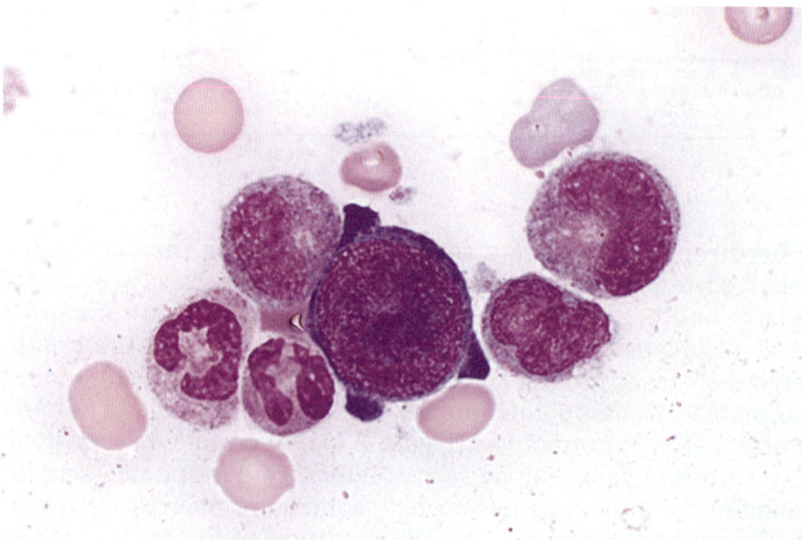

FIGURE 2.16 **The earliest recognizable precursor of erythroid and megakaryocytic cells is a large blast with basophilic cytoplasm and occasional cytoplasmic blebs, as shown here, but at this stage, morphologic distinction between these two lineages is still unreliable.**

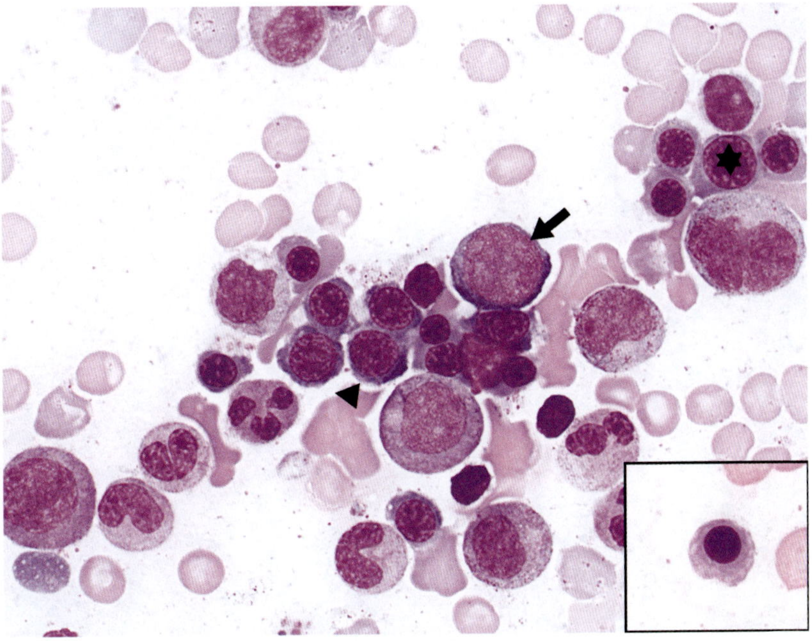

FIGURE 2.17 **As erythroid cells mature, they decrease in size and their cytoplasm becomes pinkish because of hemoglobinization.** A pronormoblast (arrow) matures into a basophilic normoblast (arrowhead), to a polychromatic normoblast (*star*), and finally to an orthochromic normoblast (*inset*).

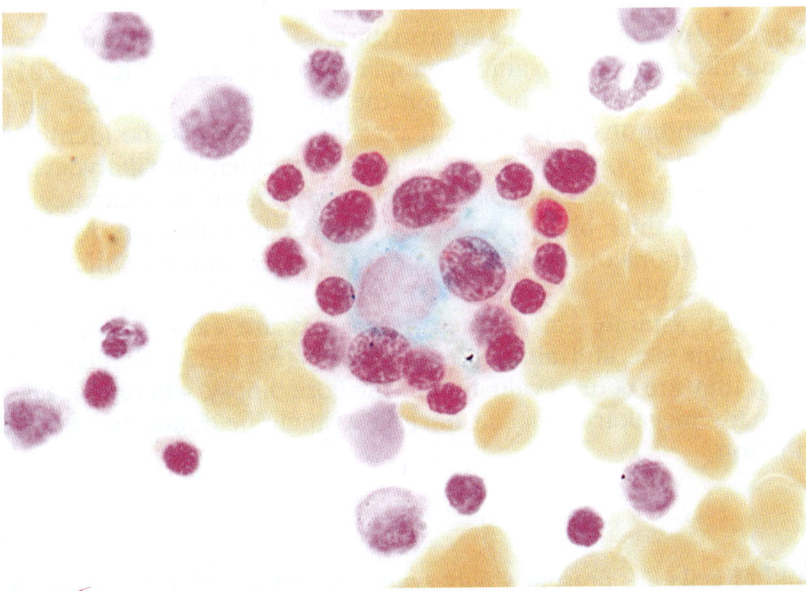

FIGURE 2.18 **This Prussian blue stain highlights an iron-containing histiocyte, sometimes called a "nurse cell," surrounded by aggregates of erythroid cells.**

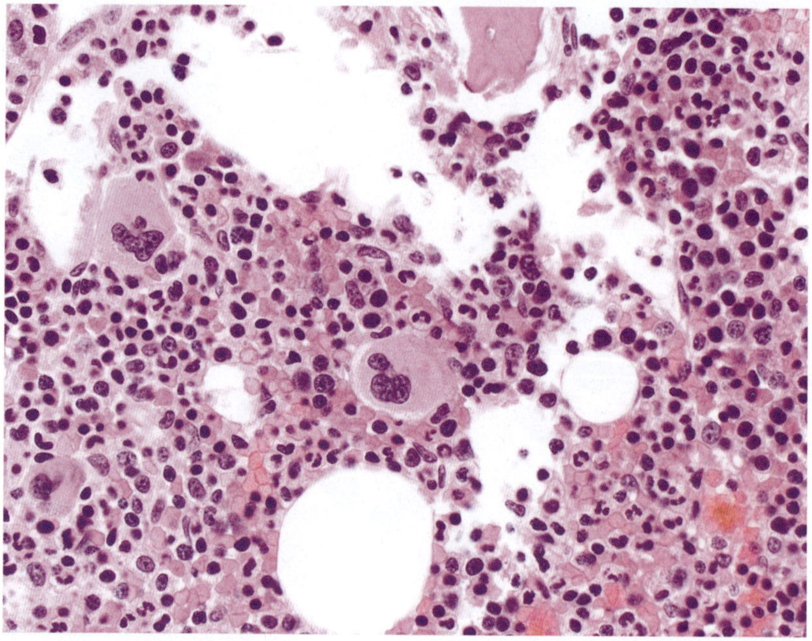

FIGURE 2.19 Normal megakaryocytes have multiple lobes and are generally singly scattered among other elements, often near sinuses.

MEGAKARYOCYTES

The largest hematopoietic cells are also the least numerous. Megakaryocytes, large, multilobed cells with ample cytoplasm (Figure 2.19; eFigure 2.21), are normally singly scattered throughout the interstitium, often near sinuses. In normal conditions, three to four megakaryocytes can be identified on the core per high-power field. Small megakaryocytes, megakaryocyte clusters of more than three cells, or hypo- or hyperlobated megakaryocytes, are abnormal, and their presence requires further investigation. Megakaryocytes shed portions of their cytoplasm into nearby sinuses, which become platelets in the PB.

On the aspirate smear, megakaryocytes are easily identifiable because of their size and abundant cytoplasm (Figure 2.20; eFigure 2.22), although they are better evaluated on the core biopsy, where it is easier to assess many megakaryocytes at once in a single field, and to assess their distribution.

LYMPHOCYTES

Lymphoid cells are present singly scattered in the BM interstitium or occasionally form small lymphoid aggregates, especially in older individuals (Figure 2.21; eFigure 2.23). Normal lymphoid aggregates are small and

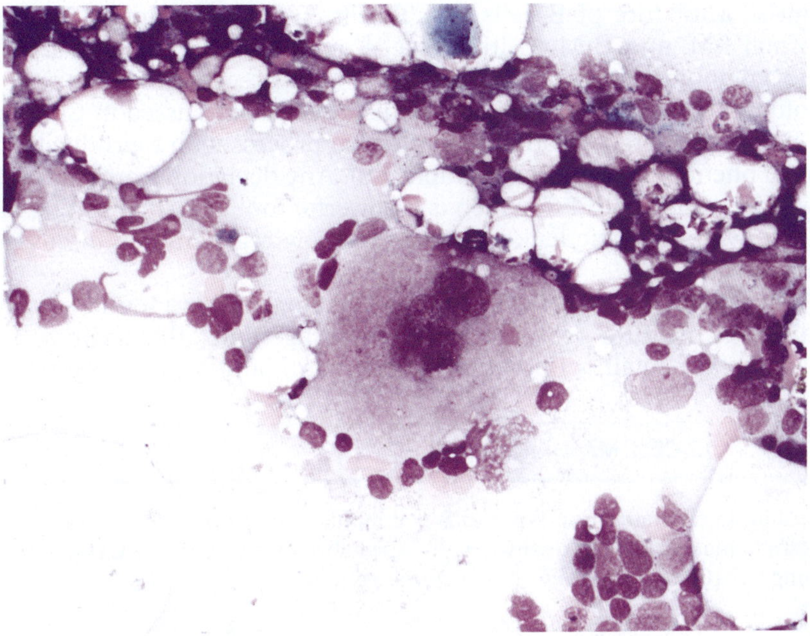

FIGURE 2.20 Wright-Giemsa stain of a single large megakaryocyte with a characteristic polylobated nucleus and fluffy blue-gray cytoplasm with RNA-containing reticular streaks.

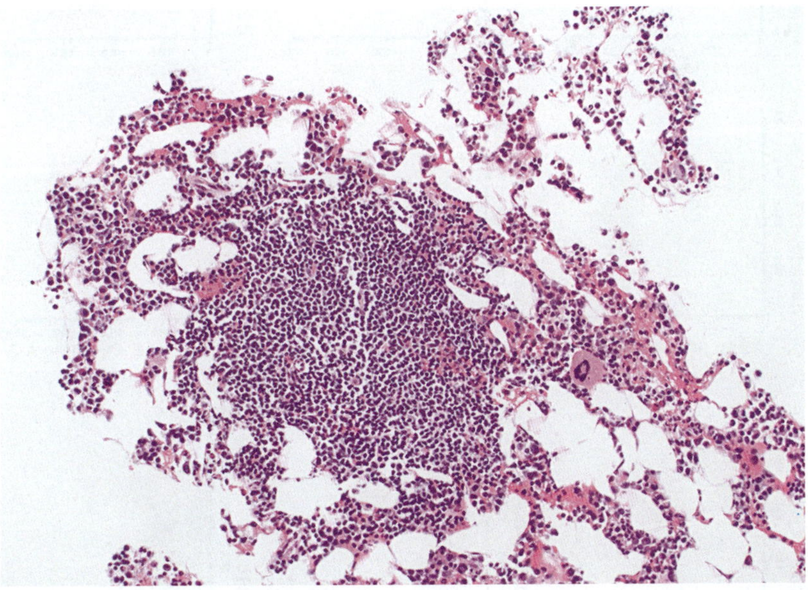

FIGURE 2.21 Small, well-demarcated lymphoid aggregates composed of mature lymphocytes with scant cytoplasm are not uncommon, especially in older individuals.

comprise a mixture of B cells and T cells. T cells outnumber B cells in a normal BM, and CD4-positive T cells outnumber CD8-positive T cells. Large lymphoid aggregates or paratrabecular aggregates are abnormal and are often seen in lymphoproliferative disorders, as discussed in Chapter 8.

B cells undergo an orderly maturation process with reproducible patterns of phenotypic expression (Table 2.6). Any deviation from this pattern may be identified with FC, which is a powerful tool in distinguishing blasts of acute lymphoblastic leukemia from marrow regeneration, discussed in Chapter 3.

Precursor B cells, also known as hematogones, are found in varying numbers in the BM, depending on patient age and other factors. These precursors are small, with compact chromatin, and have a very thin rim

TABLE 2.6 B CELL MATURATION BY FC

Normal B cell maturation Normal B cell maturation, from light to dark, shows hematogones expressing progressively brighter CD20 and CD45 while losing CD10 and CD34. FC, flow cytometry

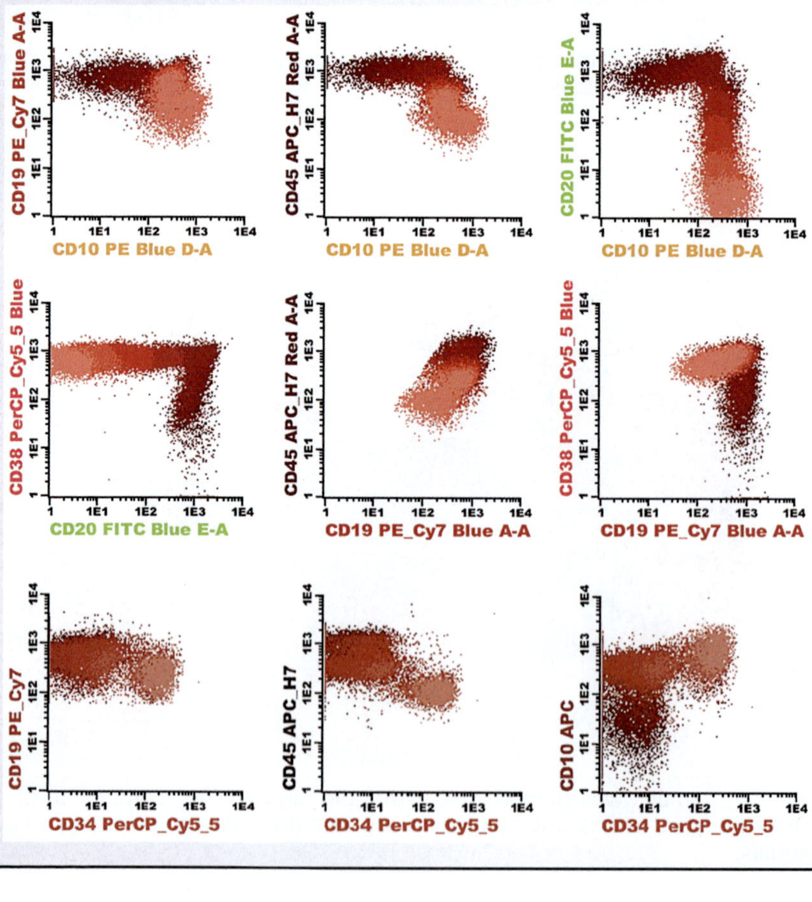

of pale cytoplasm, often requiring oil immersion examination to identify (Figure 2.22; eFigure 2.24), although at some stages these are larger with more abundant cytoplasm.

Mature B cells in the BM look identical to circulating mature lymphocytes and cannot be distinguished from T cells morphologically. Their presence and distribution in the marrow can be identified on the core biopsy by their strong CD20 expression.

Plasma cells develop in lymph nodes and other tissues and home back to the BM. Plasma cells normally comprise <10% of total BM cellularity (Figure 2.23; eFigure 2.25). On the core biopsy, they typically form a linear cluster around small vessels, best appreciated with IHC stains (Figure 2.24) but may also be scattered in the interstitium. Large clusters of plasma cells that are not associated with vessels are most likely pathologic, although not necessarily neoplastic.

Although the earliest stages of T cell development occur in the BM before these cells migrate to the thymus and further mature into mature T cells and T cell subsets, precursor T cells are essentially never seen in the marrow cannot be assessed. Scattered mature T cells (and natural killer [NK] cells) are typically present, however, and can be visualized by IHC; T cells normally outnumber B cells.

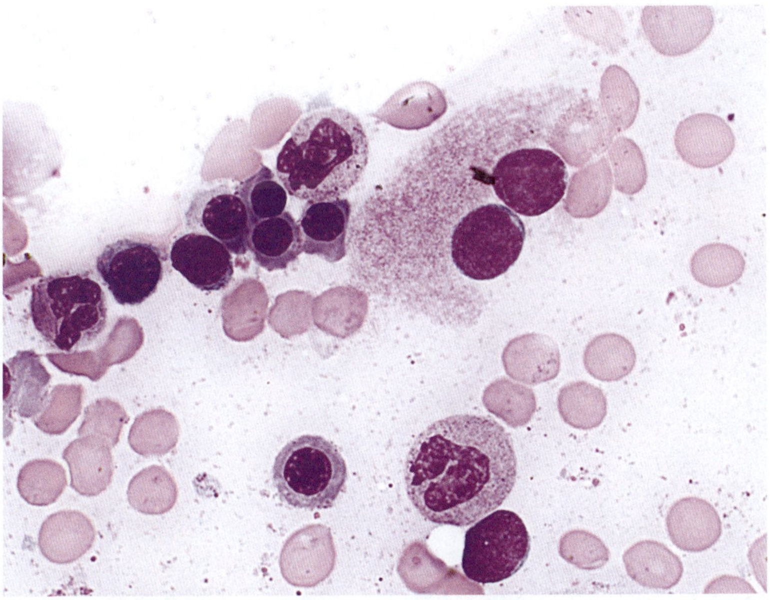

FIGURE 2.22 **Normal precursor B cells (*top right*), also known as hematogones, can be recognized as lymphoid-appearing cells with compact but not clumped chromatin and very high N/C ratios, with only a small rim of cytoplasm at one end.** Compare the lack of nuclear chromatin clumping to the red cell precursors on the left.

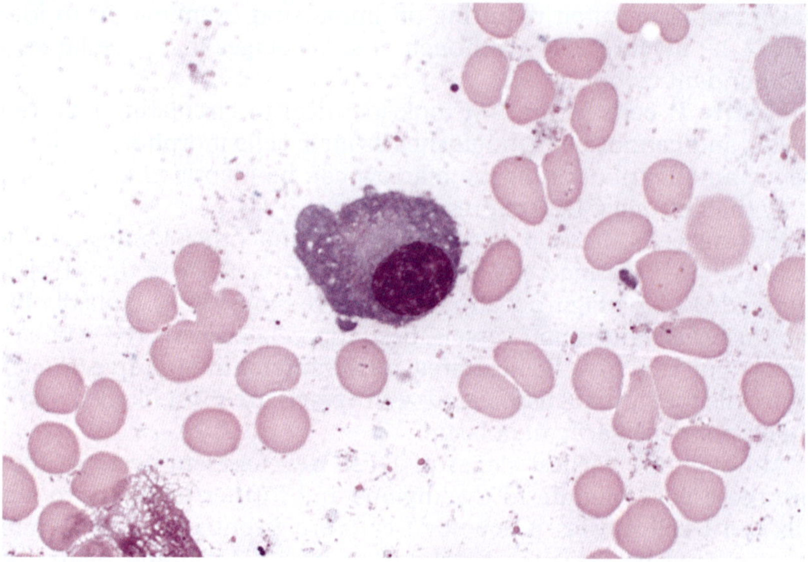

FIGURE 2.23 Plasma cells have eccentric nuclei and a cleared-out Golgi zone or cytoplasmic Hof near the nucleus.

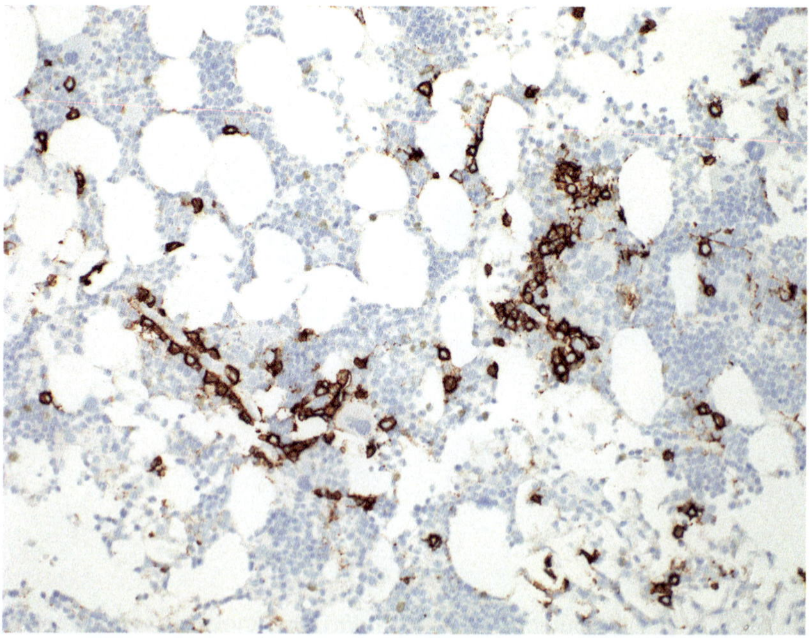

FIGURE 2.24 Plasma cells are normally found around blood vessels as shown here with an immunostain for CD138.

OTHER CELLS AND NORMAL BM CONSTITUENTS

Mast cells can be seen scattered throughout the aspirate smear. These cells may be round-to-spindled in shape, have oval nuclei and dark purple, metachromatic granules (Figure 2.25; eFigure 2.26). If there are large clusters of mast cells, a mast cell neoplasm should be considered.

Small vessels are present throughout the BM interstitium and are highlighted by vascular markers such as CD34 and ERG (Figure 2.26; eFigure 2.27). They are typically supported by a fine reticulum network that is better seen on a reticulin stain. This same stroma can be seen around vascular sinuses that are present throughout the interstitium. Mature hematopoietic cells exit the BM via these sinuses. Megakaryocytes are often positioned near sinuses and extrude cellular fragments of cytoplasm, which form platelets in the PB.

Cortical bone and bony trabecula can be identified in BM core biopsies and appear deeply eosinophilic on H&E (Figure 2.27). Cortical bone represents the outer surface of the bone; in young patients before endosteal mineralization, cartilage may be present. Bony trabeculae are composed of lamellar bone (Figure 2.28), with osteocytes visible in lacunae. Osteoblasts may be present lining the trabeculae (Figure 2.29; eFigure 2.28), especially in young patients or in patients with bone remodeling (see Chapter 10). Osteoclasts are multinucleated cells that assist in bone resorption (Figure 2.30; eFigure 2.29).

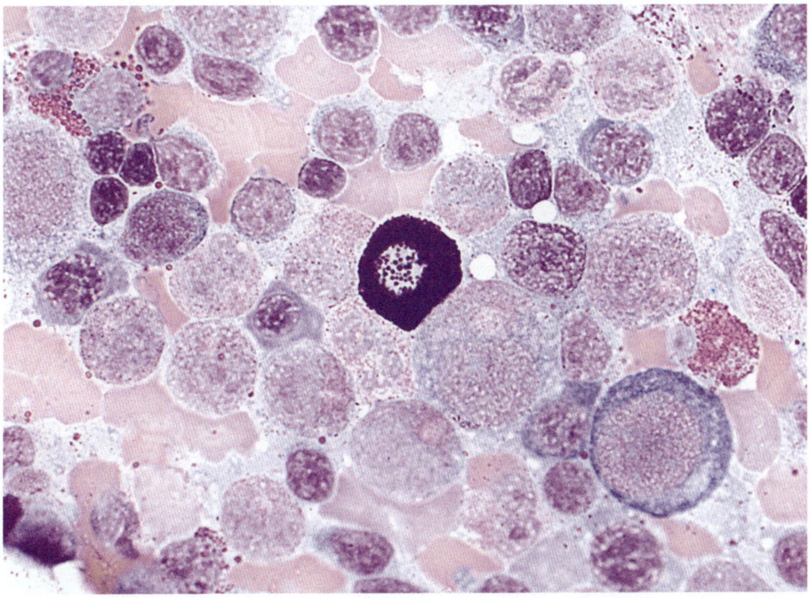

FIGURE 2.25 **Mast cells are easily recognized by their coarse dark purple granules.** Most normal mast cells are round, as shown here, but they may also have a spindle shape. They may be seen as isolated individual cells in the aspirate smear, although they are more commonly seen within spicules.

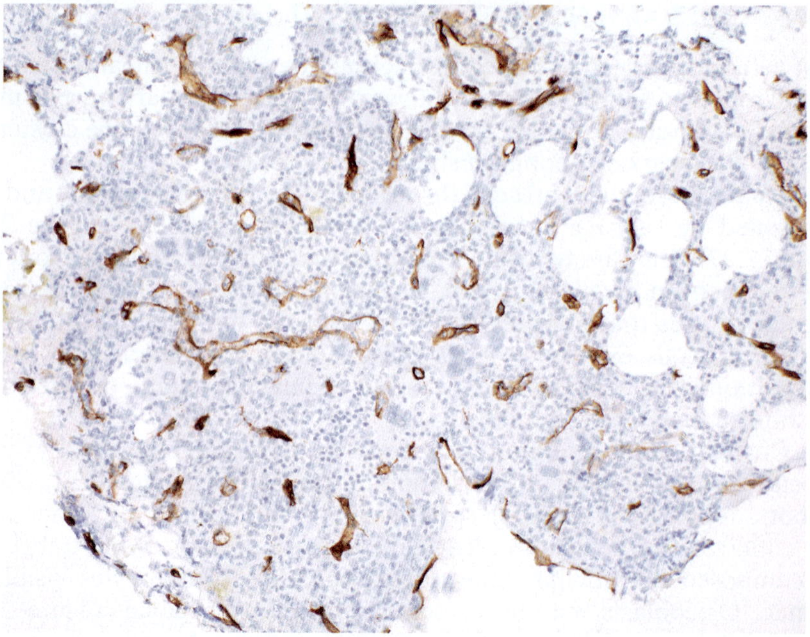

FIGURE 2.26 **In addition to staining blasts, CD34 highlights small vessels throughout the bone marrow.**

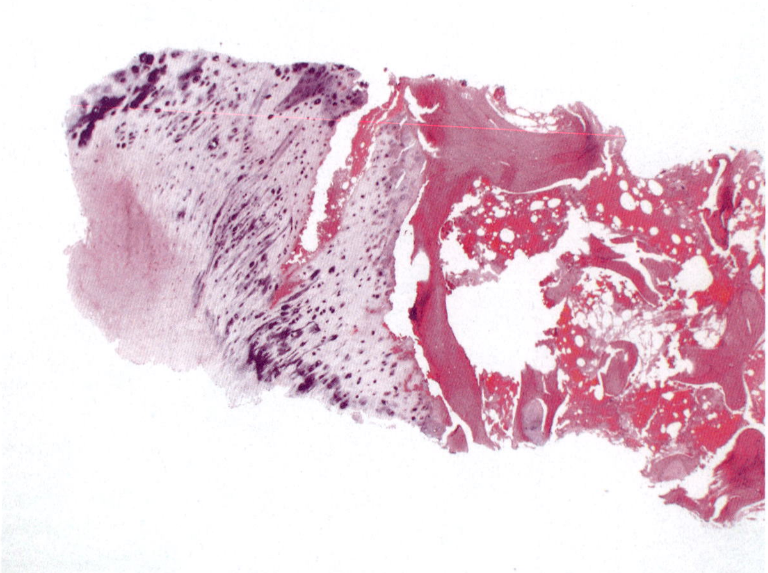

FIGURE 2.27 **Although a good marrow biopsy should not have much cortical bone, when present, it appears as dense eosinophilic material on hematoxylin and eosin (H&E).** Depending upon the age of the patient, there can be variable amounts of purple cartilage outside of the cortex.

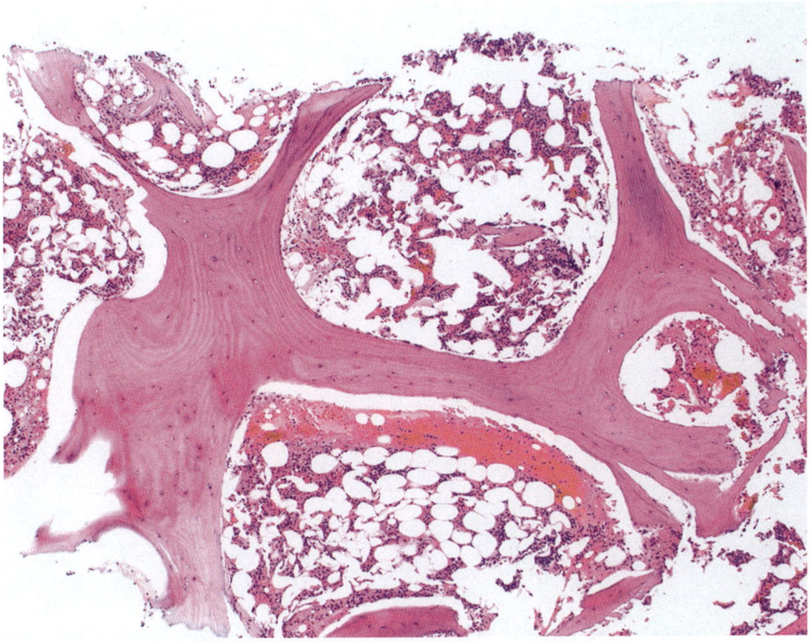

FIGURE 2.28 Bony trabeculae stain darkly eosinophilic and shows the lacunae where osteocytes reside.

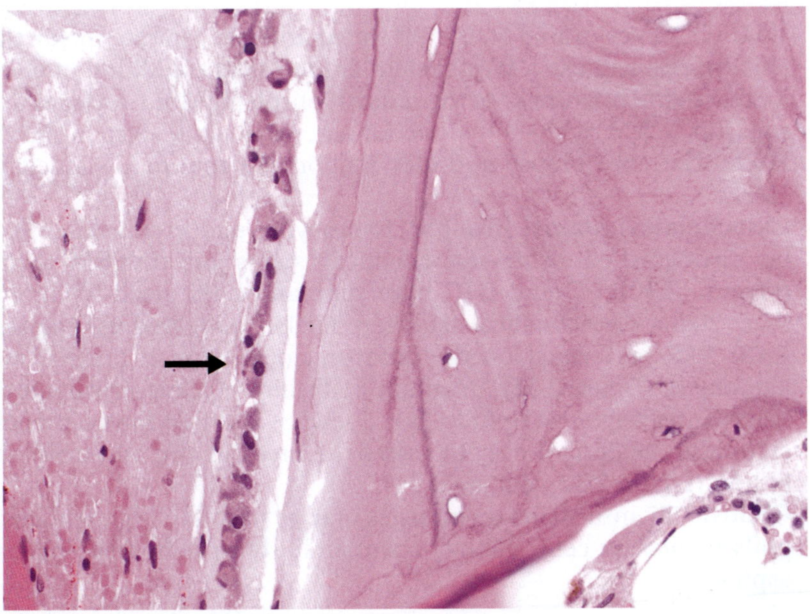

FIGURE 2.29 Osteoblasts (arrow) are cells with a single nucleus and are typically seen lining the trabeculae.

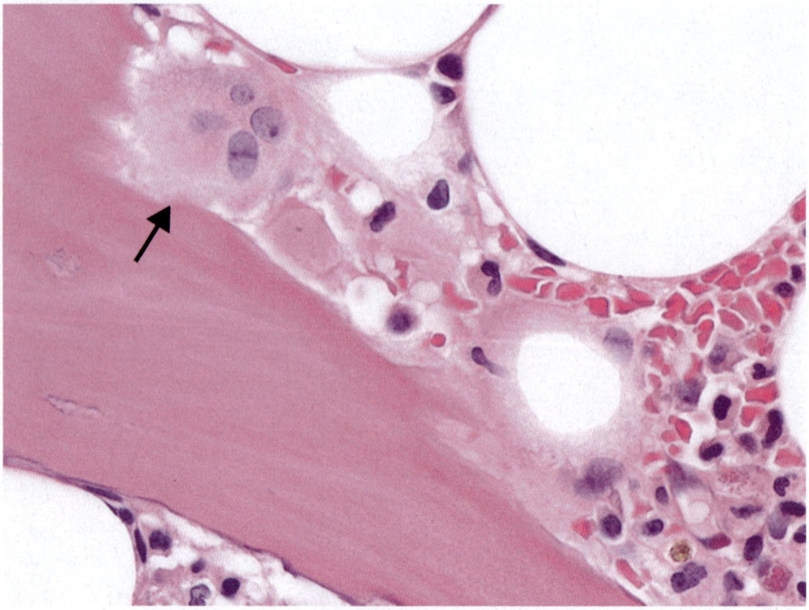

FIGURE 2.30 Osteoclasts (*arrow*) are multinucleated cells near the trabeculae and indicate that bone resorption is taking place.

STAINS

1. **WG:** WG is performed on the PB smear and BM aspirate smear. Some laboratories will use a Wright stain alone, but the addition of Giemsa increases the brightness of the reddish-purple myeloid granules and is superior to a Wright stain alone for assessing subtle dyspoiesis.
2. **H&E:** The core biopsy and clot section are routinely stained with H&E.
3. **Cytochemical stains:** Myeloid, monocytic, and erythroid cells can be distinguished using cytochemical stains on the BM aspirate (eFigure 2.30). FC and IHC have supplanted the need for many of these stains. Cytochemical stains are further discussed in Chapter 3.
4. **PAS:** PAS performed on the core or clot section highlights megakaryocytes (Figure 2.31). In addition, it stains myeloid precursor cytoplasm intensely eosinophilic, but does not stain erythroid precursor cytoplasm, making it easy to assess the myeloid and erythroid distribution (Figure 2.32; eFigure 2.31).
5. **Giemsa:** Giemsa stains on biopsies may be useful to highlight eosinophils or plasma cells, as they stain similarly to how they appear on aspirates.

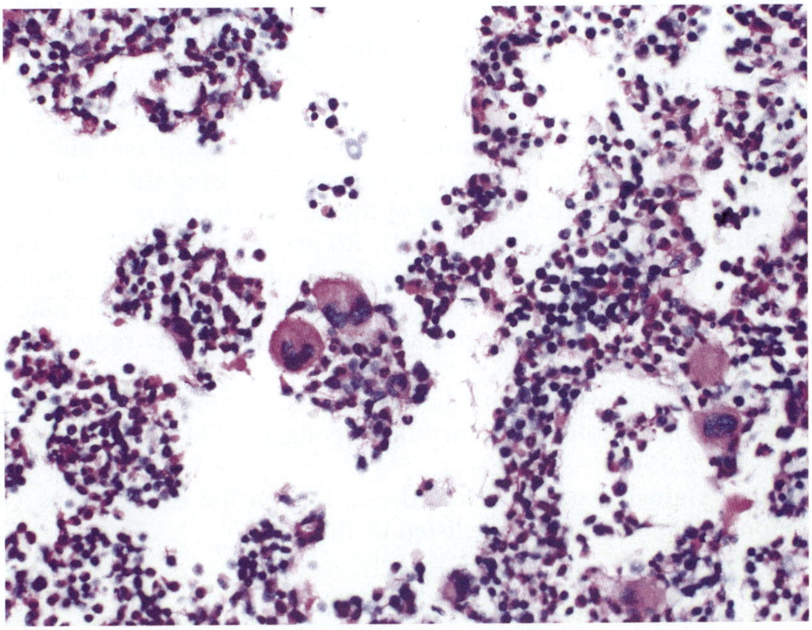

FIGURE 2.31 **A PAS stain is particularly useful for identifying megakaryocytes as the cytoplasm is intensely PAS positive.** PAS, periodic acid-Schiff.

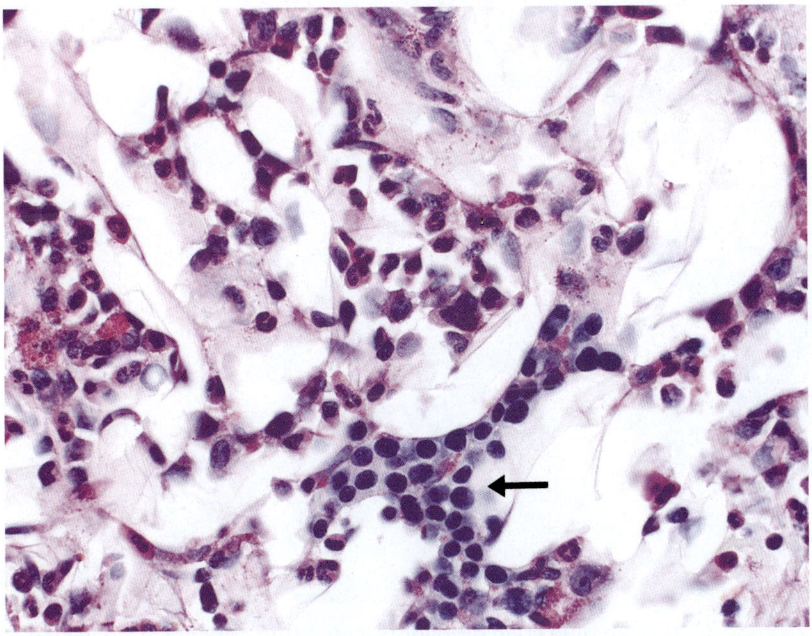

FIGURE 2.32 **A PAS stain of a marrow showing the pink staining of the myeloid cell cytoplasm and the pale or slightly blue staining of the erythroid precursor cytoplasm (arrow).** PAS, periodic acid-Schiff.

6. **Iron stain:** A Prussian blue stain for iron can be performed on the core, clot, or the aspirate smear, although decalcification may leach iron from a specimen. Iron may be increased in patients with a history of transfusions or MDS (Figure 2.33; eFigure 2.32). Sideroblasts, or RBC progeny, contain iron in their cytoplasm and can be appreciated with an iron stain (eFigure 2.33). Ring sideroblasts (RS) can also be identified because of the accumulation of iron in a ring around the nucleus (Figure 2.34). RS are found in MDS, as well as in other reactive scenarios, including alcoholism and zinc overload, although they tend to be less numerous in reactive conditions.
7. **Reticulin:** Reticulin is a special stain that highlights reticulin fibers (eFigure 2.34).[3]
8. **Trichrome** (most commonly Masson trichrome): Trichrome is a special stain utilized to highlight collagen fibrosis (Figure 2.35; eFigure 2.35).
9. **Other stains:** May be utilized depending on the BM findings. Common BM special stains are listed in Table 2.7.[4,5]

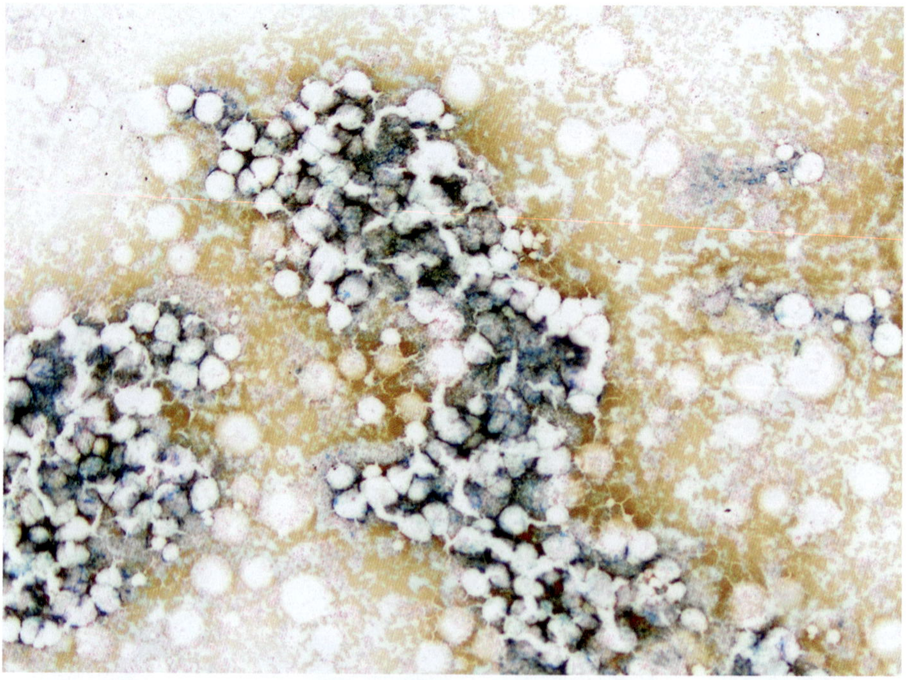

FIGURE 2.33 A Prussian blue stain highlights iron, often concentrated in spicules as on this aspirate smear from a patient with iron overload.

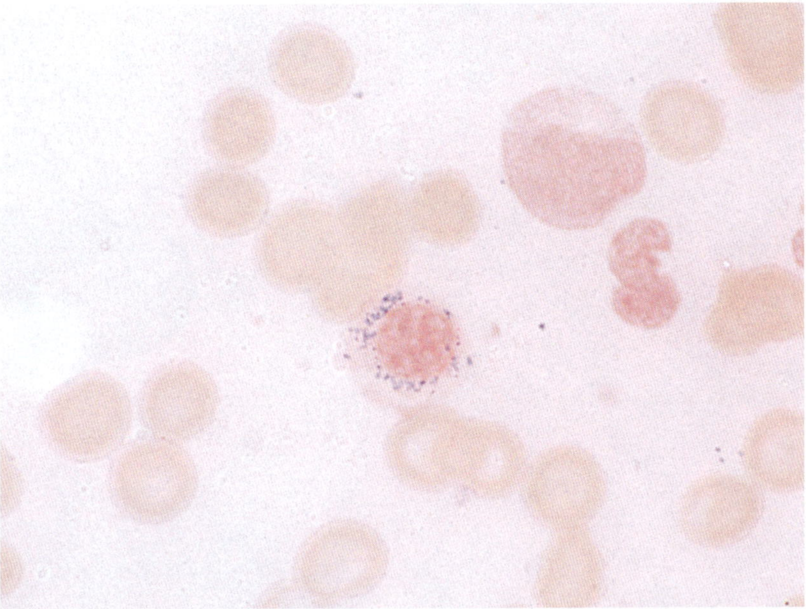

FIGURE 2.34 **Ring sideroblasts are erythroid precursors that show iron circling the nucleus.** They are always abnormal.

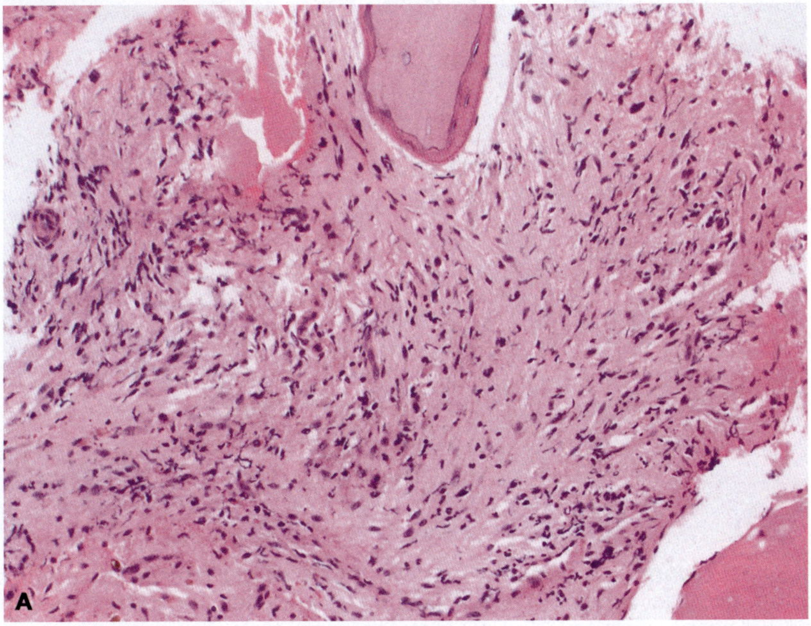

FIGURE 2.35 **This composite shows a fibrotic bone marrow stained with H&E (A);**

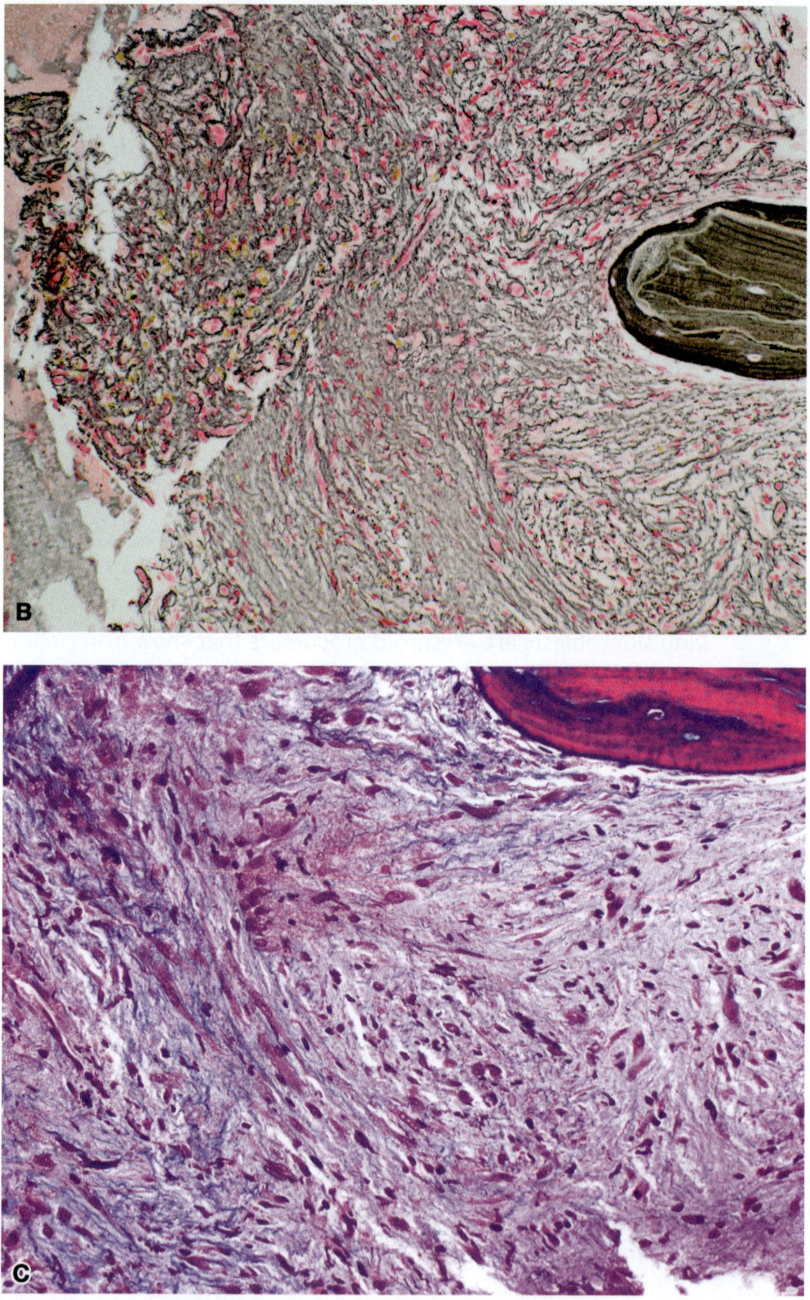

FIGURE 2.35 (*continued*) **silver stain for reticulin (B); and a Masson trichrome stain for collagen (C).** Not all marrows with fibrosis will have collagen, and early reticulin fibrosis typically will not be visible on H&E. H&E, hematoxylin and eosin.

TABLE 2.7 Special Stains Performed on Bone Marrow Biopsy

Stain	Specimen	Notes
Reticulin	Core biopsy	• Normally none or rare strands • Increased in reticulin fibrosis • Graded (MF 0-3); see Chapter 6
Trichrome (Masson, Mallory or Van Gieson)	Core biopsy	• Normally none • Increased in collagen fibrosis, late-stage fibrosis • Graded (0-3); see Chapter 6
PAS	Core or clot	• Bright pink cytoplasm in megakaryocytes • Helps differentiate between myeloid and erythroid cells
Iron	Aspirate smear	• Increased in transfusions • Decreased in iron deficiency • Decalcified specimen may affect staining

PAS, Periodic acid-Schiff.

REFERENCES

1. Chasis JA, Mohandas N. Erythroblastic islands: niches for erythropoiesis. *Blood.* 2008;112(3):470-478.
2. Rhodes MM, Kopsombut P, Bondurant MC, Price JO, Koury MJ. Adherence to macrophages in erythroblastic islands enhances erythroblast proliferation and increases erythrocyte production by a different mechanism than erythropoietin. *Blood.* 2008;111(3):1700-1708.
3. Kvasnicka HM, Beham-Schmid C, Bob R, Dirnhofer S, Hussein K, Kreipe H, et al. Problems and pitfalls in grading of bone marrow fibrosis, collagen deposition and osteosclerosis: a consensus-based study. *Histopathology*. 2016;68(6):905-915.
4. Armeanu S, Bühring HJ, Reuss-Borst M, Müller CA, Klein G. E-cadherin is functionally involved in the maturation of the erythroid lineage. *J Cell Biol.* 1995;131(1):243-249.
5. Dong HY, Wilkes S, Yang H. CD71 is selectively and ubiquitously expressed at high levels in erythroid precursors of all maturation stages: a comparative immunochemical study with glycophorin A and hemoglobin A. *Am J Surg Pathol.* 2011;35(5):723-732.

3

ANCILLARY STUDIES

In the current era, there are very few bone marrow (BM) diseases that can be diagnosed by morphology alone, and even those with highly characteristic morphologic findings generally require confirmation by some specialized technique. Ancillary studies in the broadest sense could include something as simple as a complete blood count (CBC) or a serum protein study, but in this chapter, we will discuss two major areas: immunophenotyping and genetics. The first of these includes both flow cytometry (FC) and immunohistochemistry (IHC), whereas the latter encompasses traditional genetic techniques including karyotyping and fluorescence in situ hybridization (FISH), as well as a variety of molecular genetic tests.

FLOW CYTOMETRY

FC is an especially useful ancillary tool for detecting and classifying BM disorders. Antibodies conjugated to fluorescent detectors bind to cellular proteins. These labeled cells subsequently pass by a laser in a fluid stream.

FC lends itself especially well to the field of hematopathology because hematolymphoid cells express a plethora of cellular markers (Table 3.1), and liquid hematopathology specimens naturally "flow." FC creates a snapshot of a specimen's cellular composition by assessing tens of thousands to millions of cells, far exceeding the abilities of the human eye.

FC analysis is quasi-quantitative, so it is possible to identify and enumerate different populations by comparing amounts of proteins on different cell types by the intensity of the fluorescent signal. Distinct types of hematolymphoid disorders are associated with particular patterns of antigen expression; these will be discussed in detail in specific chapters.

FC is particularly useful in the diagnosis and classification of acute leukemias, chronic lymphoproliferative disorders, and non-Hodgkin lymphoma, but classic Hodgkin lymphoma (CHL) cannot be diagnosed by routine FC and FC plays no role in the diagnosis of chronic phase chronic myeloid leukemia (CML).

The FC process can be separated into three broad categories, namely: (a) preanalytic, or specimen collection; (b) analytic, including sample processing, acquisition, and gating; and (c) postanalytic, or interpretation and reporting. All stages are important for an accurate diagnosis.

TABLE 3.1 Common Cellular Markers on Hematolymphoid Cells

Type of cell	Common cellular markers
Leukocytes	CD45
Blasts	CD34, CD38, HLA-DR, CD117 (myeloid blasts), Tdt (lymphoid blasts)
Neutrophils	MPO, CD13, CD33, CD15, CD24, CD11b, CD16, CD10
Monocytes	HLA-DR, CD13, CD33, CD4, CD64, CD14, CD16
Erythroid	CD71, CD36, CD235
T cells	CD3, CD2, CD5, CD7, CD4 or CD8
NK cells	CD7, CD16, CD56
B cells	CD19, CD79a, CD20, CD22, CD24, κ, λ
Plasma cells	CD19, CD38, CD138, cκ, cλ

Tdt, Terminal deoxynucleotidyl transferase; HLA-DR, Human leukocyte antigen-D related; κ, kappa; λ, lambda; cκ, cytoplasmic kappa; cλ, cytoplasmic lambda; MPO, myeloperoxidase; NK, natural killer.

Specimen Collection

Marrow aspirate specimens should be submitted fresh and anticoagulated, with either ethylenediaminetetraacetic acid (EDTA) or heparin; the former is preferred if a morphologic preparation is to be made from the same sample. Generally speaking, samples are best saved at ambient temperature, but if there is going to be a long delay in processing, refrigeration may help preserve the sample. When shipped overnight, refrigeration is not recommended, but insulating a sample from climate extremes can help to preserve it.

Sample Processing, Acquisition, and Gating

The specimen is adjusted to a specific cell concentration and incubated with different antibody panels, depending on the suspected disease (Tables 3.2

TABLE 3.2 Antibody Panel Determined by Suspected Disease

Finding	Suspected disease	Blast tube	Maturation tube	B-tube	T-tube
Blasts	Acute leukemia	+	+	+	+
Prolonged cytopenias/ blasts	MDS or acute leukemia	+	+	+	+
Lymphocytosis	CLL/SLL or other lymphoid malignancy	–	-	+	+

CLL/SLL, chronic lymphocytic leukemia/small lymphocytic lymphoma; MDS, myelodysplastic syndrome.

TABLE 3.3 Examples of Common Antibody Panels Performed in FC

Tube	Antibody panel
Blast tube	CD45, CD34, CD38, HLA-DR, CD117, CD15, CD123, CD7
Maturation tube	CD45, CD33, CD13, CD64, CD14, CD16, CD11b, CD10
B cell tube	CD45, CD19, CD20, CD10, CD38, CD200, κ, λ
T cell tube	CD45, CD3, CD2, CD5, CD7, CD4, CD8, CD56
Acute leukemia orientation tube	CD45, CD19, CD3, CD7, CD34, cCD3, cCD79a, cMPO

c, cytoplasmic; FC, flow cytometry; HLA-DR, human leukocyte antigen-D related; κ, kappa; λ, lambda.

and 3.3). Many of the cellular proteins of interest are expressed on the cell surface, but cytoplasmic and nuclear antigens can also be assessed following cell permeation; because intracellular markers are often most sensitive and specific, some laboratories use an intracellular tube as an initial screen in acute leukemia.

Most FC is done with direct immunofluorescence (IF) whereby each antibody is conjugated to a specific fluorochrome. Occasionally FC is performed using indirect IF with either a fluorochrome conjugated to an anti-mouse or rat immunoglobulin (Ig) as a secondary antibody or, if biotin-conjugated primary antibodies are used, with an avidin-fluorochrome conjugate for detection (Figure 3.1); indirect methods are more commonly used in IHC (see later). The cells are washed and fixed; if intracellular antigens are being detected, surface staining is done first, and after washing and special fixation to permeabilize cells, antibodies directed against the internal proteins are added subsequently.

The sample is introduced into the flow cytometer and passes through an aperture where it is illuminated by lasers of different wavelengths that specifically excite the multiple fluorochromes, which, in turn, emit light at different wavelengths (Figure 3.2), detected by specific photomultipliers with filters designed to admit only light of the appropriate wavelengths.

"Multiparameter" FC refers to multiple (4+, more commonly 8-10) color-antibody combinations. Unlike most IHC stains, FC uses multiple fluorochromes, which allows for the detection of simultaneously expressed antigens.

Various commercial software systems can display cell-by-cell data in a variety of formats. Most commonly used are "dot plots," where each cellular event is displayed on a bivariate plot that correlates one fluorescence parameter versus another or forward scatter (FSC) or side scatter (SSC) versus each other or against a single fluorochrome (Figure 3.3). Operators analyze the data utilizing various gating strategies, in which populations are identified as clusters on a bivariate plot and subsequent plots; the process is repeated on plots that limit displays to the gated regions. Pseudocolor is often applied to gated populations so that specific populations can be visualized in many different bivariate displays.

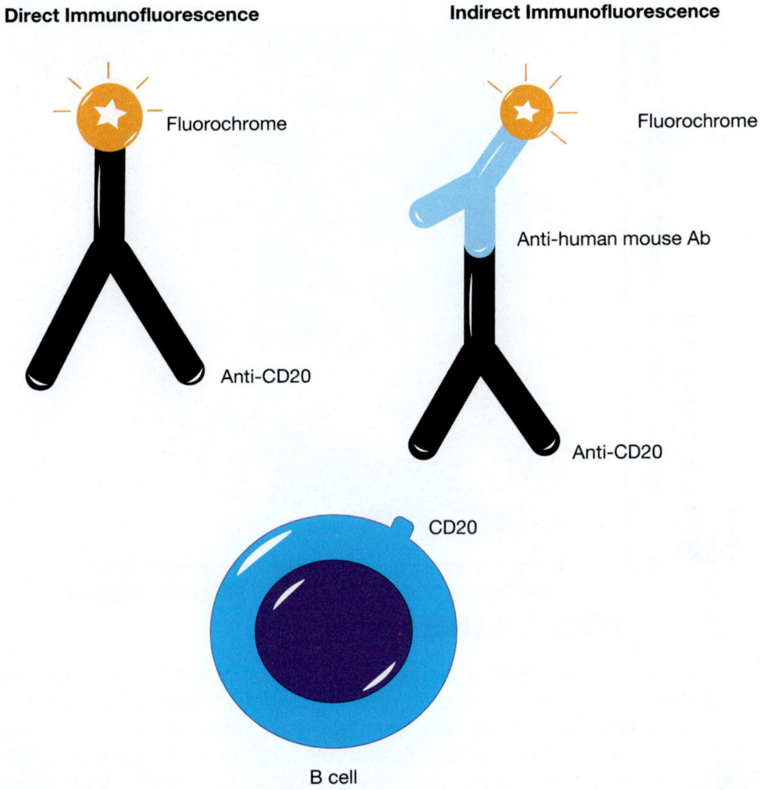

FIGURE 3.1 **Direct immunofluorescence (IF) utilizes an antibody conjugated to a specific fluorochrome.** Indirect IF, which is less commonly used in flow cytometry, utilizes an anti-mouse (or rat) immunoglobulin as a secondary antibody.

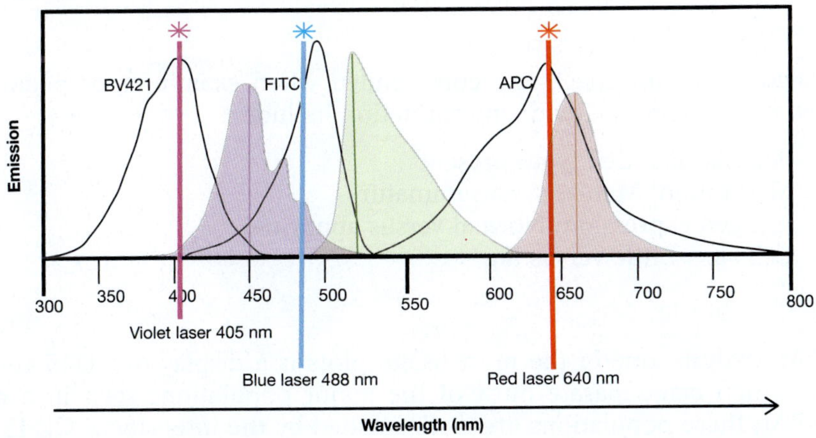

FIGURE 3.2 **The flow cytometry sample flows through an aperture and is subjected to lasers with specific wavelengths of light.** The lasers excite the fluorochromes, which emit light at different wavelengths. In this example, three fluorochromes are being used: BV421, FITC, and APC. FITC has an excitation maximum at 495 nm and an emission maximum at 519 nm.

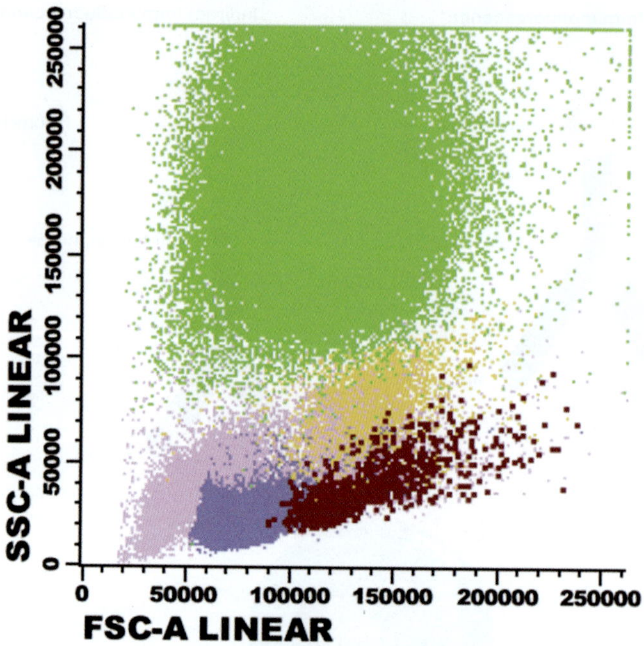

FIGURE 3.3 **Each cellular event is displayed on a bivariate dot plot that correlates one fluorescence parameter vs another, or with forward scatter (FSC) vs side scatter (SSC), as in this illustration.** Larger cells have higher FSC and cells with more granularity higher SSC. Thus myeloblasts (brown) and monocytes (orange) are larger than lymphocytes (purple) and nucleated red cells (pink), whereas myeloid cells (green) are more granular than other cells.

Interpretation

An algorithmic approach is recommended when examining a specimen. A few parameters that guide interpretation include:

1. Populations: Cell types present
2. Maturation: Mature versus immature
3. Antigen expression: Normal versus abnormal
4. Cell size: Little versus big

Cellular Populations

In BM analysis, one of the most useful plots is a display of CD45 versus SSC, which can separate most of the major populations seen in a normal BM; these populations are distinguished by the intensity of CD45 expression and the degree of SSC (Figure 3.4). The identity of the different populations is confirmed based on expression of lineage-associated and lineage-specific markers, which can also be used to determine if these populations are normal or abnormal.

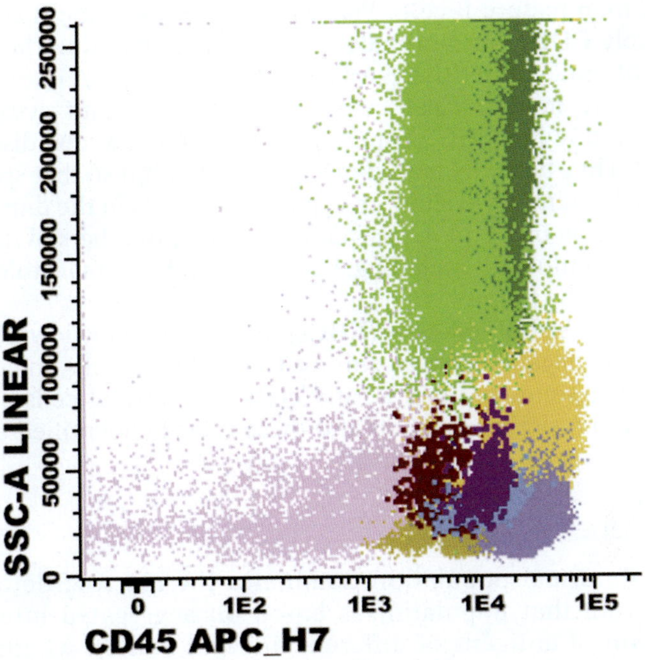

FIGURE 3.4 **The different cellular populations in a sample are distinguished by the intensity of CD45 expression and the amount of side scatter (SSC).** In this bone marrow example, the cells with the highest side scatter are myeloid cells (green), with eosinophils (dark green) showing brighter CD45; the cells with the brightest CD45 expression and low SSC are lymphocytes (light purple); monocytes (orange-yellow) have bright CD45 and higher SSC than lymphocytes; nucleated red cells (pink) are negative or very dim for CD45. The remaining cells with low CD45 and low SSC (sometimes called the "blast window") are actually a mixture of cells including myeloblasts (dark brown), basophils (dark purple), plasmacytoid dendritic cells (blue), and B cell precursors or hematogones (tan). Additional markers are needed to separate these populations.

Myeloid cells have high SSC because of their abundant cytoplasmic granules and segmented nuclei. They have moderate CD45 expression compared with other hematopoietic cells.

Monocytes have moderate SSC because of small cytoplasmic granules or cytoplasmic vacuoles, although when prominently vacuolated, SSC can be very high. They typically have brighter CD45 expression than myeloid cells.

Lymphocytes are mononuclear cells with scant cytoplasm, imparting low SSC, although they may appear larger in certain situations, discussed later. Mature lymphocytes have bright CD45. Although T cells have brighter CD45 than B cells, distinguishing them from each other and from natural killer (NK) cells requires additional markers, as noted further and in Table 3.1. Normal precursor B cells are typically seen in the BM as a population with dimmer CD45 and lower

SSC than mature B cells. Plasma cells express some B cell markers, notably CD19, but normally lack CD20 expression. They also have cytoplasmic, rather than surface, κ or λ.

Blasts are mononuclear cells with relatively scant cytoplasm and moderately low SSC properties (with some caveats, discussed further). They typically have dim CD45 expression so that specimens of acute leukemia will show an expansion of cells in the dim CD45/low SSC region of the plot, in which only small numbers of normal marrow constituents, including basophils and plasmacytoid dendritic cells, can be found.

Nucleated red blood cells (RBCs) have moderately low SSC and are typically negative or very dim for CD45. Other cells, including large platelets, some cell debris, and certain abnormal cells can also be found in a similar location and these must be identified using other markers.

Antigen Expression

When an abnormal population dominates the marrow, determining a diagnosis from that population is based on aggregated interpretation of expression of antigens of different lineages and on whether the antigens expressed are mature or immature. Because few antigens have absolute lineage specificity, large panels of markers selected from those in Table 3.1 (and others) are typically needed to classify populations accurately.

Detecting aberrancy of antigen expression is critical in helping to distinguish normal cells from neoplastic ones when there is no obvious replacement of marrow by neoplastic cells. This is particularly useful in myelodysplastic syndrome (MDS) or in the setting of minimal residual disease (MRD). This aberrancy may be a loss of a normal antigen, a gain of an unexpected antigen, or unusual antigen intensity. Normal hematopoietic precursors have predictable and reproducible patterns of maturation in the BM. Detailed discussion of these can be found in subsequent chapters. The change may be subtle and considerable experience is often required to do this well.

Clonality

B cell clonality: Detecting B cell clonality by FC is relatively straightforward. B cells should normally comprise a mixture of κ and λ in a roughly 2:1 ratio, although the standard deviation is high (Figure 3.5).

T cell clonality: Assessing T cell clonality by FC is not as straightforward as assessing B cell clonality, as T cell receptor (TCR) genes are more complex. The most common method to detect T cell clonality is via polymerase chain reaction (PCR), discussed later.[1] Many labs rely on detecting abnormal T cell antigen expression to infer an abnormal

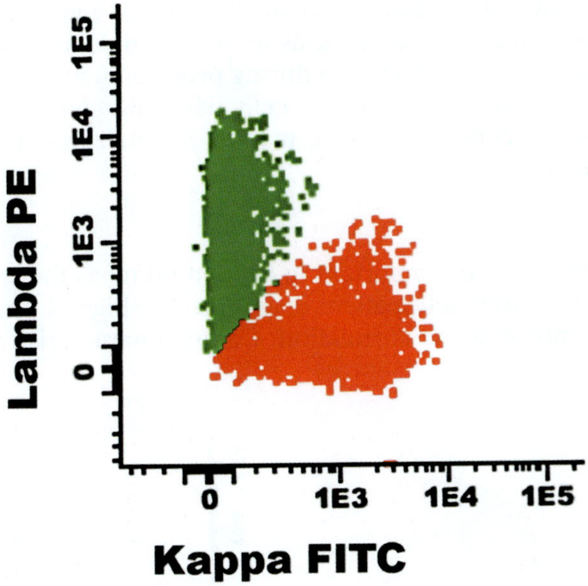

FIGURE 3.5 **B cells should normally comprise a mixture of κ and λ in about a 2:1 ratio.** This flow cytometry example illustrates a normal κ (red population) to λ (green population) ratio.

population, whereas some institutions use Vβ family repertoire analysis to detect abnormal T cell clones. This test consists of 24 antibodies that target the variable domain of the TCRβ chain, covering >65% of all Vβ domains.[2,3] Normal CD4- and CD8-positive T cells have a defined distribution of Vβ classes. Therefore, any phenotypically abnormal population with an expanded Vβ population is interpreted as a clonal population.

Another FC T cell clonality test assesses the constant domain of the TCR gene, rather than the variable domain. As discussed later, the TCRβ chain constant domain is encoded by two genes, TRBC1 and TRBC2.[4,5] Recently, an antibody to the C1 region was developed, which allows for detection of C1 distribution in a T cell population.[6] Normal T cells will show a mixture of C1 and C2, whereas a clonal population will express only C1 or C2 (Figure 3.6A and B). This test has been shown to have 97% sensitivity and 91% specificity for detecting T cell lymphomas, comparable to PCR, which detects up to 90% of all peripheral T cell lymphomas.[1]

Cell Size

Cell size can be inferred from physical properties identified on the FSC plot. Cells with high FSC are larger than those with low FSC (see Figure 3.1).

Very large cells by FSC (Figure 3.7) typically indicate a large cell neoplasm. However, in some cases, large cells, as in, for example, diffuse large B cell lymphoma (DLBCL), can break up during processing and appear as small cells or debris. Additionally, smaller cells with abundant cytoplasm, like those of marginal zone lymphoma, may be misinterpreted as large cells based on their size.

Benefits and Limitations

The limitations of FC are important to keep in mind, as they may affect interpretation and, ultimately, patient diagnosis. The biggest limitation is the lack of direct morphologic correlation: Certain characteristics or findings

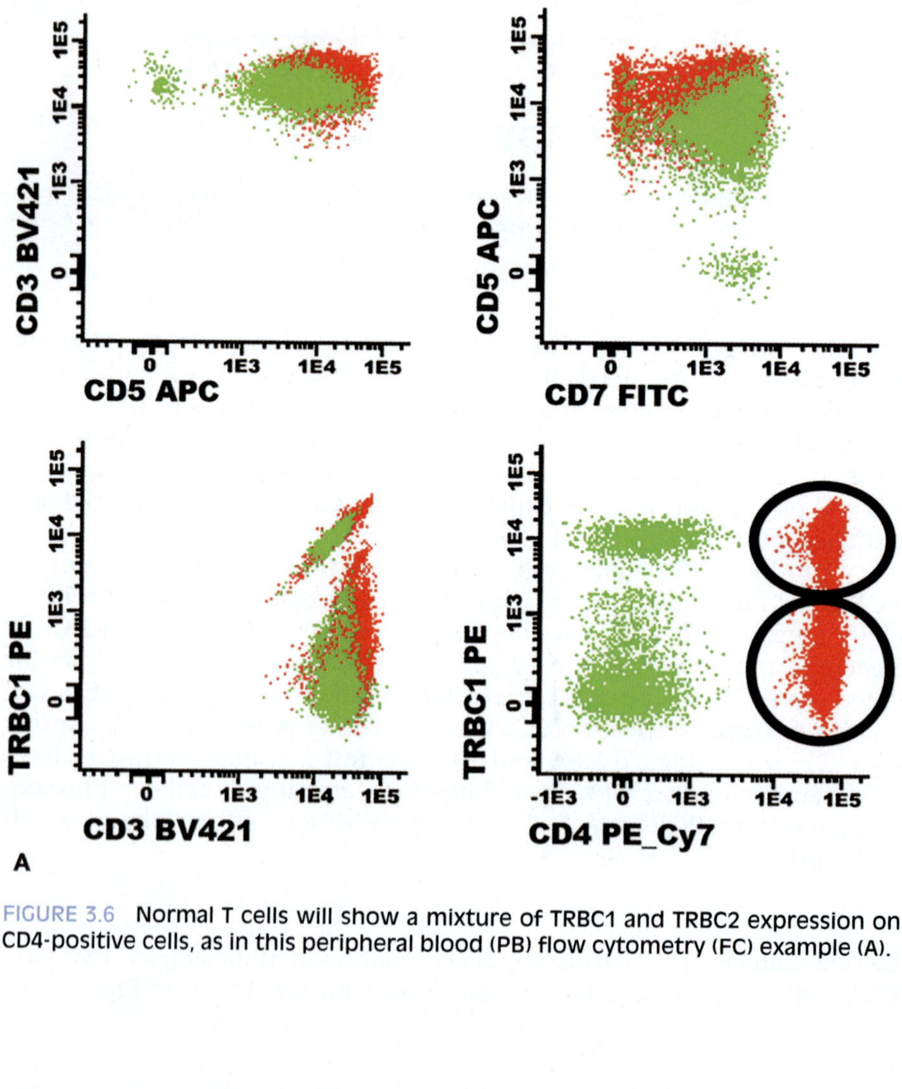

FIGURE 3.6 Normal T cells will show a mixture of TRBC1 and TRBC2 expression on CD4-positive cells, as in this peripheral blood (PB) flow cytometry (FC) example (A).

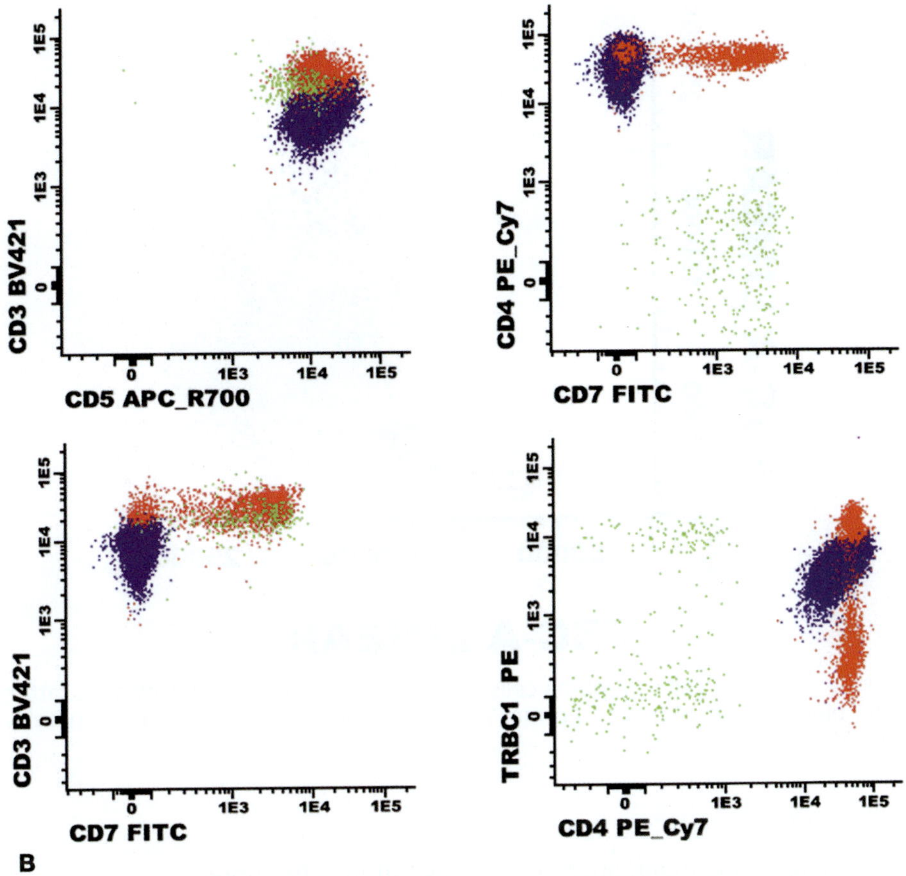

FIGURE 3.6 (*continued*) In this PB FC example from a patient with Sezary syndrome (B), there is a phenotypically abnormal CD4+ population (blue), which, compared to normal T cells, has dimmer CD3 and lacks CD7. These cells show aberrant uniform TRBC1 indicating clonality. Normal CD8+ cells (green) and residual normal CD4 cells (red) are polyclonal.

need to be corroborated by histology. Additionally, certain tumor types, like CHL, have low numbers of atypical cells that are not detectable by routine FC. Routine FC is also not a reliable method for looking at Cyclin D1 expression, so this is typically done by performing additional IHC stains on histologic specimens. The strengths of FC are its fast turnaround time; its ability to provide a comprehensive, unbiased analysis; and to identify and describe phenotypes of multiple different populations within a sample.

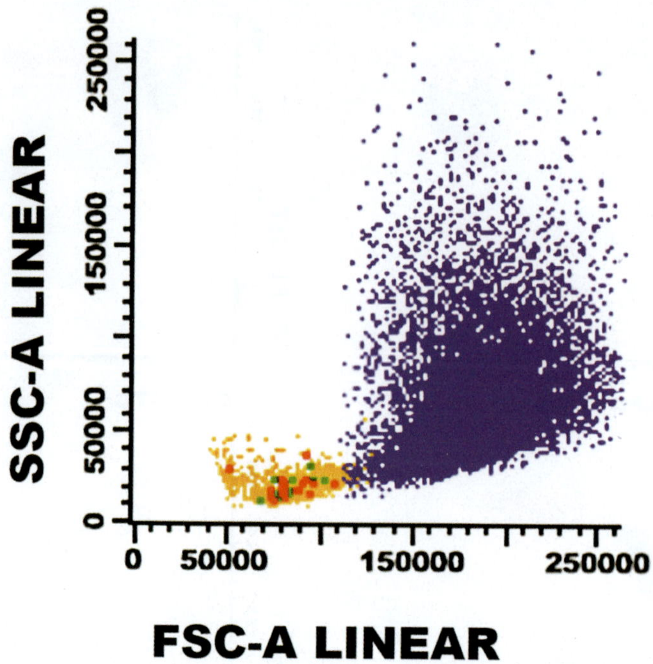

FIGURE 3.7 Large cell lymphoma cells typically have much higher forward scatter (FSC; blue) than background normal T cells (orange) and B cells (red and green). SSC, side scatter.

FC Summary

- Detecting antigen aberrancy is key but may be subtle.
- A sufficiently large panel should be used, with redundancy of markers representing different lineages, and markers expressed throughout differentiation to assess maturation abnormalities.
- Phenotypes may change over time or following treatment.
- Assessment of B cell clonality, although helpful, can be misleading; lack of light chain expression doesn't exclude lymphoma, and some clonal populations may not be neoplastic.
- False negatives may occur during cell processing. Cells that are fragile, necrotic, or large may appear as small cells or debris.
- FC results should be taken in context. FC is an ancillary test, and morphologic correlation is important.

IMMUNOHISTOCHEMISTRY

IHC detects cellular proteins for tissue classification and tumor diagnosis and is used in conjunction with hematoxylin and eosin (H&E) and/or special stains, which highlight cellular morphology and structure. In comparison with FC, IHC utilizes enzymatic chromogens to allow the visual detection of antibody-binding target tissue. Because it allows assessment of antigen expression in the context of both cellular cytomorphology and overall tissue architecture (Figure 3.8A-C), it can provide information not available by FC. Moreover, certain markers are more suitable for IHC

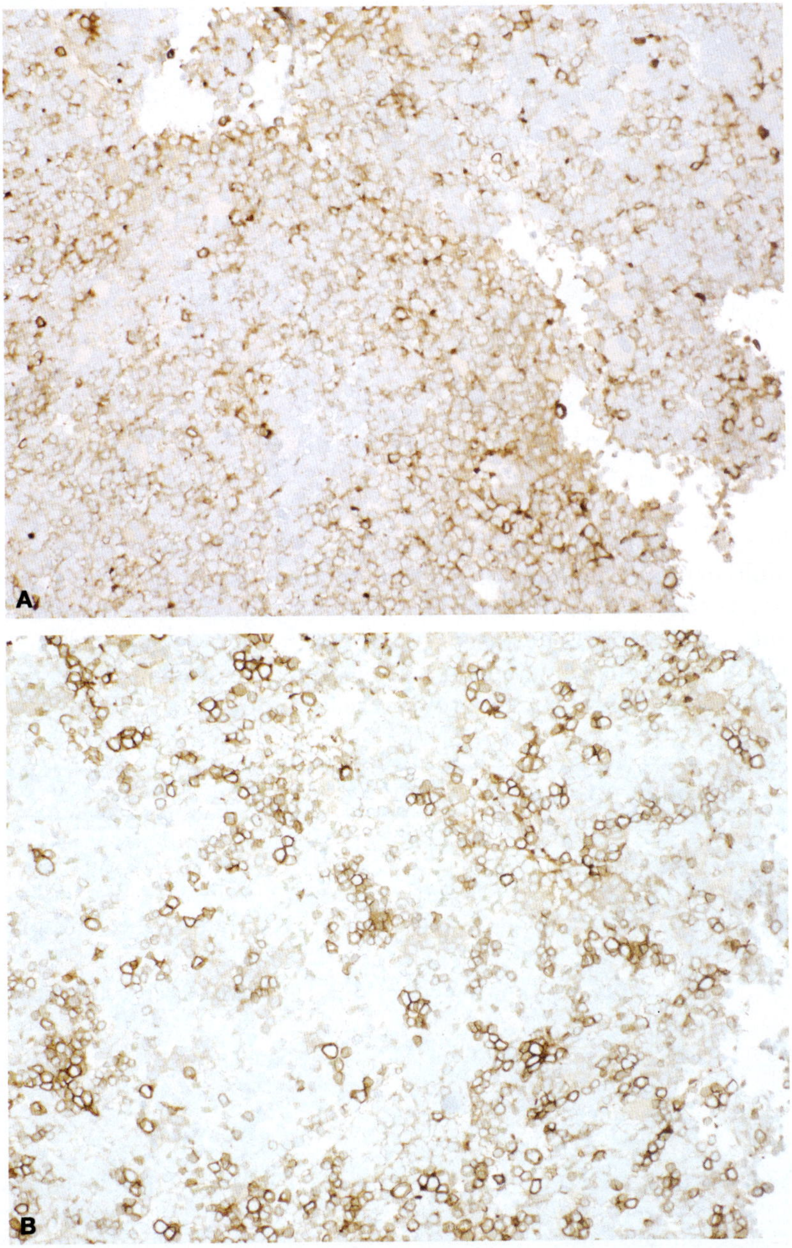

FIGURE 3.8 **Immunohistochemistry is helpful when examining bone marrow (BM) core biopsies.** Myeloperoxidase (A) weakly stains immature myeloid cells and strongly stains mature myeloid cells in the BM. E-cadherin (B) highlights erythroid progenitors in small clusters.

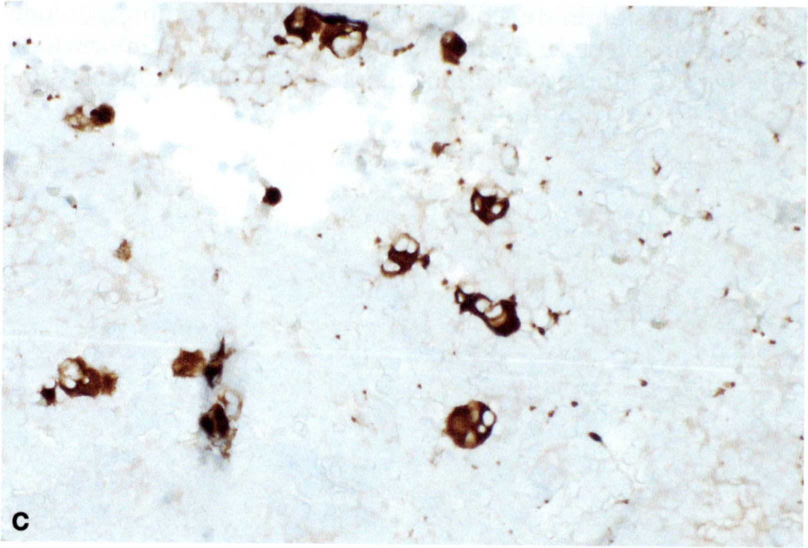

C

FIGURE 3.8 (*continued*) CD61 (C) stains scattered megakaryocytes on the core biopsy.

(Table 3.4). On the other hand, quantitation of populations or assessment of simultaneous expression of multiple markers is not possible in routine IHC (although dual color stains can look at cytoplasmic and nuclear constituents together). Tissue-based IF, especially with image analysis, does provide many of the same benefits of FC while preserving tissue architecture, but to date this is largely only a research tool.

TABLE 3.4 Additional Useful Hematopathology IHC Markers

IHC	Function	Cells positive	Pattern of staining	Useful in dx
PAX5	B cell transcription factor	B cells	Nuclear	B cell neoplasms
BCL2	Regulator of apoptosis	B cells	Cytoplasmic	B cell neoplasms (FL; DLBCL)
BCL6	Transcriptional repressor in germinal center B cells	B cells	Nuclear	B cell neoplasms (FL; DLBCL)
OCT2	B cell transcription factor for Ig production	B cells	Nuclear	B cell neoplasms (NLP)
BOB1	Transcriptional coactivator	B cells	Nuclear	B cell neoplasms (NLP)

TABLE 3.4 Additional Useful Hematopathology IHC Markers (*continued*)

IHC	Function	Cells positive	Pattern of staining	Useful in dx
MUM1	Regulation of Ig expression	Activated B cells; plasma cells	Nuclear	PCNs; B cell neoplasms
CD138	Cellular adhesion	Plasma cells	Surface	PCNs
ALK	Tyrosine receptor; constitutively active in ALCL because of fusion with *NPM*	Abnormal T cells or B cells	Nuclear	ALCL; anaplastic large B cell lymphoma
CD30	TNFR signal transducer	Immunoblasts (activated B or T cells); abnormal B or T cells; HRS cells, ALCL cells	Surface; cytoplasmic	CHL, ALCL, other lymphomas
Cyclin D1	Regulation of cell cycle	Abnormal B cells with t(11;14); also on endothelial cells	Nuclear	MCL
SOX11	Transcription factor	Abnormal B cells with t(11;14)	Nuclear	MCL
LEF1	Enhancer binding protein	Normal pre-B cells; normal T cells; abnormal B cells in CLL/SLL	Nuclear	CLL/SLL
CD43	Anti-adhesion molecule	Hematolymphoid cells	Surface	Hematolymphoid neoplasms
KI67	Nuclear protein associated with proliferation	Proliferating cells	Nuclear	Hematolymphoid neoplasms

ALCL, anaplastic large cell lymphoma; CHL, classic Hodgkin lymphoma; CLL/SLL, chronic lymphocytic leukemia/small lymphocytic lymphoma; DLBCL, diffuse large B cell lymphoma; dx, diagnosis; FL, follicular lymphoma; HRS, Hodgkin Reed Sternberg; Ig, immunoglobulin; IHC, immunohistochemistry; MCL, mantle cell lymphoma; NLP, nodular lymphocyte predominant; PCNs, plasma cell neoplasms; TNFR, tumor necrosis factor receptor.

Limitations

IHC has limitations, and a pathologist should be aware of technical artifacts that may hamper evaluation. Some of the most common include:

- Inconsistent fixation of tissues may lead to dim/false-negative IHC.
- Inconsistent application of reagents may create inhomogeneous staining of tissue.
- Cross-reactivity may cause false positives because of the presence of endogenous biotin or peroxidase. This can be prevented or at least mitigated with a blocking step.
- High background staining can make interpretation difficult but can be mitigated using a universal protein block.

Cytochemistry

These methods have been largely supplanted by IHC and FC in most laboratories. The most common cytochemical stains are listed in Table 3.5.

TABLE 3.5 Commonly Utilized Cytochemical Stains

Stain	Abbreviation	Stains	Uses
Myeloperoxidase	MPO	• Primary granules in neutrophils • May weakly stain monocytes	• Differentiate myeloid from lymphoid leukemia. • May be negative in some early AMLs
Sudan Black B	SBB	• Intracellular lipids and phospholipids of myeloid cells	• Differentiate myeloid from lymphoid leukemia.
Periodic acid Schiff	PAS	• Intracellular glycogen and mucopolysaccharides	• B lymphoblasts (block like) • Atypical erythroid precursors (diffuse pattern)
Toluidine blue	TB	• Acid mucopolysaccharides in granules of basophils and mast cells	• Highlights basophils and mast cells

TABLE 3.5 Commonly Utilized Cytochemical Stains (*continued*)

Stain	Abbreviation	Stains	Uses
Nonspecific esterase • α-Naphthyl butyrate • α-Naphthyl acetate	NSE	• Stains monocytes red • B-ALL may be positive	• Differentiate myeloid from monocytic leukemia
Chloroacetate esterase (specific esterase)	CAE	• Enzymatically hydrolyzed by specific esterases in granulocytic cells	• Differentiate myeloid from lymphoid leukemia • May be negative in AML without maturation or with minimal differentiation
Dual esterase	DE	• Both specific and nonspecific esterases utilized	• Stains myeloid cells black and monocytic cells blue • Helpful to distinguish AMML

ALL, acute lymphoblastic leukemia; AML, acute myeloid leukemia; AMML, acute myelomonocytic leukemia.

Cytogenetics

Cytogenetic studies are mainstays for BM evaluation, critical for diagnosis, classification, and prognosis of many hematologic disorders. Unlike epithelial carcinomas, many leukemias and lymphomas exhibit characteristic structural chromosomal abnormalities, which makes cytogenetics a powerful tool for detecting and classifying hematologic malignancies. Indeed, many types of leukemia are defined by their cytogenetic abnormalities.

Methods

The clinical question dictates which cytogenetic test will be most informative for diagnosis. Some questions are better answered with a karyotype, which detects the entire chromosomal complement, whereas others require FISH to detect the specific genetic alteration characteristic of specific entities. Different cytogenetic tests also vary in their levels of sensitivity of detection.

Like FC, the accuracy of cytogenetic studies relies on preanalytic, analytic, and postanalytic factors. Unlike FC, specimen collection depends on the chosen test. For instance, karyotyping requires live cells and must be performed on fresh samples, whereas FISH may be performed on fresh cells or formalin-fixed paraffin-embedded (FFPE) tissue.

CONVENTIONAL CYTOGENETICS/KARYOTYPE

A karyotype is an individual's entire complement of chromosomes, detected via a laboratory technique that produces an image, or karyogram, of the chromosomes (Figure 3.9). Karyotyping has been used in clinical and research settings since the 1950s to study different pathologic disorders by detecting numerical or structural alterations of chromosomes.

Preanalytic

Fresh peripheral blood (PB), BM, or tissue samples are required for this test. The specimen is either directly assessed or cultured over time (24-48 hours) to allow for the growth and expansion of any clones. Effective communication with clinicians is necessary, as the specific clinical question or suspected disorder will guide laboratory setup. For example, mitogens

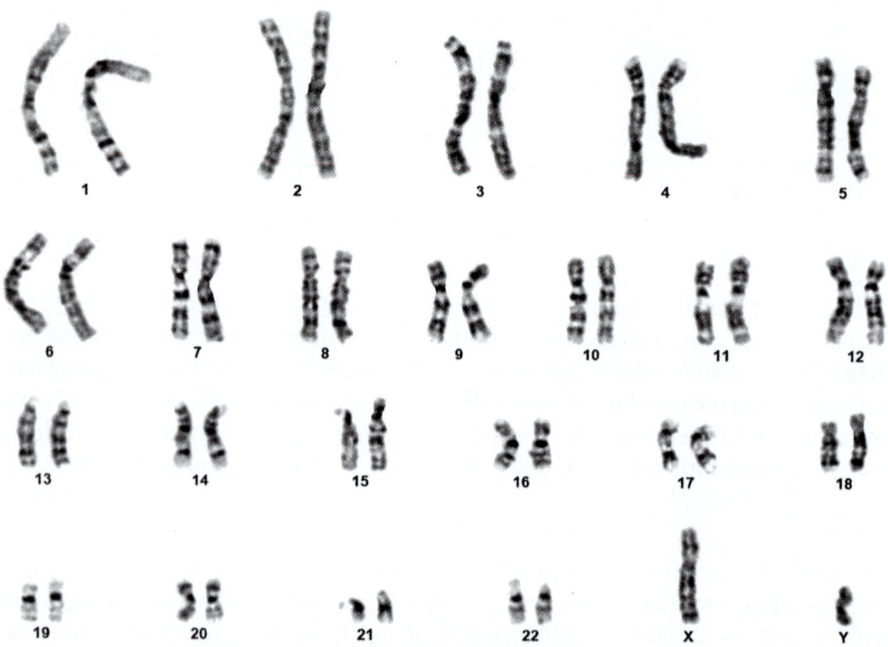

FIGURE 3.9 **A karyotype, pictured here, is an individual's entire complement of chromosomes, detected via a laboratory technique that produces an image, or karyogram, of the chromosomes.** This is a normal karyotype. Image courtesy of Dr. Ying Zou.

TABLE 3.6 The General Procedural Steps to Perform a Karyotype

Process	Description
Culturing	• Tissue sample is cultured in a growth medium • Chemicals are added to stimulate mitosis. • Specimen incubated for 1-2 days • Colcemid added to stop mitosis in metaphase
Centrifuge	• Cells are transferred to a separate tube and centrifuged to concentrate the cells in layers • Fixative is added to the cells.
Staining	• Cells pipetted onto a microscope slide • Stain is added to enhance the chromosomes
Arranging	• Chromosomes are identified, arranged in order, and photographed

may be added for growth in suspected lymphoid malignancies; interleukin (IL)-4 may be added in suspected plasma cell neoplasms. The procedure is explained in Table 3.6.

Analytic

In the 1950s, chromosomes were stained with Giemsa and Wright and categorized into seven groups based on their size and centromeric position. In the 1970s, additional staining techniques were utilized to provide precise identification of various chromosomal regions, or "bands."[7] Today, chromosomes are stained using one of a few techniques.

The most common technique in the United States is G banding, or Giemsa banding. Chromosomes are stained with Giemsa following treatment with trypsin, which removes proteins from chromatin, and defines light and dark areas. Such characteristic banding patterns help identify the chromosome and specific loci.

Chromosomes are numbered from 1 to 22 in order of descending size. Each sex chromosome is labeled either X or Y. The short arm of a chromosome is designated "p" and the long arm is designated "q." Each area of a chromosome is also numbered. The lowest numbers are proximal to the centromere, and the highest numbers are at the tips of the chromosomes.

Postanalytic

Twenty metaphase spreads are examined for structural and numerical chromosomal abnormalities. The genetic complement is documented using the International Standard for Human Chromosome Nomenclature (ISCN). ISCN is a simple, consistent form of documentation that is well-recognized throughout the medical community. The general formula includes listing the number of somatic chromosomes including the sex chromosomes, followed by a comma, the sex designation, and the number of metaphases in brackets.

Normal Karyotype

46, XX[20]/46, XY[20]: Normal female/male with 46 chromosomes in 20 metaphases

Abnormal Karyotypes

Abnormalities may only be numerical, without structural changes (hyper- or hypodiploidy) or involve either a part or a whole chromosome, and include translocations, deletions, duplications, inversions, and unusual chromosome formation like ring chromosomes and markers of unknown origin. Some of the most common abnormalities are discussed in Chapter 5.

A karyotype abnormality is considered clonal if:

- two metaphases are identified with the same additional chromosome or structural abnormalities; or
- three metaphases are identified with loss of a single chromosome (monosomy); or
- one metaphase with a significant abnormality, although not technically qualifying, should prompt additional metaphase counting and/or the addition of a note in the diagnostic interpretation.

The number of metaphases in which the abnormality is detected should be noted in the diagnosis. For example, if 15 metaphase spreads show del20, and the remainder are normal, the nomenclature is: 46, XY del(20q)[15]/46, XY[5]. If fewer than 20 metaphases are examined, this must be mentioned in the report.

Benefits and Limitations

Karyotyping is the standard of care for the diagnosis of most myeloid disorders as certain abnormalities are used to define some entities and may be associated with prognosis in certain diseases. Additionally, a patient's diagnostic karyotype can be used as a baseline and compared with new samples to assess for clonal evolution. For patients with a less clear-cut neoplastic diagnosis, a karyotype can help confirm a clonal process. However, it is important to recognize and differentiate between germline abnormalities and somatic abnormalities; in particular, in cases in which a karyotype shows the same single abnormality in all 20 metaphases, a constitutional abnormality should be excluded.

Despite these benefits, there are also some limitations, including:

- The process requires considerable experience for interpretation.
- Fresh tissue is required.

- Turnaround time is slow.
- Resolution is low (5-10 Mb DNA); cryptic abnormalities may not be detected.
- Specific genes are inferred in translocations but are not directly visualized.
- Normal cells may preferentially outgrow tumor cells. For this reason, a "normal karyotype" result is probably best interpreted as uninformative. ALL cells typically do not grow as well as those of AML, and multiple myeloma (MM) and CHL cells do not grow well.

FLORESCENCE IN SITU HYBRIDIZATION

FISH involves hybridization of DNA-specific probes onto metaphase or interphase chromosomal DNA. Unlike conventional karyotyping, FISH methods can detect small regions of DNA (0.5-1.5 kB) and can provide information about the individual genes involved in a translocation. However, this method is only informative for the interrogated portion of the chromosome, whereas a karyotype visualizes the whole chromosome complement. Some of the other differences between these two techniques are listed in Table 3.7.

Several types of FISH techniques are utilized for clinical and research studies, including whole chromosome painting, centromeric analysis for detecting aneuploidy, telomeric analysis, and FISH for specific loci. For clinical specimens, site-specific probes are the most utilized.

Preanalytic

Unlike conventional cytogenetic studies, FISH studies do not have to be performed on fresh tissue. Various types of material may be used, including FFPE tissue. However, fixatives with heavy metal constituents (zinc formalin, B5,) Zenker's fixative and standard decalcification can inhibit FISH testing.

Analytic

The probe/probe set is selected based on the specific clinical question. The general steps are listed in Table 3.8.

TABLE 3.7 The Advantages and Disadvantages of Karyotype vs FISH

Test	FISH	Karyotype
Speed	Hours	Days-weeks
Method	Fresh or FFPE	Sterile/fresh tissue
Cell phase	Metaphase or interphase	Metaphase

FFPE, formalin fixed paraffin embedded; FISH, florescence in situ hybridization.

TABLE 3.8 The General Procedural Steps to Perform FISH

Process	Description
Preparation	• The sample is prepared directly on a glass slide (or an unstained slide with FFPE tissue).
Permeabilization and denaturation	• The cells are permeabilized. • Double-stranded (ds)DNA is denatured into single-stranded (ss)DNA. • The probe and target are combined.
Labeling	• The probes are directly tagged with fluorochromes. • Unbound probe is washed away.
Examination	• The specimen is microscopically examined and 200 cells are counted.

FFPE, formalin fixed paraffin embedded; FISH, florescence in situ hybridization.

Probes

Depending on the clinical question, different probes may be indicated:

Dual color dual fusion (DCDF) probe: This probe set is designed to bind to genes at different chromosomal locations that are known to recombine. The individual probes are labeled with either a red or green fluorescent reporter (Figure 3.10). Fusion (fused red/green signal, which may appear yellow-orange) indicates combination of the loci (Figure 3.11). This type of probe is useful when the exact translocation partner is known. This type of probe has the best sensitivity ($<1\%$).

Break-apart probe (BAP): This site-specific probe is designed to bind over a region of interest. Each probe is dually labeled with red and green reporters, which hybridize with different sequences that flank a known breakpoint region. An intact probe with adjacent red/green appears yellow (Figure 3.12). If the gene or loci is rearranged, the red/green signal is disrupted or separated, forming two separate colors: red and green (Figure 3.13). It is primarily used to detect rearrangements in genes with multiple partners, like IGH or *KMT2A*, but is uninformative about the identity of the partners. This has poorer sensitivity than the DCDF (typically around 4%). Examples of BAPs and DCDFs are listed in Table 3.9.[8]

Postanalytic

FISH interpretation requires knowledge of the probe type and loci, as well as familiarity with ISCN designation.

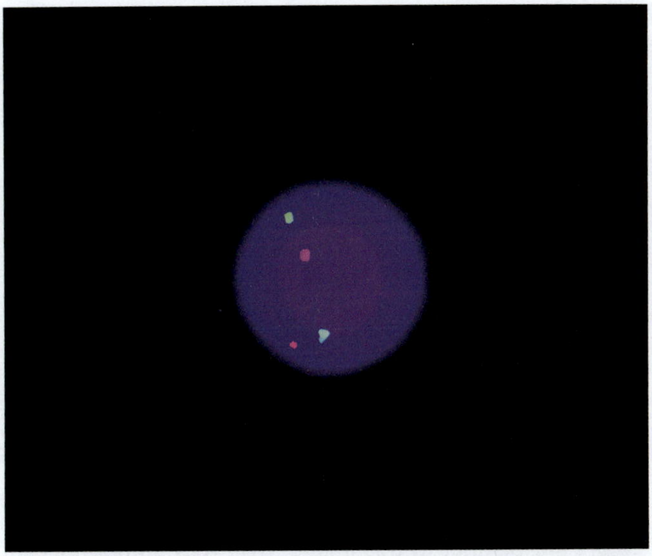

FIGURE 3.10 **A dual color dual fusion (DCDF) probe set is designed to bind genes at different chromosomal locations that are known to recombine.** In this case, a *BCR/ABL1* DCDF translocation probe is hybridized to a normal nucleus, showing a normal signal pattern (red, *ABL1*; green, *BCR*). Image courtesy of Dr. Ying Zou.

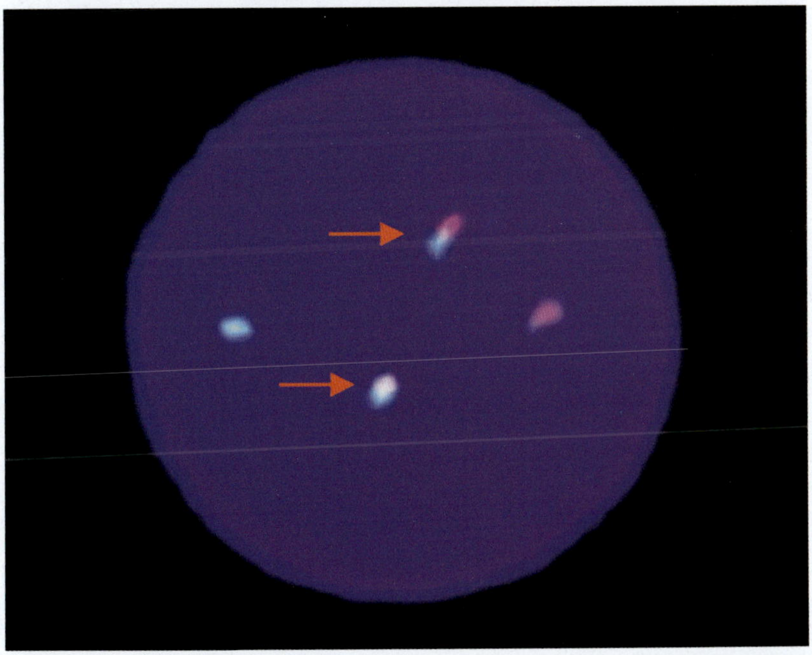

FIGURE 3.11 **In this case, the *BCR/ABL1* dual color dual fusion probe hybridized to a nucleus containing a *BCR::ABL* translocation, t(9;22).** There is one normal red signal, one normal green signal, and two red/green fusion signals, making the image appear at least focally yellow (red arrows). Image courtesy of Dr. Ying Zou.

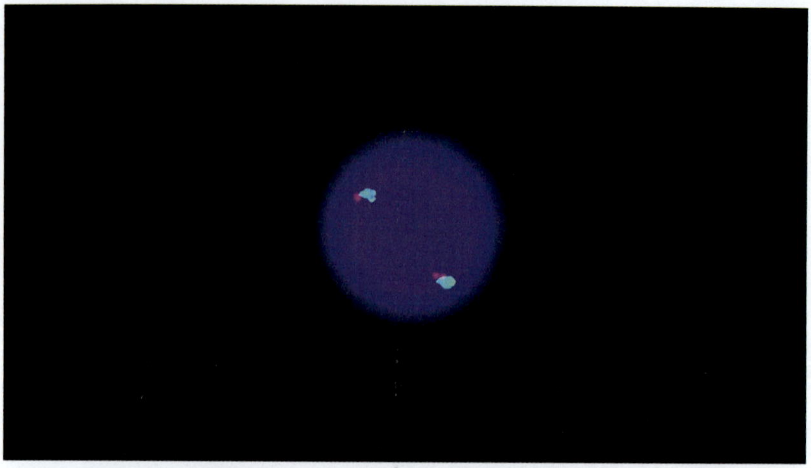

FIGURE 3.12 **In this example, an *MLL* dual color break-apart probe is hybridized to a normal nucleus showing an intact signal with adjacent red and green colors; although the colors are distinct in this image, they may sometimes appear yellow.** Image courtesy of Dr. Ying Zou.

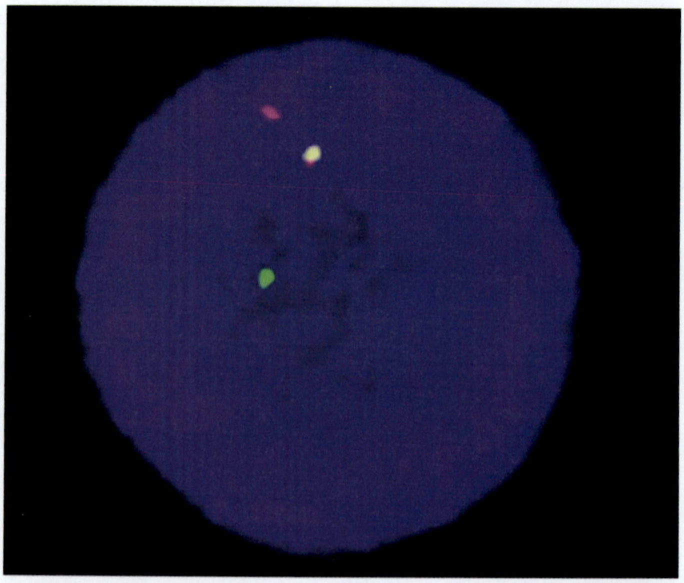

FIGURE 3.13 **In this example, the *MLL* dual color break-apart probe is hybridized to a nucleus containing a rearrangement of 11q23 (*MLL* rearrangement).** One intact signal is observed (yellow), and one rearrangement is observed (separate red and green signals). Image courtesy of Dr. Ying Zou.

TABLE 3.9 Common FISH Probes

Probe name and (location)	Type	Detects	Disease
PML (15q24); *RARA* (17q21)	DCDF	t(15;17)	APL
RUNX1T1 (8q21); *RUNX1* (21q22)	DCDF	t(8;21)	AML
MECOM (3q26)	BAP	Inv(3)	AML
MYH11 (16p13); *CBFB* (16q22)	DCDF	Inv(16)	AML
ETV6 (12p13); *RUNX1* (21q22)	DCDF	t(12;21)	AML
KMT2A (11q23)	BAP	11q23	AML; ALL
CMYC (8q24); D20S108 (20q12)	DCE	+8/20q-	MDS
TAS2R1 (5p15.31); *EGR1* (5q31)	DCE	5q-/-5	MDS
RELN (7q22); *TES* (7q31)	DCE	7q-/-7	MDS
ABL (9q34); *BCR* (22q11)	DCDF	t(9;22)	CML; ALL
PDGFRA (4q12)	BAP	4q12	MPN
PDGFRB (5q33)	BAP	5q33	MPN
FGFR1 (8q11)	BAP	8q11	MPN
BCL6 (3q27)	BAP	3q27	B cell neoplasms
CMYC (8q24)	BAP	8q24	B cell neoplasms; Burkitt; HGBCL
BCL2 (18q21)	BAP	18q21	B cell neoplasms
IGH (14q32); *BCL2* (18q21)	DCDF	t(14;18)	B cell neoplasms
IGH (14q32)	BAP	14q32	B cell neoplasms
CCND1 (11q13); IGH (14q32)	DCDF	t(11;14)	MCL
MALT1 (18q21)	BAP	18q21	B cell neoplasms
ATM (11q22); *TP53* (17p13)	DCE	11q-/17p-	CLL/SLL
FGFR3 (4p16.3); IGH (14q32)	DCDF	t(4:14)	MM/MGUS
ALK (2p23)	BAP	2p23	ALCL
TCRB (7q34)	BAP	7q34	T-ALL

ALCL, anaplastic large cell lymphoma; ALL, acute lymphoblastic leukemia; AML, acute myeloid leukemia; APL, acute promyelocytic leukemia; BAP, break-apart probe; CLL/SLL, chronic lymphocytic leukemia/small lymphocytic lymphoma; CML, chronic myeloid leukemia; DCDF, dual color dual fusion; DCE, dual color enumerate; FISH, florescence in situ hybridization; HGBCL, high-grade B cell lymphoma; MDS, myelodysplastic syndrome; MGUS, monoclonal gammopathy of undetermined significance; MCL, Mantle cell lymphoma; MM, multiple myeloma; MPN, myeloproliferative neoplasm.

Normal FISH

In normal patients, there are two nuclear in situ hybridization (ISH) signals for *ABL1* and two signals for *BCR*; if 200 cells are counted, this is documented as:

nuc ish(*ABL1*,*BCR*)×2[200]: Two separate *ABL1* and *BCR* probes in 200 nuclei counted (using ISH)

Reference ranges must be designated for both the FISH probes and the sample type to ensure correct interpretation. When used to detect numerical changes, FISH performed on FFPE is not as accurate as FISH performed on fresh tissue, as the tissue sections may artificially cut a cell in two, with subsequent loss of probe signal.

Chromosome Microarrays

Unlike FISH that targets a specific locus, array probes span the whole length of the genome, allowing for rapid detection of copy number (CN) changes and loss of heterozygosity (LOH). The two types of arrays utilized include:

Comparative genomic hybridization (CGH) array: Patient and control samples are hybridized to the same microarray and compared.

Single-nucleotide polymorphism (SNP) array: Patient sample is compared to a database of controls. This is an effective way to identify single-nucleotide changes/polymorphisms.

Because the chromosomes are not visualized, translocations cannot be detected with microarrays.

MOLECULAR STUDIES

Molecular studies are invaluable for the detection and diagnosis of hematolymphoid disorders. These techniques are sufficiently sensitive to interrogate small quantities of tissue provided there is sufficient tumor representation in the sample.

The rationale for utilizing molecular tests depends on the specific case, suspected diagnosis, and laboratory capabilities. Some of the most encountered tests in hematopathology include:

1. PCR analysis for B cell and T cell gene rearrangements
2. Reverse transcriptase (RT)-PCR for detecting RNA-based translocations associated with many myeloid malignancies
   i. Qualitative: Typically used for diagnostic purposes
   ii. Quantitative (q)PCR: Used for quantifying translocation transcripts for disease monitoring
3. DNA sequencing, now mainly via next-generation sequencing (NGS), also called high-throughput sequencing (HTS): Used for mutational analysis

Fresh specimens should be collected in EDTA rather than heparin, which can inhibit PCR. Rapid acid decalcification should be avoided. Fresh specimens should be processed in under 72 hours to prevent RNA degradation. Other samples may also be used, including FFPE tissue, but the sample quality affects the test: In general, up to 500 base pairs (bp) can be amplified by PCR using fresh or frozen tissue, whereas only about 200 bp can be amplified using FFPE as starting material.

PCR Analysis

PCR is an elegant method of analyzing a genetic locus by amplifying a specific DNA sequence.[9] The technique involves a series of cycles comprised of three steps, as described in Table 3.10.

The products are analyzed by either gel or capillary electrophoresis using fluorescent-labeled primers that are incorporated during amplification. PCR products separate as they migrate through the capillary according to their electrophoretic mobility/size. At the capillary outlet, a laser excites the fluorochromes and the products are compared with reference size standards.

"PCR" refers simply to the amplification method, but there are a variety of ways this can be employed to answer different clinical questions.

Allele-Specific PCR

Specific primers bind to variant or non-variant sequences at a particular DNA locus. This type of test is utilized to detect mutant sequences.

TABLE 3.10 The General Procedural Steps to Perform PCR

Process	Description
Denaturation	• Double-stranded (ds)DNA is separated into single-stranded (ss)DNA at an elevated temperature (95°C).
Annealing	• The temperature is lowered (55°C). • Primers attach at the 3′ end of each ssDNA. • Multiple sets of complementary primers may be used ("Multiplex" PCR).
Extension	• Heat-stable DNA polymerase (Taq polymerase) and nucleotides are added at 72°C. • The complementary DNA strands are synthesized. • Four DNA strands (two dsDNA) are produced. • The cycle is repeated 20-40 times for amplification of the product.

PCR, polymerase chain reaction.

Reverse Transcriptase PCR

This method converts RNA into complementary DNA (cDNA) using a reverse transcriptase and random primers.[10] RNA contains exons only, and therefore, using it as a starting material avoids amplification of large intron regions that are present at most translocation breakpoints in genomic DNA. This type of PCR is used to amplify translocations and fusions, with a primer specific to each partner in the translocations.

Quantitative PCR

qPCR is used to determine the amount of a particular sequence in a sample. Amplicons are detected and quantified during the exponential expansion phase in real time. This is particularly useful because the amount of a transcript can be related to the number of cells with the abnormality.[10-12] There are two main methods of qPCR:

1. A nonspecific dye (SYBT green) intercalates into any dsDNA in a sample added, and the amount of dye is measured.
2. A sequence-specific DNA probe (TaqMan) labeled with a fluorescent reporter and quencher at the 3′ end is added to the DNA sample. The quencher is hydrolyzed, and fluorescence occurs with successful PCR amplification. The products are quantified based on the cycle number at which the intensity is detected above background, known as (Ct). Absolute quantitation requires obtaining a standard dilution curve.

qPCR has a level of sensitivity of 1×10^{-6} and is used for MRD detection, as well as for gene rearrangement quantitation. Examples of clinically useful qPCR are listed in Table 3.11.[13-18]

TABLE 3.11 Examples of Clinically Useful qPCR

Abnormality	Disease
AML1::MTG8	t(8;21) AML
BCR::ABL1	CML
TEL::AML1	B-ALL
t(14;18)(q32;q21)	FL; DLBCL
MYC rearrangements	BL; DLBCL; HGBCL
BCL2 rearrangements	FL; DLBCL; HCBCL
BCL6 rearrangements	FL; DLBCL; HGBCL

AML, acute myeloid leukemia; B-ALL, B-acute lymphoblastic leukemia; BL, Burkitt lymphoma; CML, chronic myeloid leukemia; DLBCL, diffuse large B cell lymphoma; FL, follicular lymphoma; HGBCL, high-grade B cell lymphoma; qPCR, quantitative polymerase chain reaction.

Digital Droplet PCR

Digital droplet PCR (ddPCR) uses small independent PCR reactions to detect and quantitate nucleic acids. A patient sample is divided into small compartments and combined with a water-oil emulsion droplet system. The amount of the target nuclei acid in each compartment depends on the initial concentration and is estimated using a Poisson distribution. After the PCR reaction, the number of compartments with the amplified targets is used to calculate the original concentration. This type of test is useful especially in samples with very little tissue or low tumor burden. It is used to detect alterations like *NPM1*, *KIT*, or *IDH1/2* mutations.[19-21]

Clonality Testing With PCR

In the early 1980s, restriction fragment length analysis (RFLA), also known as "Southern blot," was used for detecting B cell and T cell gene rearrangements,[22] but it has largely been replaced by PCR analysis in most clinical laboratories. Currently, B cell and T cell clonality tests are some of the most ordered molecular tests in hematopathology.

B Cell Receptor

B cell receptors (BCRs), or Igs, are responsible for identifying a myriad of foreign antigens, and therefore, they must be capable of extreme diversity.

Igs are comprised of two heavy chains (IgH) and two light chains, either κ (IgK) or λ (IgL). Both heavy chains and light chains have variable domains and constant domains.

The end portion of the constant domain is attached to the B cell surface or, in the case of soluble Igs/antibodies, the fragment crystallizable region (FC region) of the molecule activates other cells by binding their FC receptor, or triggers phagocytosis or complement activation, depending on the isotype.

The variable domain is comprised of gene segments (VDJ on the heavy chains and VJ on the light chains) that combine to form unique sequences that comprise the specific regions where antigens bind, known as complementarity determining regions (CDRs). Each chain has a total of 3 CDRs, for a total of 12 CDRs per molecule. CDRs are flanked by consensus sequences, recombination signal sequences (RSSs), and interspersed with framework regions (FRs), which are conserved DNA sequences.

The Ig heavy chain, IGH, located on 14q32, rearranges first, as the B cell matures in the BM, using enzymes that recognize RSS. This results in a functional heavy chain and a surrogate light chain, known as the pre-BCR. Next, the light chain is rearranged, starting with the κ loci. If this is not productive, the second κ allele is rearranged, following the principle of allelic exclusion. Finally, if there is no productive κ rearrangement, the λ loci rearrange; this phenomenon is what accounts for the skewed 2:1 κ:λ ratio in B cells.

When the complete Ig molecule is formed, the naïve B cell exits the BM and travels throughout the body to the lymph nodes. After encountering antigen compatible with its CDR3 region, it undergoes class (isotype) switch and somatic hypermutation (SHM) in the germinal center, which adds even more variation to the variable domain. SHM increases the diversity of all three CDRs of both heavy and light chains.

To assess B cell clonality using PCR methods, premade primers bind to RSS near three different regions, FR3, FR2, FR1, as well as the heavy chain joining region (JH) consensus sequence. FR3 corresponds to CDR3.

Normally, PCR products show a normal Gaussian distribution for all three FRs, reflecting a variety of rearrangement products (Figure 3.14). A clonal B cell population, however, with identically rearranged Igs, will appear on the electropherogram as a tall peak. This peak should be at least twice the height of the background polytypic peaks (Figures 3.15A-C).

T Cell Receptor

Precursor NK/T cells exit the BM and develop in the thymus, after differentiating into either an NK cell or a T cell. T cells undergo several changes during maturation, including expression of a surface TCR. TCRs are part of the CD3 complex on the surface of T cells along with three other dimeric signaling modules: CD3εγ, CD3εδ, and CD3ζζ.

The TCR is comprised of heterodimers, either an α and β subunit pair (TCRαβ) or a γ and δ subunit pair (TCRγδ). Four genes rearrange to form these two types of receptors. The δ gene, which resides within the α gene on chromosome 14, rearranges first, followed by the γ gene. If this is successful, a TCRγδ cell is formed. If it is not successful, the β gene is rearranged followed by the α gene, to make a functional TCRαβ receptor.

Although TCRαβ is the most prevalent TCR type, TCRγ is the usual target of PCR analysis, mostly because it is a simpler gene to assess. Importantly, gene rearrangement does not predict surface expression: because αβ T cells rearrange the γ gene before the β gene, a clonal γ gene rearrangement does not inform which TCR receptor subtype is utilized; only that it is clonal.

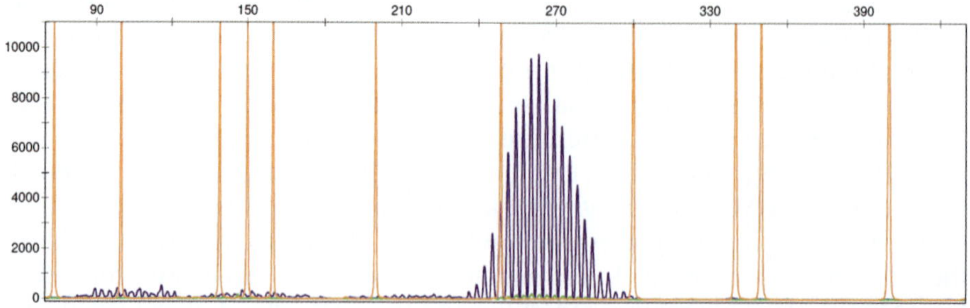

FIGURE 3.14 **Normally, polymerase chain reaction products show a normal Gaussian distribution for all three framework regions, reflecting a variety of rearrangement products.** Figure courtesy of Dr. Rena Xian.

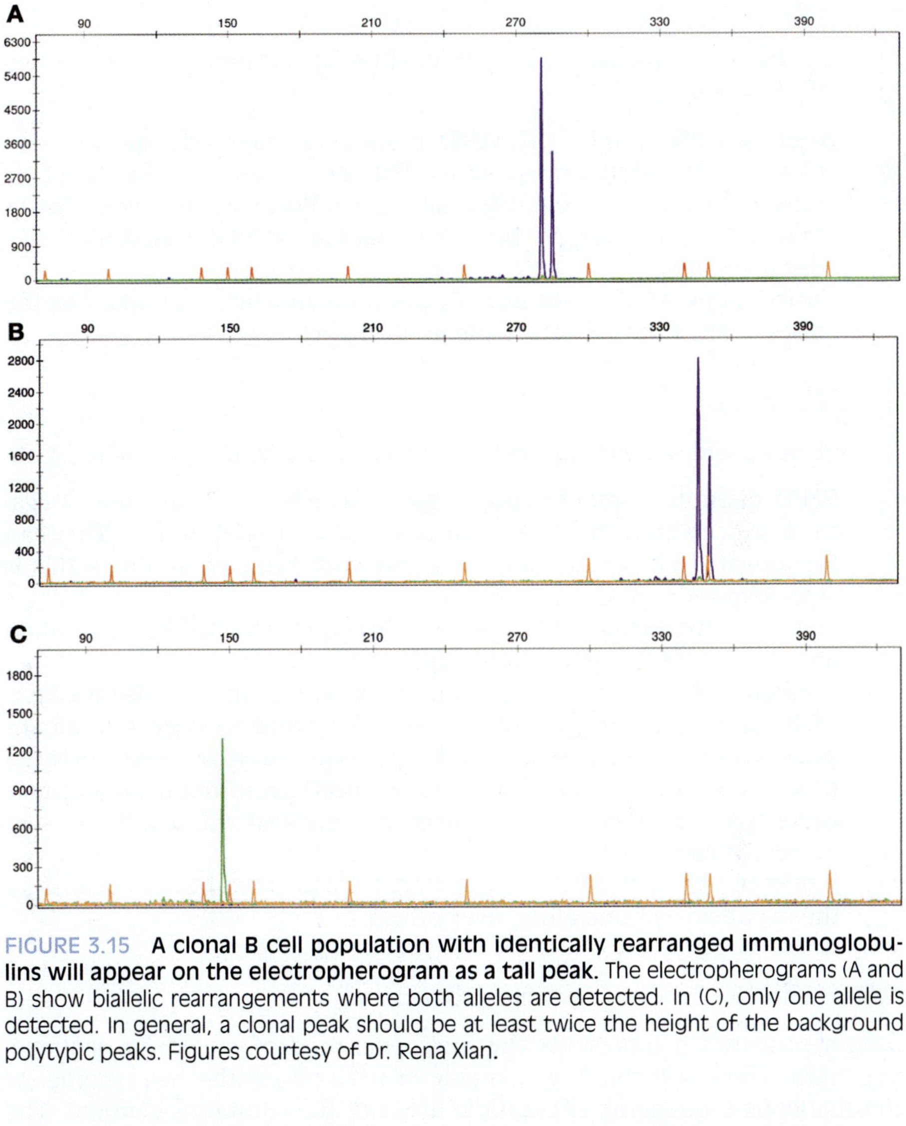

FIGURE 3.15 **A clonal B cell population with identically rearranged immunoglobulins will appear on the electropherogram as a tall peak.** The electropherograms (A and B) show biallelic rearrangements where both alleles are detected. In (C), only one allele is detected. In general, a clonal peak should be at least twice the height of the background polytypic peaks. Figures courtesy of Dr. Rena Xian.

Although the B cell Ig is responsible for identifying epitopes on foreign antigens, the TCR is responsible for recognizing peptides presented by self-MHC molecules (MHCI or MHCII). Structurally, TCR has many similarities with Ig, but they do not vary as much as Ig and do not undergo SHM.

To detect a T cell clone, primers are utilized to assess various sequences in the γ gene. The products are analyzed and compared with the background polytypic T cells.

PCR MRD Detection

PCR is extremely sensitive, making it ideal for MRD testing. There are two types of MRD testing:

Allele-specific IGH/TCR MRD requires a diagnostic specimen to compare clonal rearrangements. Patient-specific reagents must be synthesized and validated for each case. Because of its complexity, this technique is largely being supplanted by NGS-based methods, discussed later.

Fusion gene MRD does not require a diagnostic specimen, but the disease must have a detectable abnormality.

Benefits and Limitations

In spite of its widespread applicability, there are some limitations to PCR:

- SHM disrupts primer-binding regions, which may cause false negatives, especially in postgerminal center B cell lymphomas. This can be mitigated by the use of more framework primers, although this is more expensive and more complex.
- False negatives may occur when clones go undetected because of an abundance of background polytypic cells.
- Limited cell numbers or degraded DNA may result in a false positive. PCR may amplify only a few DNA templates and produce a dominant peak, which may be mistaken for a clone. However, this potential pitfall is routinely avoided by running reactions in duplicate because these "pseudo-clones" are not reproducible and will not be present on repeat runs.
- Florid hyperplasia can also produce false-positive peaks because of the expansion of one clone over others.

NEXT-GENERATION SEQUENCING

Sanger sequencing represents the first generation of molecular sequencing. NGS refers to technology capable of massive parallel sequencing, or simultaneous sequencing of multiple areas of the exome or genome. The process involves sequencing several short overlapping DNA sequences, or "reads," and then reconstructing the continuous DNA sequences using bioinformatics.

NGS is a powerful tool often used in reference labs and academic centers for diagnosing and classifying hematologic malignancies. NGS can detect base substitutions, deletions, and insertions to identify driver mutations and mutational pathways in diseases that can be treated with targeted therapy. Although capable of sequencing the whole genome, many NGS tests used in clinical settings only target "panels" of genes commonly

TABLE 3.12 Panels of Commonly Mutated Genes in Certain Hematologic Disorders

Myeloid neoplasm panel
ABL1, ASXL1, ATM, BCOR, BCORL1, BIRC3, BRAF, BRINP3, CALR, CBL, CDKN2A, CEBPA, CSF1R, CSF3R, DDX3X, DNMT3A, ETV6, EZH2, FAM5C, FBXW7, FLT3, GATA1, GATA2, GNAS, HNRNPK, IDH1, IDH2, IKZF1, IL7R, JAK1, JAK2, KDM6A, KIT, KLHL6, KRAS, MPL, NFE2, NOTCH1, NPM1, NRAS, PFH6, PTPN11, RAD21, RUNX1, SETBP1, SF3B1, SH2B3, SMC1A, SMC3, SRSF2, STAG2, SUZ12, TET2, TP53, U2AF1, WT1, ZRSR2
Lymphoid neoplasm panel
ARID1A, BCL2, BIRC3, BRAF, BTK, B2M, CARD11, CCND1, CDKN2A, CD79A, CD79B, CREBBP, CXCR4, EP300, EZH2, FOXO1, ID3, KCF2, MEF2B, MYC, MYD88, NFKBIE, NOTCH1, NOTCH2, PLC62, PTPRD, SF3B1, STS6, TCF3, TNFAIP3, TP53, TRAF2, XPO1

mutated in certain disorders (Table 3.12). The general workflow is listed in Table 3.13.[23-25]

Variant calling is complex and requires a sophisticated bioinformatics system and expert molecular pathologists. The bioinformatics pipeline identifies multiple variants and filters out inferior quality reads and germline variants to eliminate common polymorphism. However, interpreters must be aware that some polymorphisms escape this filtration.

TABLE 3.13 Next-Generation Sequencing Procedure

Process	Description
Target enrichment	• Nucleic acid is isolated and purified.
Creating library DNA	• DNA is fragmented. • Specialized adapters are added to both ends (to be compatible with a sequencer).
Sequencing	• Libraries are sequenced through SBS.
Variant calling	• Software identifies the nucleotides that are added. • Software checks the accuracy.
Tier listing	• Various pipelines are utilized to determine detrimental changes. • Molecular pathologist interprets findings.

SBS, sequencing by synthesis.

Variants are annotated with cDNA (c.) and protein (p.) nomenclature as in these examples:

c.1799T>A = substitution at position 1799, the nucleic acid thymine is replaced by adenine
p.V600E = missense substitution at position 600, the amino acid valine is replaced by glutamic acid

In addition to analyzing the specific abnormality in the gene, the mutant variant allele frequency (VAF) is noted, which is approximately proportional to the amount of variant DNA in the sample for that gene. In theory, germline or heterozygous somatic alterations have a VAF of 50%, but this may vary based on other technical or biologic factors.

Variants are categorized into tiers or "levels" on the final molecular report based on the likelihood of their pathogenicity (Table 3.14).[26] Public databases like COSMIC[26] or published literature and guidelines from the Association of Molecular Pathology (AMP), American Society of Clinical Oncology (ASCO), and College of American Pathologists (CAP) are useful when interpreting and reporting variants.

NGS for MRD

The presence of MRD is one of the most important predictors of relapse and patient survival in many hematologic disorders, including ALL, AML,

TABLE 3.14 Tiers of Variants Are Often Categorized Based on Their Likely Pathogenicity

Tiers	Description	Level of evidence
Category 1	Variants of strong clinical significance	• Diagnostic for a specific tumor type • Predicts response or resistance to therapies for specific tumors
Category 2	Variants of potential clinical significance	• Diagnostically significant/may assist in diagnosis • May be therapeutically relevant
Category 3	Variants of unknown clinical significance	• Not seen at a significant allele frequency in the general population • No convincing published evidence
Category 4	Benign or likely benign variants	• Observed at frequent allele frequency in the general population • No published evidence of association with cancer

MM, and CLL, to the extent that it is incorporated into the clinical algorithms of these diseases.

Although MRD is commonly assessed via FC and PCR methods, NGS has a higher sensitivity (~10^{-6}) than these methods and is an increasingly important technique in diseases in which high sensitivity is critical. However, it is costly and requires specific expertise, making it unfeasible for some labs.

NGS for lymphoid MRD most often targets the Ig gene.[20] In AML or MDS, mutations/single-nucleotide variants (SNVs) or insertions/deletions are quantified for monitoring disease. However, interpreting NGS MRD in myeloid malignancies must be done with caution because clonal hematopoiesis of indeterminate potential (CHIP) can occur in healthy individuals with no evidence of hematopoietic disease (See Chapter 5). Distinguishing CHIP from leukemic clones in patients at first remission may be difficult. Because the most common mutations in CHIP overlap with the most common mutations in MDS, including *DNMT3*, *TET2*, and *ASXL1* (also known as "DTA" mutations),[21] most studies exclude these mutations when assessing for MRD. One study showed that persistent DTA mutations after first remission were not associated with a higher relapse rate, whereas patients with persistent non-DTA mutations had a higher rate of relapse.[22]

Benefits of NGS for MRD detection:

- High sensitivity
- Patient-specific primers not necessary

Limitations of NGS for MRD detection:

- Diagnostic specimen needed to compare mutations
- High expertise needed
- Expensive

FUTURE APPROACHES

Many new important genetic lesions in leukemia are intragenic or involve transcriptional alterations. As sequencing becomes cheaper and more accessible, techniques such as whole-genome sequencing and whole-transcriptome sequencing ("RNA-seq") will be important tools for the clinical laboratory.

CONCLUSION

In summary, ancillary testing is a critical part of diagnosing BM specimens, and each of the aforementioned methods has its own benefits and limitations. The best method utilized depends on the sample and clinical question.

REFERENCES

1. Novikov ND, Griffin GK, Dudley G, et al. Utility of a simple and robust flow cytometry assay for rapid clonality testing in mature peripheral T-cell lymphomas. *Am J Clin Pathol.* 2019;151(5):494-503.
2. van den Beemd R, Boor PPC, van Lochem EG, et al. Flow cytometric analysis of the Vβ repertoire in healthy controls. *Cytometry.* 2000;40(4):336-345.
3. Morice WG, Kimlinger T, Katzmann JA, et al. Flow cytometric assessment of TCR-Vbeta expression in the evaluation of peripheral blood involvement by T-cell lymphoproliferative disorders: a comparison with conventional T-cell immunophenotyping and molecular genetic techniques. *Am J Clin Pathol.* 2004;121(3):373-383.
4. Sims JE, Tunnacliffe A, Smith WJ, Rabbitts TH. Complexity of human T-cell antigen receptor beta-chain constant and variable-region genes. *Nature.* 1984;312(5994):541-545.
5. Tunnacliffe A, Kefford R, Milstein C, Forster A, Rabbitts TH. Sequence and evolution of the human T-cell antigen receptor beta-chain genes. *Proc Natl Acad Sci USA.* 1985;82(15):5068-5072.
6. Maciocia PM, Wawrzyniecka PA, Philip B, et al. Targeting the T-cell receptor β-chain constant region for immunotherapy of T-cell malignancies. *Nat Med.* 2017;23(12):1416-1423.
7. Yunis JJ, Sanchez O. G-banding and chromosome structure. *Chromosoma.* 1973;44(1):15-23.
8. Cui C, Shu W, Li P. Fluorescence in situ hybridization: cell-based genetic diagnostic and research applications. *Front Cell Dev Biol.* 2016;4:89.
9. Mullis KB. The unusual origin of the polymerase chain reaction. *Sci Am.* 1990;262(4):56-61, 4-5.
10. Waters DL, Shapter FM. The polymerase chain reaction (PCR): general methods. *Methods Mol Biol (Clifton, NJ).* 2014;1099:65-75.
11. Sanchez-Vega B, Vega F, Hai S, Medeiros LJ, Luthra R. Real-time t(14;18)(q32;q21) PCR assay combined with high-resolution capillary electrophoresis: a novel and rapid approach that allows accurate quantitation and size determination of bcl-2/JH fusion sequences. *Mod Pathol.* 2002;15(4):448-453.
12. Luthra R, Medeiros LJ. TaqMan reverse transcriptase-polymerase chain reaction coupled with capillary electrophoresis for quantification and identification of bcr-abl transcript type. *Methods Mol Biol (Clifton, NJ).* 2006;335:135-145.
13. Marcucci G, Livak KJ, Bi W, Strout MP, Bloomfield CD, Caligiuri MA. Detection of minimal residual disease in patients with AML1/ETO-associated acute myeloid leukemia using a novel quantitative reverse transcription polymerase chain reaction assay. *Leukemia.* 1998;12(9):1482-1489.
14. Krauter J, Heil G, Ganser A. The AML1/MTG8 fusion transcript in t(8;21) positive AML and its implication for the detection of minimal residual disease. *Hematology (Amsterdam, Netherlands).* 2001;5(5):369-381.
15. Barthe C, Mahon Fo-X, Gharbi M-J, et al. Expression of interferon-α (IFN-α) receptor 2c at diagnosis is associated with cytogenetic response in IFN-α–treated chronic myeloid leukemia. *Blood.* 2001;97(11):3568-3573.
16. Pongers-Willemse MJ, Verhagen OJ, Tibbe GJ, et al. Real-time quantitative PCR for the detection of minimal residual disease in acute lymphoblastic leukemia using junctional region specific TaqMan probes. *Leukemia.* 1998;12(12):2006-2014.
17. Luthra R, McBride JA, Cabanillas F, Sarris A. Novel 5′ exonuclease-based real-time PCR assay for the detection of t(14;18)(q32;q21) in patients with follicular lymphoma. *Am J Pathol.* 1998;153(1):63-68.
18. Ginzinger DG. Gene quantification using real-time quantitative PCR: an emerging technology hits the mainstream. *Exp Hematol.* 2002;30(6):503-512.

19. Beck RC, Kim AS, Goswami RS, Weinberg OK, Yeung CCS, Ewalt MD. Molecular/cytogenetic education for hematopathology fellows. *Am J Clin Pathol.* 2020;154(2):149-147.
20. Dogliotti I, Drandi D, Genuardi E, Ferrero S. New molecular technologies for minimal residual disease evaluation in B-cell lymphoid malignancies. *J Clin Med.* 2018;7(9):288.
21. Quan PL, Sauzade M, Brouzes E. dPCR: a technology review. *Sensors (Basel, Switzerland).* 2018;18(4):1271.
22. Southern EM. Detection of specific sequences among DNA fragments separated by gel electrophoresis. *J Mol Biol.* 1975;98(3):503-517.
23. Kuo FC. Next generation sequencing in hematolymphoid neoplasia. *Semin Hematol.* 2019;56(1):2-6.
24. Yohe S, Thyagarajan B. Review of clinical next-generation sequencing. *Arch Pathol Lab Med.* 2017;141(11):1544-1557.
25. Johnsen JM, Nickerson DA, Reiner AP. Massively parallel sequencing: the new frontier of hematologic genomics. *Blood.* 2013;122(19):3268-3275.
26. Li MM, Datto M, Duncavage EJ, et al. Standards and guidelines for the interpretation and reporting of sequence variants in cancer: a joint consensus recommendation of the Association for Molecular Pathology, American Society of Clinical Oncology, and College of American Pathologists. *J Mol Diagn.* 2017;19(1):4-23.

4

ACUTE MYELOID LEUKEMIA

Acute myeloid leukemia (AML) represents a group of diseases with phenotypic and genetic heterogeneity. These clonal neoplasms affect stem cells or myeloid progenitors and result in (a) a block in normal hematopoietic maturation as well as (b) increased clonal proliferation and/or survival advantage. These diseases are characterized by accumulation of blasts (or blast equivalents) in the bone marrow (BM) and/or peripheral blood (PB), typically resulting in ineffective hematopoiesis.

DIAGNOSIS

A diagnosis of AML requires the morphologic detection of 20% or more blasts/blast equivalents in the PB or BM except when certain genetic abnormalities are present (see later).

AML CLASSIFICATION

Historically, AML classification schemes were based on blast percentages and morphologic features; the French-American-British (FAB) classification categorized AML based on the degree and lineage of blast maturation as identified by morphologic and cytochemical features.[1] Subsequent World Health Organization (WHO) classifications categorized AML based on (a) recurrent genetic abnormalities, recognizing that these alterations have unique clinical, pathologic, and prognostic significance,[2] as well as (b) other specific entities with prognostic implications. This approach has recently been revised and extended[3]; current nomenclature used in the International Consensus Classification (ICC) is presented in Table 4.1.

EPIDEMIOLOGY AND CLINICAL PRESENTATION

AMLs are rare, comprising only 1% of all cancers. Approximately 3.4/100,000 people are diagnosed with AML each year in the United States, with a similar sex distribution (M:F=1.3:1) and a bimodal age distribution.[4] Although this disease occurs in patients of every age, the median age at diagnosis is 68 years; incidence increases with age, likely because of increased incidence of myelodysplasia and clonal hematopoiesis with age.

TABLE 4.1 The International Consensus Classification of AML

Entity
APL with *PML::RARA*
APL with other *RARA* rearrangements
AML with t(8;21)(q22;q22.1)/*RUNX1::RUNX1T1*
AML with inv(16)(p13.1q22) or t(16;16)(p13.1;q22)/*CBFB::MYH11*
AML with t(9;11)(p21.3;q23.3)/*MLLT3::KMT2A*
AML with other *KMT2A* rearrangements
AML with t(6;9)(p22.3;q34.1)/*DEK::NUP214*
AML with inv(3)(q21.3q26.2) or t(3;3)(q21.3;q26.2)/*GATA2::MECOM(EVI1)*
AML with other *MECOM* rearrangements
AML with other rare recurring translocations
AML with t(9;22)(q34.1;q11.2)/*BCR::ABL1*
AML with mutated *NPM1*
AML with in-frame bZIP *CEBPA* mutations
AML with mutated *TP53*
AML with myelodysplasia-related gene mutations
AML with myelodysplasia-related cytogenetic abnormalities
AML not otherwise specified
Myeloid sarcoma

AML, acute myeloid leukemia; APL, acute promyelocytic leukemia.

AML arises as a result of accumulated genetic abnormalities that cooperate to produce the disease phenotype. In pediatric patients and young adults, the disease is associated with certain inherited disorders, like Down syndrome, congenital neutropenia, Fanconi anemia, and others.[5] Certain chemotherapies are also associated with increased risk, most notably topoisomerase II inhibitors, alkylating agents, anthracyclines, and anti-tubulin agents.[6]

Clinically, patients typically present with symptoms related to ineffective hematopoiesis, including excessive bruising, bleeding, infections, and fatigue.

A proper initial lab workup is critical to the diagnosis of AML. A complete blood count (CBC) typically reveals cytopenias, including anemia and thrombocytopenia, and variable numbers of white blood cells (WBCs) and blasts. The diagnosis requires a combination of findings, including morphologic and immunophenotypic assessment, as well as genetic testing. Additional laboratory information is helpful, including assessment of lactate dehydrogenase (LDH) levels, which may be a marker of high cell turnover. Coagulation studies including prothrombin time (PT), partial thromboplastin time (PTT), fibrinogen, and D-dimer are important to assess for bleeding or clotting risk.

MORPHOLOGY

Diagnostic workup for AML requires morphologic assessment of a well-prepared PB smear or BM aspirate stained with Wright-Giemsa or May-Grünwald-Giemsa. A BM trephine biopsy is also recommended and is essential in cases of an inaspirable marrow ("dry tap"), with touch imprints aiding in morphologic evaluation of blast count and potential dysplasia.

On the core biopsy, the BM appears hypercellular for age with increased immature cells (Figure 4.1A and B; eFigure 4.1).

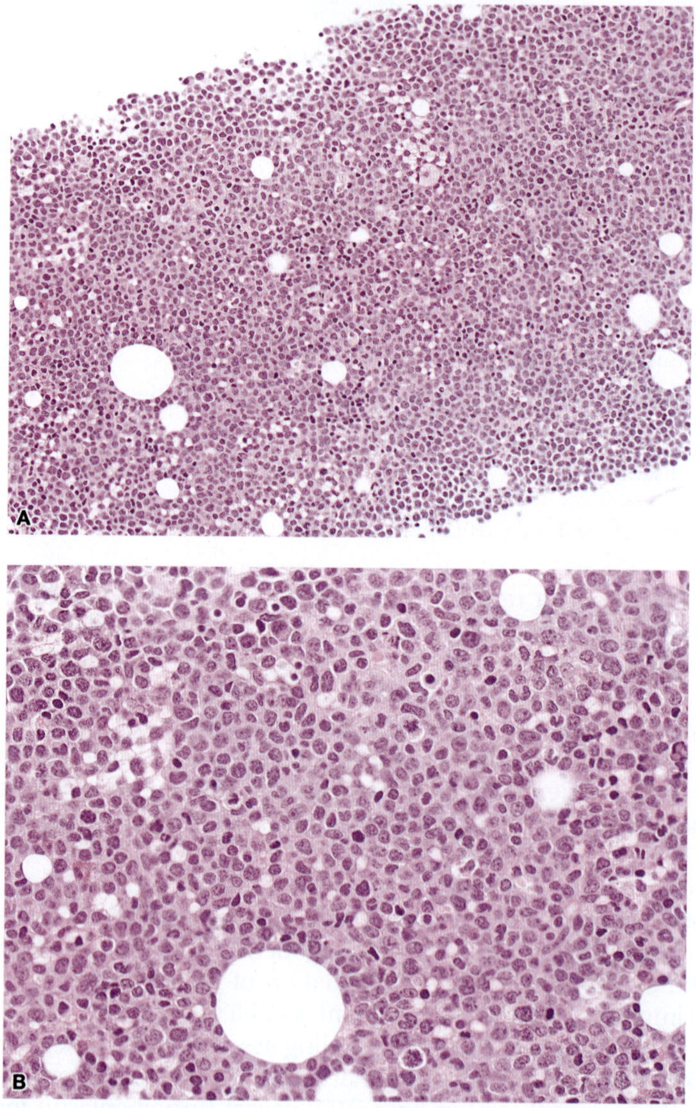

FIGURE 4.1 **Although bone marrow cellularity can vary in acute myeloid leukemia, the marrow is most often hypercellular, with little-to-no residual normal hematopoiesis, as seen here (A).** The blasts are large, with irregular nuclei, fine chromatin, a small amount of eosinophilic cytoplasm, and variably prominent nucleoli (B).

The aspirate smear often appears hypercellular with abundant blasts (Figure 4.2A and B; eFigure 4.2). It is recommended that 200 nucleated cells be counted on the PB smear, and 500 nucleated cells be counted on a spiculated BM aspirate to accurately determine the percentage of blasts.

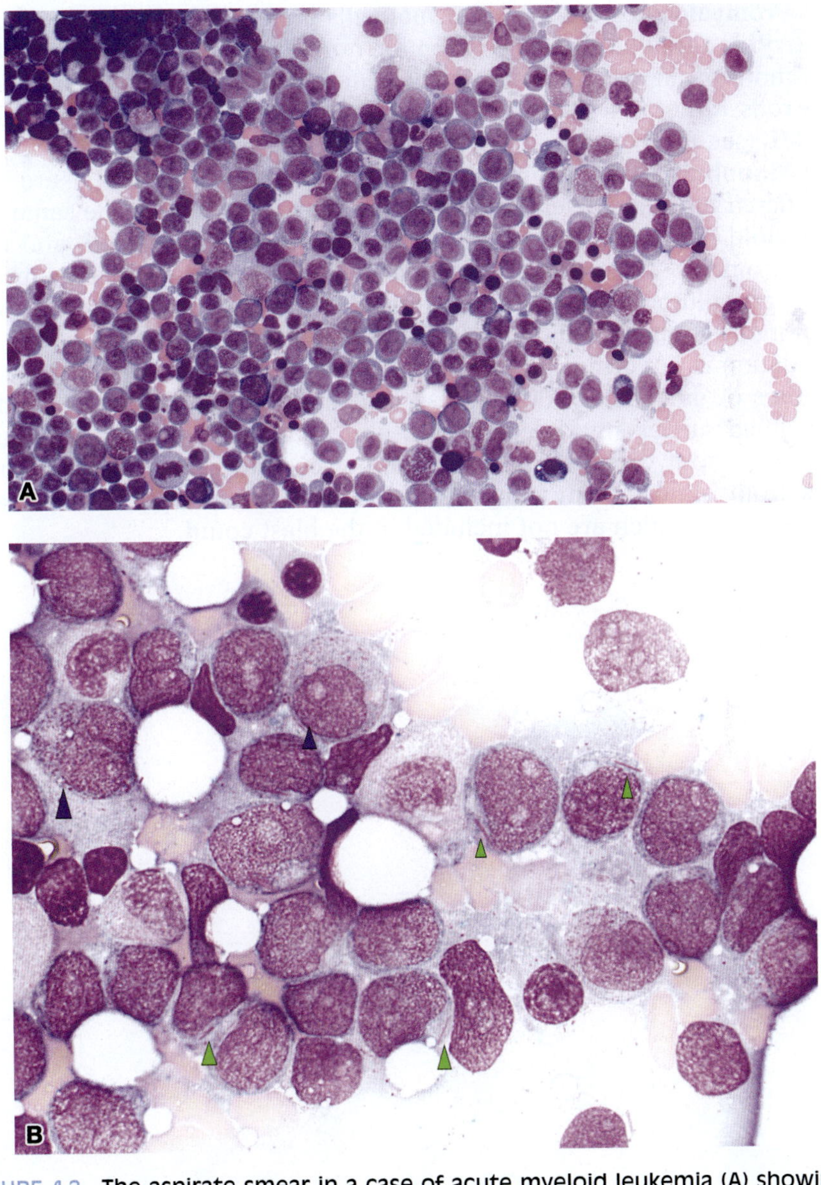

FIGURE 4.2 **The aspirate smear in a case of acute myeloid leukemia (A) showing a relatively homogeneous population comprised of myeloblasts with a small amount of cytoplasm with little background maturation.** At higher power (B), blasts show fine chromatin, prominent nucleoli, and scant cytoplasm. There are often admixed early maturing cells with granules (dark blue arrowhead), and Auer rods may be seen in blasts (green arrowheads).

Myeloblasts, described in Chapter 2 (arrowhead), are the hallmark of AML, and these generally resemble those seen in a normal BM, except that some cases may show Auer rods, which are collections of azurophilic crystalline cytoplasmic inclusions (Figure 4.3). Other types of so-called blast equivalents either do not have a normal marrow counterpart or are sufficiently different from normal to require further description.

Promyelocytes are the abnormal cells in acute promyelocytic leukemia (APL); although they may resemble normal promyelocytes, they often have more prominent granules and are notable for prominent bundles of Auer rods, rather than the single cytoplasmic Auer rods seen in other forms of AML (see Figure 4.12).

Monoblasts and **promonocytes** (Figure 4.4; eFigure 4.3) are also considered blast equivalents. Monoblasts are approximately the same size as myeloid blasts with oval-shaped nuclei, one to two nucleoli, and delicate chromatin. The cytoplasm is typically more abundant than in myeloblasts, gray-blue, and may contain fine eosinophilic granules or vacuoles. Promonocytes may be difficult to differentiate from monoblasts, but differentiation is not critical, as both are considered blast equivalents for the purposes of diagnosing AML. These cells are large, with bean-shaped or convoluted nuclei, multiple nucleoli, and abundant gray-blue cytoplasm with or without vacuoles. It is critical, however, to distinguish promonocytes from abnormal monocytes, which have more nuclear chromatin clumping and which are not included in the blast count.

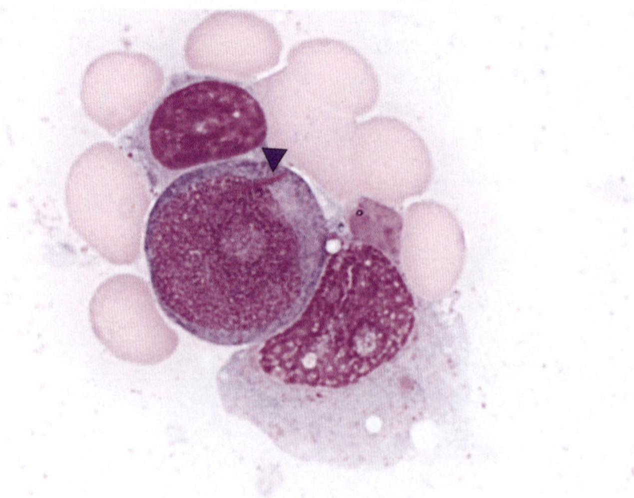

FIGURE 4.3 Higher power view of a myeloblast with a single prominent Auer rod (arrowhead).

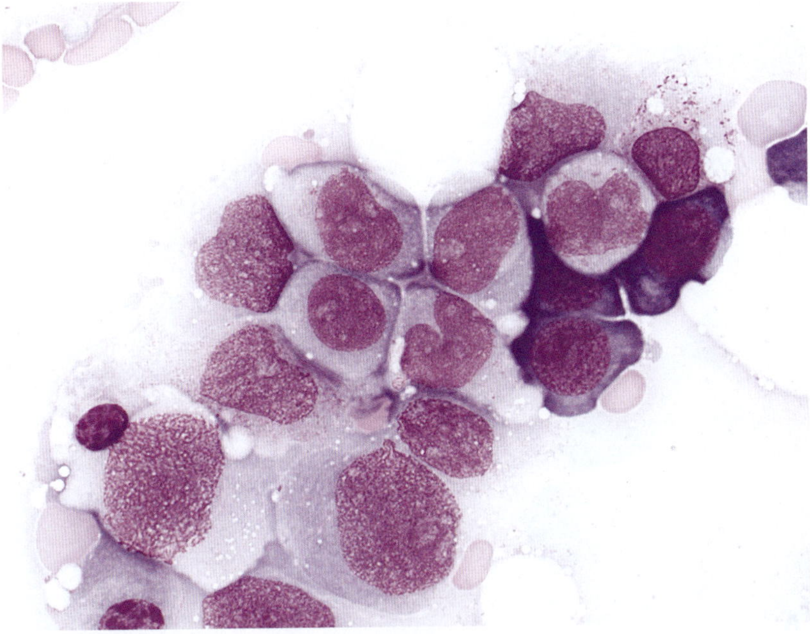

FIGURE 4.4 **In this case of acute myeloid leukemia with monocytic differentiation, both abnormal monoblasts and promonocytes are present.** Monoblasts have round to oval nuclei, whereas the promonocytes have bean-shaped or delicately folded nuclei, but still have immature chromatin and nucleoli.

Megakaryoblasts are also included as blast equivalents, identifiable in the BM as medium-sized cells with high N:C ratios, one to two nucleoli, and darkly basophilic cytoplasm, sometimes with cytoplasmic blebs or pseudopods (Figure 4.5A-C; eFigure 4.4). Morphologically, it may be difficult to differentiate a megakaryoblast from a pronormoblast (erythroblast), which is not considered a blast equivalent.

PHENOTYPE

In many cases, morphologic similarities between myeloid blasts and lymphoid blasts make it necessary to use immunophenotyping to distinguish them. Blast phenotyping may be accomplished by one of several methods: cytochemical stains, immunohistochemical (IHC) stains, or flow cytometry (FC).

1. Cytochemical stains, both enzymatic and non-enzymatic, are performed on unfixed/unstained BM aspirates to assess blast lineage, as described in Chapter 2.[7] They are rarely used in current practice because of the efficiency of IHC stains and FC (see Chapter 3).
2. IHC stains are used to assess the phenotype of blasts on the core biopsy, clot section, or other formalin-fixed paraffin-embedded (FFPE)

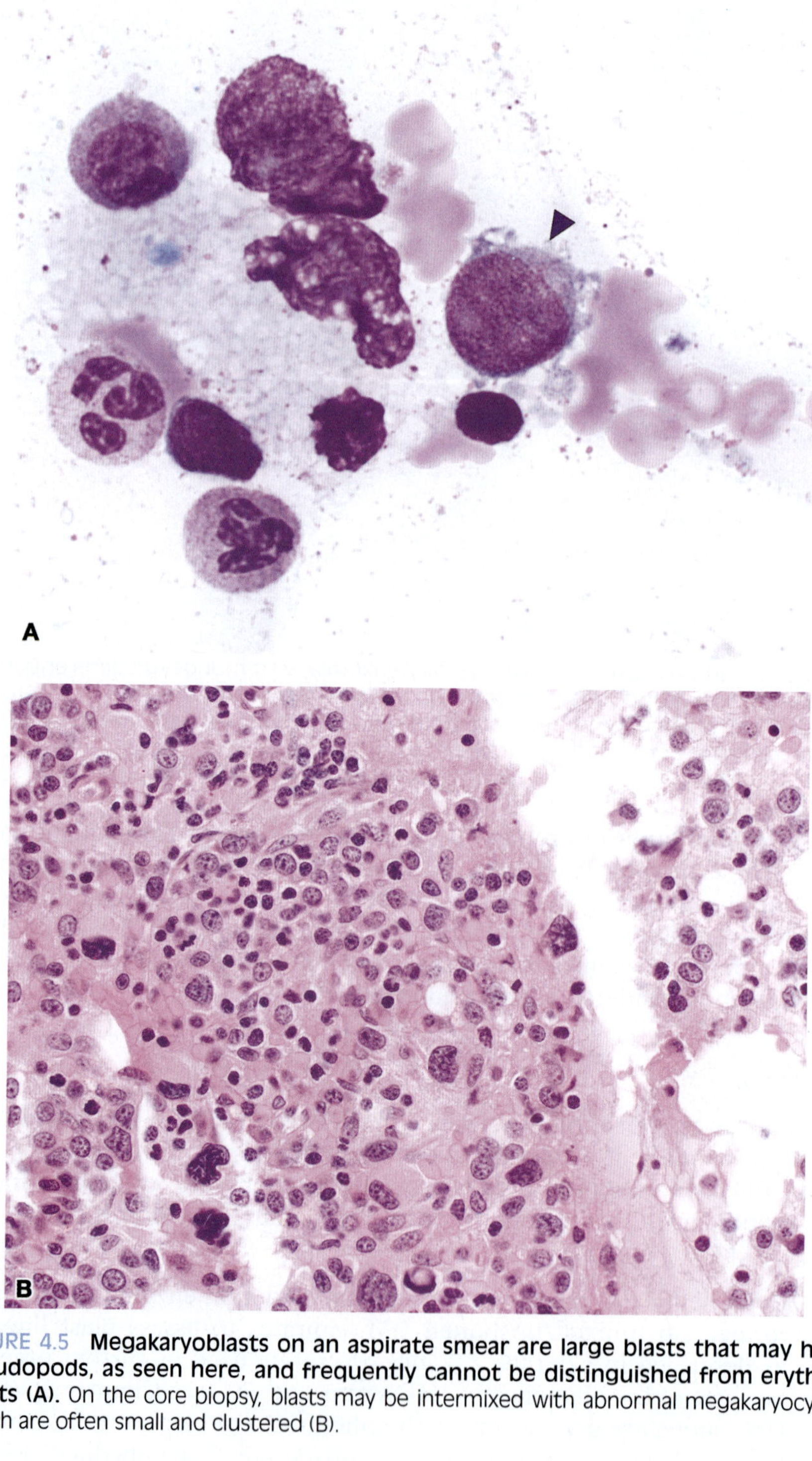

FIGURE 4.5 **Megakaryoblasts on an aspirate smear are large blasts that may have pseudopods, as seen here, and frequently cannot be distinguished from erythroblasts (A).** On the core biopsy, blasts may be intermixed with abnormal megakaryocytes, which are often small and clustered (B).

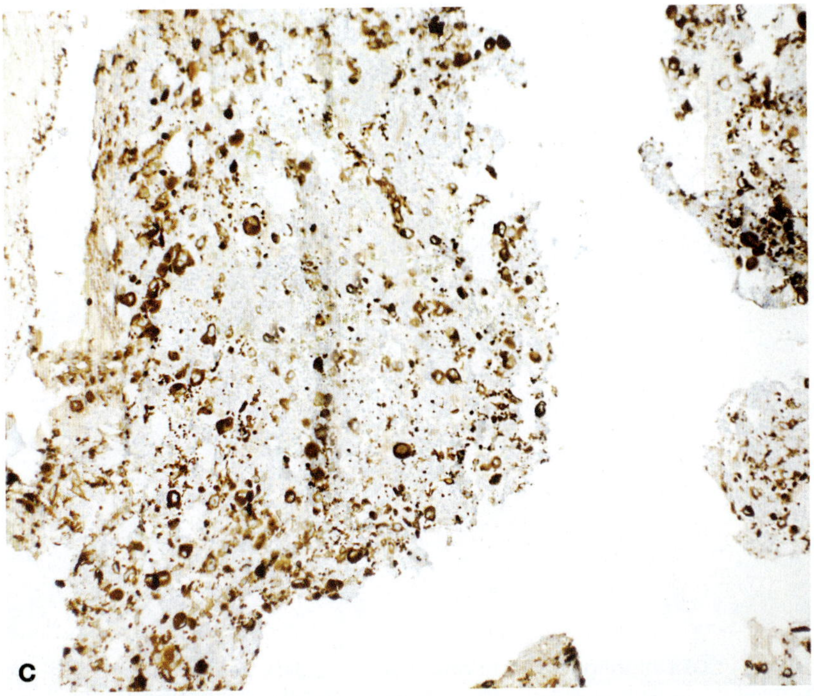

FIGURE 4.5 (*continued*) Immunohistochemical stains or flow cytometry may be necessary to help determine the lineage of the blasts. Megakaryoblasts are highlighted on this core biopsy with CD61.

tissue. This is especially useful in cases of "dry tap" aspirates. CD34 (Figure 4.6) is useful to identify blasts but in practice, leukemia classification by IHC generally requires comprehensive panels of B, T, and myeloid markers because no single marker is sufficiently lineage specific enough to stand on its own.

3. Immunophenotyping by multiparameter FC has become the gold standard for most labs in assessing AML because of its sensitivity and quick turnaround time. FC has the benefit of assessing not only normal and abnormal surface and cytoplasmic cellular markers, but also the intensity of expression relative to other populations, as well as the patterns of cellular maturation, features that can help distinguish leukemic cells from normal cells. FC is also a powerful tool to assess the BM for minimal residual disease (MRD), defined as disease below the threshold of detection by the naked eye. Although FC is critical to determine the blast phenotype, it is not a substitute for morphologic evaluation of blast percentage, as FC may over- or underrepresent the number of blasts because of hemodilution, degeneration, relative hypersensitivity of red cell precursors to lysis during preparation, or other preanalytical factors. Table 4.2 lists markers commonly used in AML FC and their characteristics.

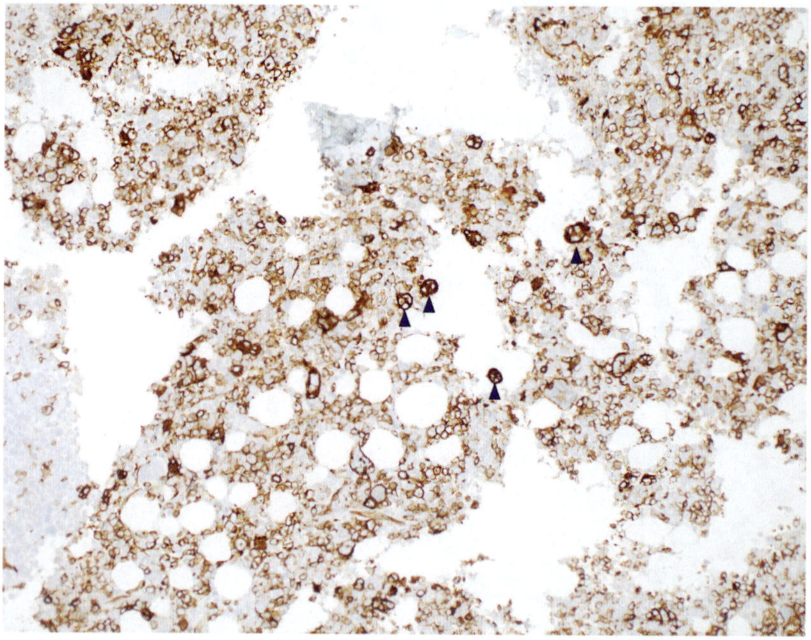

FIGURE 4.6 **CD34 highlights abundant myeloid blasts in this biopsy in a case of acute myeloid leukemia arising from myelodysplastic syndrome (MDS).** Abnormal small megakaryocytes in MDS will also frequently stain with CD34 (arrowheads).

TABLE 4.2 Markers Used in Flow Cytometric Analysis of AML

Marker	Comment
CD45	Not lineage specific; used to identify blast pocket
CD34	Present on blasts in most AML, but not reliably in APL or monocytic leukemias
CD117	Commonly present; often over- or underexpressed vs normal. On some T-ALL
CD33	Sensitive but not specific; may be aberrantly lost; higher in monocytic leukemias and APL
CD13	Sensitive but not specific; often discordant intensity with CD33
CD7	Often positive on blasts but on regenerating marrow as well
CD56	Aberrantly expressed, often with *KIT* mutation, but on regenerating marrow as well
CD38	Not lineage specific; often underexpressed or lost
CD123	Not lineage specific; higher in monocytic leukemias; may be a target for therapy
CD64	High expression in monocytic leukemias
CD14	Usually negative in acute monocytic leukemias, but may have high expression
CD36	Monocytic leukemia and erythroblasts
CD11b/c	Monocytic leukemias; rare on other AML

TABLE 4.2 Markers Used in Flow Cytometric Analysis of AML (*continued*)

Marker	Comment
HLA-DR	Usually positive; intensity often abnormal; negative in APL and some *NPM1*-mutated AML
CD71	Usually positive but brightest on erythroid cells
CD41,61	Megakaryocytic leukemia but not absolutely specific
CD42b	More mature platelet marker less common on megakaryocytic leukemia
MPO	Myeloid specific but often negative

ALL, acute lymphoblastic leukemia; AML, acute myeloid leukemia; APL, acute promyelocytic leukemia; HLA-DR, human leukocyte antigen-D related; MPO, myeloperoxidase.

BLAST IDENTIFICATION BY FC

Blasts in cases of AML are typically, but not invariably, detected in the "blast pocket" or "blast window" (Figure 4.7A and B) and, occasionally, exhibit higher side scatter (SSC), especially in the case of blast equivalents

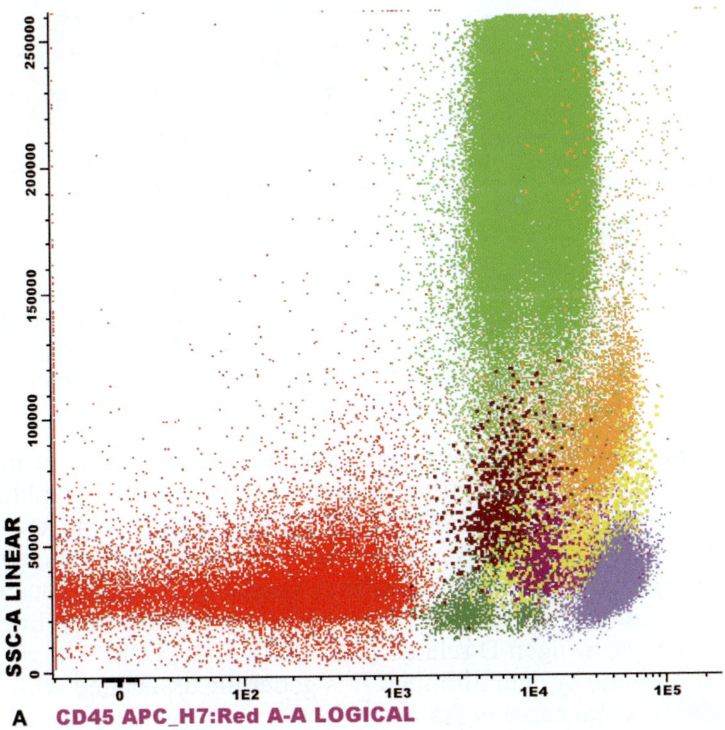

FIGURE 4.7 In flow cytometry (A), the "blast pocket" refers to the area immediately below the myeloid cells in light green and encompasses blasts (brown) with low side scatter (SSC) and dim CD45.

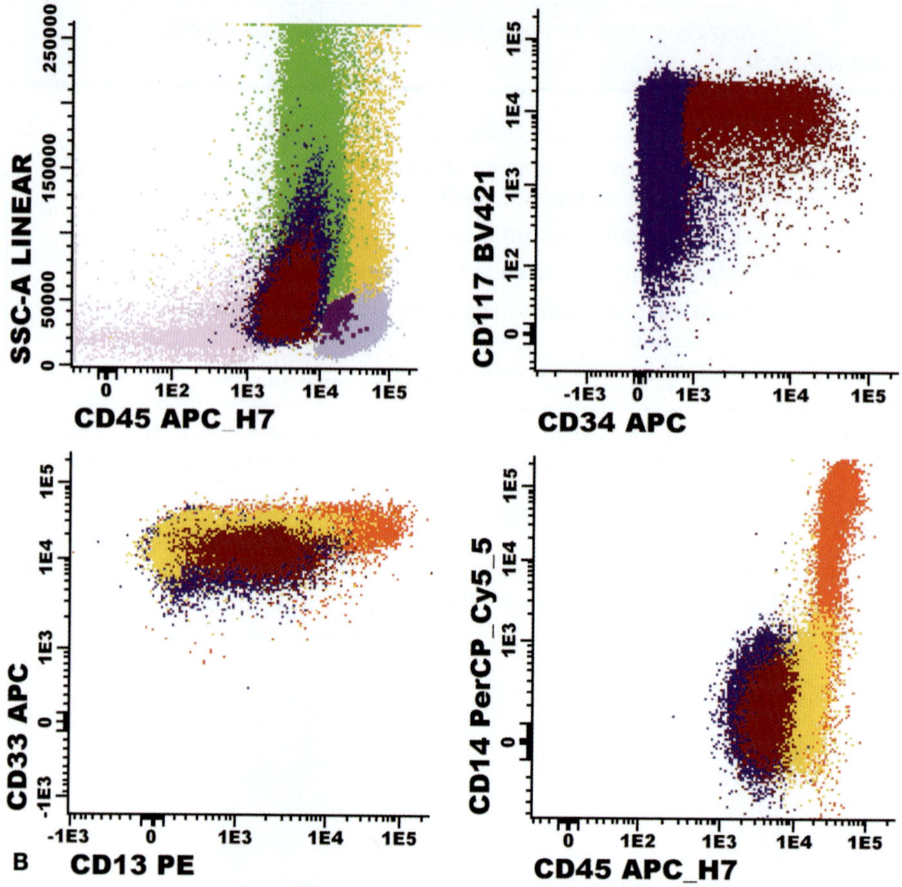

FIGURE 4.7 *(continued)* The blast pocket may also contain basophils (purple), hematogones (dark green), and plasmacytoid dendritic cells (yellow). In (B), the blast pocket contains an expanded population of myeloid blasts (both the brown and blue populations), consistent with acute myeloid leukemia. A subset of blasts expresses CD34 (brown) and also CD117 and CD33. Also shown are lymphocytes (gray), nucleated red cells (pink), basophils (purple), and both immature and mature monocytes (light and dark orange, respectively).

of APL (see Figure 4.16) or monoblastic leukemia (Figure 4.8), or may have dim or even negative CD45, as with erythroblasts or megakaryoblasts and some cases of B cell acute lymphoblastic leukemia (ALL). Moreover, cytoplasmic vacuoles or granularity (eg, in APL) can cause SSC characteristics to vary considerably. Because blasts may be seen in various locations on dot plots, it is important to assess markers of immaturity, including CD34, human leukocyte antigen-D related (HLA-DR), and CD38. Tdt is a reliable marker of immaturity, and although it is generally associated with ALL, it is also seen in some cases of AML.

Once blasts are identified, a variety of markers can be used to help determine the subtype of myeloid leukemia.

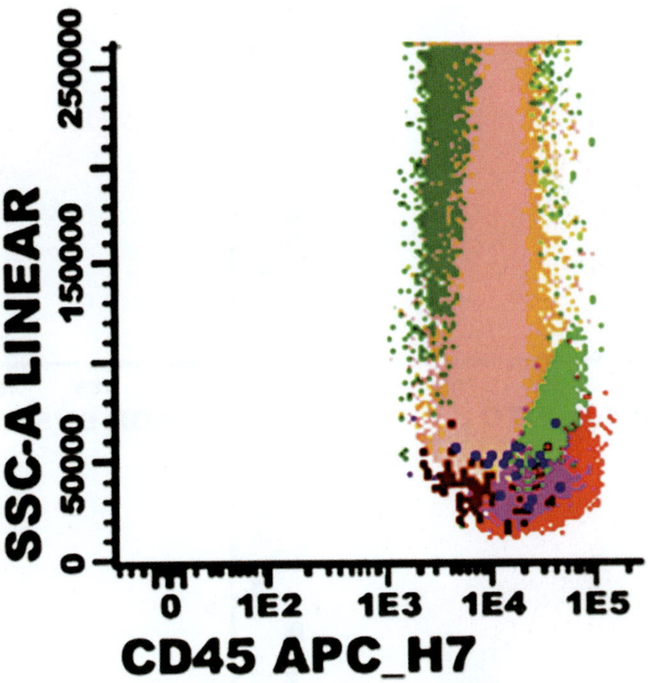

FIGURE 4.8 By flow cytometry, blasts in acute myeloid leukemia with monocytic features typically do not appear in the blast pocket and show higher light side scatter (SSC) on CD45 versus SSC than normal myeloid blasts (peach population).

Myeloid markers: Lineage is assigned based on typical "myeloid" markers, including CD117, CD33, CD13, and myeloperoxidase (MPO), although, with the exception of MPO, none are myeloid specific. However, many cases of AML will lack MPO. CD117 is relatively specific, although it may be expressed in T-ALL but not B-ALL. It is also positive on erythroid progenitors and some early promyelocytes as well as mast cells but is at least 10-fold brighter in the latter. Markers associated with more mature differentiated myeloid-lineage cells such as CD15, CD16, or CD11b are uncommonly positive on the blasts of AML.

Monocytic markers: Markers characteristic of monocytic leukemias include CD4, CD11b, CD11c, CD14, CD33, CD36, CD64, CD65, HLA-DR, and lysozyme (Figure 4.9). However, with the exception of CD36 and CD11c, these are also seen on granulocytic leukemias; bright intensity of expression of many of these, notably CD14, CD33, and CD64, is generally more specific. Monoblasts are generally negative for CD34 and may also lack CD117; there is no single reliable phenotypic marker for a monoblast, which makes morphologic blast evaluation critical.

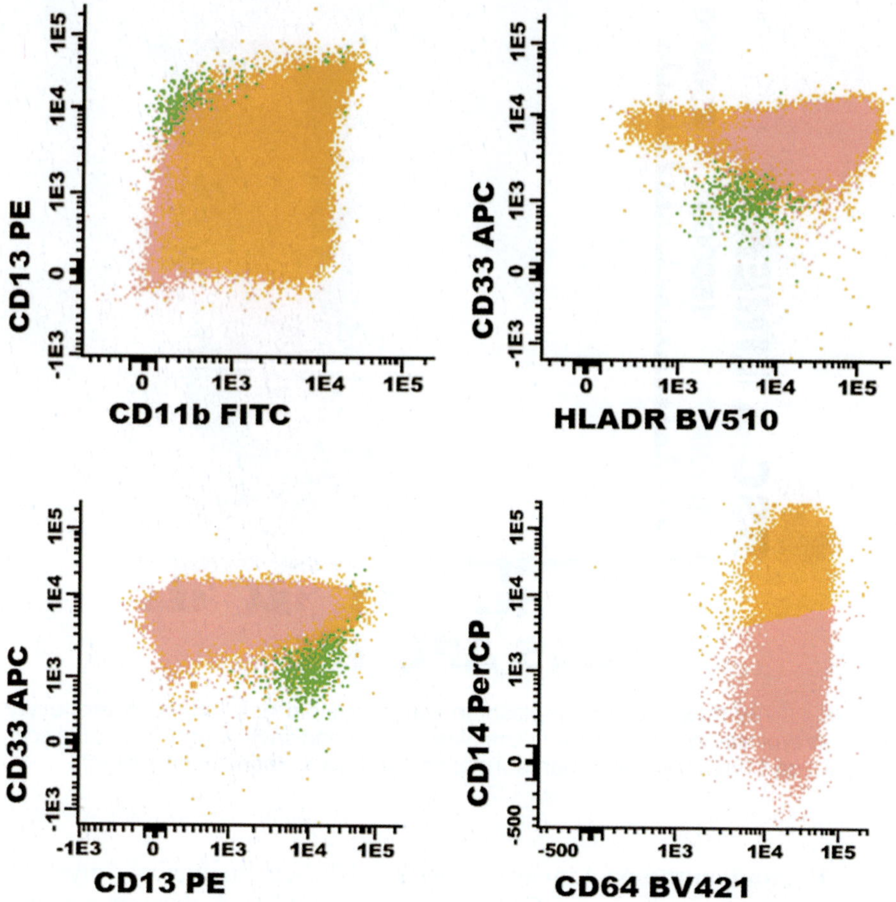

FIGURE 4.9 **Monocytes in acute monocytic leukemia can show a range of maturation.** In most cases of acute monocytic leukemia, the immature population is expanded, but both mature and immature forms express bright CD33. However, there is variable expression of CD11b and CD13, with the mature monocytic forms (orange) showing dimmer than normal expression of these markers (upper left panel).

Erythroid markers: Erythroid blasts can be recognized based on expression of CD117 and/or bright CD71 and typically lack CD34, HLA-DR, or other myeloid-associated markers. They may or may not express more mature erythroid markers such as glycophorin. They also express CD36 but are readily distinguished from monocytes.

Megakaryocytic markers: Megakaryoblasts are generally positive for CD36, CD41, and CD61 and may or may not express the more mature platelet-associated marker CD42b (Figure 4.10).

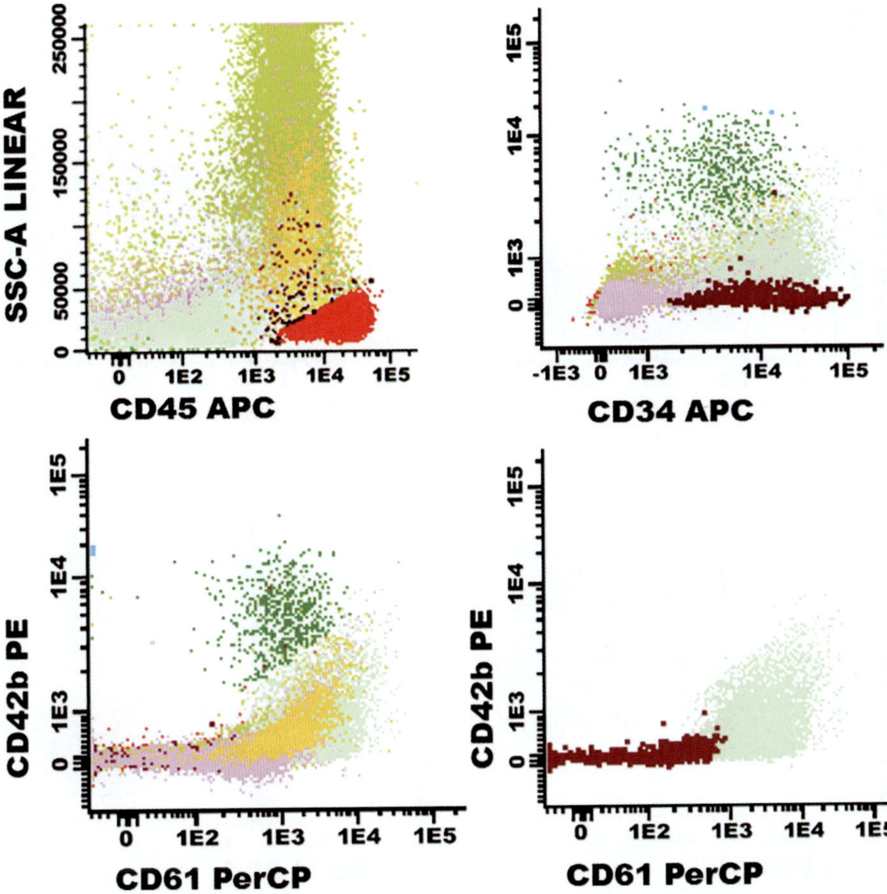

FIGURE 4.10 **In this case of acute megakaryoblastic leukemia, the blasts (light green) express dim CD45, CD34, and CD61, but have little, if any, CD42b.** The brighter CD42b-positive cells (dark green) likely represent platelets adherent to blasts.

Abnormal markers: Markers that are not expressed on typical myeloid blasts may be helpful to identify the population as abnormal (Figure 4.11). These markers include CD7 and CD56 expression. A loss of markers is another way to identify abnormal populations, including a loss of CD38 and/or HLA-DR expression.

Many, although not all, of the markers listed earlier are also available for classifying leukemias by IHC, and some markers, including E-cadherin, CD71, or Spectrin for red cells and MPO or lysozyme for myelomonocytic cells, are more frequently used in IHC. In cases where leukemia replaces the marrow, IHC is generally reliable for classification, although when blasts are in the minority, accurately distinguishing blasts from background myeloid cells may be more challenging.

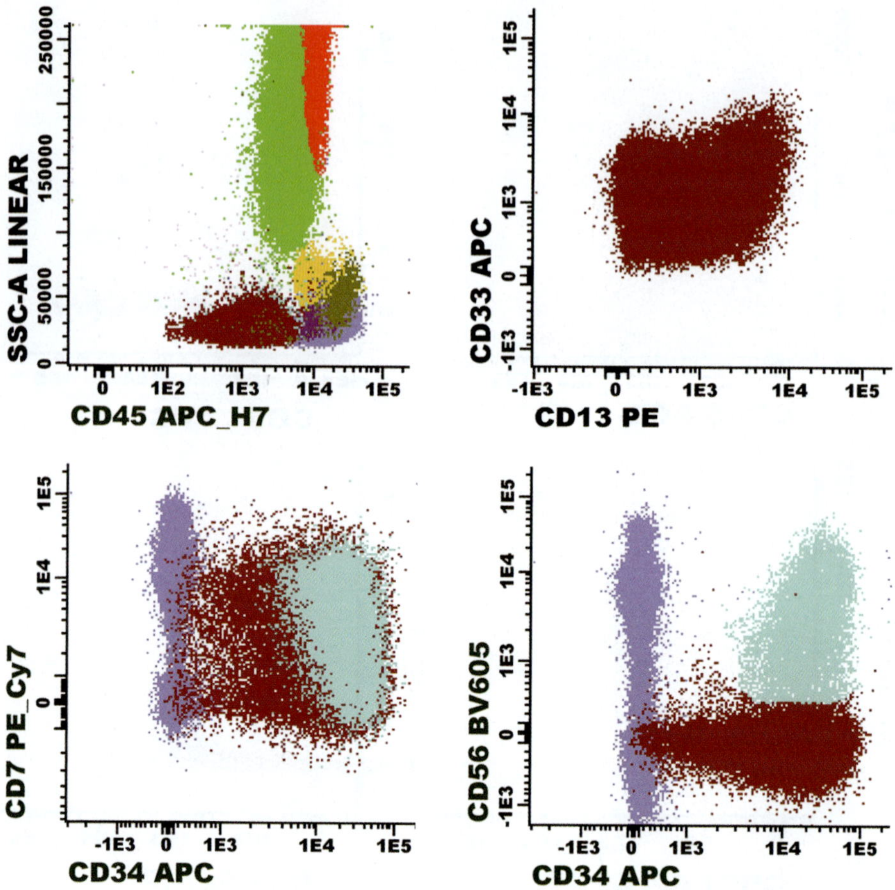

FIGURE 4.11 The myeloid blast population (brown) in this case expresses an abnormal phenotype; in addition to myeloid-associated markers CD33 and CD13, a subset of the blasts also expresses CD56 (cyan) and there is also partial CD7, although these are not exactly the same subpopulations.

GENETICS

All cases of AML have genetic alterations. These commonly include chromosomal translocations or inversions, as well as deletions or additions, generally detected by conventional karyotyping or fluorescence in situ hybridization (FISH). Essentially all cases of AML also have gene mutations, typically detected nowadays by next-generation sequencing (NGS). The latter include numerous recurrent driver mutations known to be important in leukemogenesis as well as passenger mutations whose function is not entirely known.

The most common lesions detectable by cytogenetic techniques were discovered much earlier than individual gene mutations; many of these were associated with distinct morphologic and phenotypic findings, and these formed the basis for the first genetic subclassification of AML. It was later discovered, however, that these translocations were not sufficient to produce leukemia but require cooperating gene mutations. With a few exceptions mentioned later, these mutations do not define distinct entities and so are not primarily included in the classification, although they affect prognosis, and in many cases represent targets for therapy.

SUBCLASSIFICATION OF AML

The specific entities currently recognized by the ICC are defined in whole or in part by genetic lesions, although some are closely related and could be thought of as variants. The most common of these are discussed in detail below, and key distinguishing features of some of the other entities are briefly noted. The "AML with rare translocations" subcategory includes an additional 12 types of AML with rare recurring translocations. Some, such as AML with t(1;22)(p13.3;q13.1)/*RBM15::MRTF1*, a rare megakaryoblastic leukemia seen in infants, have long been known, whereas many others are newly discovered. In the ICC, lesions defined by specific translocations or gene mutations now require 10% blasts to establish the diagnosis, although there is no requirement for minimal blast percentage for these subtypes in the WHO 5th edition. However, in both classifications, AML with *BCR::ABL1* still requires ≥20% blasts. Cases that lack any of the defined genetic lesions are referred to as AML not otherwise specified (NOS) and still require ≥20% BM or PB blasts; tissue presentations of AML are considered myeloid sarcoma (eFigure 4.5).

AML WITH RECURRENT TRANSLOCATIONS

APL With *PML::RARA*

Epidemiology and Presentation

This represents approximately 5% of all AMLs, mostly occurring in young to middle-aged adults (eFigure 4.6). The gold standard for the diagnosis of this entity is the identification of the *PML::RARA* fusion. Notorious for triggering disseminated intravascular coagulation (DIC), this acute leukemia is considered a medical emergency.

Morphology

Two well-known morphologic variants are recognized[2]: the hypergranular (typical) variant (Figure 4.12 A-C) and the hypogranular (microgranular) variant (Figure 4.13A and B), which has few, if any, cytoplasmic granules, but can often be recognized by the cell's bilobed, or "wasp-waisted" nuclei (Figure 4.14). Both variants are associated with DIC. The hypergranular variant often has low WBC counts and the diagnostic cells are difficult to find in the blood, whereas the hypogranular variant may mimic acute monocytic leukemia.

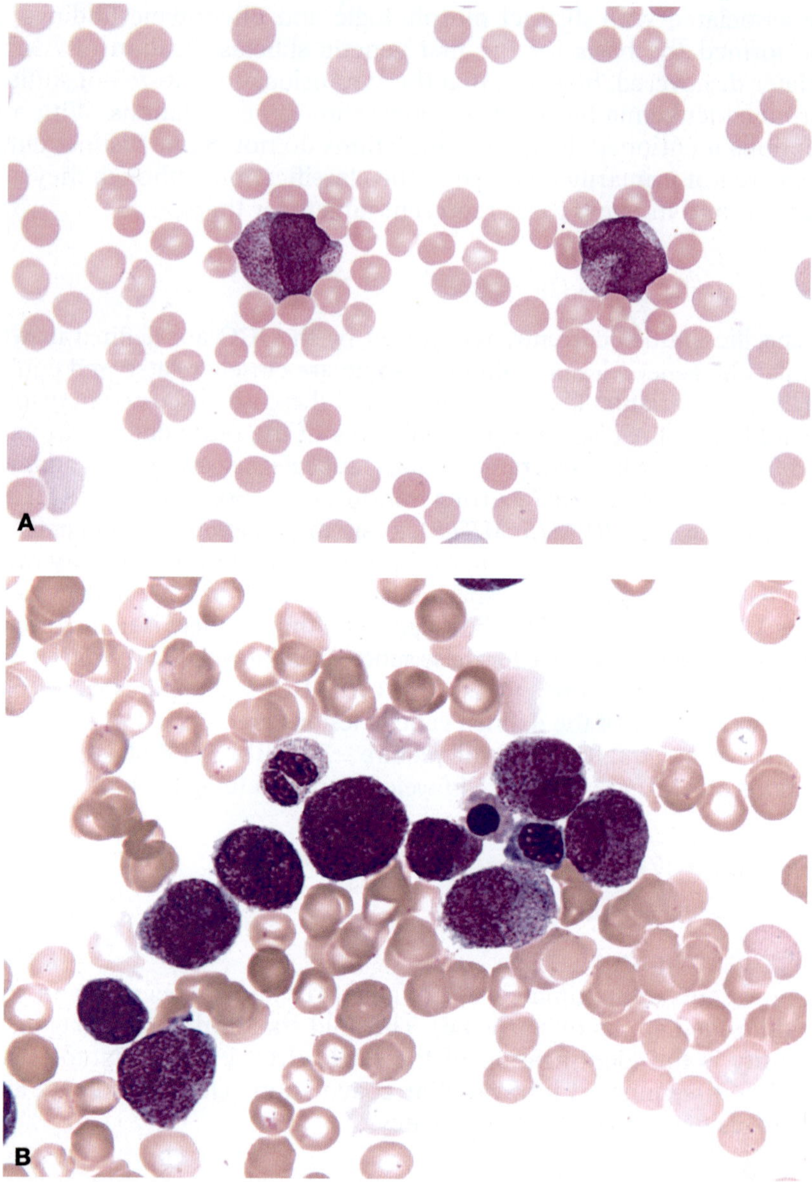

FIGURE 4.12 **In this example of acute promyelocytic leukemia, two abnormal promyelocytes can be seen circulating in the peripheral blood (A).** The marrow aspirate (B) shows a cluster of several abnormal promyelocytes with abundant granules (B); these abnormal cells also often have multiple Auer rods (arrowhead) (C).

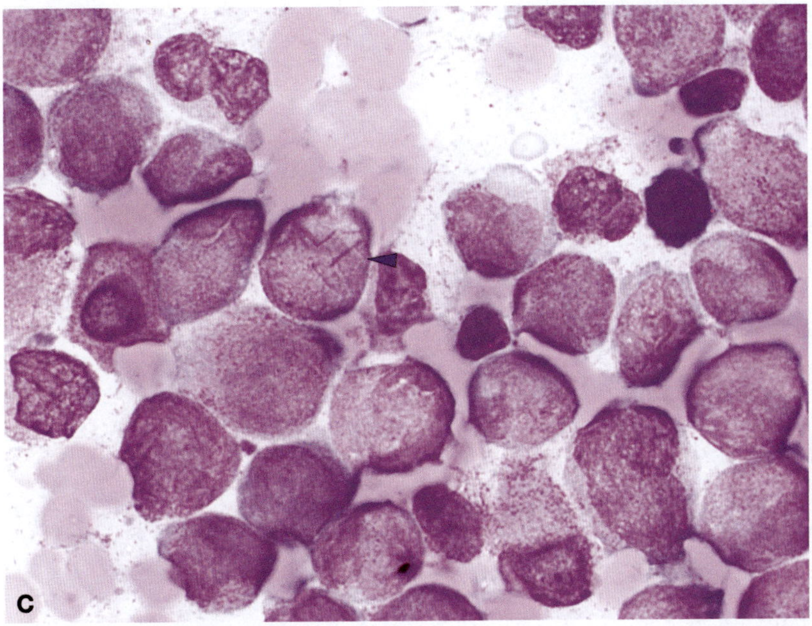

FIGURE 4.12 (*continued*)

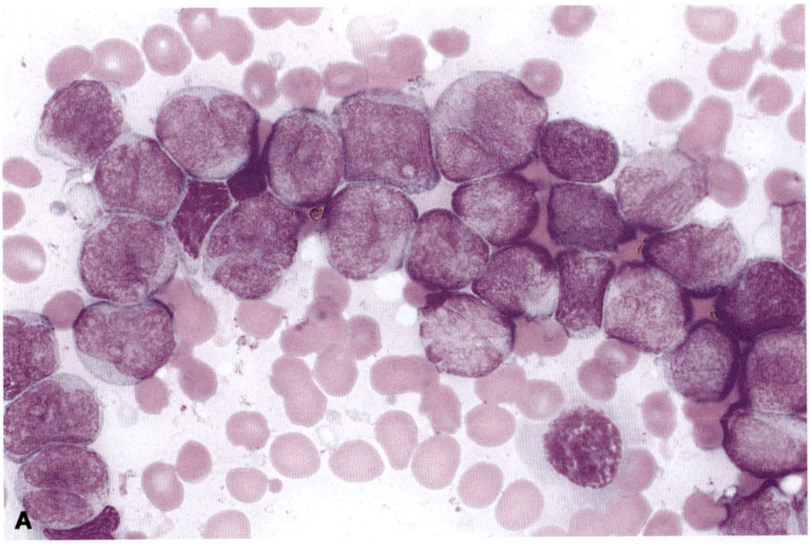

FIGURE 4.13 In contrast to the promyelocytes in cases of classical hypergranular acute promyelocytic leukemia (APL; Figure 4.12), the hypo-/microgranular variant of APL shows blasts with bilobed or complex nuclei, often confused with monoblasts (A).

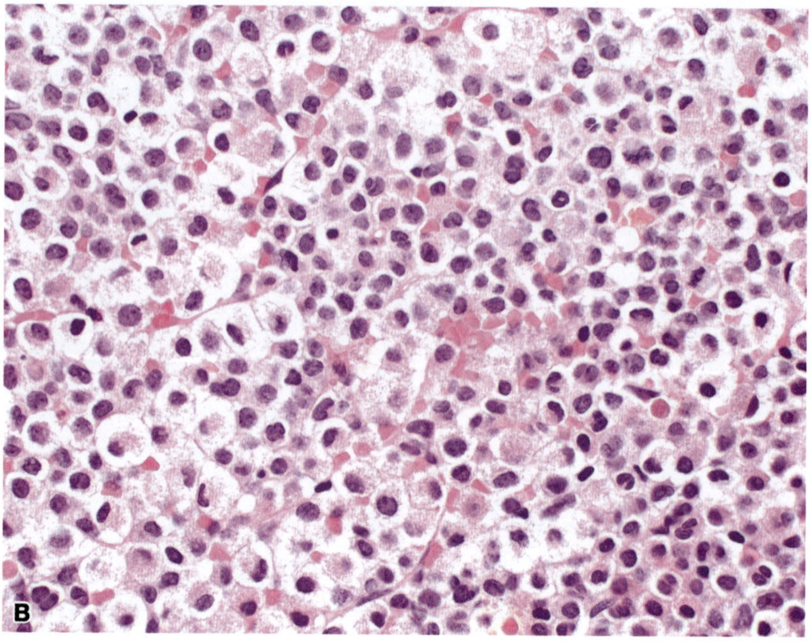

FIGURE 4.13 **(*continued*)** On a core biopsy (B), many cells have bean-shaped nuclei or otherwise irregular nuclei and abundant cytoplasm that is typically more eosinophilic than in cases of monocytic leukemia.

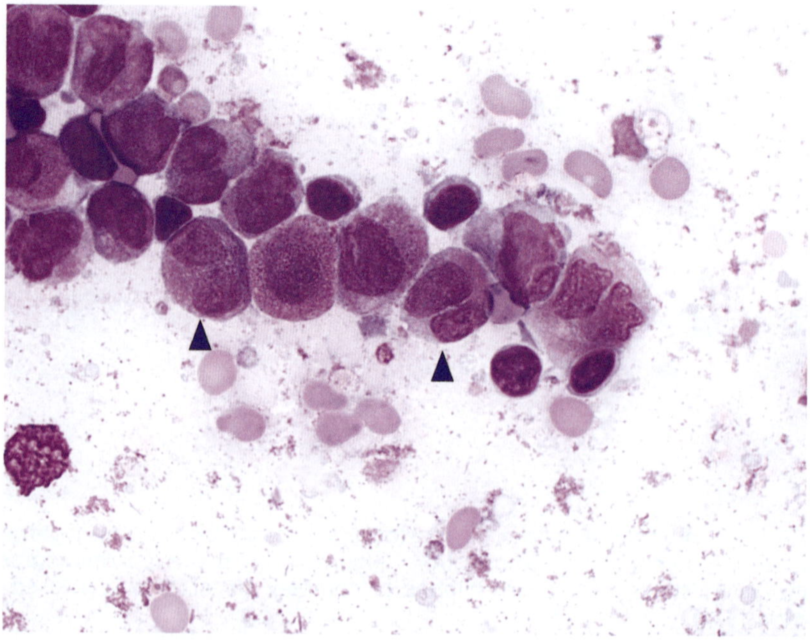

FIGURE 4.14 **The most distinctive cell in microgranular acute promyelocytic leukemia is the so-called "wasp-waisted" blast (arrowheads), which has nuclei with equal-sized lobes that appear to be separated.** There is also often an eosinophilic cytoplasm blush in these blasts equivalents, as shown here.

PHENOTYPE

By FC, APL has characteristic high Side scatter (SSC) and high autofluorescence (Figure 4.15) because of the abundant cytoplasmic granules. APL is classically negative for CD34 and HLA-DR (Figure 4.16), although it may have partial expression of either or both of these, most often in the hypogranular/microgranular variant; this variant also may express aberrant CD2.[8] Detection of CD117 and/or MPO in the abnormal promyelocytes confirms their myeloid lineage. Usually CD33 expression is bright, at the same level of intensity as the background monocytes, whereas CD13 is variably expressed. The abnormal promyelocytes may express CD64, but unlike normal promyelocytes, are negative for the granulocytic differentiation marker CD15. It is important to remember that the CD34/HLA-DR-negative immunophenotype is not specific to APL, as a subset of AML without differentiation also lacks expression of CD34 and HLA-DR. In a case with these findings, it behooves the pathologist to suggest the diagnosis of APL, alert the clinician, and request stat FISH studies to assess for *PML::RARA*.

GENETICS

The t(15;17) results in the formation of the fusion mRNA *PML::RARA* and the translated fusion protein disrupts promyelocyte maturation.[9] In most cases, t(15;17) is detectable by karyotype and/or FISH. However, occasionally, a cryptic or complex translocation may result in a false negative.[10] In

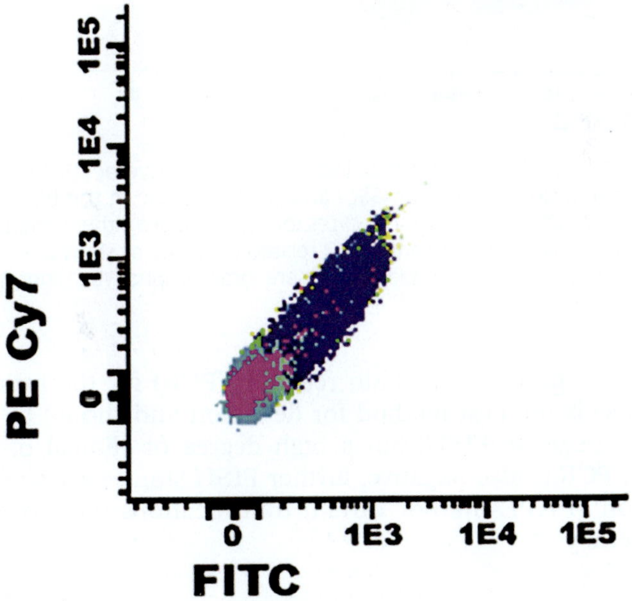

FIGURE 4.15 By flow cytometry, the leukemic cells in acute promyelocytic leukemia (dark blue) show high background autofluorescence, as seen in this unstained control.

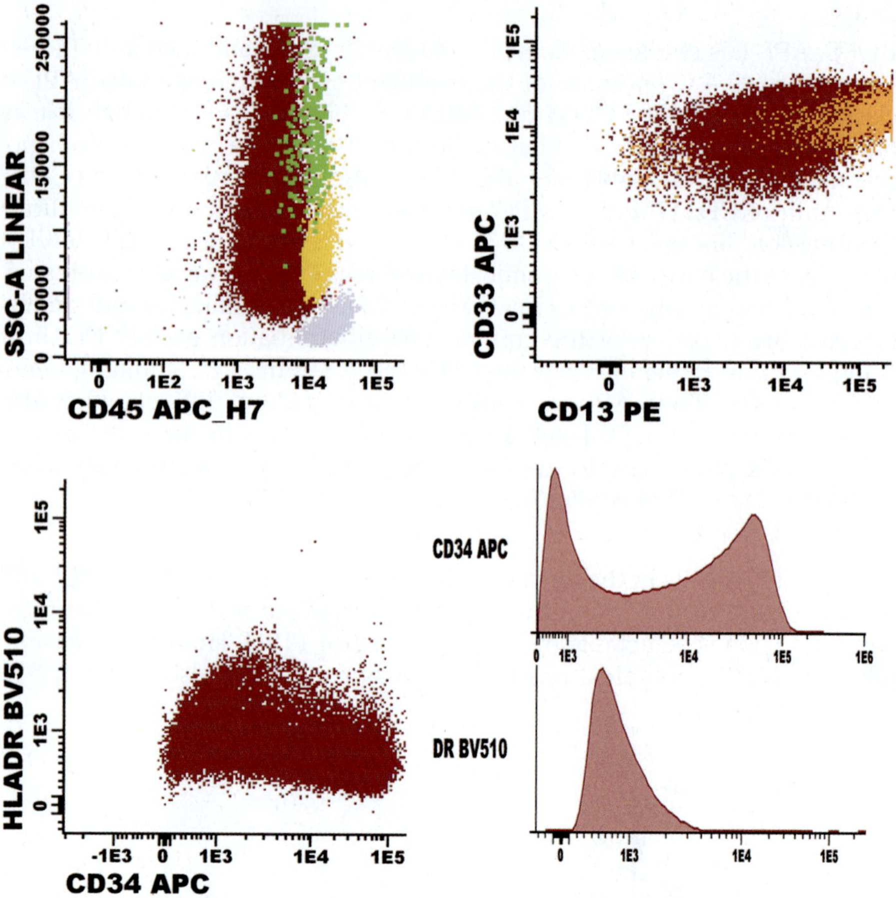

FIGURE 4.16 **The abnormal promyelocytes in acute promyelocytic leukemia (brown population) have high side scatter (SSC) and do not reside in the blast pocket.** They express bright CD33 at the level of monocytes (orange) and are either completely negative for CD34 and/or human leukocyte antigen-D related (HLA-DR), or show only partial expression, as in the flow cytometry example shown here (gray, lymphocytes; light green, residual normal neutrophils).

those instances, polymerase chain reaction (PCR) for the fusion product (*PML::RARA*) is the best method for detection and should be ordered in cases with a negative FISH, but a high degree of clinical or pathologic suspicion. If PCR is also negative, further FISH studies are warranted as a small fraction of APLs harbor variant translocations that are resistant to standard therapy.

Prognosis

APL with *PML::RARA* has a good prognosis, mainly because of its responsiveness to therapy. APL is very sensitive to treatment with all-trans retinoic acid (ATRA), which acts as the differentiating agent. ATRA must be administered immediately and for at least 5 days to be effective in reducing the risk of hemorrhage associated with DIC. Together, ATRA and arsenic trioxide achieve >90% cure rate when combined with anthracycline chemotherapy.[11]

A number of other genes, most commonly *ZBTB16* at 11q23.2, have been discovered as alternative partners with *RARA*; such cases are classified as APL with other *RARA* rearrangements. Compared to APL with *PML::RARA*, these can vary in morphology, phenotype, and response to ATRA. Cases with t(11;17)/*ZBTB16::RARA* have blasts with generally oval nuclei, less prominent granules, and lack Auer rods. It is also resistant to ATRA and has a poor prognosis. By contrast, the rare t(5;17)(q35.1;q21)/*NPM1::RARA* variant does appear to be ATRA responsive.

AML With t(8;21) (q22;q22)/*RUNX1::RUNX1T1*

Epidemiology and Presentation

This translocation represents approximately 4% to 8% of all AML cases and often presents with a low percentage of blasts (eFigure 4.7).[2] Although patients of any age may be affected, this is typically a disease of younger adults. Patients present as with other AMLs, but may also present as myeloid sarcoma, which in children commonly occurs within the orbits. In addition to anemia and thrombocytopenia, patients may have monocytopenia, which is evident on routine CBC and by FC.

Morphology

The PB or BM shows varying numbers of blasts with distinct Golgi zones (Hofs) and large azurophilic or salmon-colored granules (Figure 4.17). Occasionally, blasts in this type of AML are morphologically distinct, with the granules coalescing to form a bright Golgi space that appears as an orange sun and peripheral basophilic cytoplasm representing the residual sky, earning them the nickname "sunset cells." Auer rods are commonly seen in blasts and in differentiating cells even in mature neutrophils. In contrast with APL with *PML::RARA*, which presents with abundant cytoplasmic Auer rods in bundles, the Auer rods in t(8;21) are typically single, long, and slender with sharply pointed ends (see Figure 4.3). Occasionally, blasts may have very large coarse cytoplasmic granules, often referred to as pseudo-Chédiak-Higashi granules (Figure 4.18; eFigure 4.8). Eosinophilic precursors may be increased, but they do not exhibit the same abnormalities seen in AML with t(16;16)/inv(16) (see later). Myeloid dysplasia is common, most often identified as dysplastic neutrophils in the BM and PB (Figure 4.19A and B),[12] but there is no significant dysplasia in the other lineages.

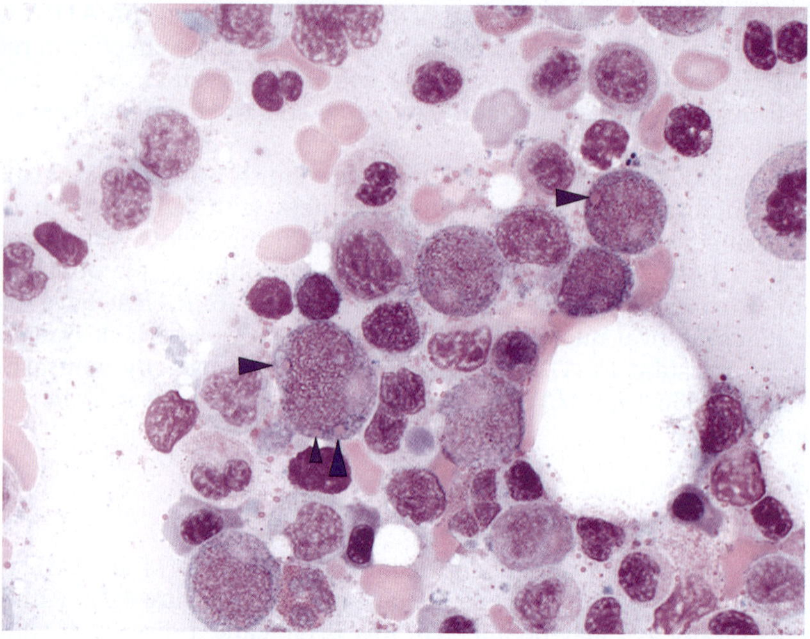

FIGURE 4.17 **This is an example of acute myeloid leukemia with t(8;21).** Leukemic cells show evidence of differentiation and often have distinct Golgi zones and azurophilic or salmon-colored granules (arrowheads). Blasts are not present in this field and will often be <20% of cells.

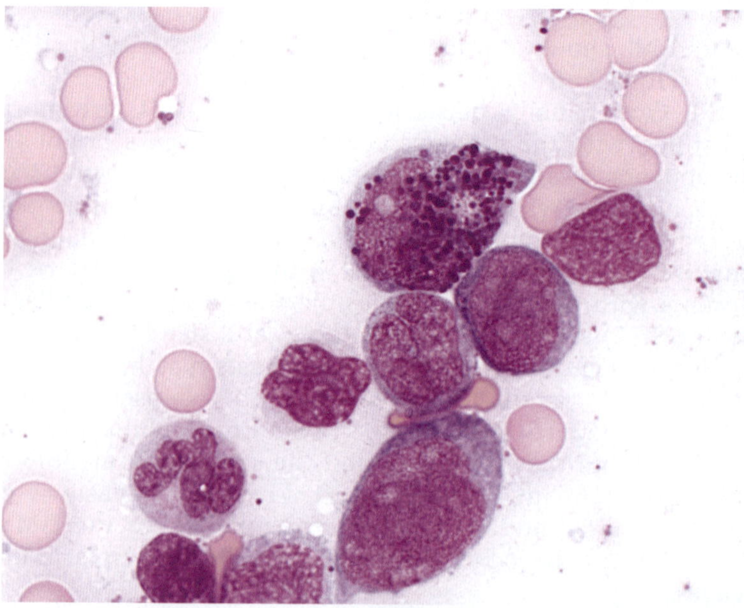

FIGURE 4.18 **Large coarse cytoplasmic granules, known as "pseudo-Chédiak-Higashi granules," are also sometimes seen in cases of acute myeloid leukemia with t(8;21).**

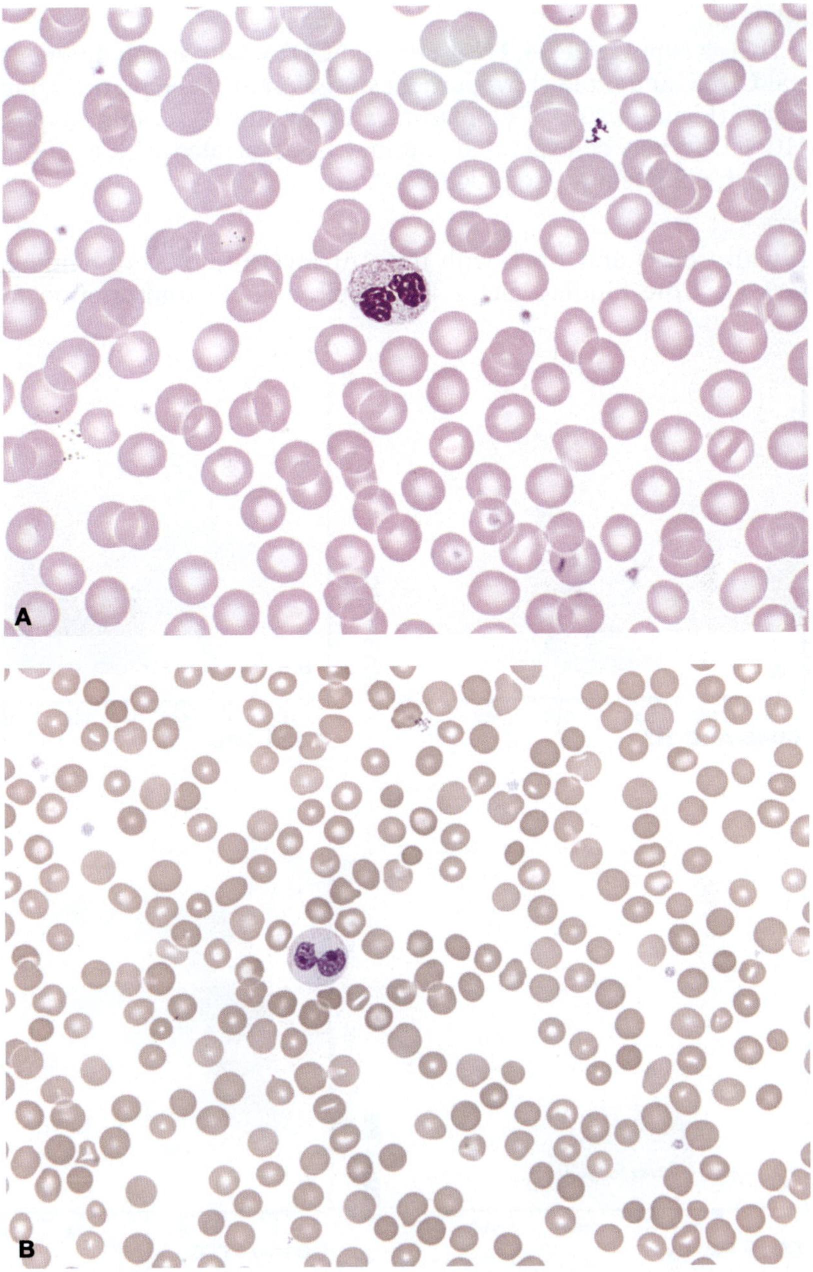

FIGURE 4.19 **Peripheral blood from a patient with acute myeloid leukemia with t(8;21) illustrating a dysplastic, bilobed neutrophil with abnormally clumped chromatin and prominent granules (A).** In some cases, the cytoplasm of the dysplastic neutrophils may be hypogranular (B).

Phenotype

By FC, blasts express CD34, HLA-DR, and CD13, with much dimmer than normal CD33, and often show partial expression of B cell markers, including CD19 (Figure 4.20).[13] Cytoplasmic CD79a and PAX5 may be positive by IHC. CD56 may be expressed and may be associated with a *KIT* mutation, which confers a worse prognosis.[14]

Genetics

AML with t(8;21) and AML with t(16;16)/inv(16) are "core binding factor" AMLs. Core binding factor is a heterodimeric transcription factor

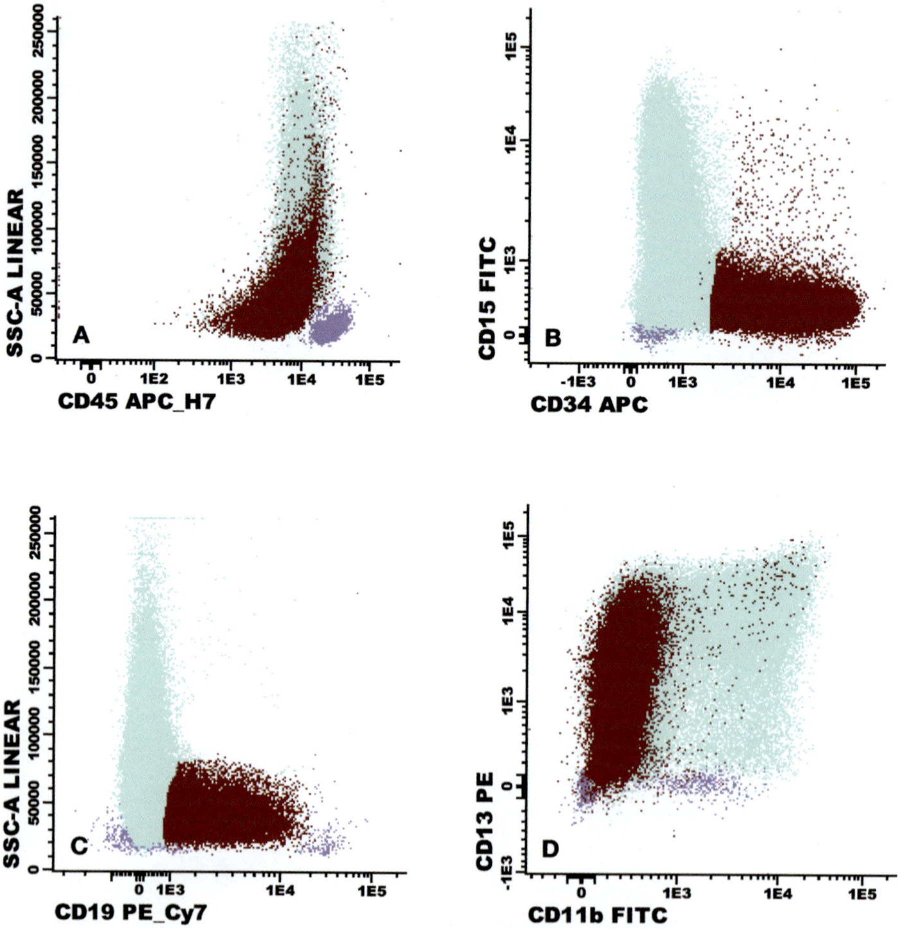

FIGURE 4.20 **On a CD45 versus side scatter (SSC) plot by flow cytometry, acute myeloid leukemia with t(8;21) will typically show a "vertical" pattern of myeloid maturation.** The lower SSC blasts (brown) will express CD34, often quite brightly, whereas the more differentiated granulocytes (light blue) will lack CD34 and express CD15 and CD11b. Blasts, but not the more mature cells, will characteristically show variable expression of CD19. Other markers present on the blasts include HLA-DR and CD13, whereas CD33 is typically dimly expressed.

composed of DNA-binding subunit CBFα and its partner, CBFβ. These subunits interact to form a transcriptionally active nuclear complex.[15]

CBFα is encoded by *RUNX1* and is important for hematopoietic differentiation and myeloid development. The *RUNX1T1* portion of the novel fusion gene that results from t(8;21) mediates the recruitment of repressors (including the histone deacetylase [HDAC] complex) to the *RUNX1* portion. This results in the blocking of *RUNX1* target genes, which prevents cell differentiation, increases cell survival, and ultimately promotes leukemogenesis.[15] The *RUNX1::RUNX1T1* fusion transcript may be detected in the PB or BM by FISH or reverse transcription (RT)-PCR and can be used to detect MRD.

Prognosis

Patients with t(8;21) usually have a good response to therapy, which is reflected in the favorable prognosis of this disease. Patients have high complete remission (CR) rate and long-term survival when treated with intensive chemotherapy.[16]

AML With t(16;16)(p13.1;q22), or inv(16)(p13.1q22)/ *CBFB::MYH11*

Epidemiology and Presentation

This comprises approximately 5% to 7% of all AMLs; it is relatively more common in children and young adults (eFigure 4.9).

Morphology

Blasts typically display myelomonocytic (FAB M4) features and may have cytoplasmic granules. Classically, this AML is known for having abundant abnormal eosinophils in the BM with both eosinophilic granules and large basophilic inclusions, earning these cells the moniker “eo-basos” (Figure 4.21). “Eo-basos” are not absolutely specific because they may be seen in some cases of myelodysplasia. In a subset of cases, abnormal eosinophils are scarce or absent, and the diagnosis can be made only with the detection of the genetic abnormality.

Phenotype

By FC, the blasts express CD34 and HLA-DR. They may express CD15 or other markers of granulocytic maturation, or show monocytic markers, CD4, CD11b, and CD64. CD2 is occasionally expressed on the monocytic cells.

Genetics

Like t(8;21), t(16;16)/inv(16) is a “core binding factor” AML. Rearrangements between *CBFB*, which encodes the β subunit of core binding factor, and *MYH11*, which encodes the smooth muscle myosin heavy chain, inhibits differentiation of hematopoietic cells. FISH and/or RT-PCR may be required to rule out this abnormality, as the karyotypic rearrangement can be difficult to detect. Additional mutations are common in this type of AML, with 70% of cases showing mutations in *NRAS*, *KRAS*, *KIT*, or *FLT3*.[17]

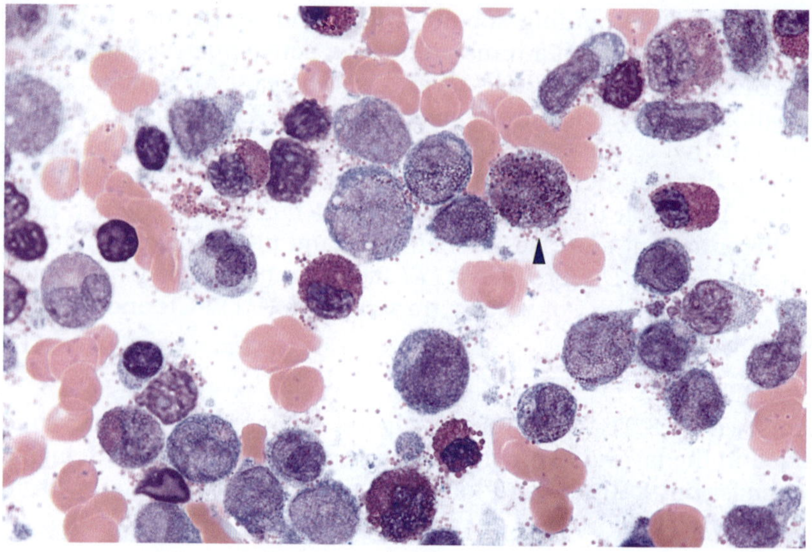

FIGURE 4.21 **Abnormal eosinophils with both eosinophilic granules and large basophilic inclusions, known colloquially as "eo-basos," are a characteristic feature of acute myeloid leukemia with t(16;16)/inv(16).** They are not absolutely specific, however, as they may be seen in some cases of myelodysplastic syndrome.

Prognosis

This leukemia is associated with a favorable prognosis unless it also harbors a *KIT* mutation. CR rates are high, especially when treated with multiple cycles of cytarabine. However, approximately 30% to 40% of patients will experience a relapse.

AML With t(9;11)(p21.3;q23.3)(*MLLT3::KMT2A*)

Epidemiology and Presentation

These cases are more common in pediatric than adult patients. Patients may present with extramedullary disease, especially gingival or soft tissue infiltrates, and DIC is not uncommon.

Morphology and Phenotype

Blasts typically have a monocytic morphology (Figure 4.22) and phenotype, with expression of CD14, CD4, CD11b, and CD64. Cases may lack CD34, particularly in children.

Genetics and Prognosis

KMT2A at 11q23 is a histone methyltransferase that assists in chromatin remodeling. It has >80 translocation partners that can produce AML, ALL, or mixed phenotype leukemias. Six recurrent alternative translocation partners (*AFF1*, *AFDN*, *MLLT10*, *TET2*, *ELL*, and *MLLT1*) are recognized in the ICC as AML-producing entities and are collectively designated as AML with other *KMT2A* rearrangements. In general, these have a prognosis that is

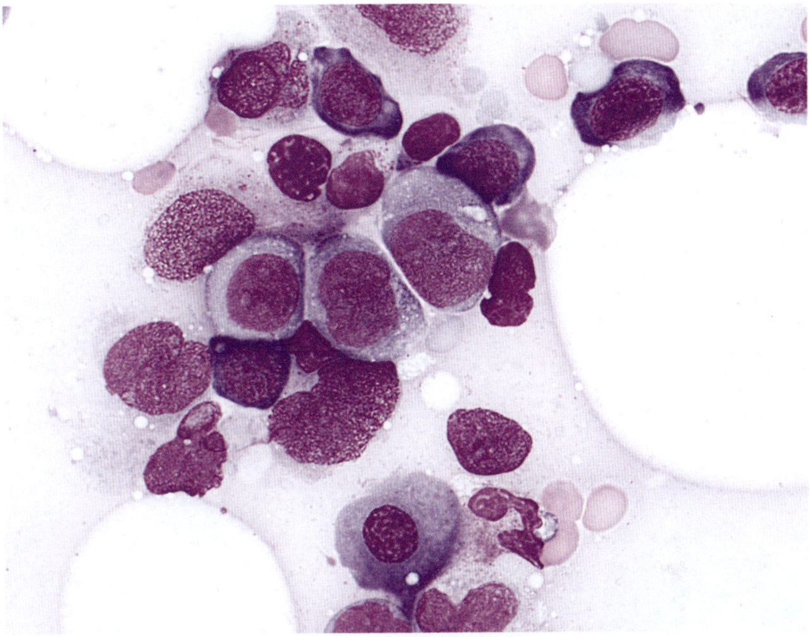

FIGURE 4.22 In this example of acute myeloid leukemia with t(9;11), the blasts have a monocytic appearance, with oval nuclei, and relatively abundant light blue cytoplasm.

not as good as the t(9;11), which involves *MLLT3*.[18] Secondary cytogenetic abnormalities, especially gain of chromosome 8, are common in this entity.

OTHER ENTITIES

- **AML with inv(3)(q21.3 q26.2) or t(3;3)(q21.3;q26.2)/*GATA2::MECOM*** (*EVI1*) (also known as AML with *MECOM* rearrangements in the WHO 5th edition) is rare, comprising 1.4% to 1.6% of AML. It is notable for characteristic atypical megakaryocytes (Figure 4.23A-C; eFigure 4.10). Platelets are typically preserved or may be increased and this AML is often associated with multilineage dysplasia; in such cases, genetic changes associated with MDS are often present. Pathogenesis involves activation of the *MECOM* gene at 3q26 because of translocation of a *GATA* enhancer. It is a very aggressive disease with CR rates of around 30% and a 5-year survival on the order of 5%. Rarely can there be an activating translocation involving *MECOM* that produces an AML with the identical characteristic morphology (eFigure 4.11).
- **AML with t(6;9)(p23;q34.1)(*DEK::NUP214*)** is also rare, accounting for 1% of AML cases, typically occurring in patients <35 years of age. Morphologically, the blasts are usually monocytic, but there is a frequent associated basophilia, and background dysplasia in any or all lineages, including ring sideroblasts. Prognosis is very poor, with median survival <1 year.

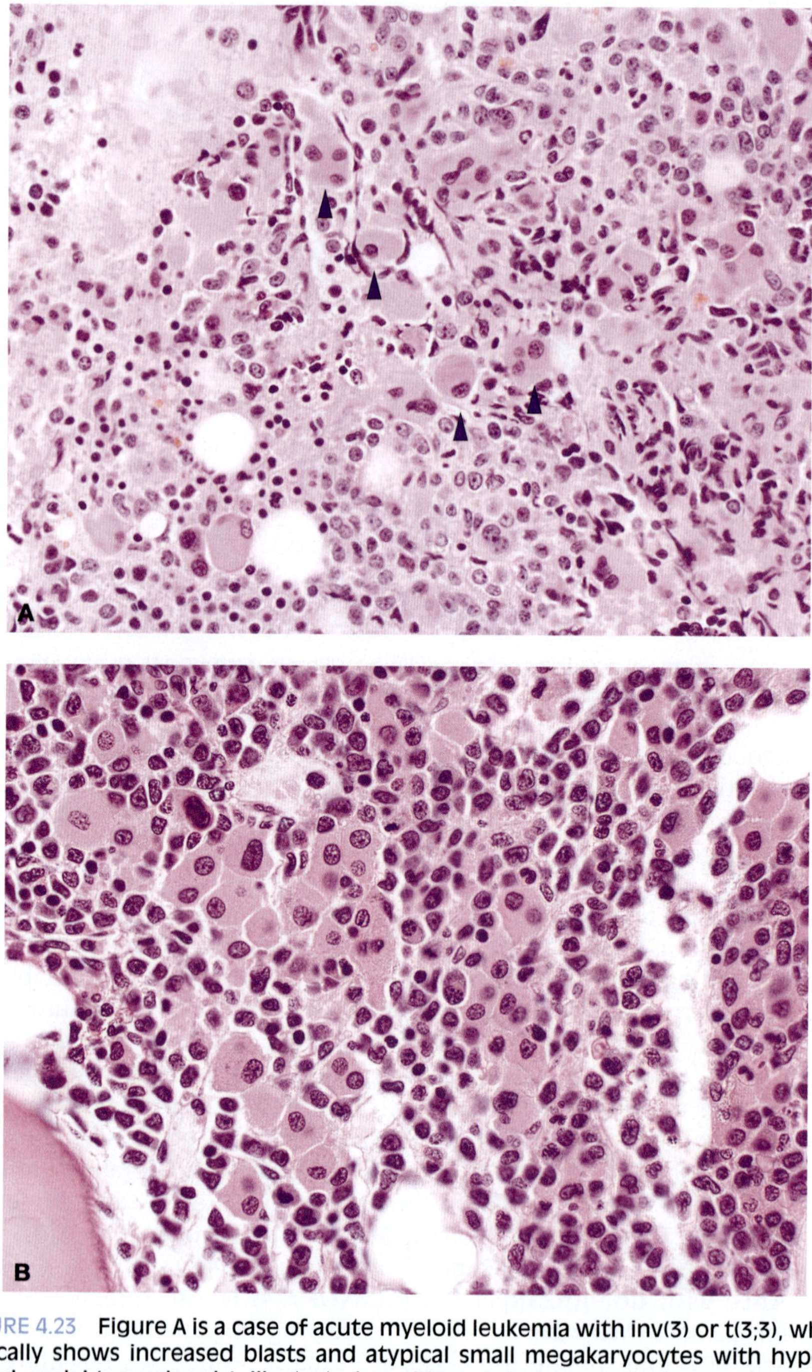

FIGURE 4.23 **Figure A is a case of acute myeloid leukemia with inv(3) or t(3;3), which typically shows increased blasts and atypical small megakaryocytes with hypolobated nuclei (arrowheads), illustrated on this core biopsy.** The leukemogenic mechanism involves dysregulation of *MECOM* and, less commonly, translocations of *MECOM* to other partner genes, which can produce a phenocopy of the leukemia with identical morphology (B, C).

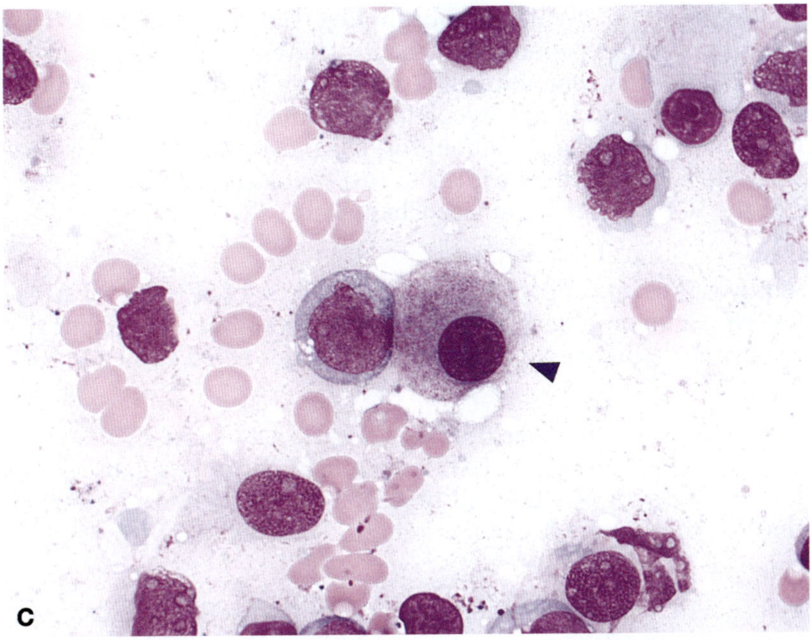

FIGURE 4.23 **(*continued*)** The aspirate in figure C shows a characteristic small monolobated megakaryocyte (arrowhead) adjacent to a myeloblast.

- **AML with *BCR::ABL1***: This AML diagnosis is difficult to distinguish from chronic myeloid leukemia (CML) in myeloid blast phase, which also harbors *BCR::ABL1*, and therefore it is essentially a diagnosis of exclusion. Blast counts ≥20% are required. Unlike CML, marrow cellularity is typically <100%, and basophilia is also less common. Some cases may have AML-associated gene mutations, such as FLT3-ITD, or NPM1 mutations, or deletion of IKZF1, which are not seen in blast phase CML. Prognosis is poor even with tyrosine kinase inhibitors.

The ICC also recognizes additional recurring translocations, discussion of which is outside the scope of this chapter. The WHO 5th edition recognizes all the entities mentioned earlier as well as a subset of the rare lesions in the ICC.

AML With MDS-Related Gene Mutations or Cytogenetic Abnormalities (AML, Myelodysplasia Related)

It has long been recognized that MDS has the propensity to transform to AML, but also that some patients presenting with acute leukemia have features in common with those patients with MDS. Although dysplastic morphology was previously required to recognize these cases, this presented difficulty for a number of reasons. For example, some AML cases with genetic lesions have dysplastic morphology, but lack the expected poor prognosis, and some patients with acute leukemia that belonged in this category had too few remaining differentiating cells to recognize dysplasia. This group of diseases is now recognized on the basis of either certain cytogenetic alterations or gene mutations. Diagnosis of AML in this category requires ≥20% blasts; cases with 10% to 19% blasts are now called MDS/AML in the ICC classification (see Chapter 5).

Epidemiology and Presentation

This entity represents approximately 25% to 35% of all cases of AML and most often occurs in elderly patients. There should be no evidence of the AML subtype–defining cytogenetic abnormalities listed earlier.

Morphology and Phenotype

Most cases show multilineage dysplasia (Figure 4.24A and B; eFigure 4.12). In cases evolving from MDS, CD34 may highlight only a subset of blasts. Aberrant expression of CD7 and/or CD56 is common, as is aberrant expression of other B and T cell markers (CD10, CD5, etc).

Genetics

The cytogenetic abnormalities and mutations that define this category can be found in Table 4.3.

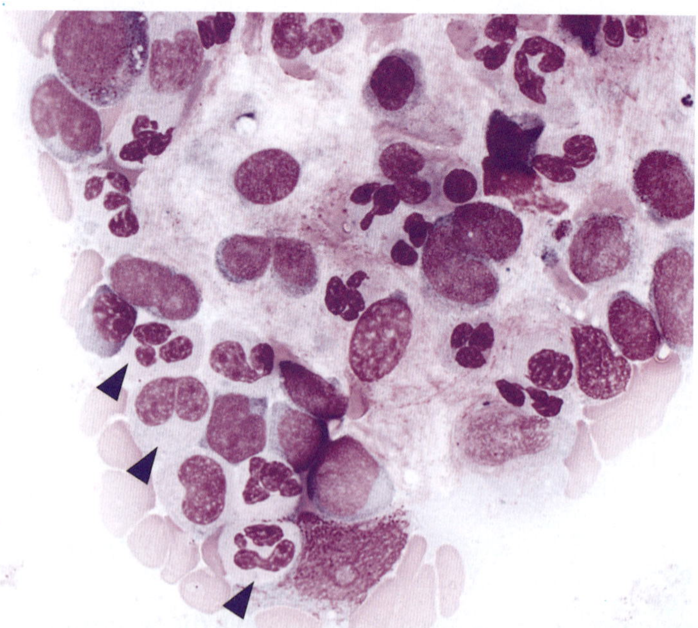

A

FIGURE 4.24 In addition to the increased blasts, acute myeloid leukemia with MDS-related gene mutations or cytogenetic abnormalities often show dysplastic morphologic features, including hypogranular myeloid cells (arrowheads; A) and small, hypolobated, atypical megakaryocytes (arrowheads; B).

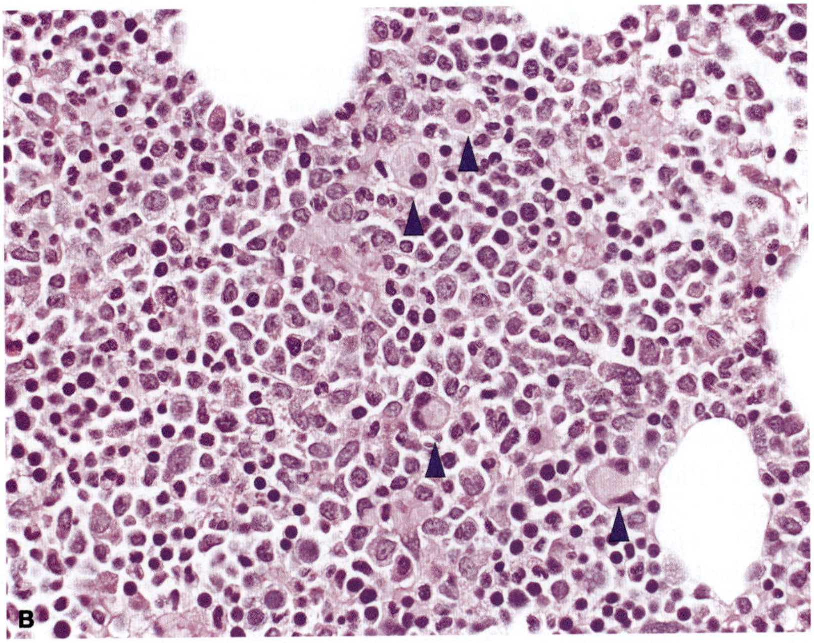

FIGURE 4.24 *(continued)*

PROGNOSIS

AML with any of the lesions mentioned earlier have a poor prognosis, and compared with AML-NOS, they have a worse overall survival.[19]

TABLE 4.3 AML with MDS-related gene mutations or cytogenetic abnormalities

Cytogenetic	Mutation
Complex (>3 clones) karyotype (in the absence of a *TP53* mutation)	*ASXL1*
del(5q)/t(5q)/add(5q)	*BCOR*
-7/del(7q)	*EZH2*
+8	*RUNX1*
del(12p)/t(12p)/add(12p)	*SF3B1*
i(17q)	*SRSF2*
-17/add(17p) or del(17p)	*STAG2*
del(20q)	*UA2F1*
idic(X)(q13)	*ZSR2*

AML, acute myeloid leukemia; MDS, myelodysplastic syndrome.

SUBTYPES OF AML WITH UNIQUE GENE MUTATIONS

There are three unique AML entities defined by mutations that have distinctive clinical characteristics and prognosis. Although these may also occasionally harbor the MDS-like morphologic changes, clinical behavior is defined by these mutations, supporting the idea of keeping such cases within the separately defined category. With the exception of AML with *TP53* mutations, a blast threshold of 10% is required by the ICC to make the diagnosis of AML in these cases; although the WHO 5th edition does not have a blast cutoff for AML with mutated *NPM1*, it still requires 20% blasts for AML with mutated *CEBPA*.

AML With Mutated *Nucleophosmin 1*

Epidemiology and Presentation

Mutation of the *NPM1* gene is one of the most common recurrent genetic alterations found in AML, present in 35% of cases of primary adult AML and in 50% to 60% of cases of cytogenetically normal (CN) AML.[20] Presentation is similar to other patients with AML, although some patients have preserved platelet counts.

Morphology

Blasts often show monocytic features both morphologically and phenotypically. Blasts may display a characteristic "cup-like" nuclear morphology (Figure 4.25; eFigure 4.13).

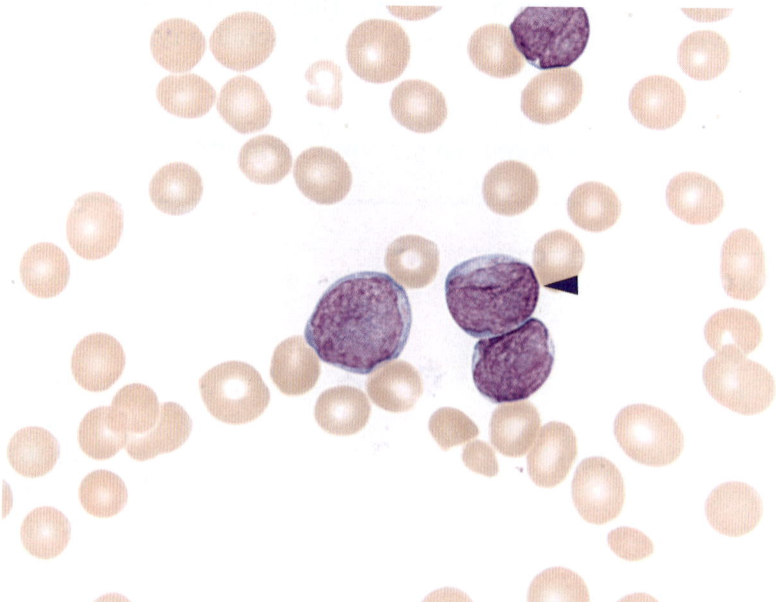

FIGURE 4.25 The blasts in acute myeloid leukemia with *NPM1* mutation often have nuclear invaginations, imparting what is sometimes called "cup-like" morphology (arrow heads).

Phenotype

The blasts in this subcategory of AML are often entirely or partially negative for CD34 (Figure 4.26), and if monocytic features are present, it is not possible to distinguish AML with *NPM1* mutation from other monocytic leukemias without genetic testing. The phenotype can also mimic the CD34 and HLA-DR-negative phenotype of APL, but *NPM1*-mutated AML cases have lower autofluorescence.

Genetics

The NPM1 protein acts as a nuclear-to-cytoplasmic shuttle for proteins and helps facilitate orderly mitosis.[21] An *NPM1* mutation represents a late event in leukemogenesis, frequently secondary to mutations in epigenetic modifiers such as *DNMT3A*, *TET2*, *IDH1*, and *IDH2*, but usually preceding any *FTL3* mutations.

Prognosis

NPM1 mutations vary in prognosis based on whether there is an accompanying *FLT3-ITD* mutation and differ based on patient age; elderly patients have better prognosis with *NPM1* without *FLT3-ITD* than younger patients.[22]

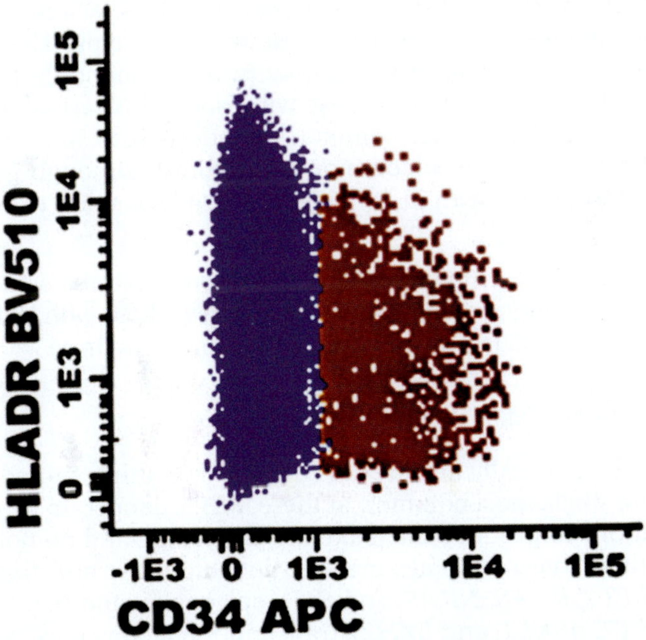

FIGURE 4.26 **By flow cytometry, the blasts in acute myeloid leukemia with *NPM1* mutation will either be CD34 negative or have a small subset expressing CD34 (brown, compared to the major population in blue).** HLA-DR is similarly also either negative or variable, as shown here, and can thus sometimes be confused immunophenotypically with acute promyelocytic leukemia with *PML-RARA*.

AML With In-Frame bZIP *CEBPA* Mutations

Mutations in the *CEBPA* gene are relatively common in AML, but those patients who had a biallelic *CEBPA* mutation were recognized to have an excellent prognosis. More recently, it was recognized that it is not the presence of a biallelic mutation but rather the particular type of mutation that confers the excellent prognosis (see later).[23]

Epidemiology and Presentation

AML with in-frame basic leucine zipper (bZIP) *CEBPA* mutations represents 4% to 9% of childhood/young adult AML.

Morphology and Phenotype

Although blasts may appear monocytic, by FC, the blast immunophenotype often shows both granulocytic maturation markers in addition to blastic markers, including expression of CD34, CD117, CD33, and CD13; monocytic markers are usually absent.

Genetics

CEBPA encodes a transcription factor that is essential for granulocytic maturation.[24] Mutations occur in either the N-terminal or C-terminal region, the latter involving the bZIP region; leukemias with biallelic mutations have both. However, patients with biallelic mutations and those with only bZIP mutations have similar characteristics, whereas those with N-terminal mutations are similar to those with wild type. The former are younger, present with higher white counts, and commonly have associated *GATA2* mutations, whereas those with isolated N-terminal mutations are more likely to have other common mutations seen in AML. Isolated N-terminal mutations are uncommon in children, although germline N-terminal mutations are seen in patients with predisposition to AML.

Prognosis

Patients with AML with in-frame bZIP mutations have the same favorable prognosis whether monoallelic or biallelic, whereas those with isolated N-terminal mutations have a less favorable outcome, similar to those with wild type.

OTHER GENE MUTATIONS IN AML

As noted earlier, virtually all cases of AML have multiple mutations. Most, including the single most common of these, *FLT3*, cooperate with other genetic alterations to produce the leukemic phenotype and do not represent distinct entities. Types of genes involved include those affecting signaling pathways (*FLT3*, *KRAS*, *NRAS*, and *KIT*), epigenetic modifiers (*DNMT3A*, *IDH1/2*, *TET2*, *ASXL1*, and *EZH2*), transcription factors (*GATA2*, *CEBPA*, and *RUNX1*), or tumor suppressors (*TP53* and *WT1*). Some of these genes define cases of AML with MDS-related genetic lesions, discussed earlier, and others, as discussed later, define unique entities in and of themselves. Others, including *FLT3-ITD* and *KIT*, confer adverse prognosis in whichever entity they are found, whereas still others (*IDH1/2*) may be specifically targeted with small molecule biologics.

Germline mutations in an increasingly large number of genes have been shown to be associated with an increased risk of developing AML, and when AML arises in such situations the ICC recommends adding the qualifier "germline predisposition" to the diagnosis. Although a detailed discussion of all of these is outside the scope of this chapter, AML associated with Down syndrome is common enough that it is discussed in some detail below.

MYELOID NEOPLASMS ASSOCIATED WITH DOWN SYNDROME

Myeloid proliferations associated with Down syndrome (trisomy 21) fall into two general categories: transient abnormal myelopoiesis (TAM) and myeloid leukemia associated with Down syndrome (MLADS).[2]

Transient Abnormal Myelopoiesis

Transient abnormal myelopoiesis, which may be present at birth, resembles AML, with increased blasts in the PB or BM, although it is typically more heterogeneous. Blasts often have a megakaryocytic phenotype (Figure 4.27; eFigure 4.14). Unlike normal AML, this phenomenon typically spontaneously resolves within 1 to 2 months. However, 20% to 30% of patients with TAM may develop non-remitting acute megakaryoblastic leukemia within 1 to 3 years.

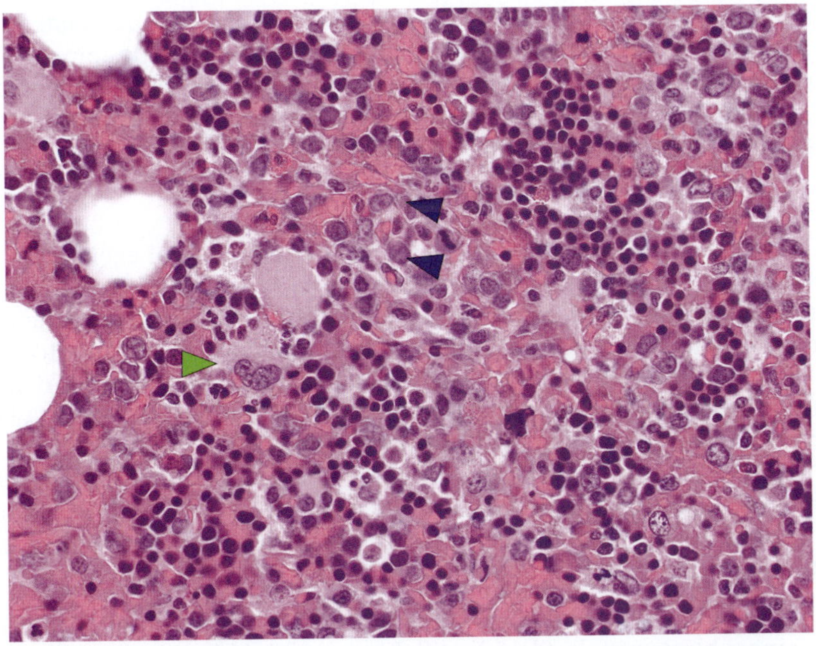

FIGURE 4.27 Bone marrow core biopsy from an infant with transient abnormal myelopoiesis, showing a panmyelosis with increased blasts and immature myeloid cells (blue arrowheads) and small atypical megakaryocytes (green arrowhead) along with numerous clusters of erythroid precursors.

Myeloid Leukemia Associated With Down Syndrome

Myeloid leukemia associated with Down syndrome (MLADS) usually presents in patients with Down syndrome <5 years of age following an MDS-like phase. In MLADS, a specific blast count is not required for the diagnosis, and thus there is no subclassification of MLADS into MDS versus AML. Like TAM, MLADS has a megakaryoblastic morphology and immunophenotype.

GATA1 mutations are associated with both disorders. GATA1 is part of a family of proteins with zinc finger domains that bind DNA at certain sequences and act as either activators or repressors of transcription factors that affect erythroid and megakaryocytic maturation.[2,25]

AML Following Chemotherapy

Although previously such cases were classified together with MDS or myeloproliferative neoplasms (MPNs) that occurred following therapy under the term "therapy-related myeloid neoplasms," the ICC now recommends subclassifying cases of AML as usual and to append the term "therapy-related" as a diagnostic qualifier. Of note, the types of AML most likely to occur following therapy are those with MDS-related genetic lesions, including *TP53* mutations, and those with *KMT2A* translocations. The former occur most often following alkylating agent therapy or ionizing radiation, usually with a latency of 5 to 7 years, and often follow a period of MDS.

Cases without features of MDS occur with much shorter latency, sometimes as short as a year, and present abruptly. They are associated with intercalating agents such as adriamycin and especially with epipodophyllotoxins. These agents may also occasionally give rise to therapy-related APL with *PML::RARA*. Therapy-related leukemias tend to have a worse prognosis than the equivalent *de novo* AML.

AML Not Otherwise Specified

AML not otherwise specified (AML-NOS) is a diagnosis of exclusion, only after cytogenetic and molecular studies fail to reveal specific cytogenetic or molecular alterations, either acquired or congenital. In spite of the large number of subcategories, AML-NOS is still relatively common. However, the term should preferably not be used as a placeholder in a report while awaiting genetic information, but rather simply call those cases "AML," with a note reserving the need for more information.

Although there is generally no clinical significance to subclassifying AML-NOS based on the degree and type of lineage differentiation, this is often still done for historical reasons. The most common types of the antiquated FAB classification include the following:

AML without maturation (M0) has <10% mature granulocytes and most blasts may not be identifiable as myeloid in the absence of special stains or FC.

AML with maturation (M1 and M2) includes blasts with and without identifiable granules and may show more maturation, but monoblasts and promonocytes account for <20% of cells. It should be noted that because FC has supplanted cytochemistry in most institutions, distinguishing between M1 and M0 may be moot.

Acute myelomonocytic leukemia (M4) contains both myeloblasts and monoblast equivalents to at least 20% in the BM, but monoblasts are <80%; blood may not be reliable because monocytic cells preferentially circulate and may be the dominant cell. By FC separate populations are typically seen, one with granulocytic and the other with monocytic markers.

Acute monocytic leukemia (M5) requires 80% or more of the blasts to be monoblasts or equivalent. Some cases may contain a relatively homogeneous population of monoblasts, whereas others are more heterogeneous with varying degrees of monocytic maturation present. In contrast to most other AMLs, CD34 is often negative and monocytic antigens including bright CD64, CD11c, and CD36 are positive. CD33 is also typically very bright. The more mature monocyte marker CD14 is often negative but may be partly expressed in cases in which there is more maturation, and because blood often contains more mature differentiated monocytic cells, distinction from chronic myelomonocytic leukemia (CMML) may be difficult; morphologic assessment of the BM is critical in such cases.

Acute erythroid leukemia (M6) (Figure 4.28A-D; eFigure 4.15) typically will have *TP53* mutations and is not included as a separate subtype of AML in the ICC, although the term is retained in the WHO 5th edition. Similarly, most cases of acute megakaryocytic leukemia (M7) will either have a defined translocation, particularly in pediatrics, or evolve as a blast phase from another myeloid neoplasm or have other genetic changes that allow classification in another category.

Acute basophilic leukemia is exceptionally rare and can be recognized morphologically by the presence of immature basophils (Figure 4.29A and B; eFigure 4.16), although these may only be a subset of the blasts. Mature basophils have a characteristic phenotype of bright CD123 and CD117 without HLA-DR, although the latter may be expressed in some cases, causing confusion with plasmacytoid dendritic cells. Acute eosinophilic leukemia or acute leukemias of myeloid dendritic cells also exist but are so rare as to not have formal diagnostic criteria.

Acute panmyelosis with fibrosis this is the rarest type of AML-NOS. Patients present with cytopenias, fever, and bone pain and are typically quite sick. Despite abundant fibrosis in the marrow, the PB smear does not show many tear-drop red blood cells (RBCs), most likely because of the acute nature of the disease.

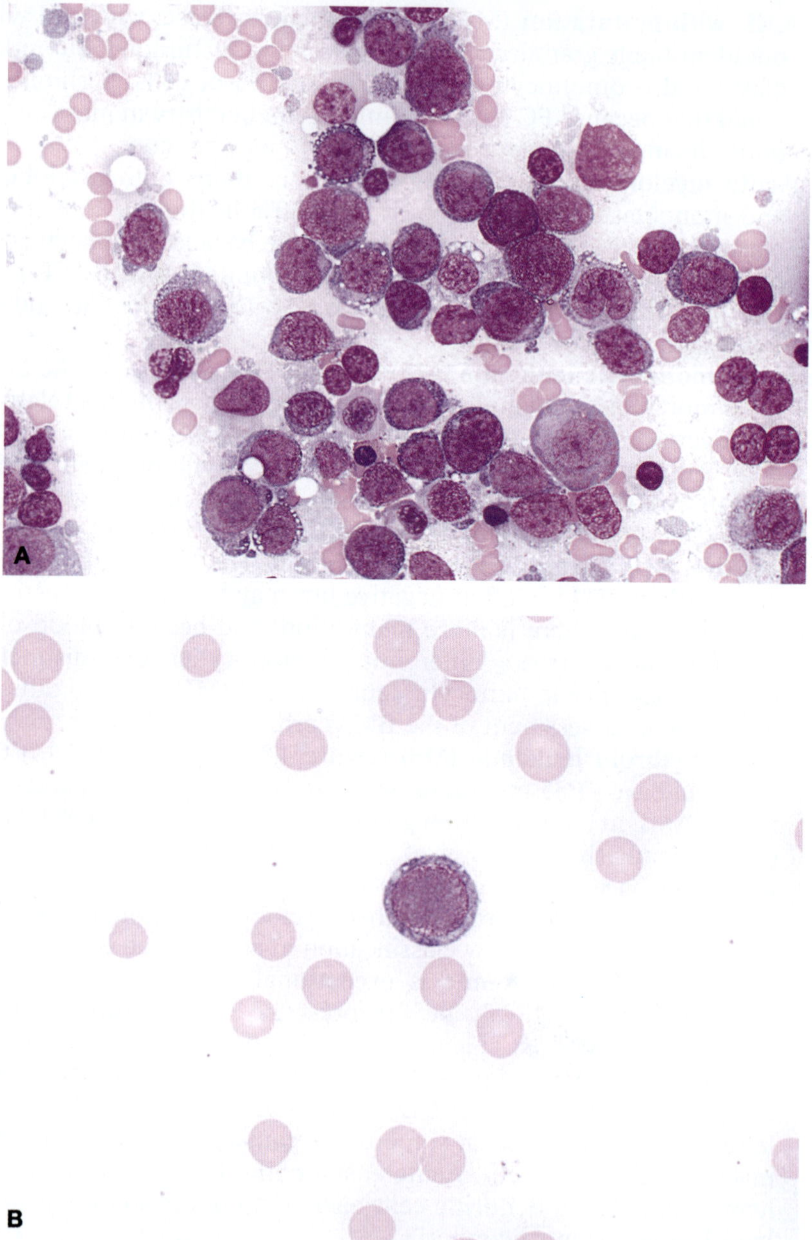

FIGURE 4.28 **Bone marrow aspirate from a patient with acute erythroid leukemia showing abundant erythroid blasts with dark blue cytoplasm and limited maturation, which can appear megaloblastic (A).** The blasts may also be seen in the peripheral blood (B). On the core biopsy, erythroblasts may be indistinguishable from other myeloid blasts (C), and immunophenotyping, in this case with E-cadherin(D), is essential to recognize these. This case was classified as acute erythroid leukemia because cytogenetic and molecular information was not available.

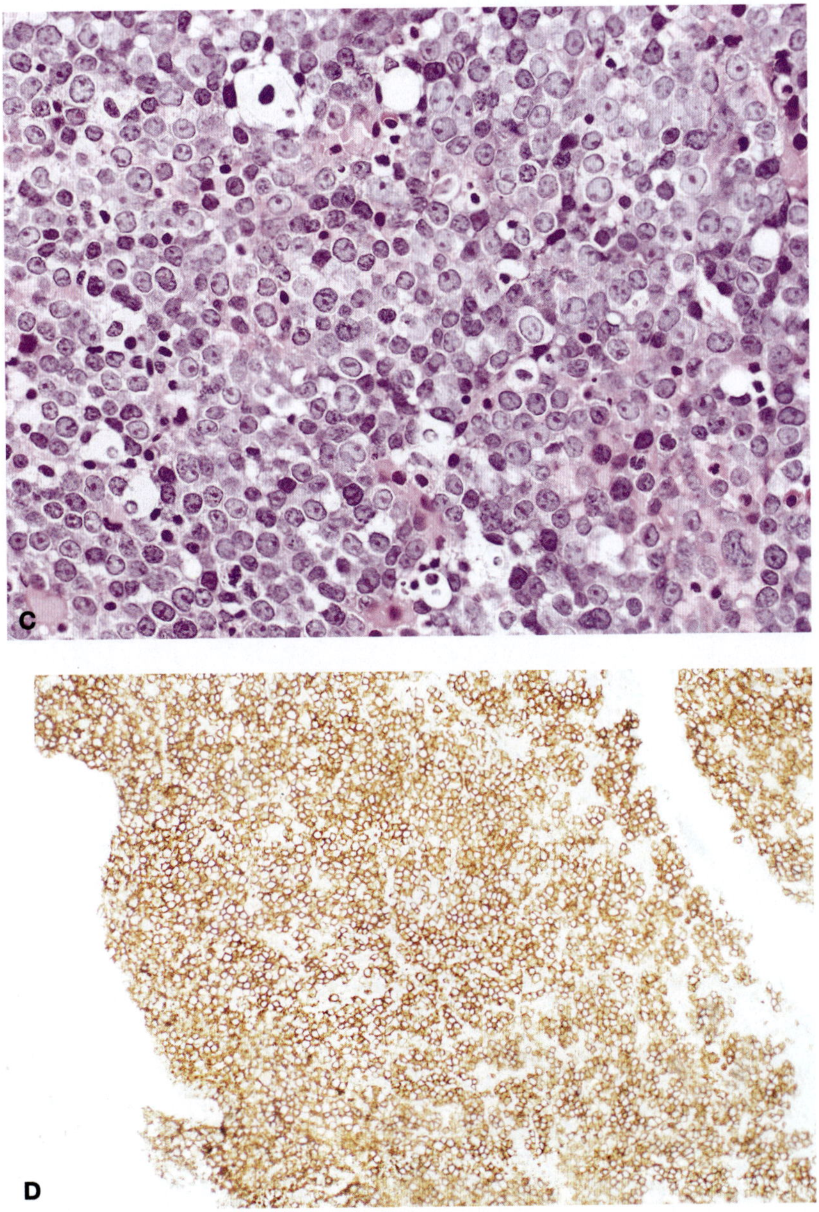

FIGURE 4.28 *(continued)*

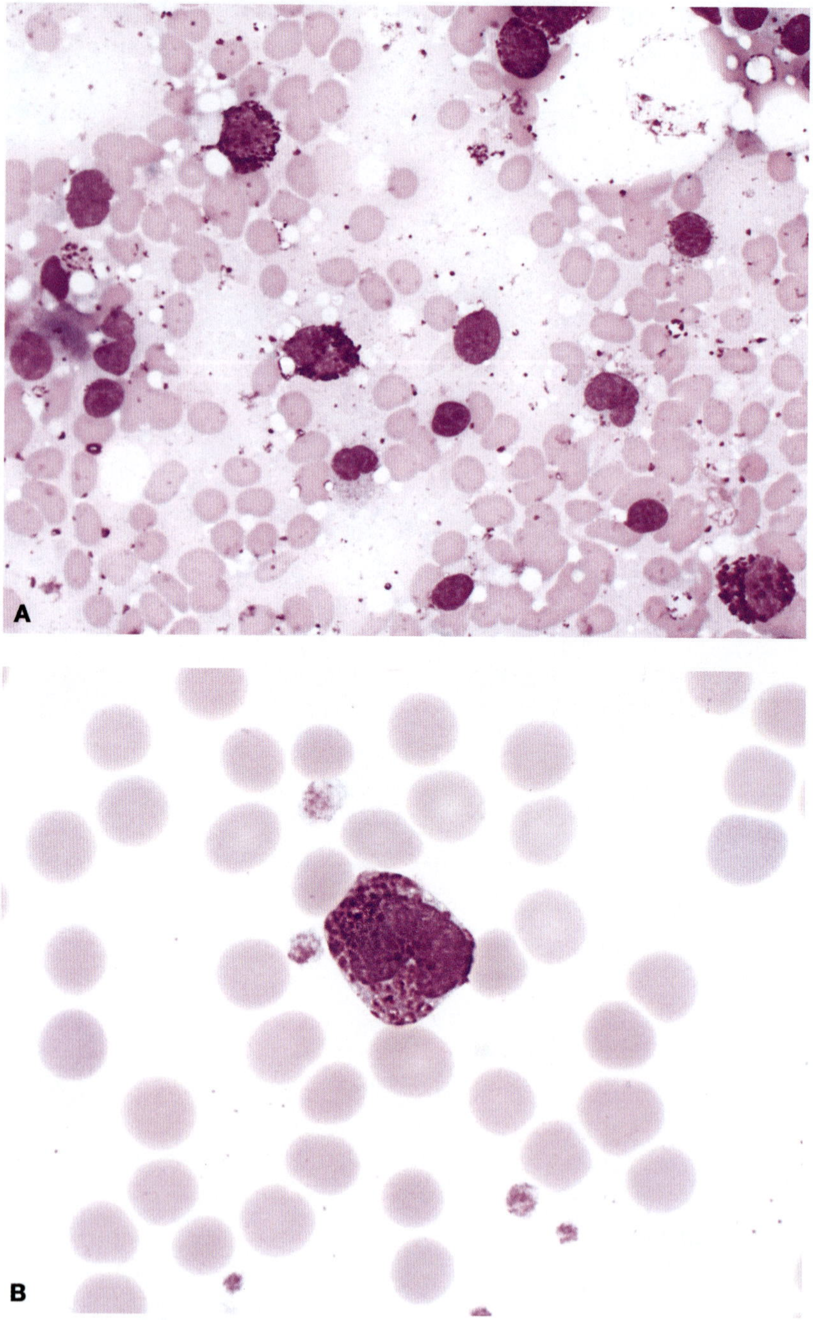

FIGURE 4.29 **A case of the very rare acute basophilic leukemia.** Although there are several naked nuclei, there are also intact blasts with abnormal basophilic granules (A). There may also be circulating immature basophils (B).

This is a unique disease, with the BM biopsy showing panmyelosis (increase in all three hematopoietic lineages), as well as abnormal megakaryocytic morphology with a markedly fibrotic marrow (Figure 4.30A-D; eFigure 4.17). This fibrosis is acute, presenting in patients without a history

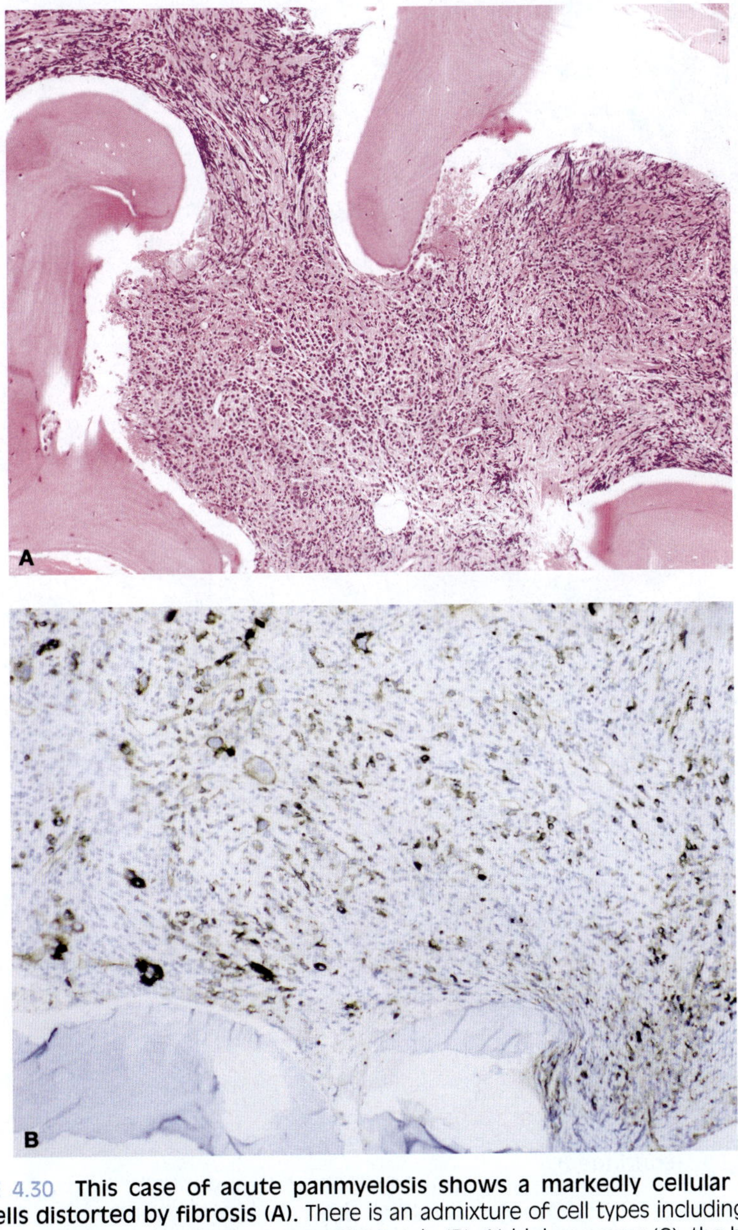

FIGURE 4.30 **This case of acute panmyelosis shows a markedly cellular marrow with cells distorted by fibrosis (A).** There is an admixture of cell types including numerous immature blast forms, best seen on CD34 stain (B). At higher power (C), the blasts can appear crushed and are admixed with atypical, large megakaryocytes with hyperchromatic nuclei. A reticulin stain shows a marked increase in reticulin fibrosis (D).

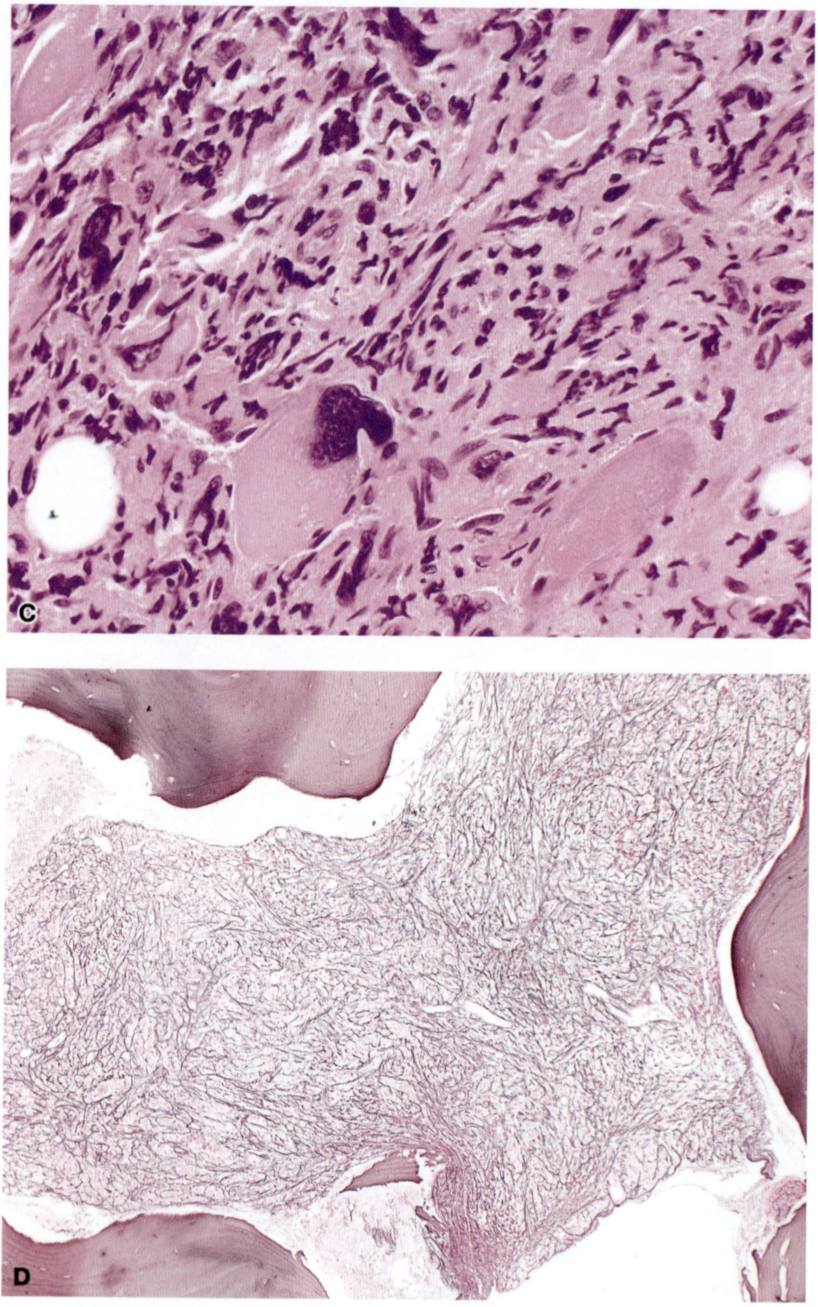

FIGURE 4.30 *(continued)*

of an antecedent MPN. The fibrosis is overtly present on hematoxylin and eosin (H&E) but is exemplified by a reticulin stain. There is usually no prominent collagen fibrosis and unlike most patients with MPN, splenomegaly is typically absent.

Diagnosis requires ≥20% blasts in the BM. However, because of the abundant associated fibrosis, the aspirate is often a dry tap, and blasts must be identified by IHC stains, generally CD34, although CD61 may sometimes help identify megakaryoblasts. CD117 and other myeloid markers are also often present on the blasts but because these markers are not blast specific they are not useful for enumeration.

The differential diagnosis includes metastatic carcinoma with a desmoplastic reaction, an MPN with fibrosis, and AML/MDS. The prognosis is poor, and patients typically have a short survival.

Posttreatment BM and MRD

AML patients are treated with cytotoxic chemotherapy regimens based on clinical protocols. Serial BM examinations are performed to assess therapy response and to glean prognostic information.[7] The morphologic spectrum of the BM depends on the time of assessment and on certain patient characteristics, including age and other factors.

Two main morphologic processes occur following myeloablative therapy:

Cellular death: This process occurs immediately and continues throughout the administration of chemotherapy. The BM appears markedly hypocellular with cellular necrosis. The marrow cellularity is comprised of adipose tissue, stromal cells, rare lymphocytes, plasma cells, and scattered macrophages.[26] Stromal and cellular damage results in the accumulation of a fibrinoid eosinophilic substance (Figure 4.31A and B; eFigure 4.18).

Reconstitution: BM reconstitution occurs several weeks after therapy (eFigure 4.19). During this phase, the BM repopulates starting with erythroid and myeloid progenitors, followed by megakaryocytic progenitors (Figure 4.32).[27] This process may be disorderly, with some accumulation of immature myeloid precursors in a non-paratrabecular distribution. There may also be a marked erythroid hyperplasia, which can lead to mild dyserythropoiesis, which is considered normal in these circumstances.

A unique phenomenon known as therapy-induced leukemic maturation may occur, especially in patients with APL treated with ATRA, wherein the abnormal leukemic clone shows morphologic maturation: The promyelocytes may appear to be maturing into myelocytes and mature granulocytes, but these cells still harbor the t(15;17) and represent residual disease.[28] Conversely, regenerating normal promyelocytes may proliferate after chemotherapy, thus mimicking persistent disease. In addition, other

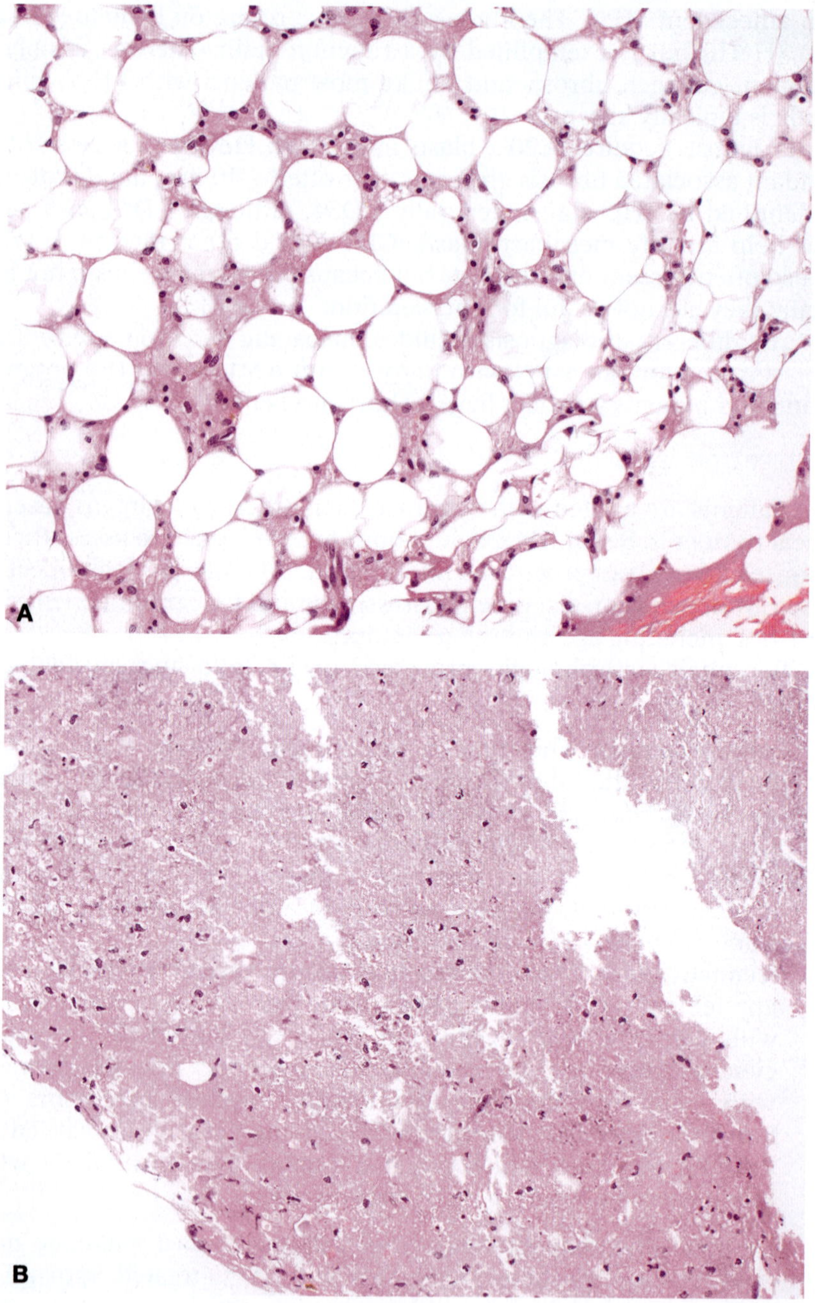

FIGURE 4.31 **A bone marrow following chemotherapy is typically hypocellular with interstitial edema.** Cellular elements are mostly only stromal cells, lymphocytes, and plasma cells, whereas hematopoietic cells are rare (A). In some cases, as in this example, there is also focal fibrinoid necrosis (B).

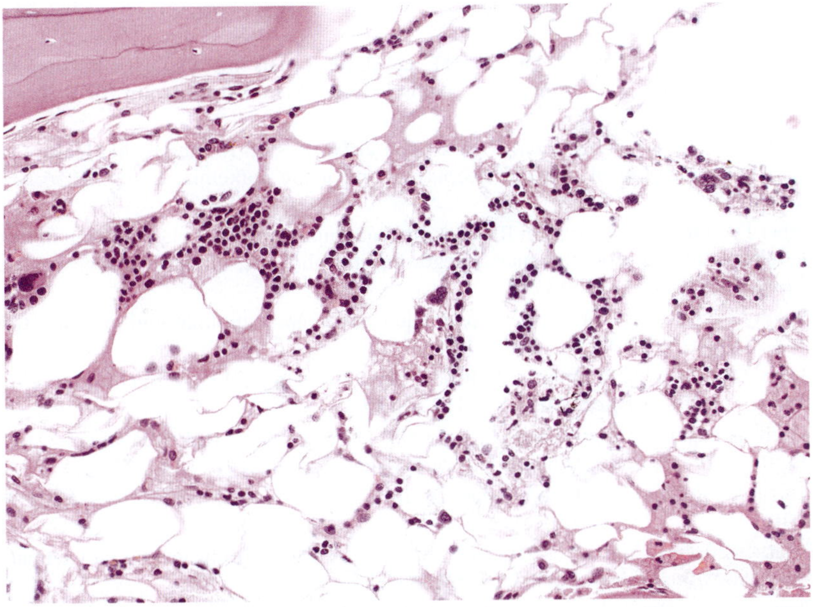

FIGURE 4.32 **Bone marrow showing regeneration following chemotherapy.** Most of the cells here are erythroid cells, as they are usually the first lineage to reconstitute.

biologics, like IDH inhibitors, may produce unusual morphologic changes, including a delayed blast clearance and evidence of leukemia cell differentiation,[29] as well as unusual morphologic and immunophenotypic populations not seen at diagnosis.[30]

Minimal residual disease (MRD) in AML can be detected either by FC or by molecular techniques, although generally speaking, these approaches are more complex than in ALL. The former approaches have utilized detection of so-called leukemia-associated immunophenotypes (LAIPs),[31] although because leukemic phenotypes may change with therapy, others have used a "different from normal" approach.[32] In either case, extensive study of regenerating and other nonneoplastic marrows is required because some of the markers considered "aberrant" can also be expressed on regenerating or other reactive myeloid populations.

A variety of molecular methods can also be used. AML with translocations, particularly *PML::RARA*, is the most straightforward and clearly clinically relevant, although others have been used as well. Gene mutations have also been used as MRD markers, although certain genes mutated in clonal hematopoiesis of indeterminate potential (CHIP) are typically avoided as markers of MRD as interpretation of a low-level positive can be misleading (See Chapter 5). The most well-established MRD methods for detecting mutated genes are for *NPM1*-mutated AML.

REFERENCES

1. Bennett JM, Catovsky D, Daniel MT, et al. Proposals for the classification of the acute leukaemias. French-American-British (FAB) co-operative group. *Br J Haematol.* 1976;33(4):451-458.
2. Arber DA, Orazi A, Hasserjian R, et al. The 2016 revision to the World Health Organization classification of myeloid neoplasms and acute leukemia. *Blood.* 2016;127(20):2391-2405.
3. Arber DA, Orazi A, Hasserjian RP, et al. International consensus classification of myeloid neoplasms and acute leukemias: integrating morphologic, clinical, and genomic data. *Blood.* 2022;140(11):1200-1228.
4. Deschler B, Lübbert M. Acute myeloid leukemia: epidemiology and etiology. *Cancer.* 2006;107(9):2099-2107.
5. Belson M, Kingsley B, Holmes A. Risk factors for acute leukemia in children: a review. *Environ Health Perspect.* 2007;115(1):138-145.
6. Leone G, Pagano L, Ben-Yehuda D, Voso MT. Therapy-related leukemia and myelodysplasia: susceptibility and incidence. *Haematologica.* 2007;92(10):1389-1398.
7. Foucar K, Reichard K, Czuchlewski D. *Bone Marrow Pathology.* 3rd ed. ASCP Press; 2010.
8. Paietta E. Expression of cell-surface antigens in acute promyelocytic leukaemia. *Best Pract Res Clin Haematol.* 2003;16:369-385.
9. Grimwade D, Howe K, Langabeer S, et al. Establishing the presence of the t(15;17) in suspected acute promyelocytic leukaemia: cytogenetic, molecular and PML immunofluorescence assessment of patients entered into the M.R.C. ATRA trial. M.R.C. Adult Leukaemia Working Party. *Br J Haematol.* 1996;94(3):557-573.
10. Grimwade D, Biondi A, Mozziconacci M-JL, et al. Characterization of acute promyelocytic leukemia cases lacking the classic t(15;17): results of the European Working Party. *Blood.* 2000;96(4):1297-1308.
11. Wang ZY, Chen Z. Acute promyelocytic leukemia: from highly fatal to highly curable. *Blood.* 2008;111(5):2505-2515.
12. Nakamura H, Kuriyama K, Sadamori N, et al. Morphological subtyping of acute myeloid leukemia with maturation (AML-M2): homogeneous pink-colored cytoplasm of mature neutrophils is most characteristic of AML-M2 with t(8;21). *Leukemia.* 1997;11(5):651-655.
13. Kita K, Nakase K, Miwa H, et al. Phenotypical characteristics of acute myelocytic leukemia associated with the t(8;21)(q22;q22) chromosomal abnormality: frequent expression of immature B-cell antigen CD19 together with stem cell antigen CD34. *Blood.* 1992;80(2):470-477.
14. De J, Zanjani R, Hibbard M, Davis BH. Immunophenotypic profile predictive of KIT activating mutations in AML1-ETO leukemia. *Am J Clin Pathol.* 2007;128(4):550-557.
15. Al-Harbi S, Aljurf M, Mohty M, Almohareb F, Ahmed SOA. An update on the molecular pathogenesis and potential therapeutic targeting of AML with t(8;21)(q22;q22.1);RUNX1-RUNX1T1. *Blood Adv.* 2020;4(1):229-238.
16. Marcucci G, Mrózek K, Ruppert AS, et al. Prognostic factors and outcome of core binding factor acute myeloid leukemia patients with t(8;21) differ from those of patients with inv(16): a Cancer and Leukemia Group B study. *J Clin Oncol.* 2005;23(24):5705-5717.
17. Boissel N, Leroy H, Brethon B, et al. Incidence and prognostic impact of c-Kit, FLT3, and *Ras* gene mutations in core binding factor acute myeloid leukemia (CBF-AML). *Leukemia.* 2006;20(6):965-970.
18. Balgobind BV, Raimondi SC, Harbott J, et al. Novel prognostic subgroups in childhood 11q23/MLL-rearranged acute myeloid leukemia: results of an international retrospective study. *Blood.* 2009;114(12):2489-2496.

19. Weinberg OK, Seetharam M, Ren L, et al. Clinical characterization of acute myeloid leukemia with myelodysplasia-related changes as defined by the 2008 WHO classification system. *Blood.* 2009;113(9):1906-1908.
20. Falini B, Mecucci C, Tiacci E, et al. Cytoplasmic nucleophosmin in acute myelogenous leukemia with a normal karyotype. *N Engl J Med.* 2005;352(3):254-266.
21. Falini B, Nicoletti I, Martelli MF, Mecucci C. Acute myeloid leukemia carrying cytoplasmic/mutated nucleophosmin (NPMc+ AML): biologic and clinical features. *Blood.* 2007;109(3):874-885.
22. Juliusson G, Jädersten M, Deneberg S, et al. The prognostic impact of FLT3-ITD and NPM1 mutation in adult AML is age-dependent in the population-based setting. *Blood Adv.* 2020;4(6):10941101.
23. Tarlock K, Lamble AJ, Wang Y-C, et al. CEBPA-bZip mutations are associated with favorable prognosis in de novo AML: a report from the Children's Oncology Group. *Blood.* 2021;138(13):11371147.
24. Koschmieder S, Halmos B, Levantini E, Tenen DG. Dysregulation of the C/EBPα differentiation pathway in human cancer. *J Clin Oncol.* 2009;27(4):619-628.
25. Xavier AC, Ge Y, Taub JW. Down syndrome and malignancies: a unique clinical relationship: a paper from the 2008 William Beaumont hospital symposium on molecular pathology. *J Mol Diagn.* 2009;11(5):371-380.
26. Dick FR, Burns CP, Weiner GJ, Heckman KD. Bone marrow morphology during induction phase of therapy for acute myeloid leukemia (AML). *Hematol Pathol.* 1995;9(2): 95-106.
27. Wittels B. Bone marrow biopsy changes following chemotherapy for acute leukemia. *Am J Surg Pathol.* 1980;4(2):135-142.
28. Petrie K, Zelent A, Waxman S. Differentiation therapy of acute myeloid leukemia: past, present and future. *Curr Opin Hematol.* 2009;16(2):84-91.
29. Mason EF, Pozdnyakova O, Roshal M, et al. Bone marrow morphologic findings in patients receiving IDH inhibitor therapy in combination with intensive induction chemotherapy: challenges with interpretation of the day 14 bone marrow biopsy. *Blood.* 2019;134(Supplement_1):1442.
30. Hagiya A, Vaidya P, Khedro T, Yaghmour B, Siddiqi I, Yaghmour G. Bone marrow features in patients with acute myeloid leukemia treated with novel targeted isocitrate dehydrogenase 1/2 inhibitors. *World J Oncol.* 2019;10(6):226-230.
31. Zeijlemaker W, Kelder A, Cloos J, Schuurhuis GJ. Immunophenotypic detection of measurable residual (stem cell) disease using LAIP approach in acute myeloid leukemia. *Curr Protoc Cytom.* 2019;91(1):e66.
32. Wood BL. Acute myeloid leukemia minimal residual disease detection: the difference from normal approach. *Curr Protoc Cytom.* 2020;93(1):e73.

5

MYELODYSPLASTIC SYNDROME (MDS) AND MYELODYSPLASTIC SYNDROME/MYELOPROLIFERATIVE NEOPLASM (MDS/MPN)

In this chapter, we discuss myelodysplastic syndrome (MDS), a clonal neoplasm that results in cytopenias and bone marrow (BM) failure, and myelodysplastic syndrome/myeloproliferative neoplasm (MDS/MPN), rare diseases that have overlapping features with MDS and MPN, which are discussed in Chapter 6.

MYELODYSPLASTIC SYNDROME/MYELODYSPLASTIC NEOPLASM

MDS is an umbrella category encompassing a variety of clonal neoplastic diseases characterized by ineffective hematopoiesis and recognized by the presence of cytopenia(s), morphologic dysplasia, and/or recurrent genetic abnormalities.[1] MDS neoplasms are a form of bone marrow (BM) failure with an increased risk of transformation to acute myeloid leukemia (AML).

The term *myelodysplastic syndrome* is retained in the International Consensus Classification (ICC) although the World Health Organization (WHO) fifth edition uses the term *myelodysplastic neoplasm* but still retains MDS as an abbreviation. Both systems subclassify these based on (a) the presence of certain genetic abnormalities; (b) the number of morphologically dysplastic cell lineages; and (c) the percent blasts (Table 5.1).[2,3] Clinically, as discussed further, many scoring systems categorize MDS based on projected survival and risk of transformation to AML.

Epidemiology

MDS is the most common myeloid neoplasm with an incidence of 4 to 5/100,000 individuals and is a disease of the elderly, affecting about 20 to 75/100,000 people over age 65.[4] It is rare in children, except in rare genetic disorders or following cytotoxic therapy. Refractory cytopenia of

TABLE 5.1 Classification of Myelodysplastic Syndromes

International classification consensus	WHO fifth edition
Low grade • MDS with mutated *SF3B1* • MDS with del(5q) • MDS, NOS without dysplasia • MDS, NOS with SLD • MDS, NOS with MLD	Genetically defined • MDS with mutated *SF3B1* • MDS with del(5q) • MDS with mutated biallelic *TP53*

High grade
• MDS with excess blasts (MDS-EB)
• MDS/AML
• MDS with mutated biallelic *TP53*
	Morphologically defined
	• MDS with low blasts
	• MDS, hypoplastic
	• MDS with increased blasts (MDS-IB)
	  • MDS with IB-1
	  • MDS with IB-2
	• MDS with fibrosis

AML, acute myeloid leukemia; del, deletion; MDS, myelodysplastic syndrome; MLD, multilineage dysplasia; NOS, not otherwise specified; SLD, single lineage dysplasia; WHO, World Health Organization.

childhood (see later) is a related form of BM failure, but is considered different from MDS.

Causes of *de novo* MDS include exposure to benzene, cigarettes, agricultural products, and other toxins. Familial syndromes also associated with MDS include Fanconi anemia, Shwachman-Diamond syndrome, Diamond-Blackfan anemia, and dyskeratosis congenita, among others. Therapy-related MDS increases with an aging population, as effective cancer treatments continue to prolong patient survival.

Presentation

The diagnosis of MDS relies on a thorough patient history, including drug and medication use, physical exam, laboratory data, and morphologic assessment of the peripheral blood (PB) and BM.

Patients present with symptoms of ineffective hematopoiesis, namely, fatigue, bleeding disorders, and increased susceptibility to infections.

Cytopenia(s), defined in Table 5.2, are nearly always present, although the categories of MDS defined by genetic abnormalities do not require the presence of cytopenias for a diagnosis. The most common cytopenia is anemia (Figure 5.1), and many patients are transfusion dependent at diagnosis.

TABLE 5.2 Criteria for Cytopenia for Each Lineage

Lineage	Criterion for cytopenia
Red cells	Hgb <13 g/dL (men) and <12 g/dL (women)
White cells	Absolute neutrophil count <1800/µL
Platelets	<150,000/µL

dL, deciliters; Hgb, hemoglobin; g, grams; uL, microliters.

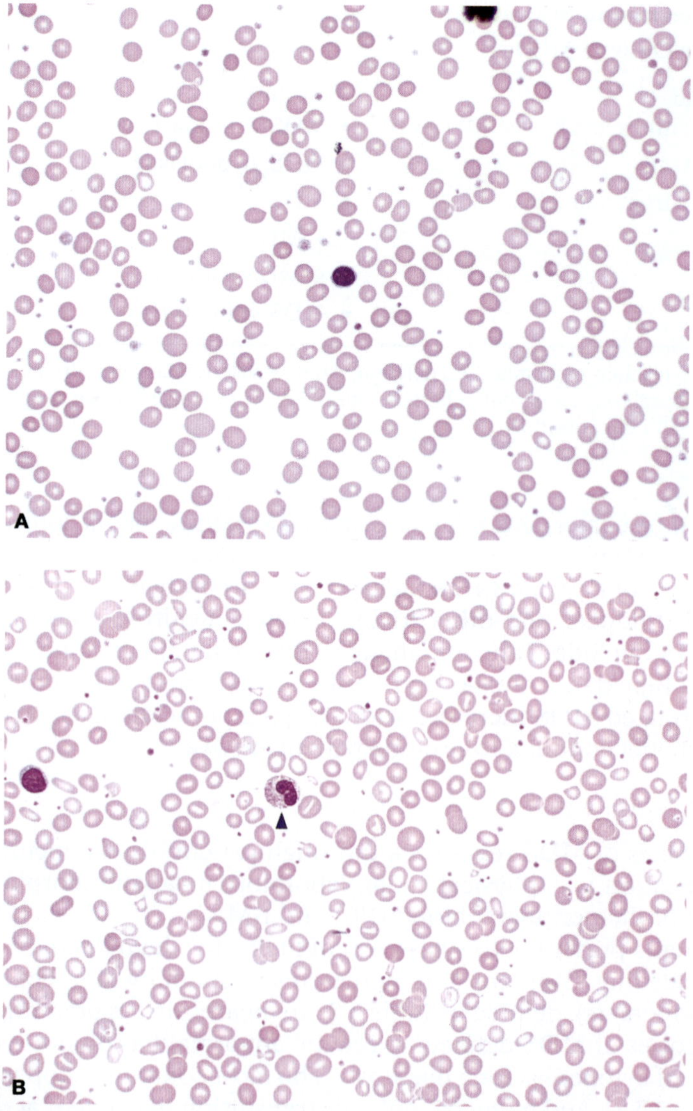

FIGURE 5.1 Patients with myelodysplastic syndrome typically present with macrocytic anemia, as seen in this peripheral blood (PB) smear (A). Occasionally, the PB may show anisopoikilocytosis, or variation in red blood cell (RBC) size and shape (B). In this case, there is also a dysplastic-appearing neutrophil with hyposegmentation (arrowhead).

In fact, some MDS scoring systems incorporate transfusion dependence in their prognostic modeling.

Cytoses are not seen in MDS, except in cases of MDS with del(5q) and inv(3), which may have high platelet counts. Otherwise, patients with cytopenia in one lineage and cytosis in another should be assessed for MDS/MPN, discussed later. Significant monocytosis is not common in MDS, and if the monocyte count is >1000/μL and dysplasia is present, a diagnosis of chronic myelomonocytic leukemia (CMML) is likely.

In many cases, blasts may be present in the blood and a careful manual 200-cell differential of all leukocytes in the PB (not including nucleated red blood cells [RBCs]) is necessary. Evaluation using buffy coat smears may be useful if the patient has marked pancytopenia. Approximately 10% to 15% of patients have higher PB blasts than BM blasts, and these may be more aggressive.[5]

Morphology

Evaluation of the BM includes assessment of the core biopsy and aspirate smear.

Evaluation of the core biopsy helps determine the overall cellularity, the cellular composition and architecture, and the megakaryocytic morphology. In most cases, the BM core biopsy is hypercellular for age with uni- or multilineage proliferation and increased apoptosis because of ineffective hematopoiesis (Figure 5.2).

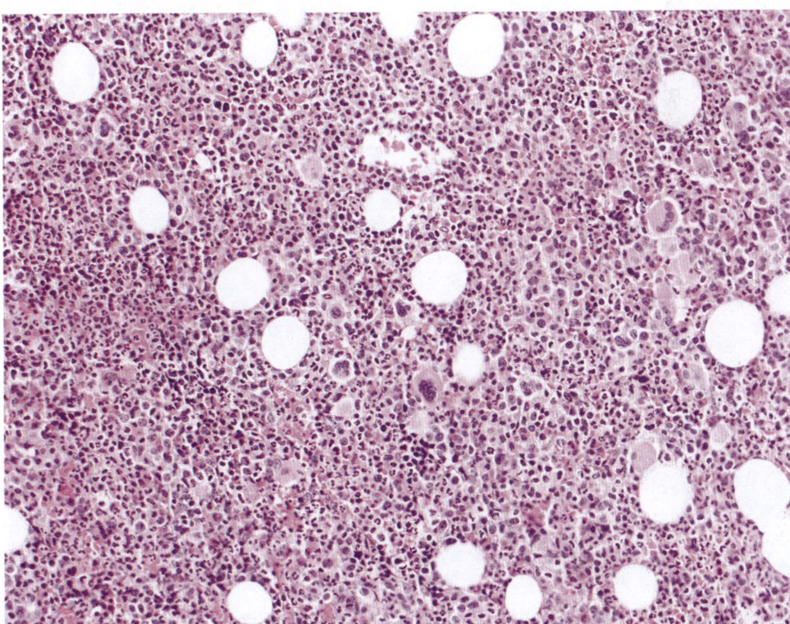

FIGURE 5.2 The core biopsy of this elderly patient with myelodysplastic syndrome shows a markedly hypercellular bone marrow for age with increased atypical megakaryocytes.

Rarely, the BM may be hypocellular for age (10% of MDS cases), mimicking aplastic anemia (AA). Careful morphologic evaluation for dysplasia (particularly outside of the red cell lineage) and blast enumeration are necessary in these circumstances. T cell large granular lymphocytic (T-LGL) leukemia can produce a similar clinical picture to MDS and should be excluded, although it may also coexist with MDS.

Architectural and morphologic features associated with MDS on the core biopsy include (a) abnormal localization of immature precursors (ALIPs), with small clusters of immature myeloid cells scattered away from the trabeculae in the interstitium; (b) disruption of erythroid islands; (c) increased small, hypolobated megakaryocytes; (d) decreased or inverted myeloid to erythroid (M:E) ratio; and (e) significant left shift or increase in blasts. Low-grade MDS commonly shows a decreased or inverted M:E ratio (Figure 5.3A and B). In high-grade MDS, there may be either myeloid or erythroid predominance and increased blasts (Figure 5.4).

A good-quality spiculated BM aspirate smear is important to evaluate morphologic features, and a 500-cell differential count of all nucleated cells must be performed to assess blast percentage. The sample should be collected and either a direct smear made at the bedside or an ethylenediaminetetraacetic acid (EDTA) anticoagulated specimen evaluated as soon as possible. Poor-quality smears make morphologic assessment difficult, especially when evaluating myeloid granulation.

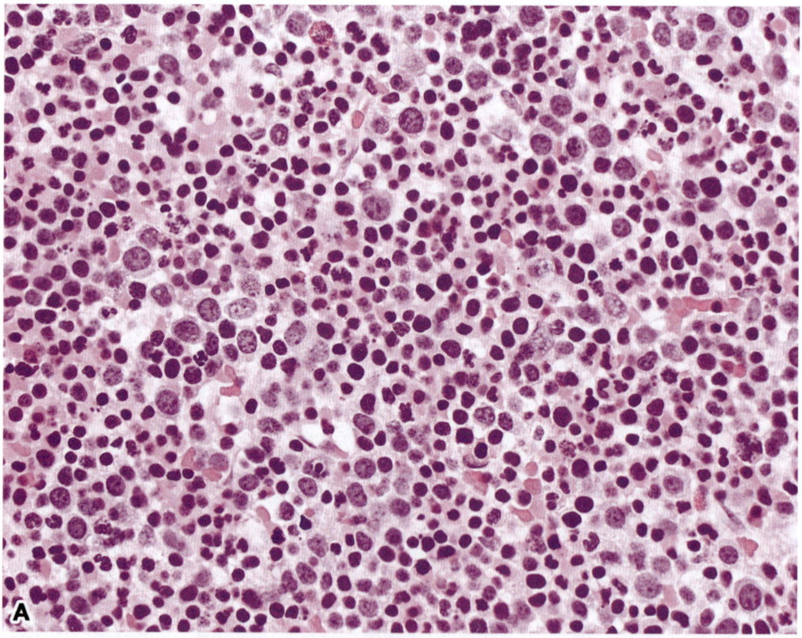

FIGURE 5.3 **The bone marrow biopsy of this patient with MDS was markedly hypercellular for age.** At high power, the majority of cells are erythroid (A), highlighted with an E-cadherin (B). An inverted myeloid to erythroid (M:E) ratio is common in myelodysplastic syndrome (MDS), especially in low-grade MDS.

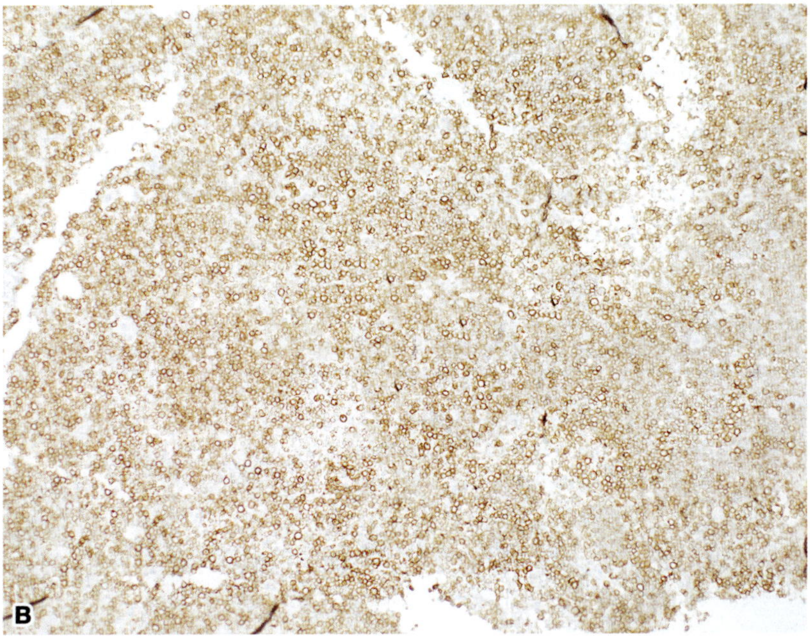

FIGURE 5.3 *(continued)*

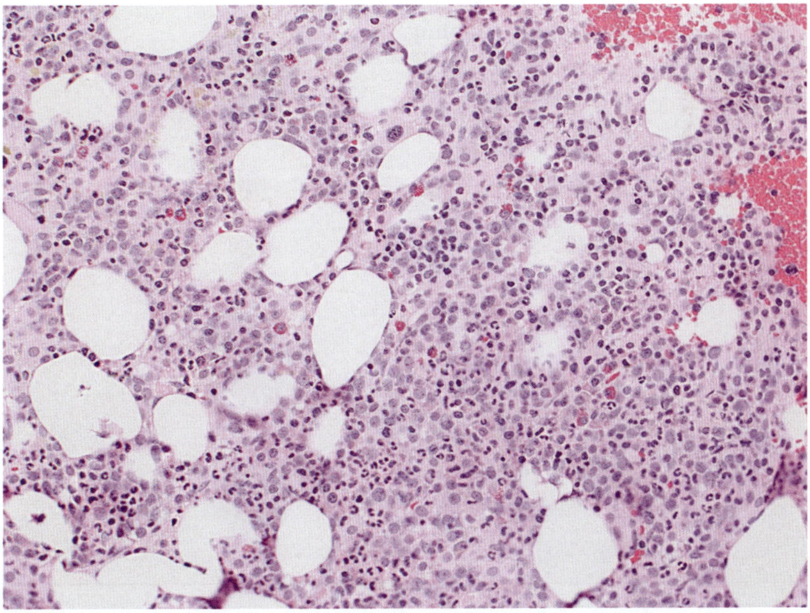

FIGURE 5.4 This core biopsy from a patient with myelodysplastic syndrome with excess blasts shows a marked myeloid predominance in addition to the increased blasts.

Dysplasia

Dysplastic features are present in one or more of the hematopoietic lineages (Table 5.3), which may or may not correlate with the PB cytopenia. The dysplastic cells must represent >10% of cells in the erythroid or myeloid lineage, and at least 30% of megakaryocytes; there are other strict criteria to diagnose dysplasia in order to minimalize interobserver variability (see later).

TABLE 5.3 Dysplastic Morphologic Features

Lineage	Feature	Morphology
Red blood cells	Nuclear budding, blebbing, and bridging	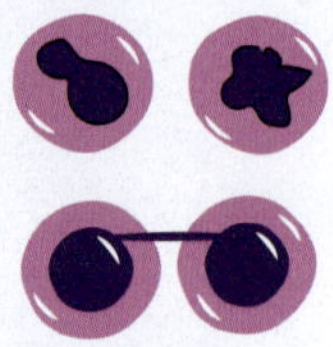
	Karyorrhexis	
	Basophilic stippling	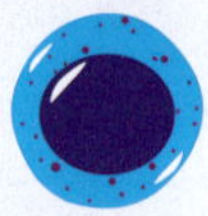
	Ring sideroblasts	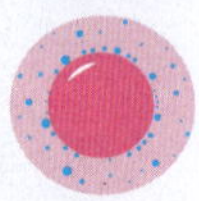
	Vacuoles	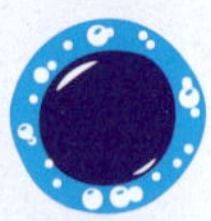
	Megaloblastic	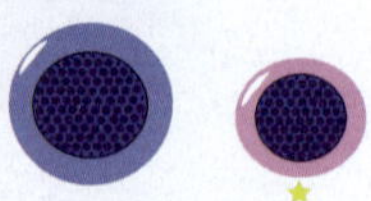

TABLE 5.3 **Dysplastic Morphologic Features (*continued*)**		
Lineage	Feature	Morphology
Neutrophils	Hypo-/hypersegmented nuclei	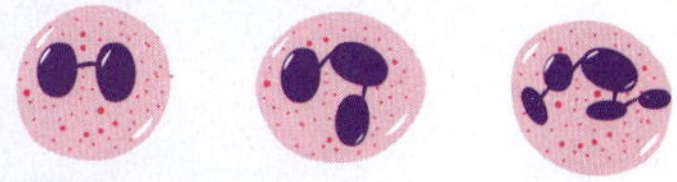
	Hypo-/hypergranular myeloid cells	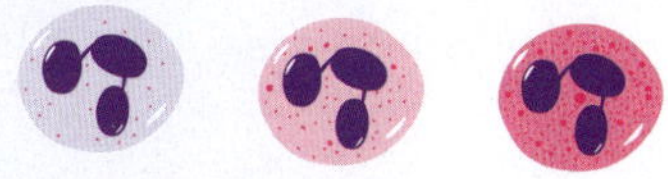
Megakaryocytes	Separated nuclear lobes ("Pawn ball nuclei")	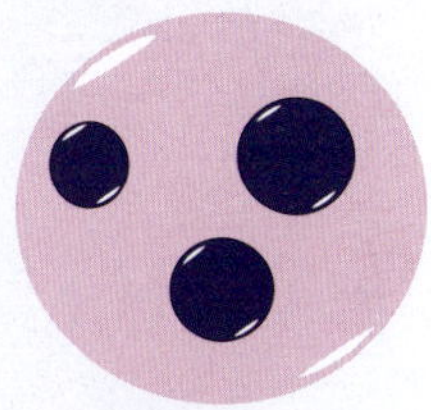
	Small, hypolobated megakaryocytes ("micromegakaryocytes")	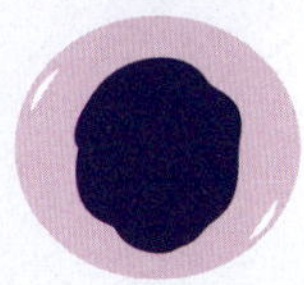

Approximately 10% to 15% of MDS cases have significant fibrosis at diagnosis, which may preclude obtaining a good aspirate smear and limit morphologic evaluation. In those cases, a touch-prep should be submitted to assess morphology. Increased fibrosis imparts an independently worse prognosis.[6]

Myeloid Dysplasia

Myeloid dysplasia is best appreciated in the PB smear and BM aspirate smears. The most common features include hypo-/hypergranulation or hypo-/hypersegmentation (eFigure 1). Pseudo Pelger-Huet cells (Figure 5.5), uni- or bisegmented neutrophils with abnormal cytoplasmic granulation, may be present. Hypogranular neutrophils appear pale in comparison to normal neutrophils, as they lack the pinkish cytoplasmic blush imparted by secondary granules and look pale in comparison (Figure 5.6). Rarely, large eosinophilic cytoplasmic granules (pseudo Chediak-Higashi granules)

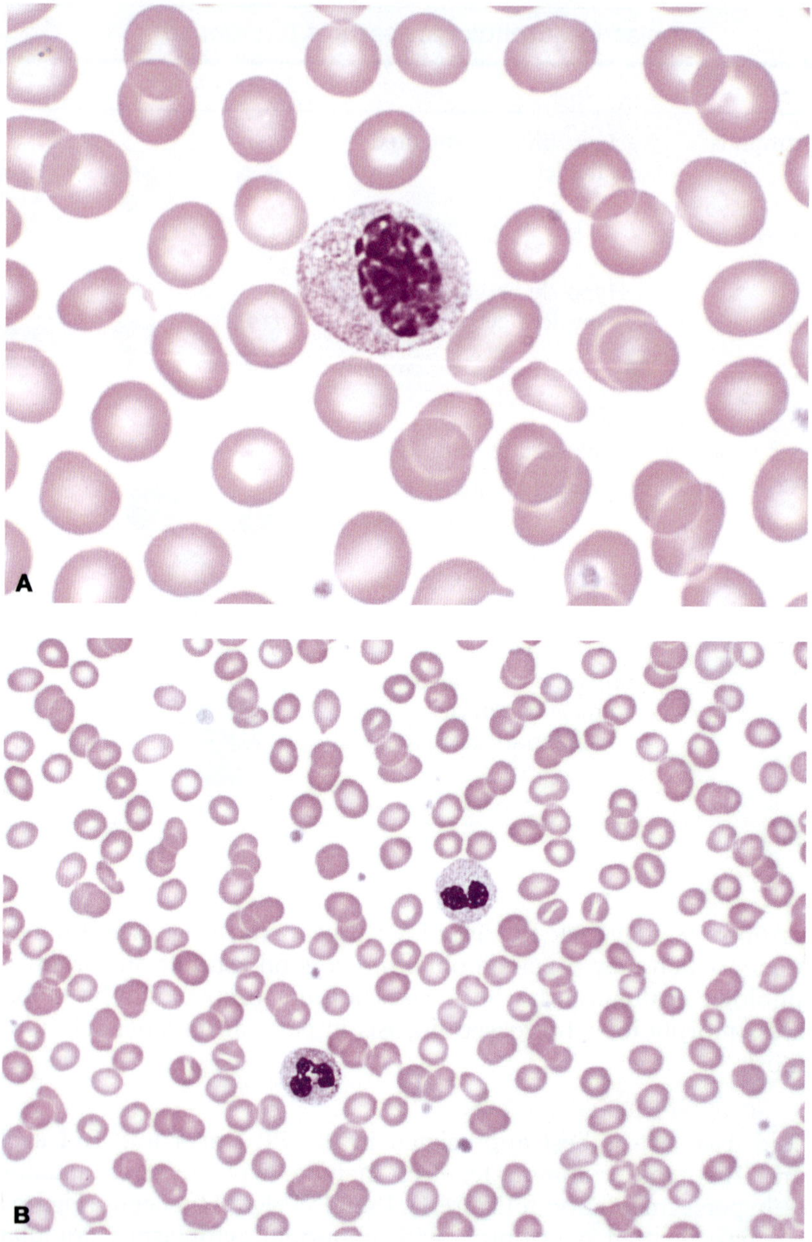

FIGURE 5.5 Pseudo Pelger-Huet cells, seen in this peripheral blood (PB) sample, are mature neutrophils with abnormal segmentation of the nucleus, either nonsegmented (A) or hyposegmented, typically with only two segments (B). These cells can be differentiated from left-shifted myeloid cells (myelocytes, metamyelocytes) because they have mature, clumped nuclear chromatin and cytoplasmic secondary granules.

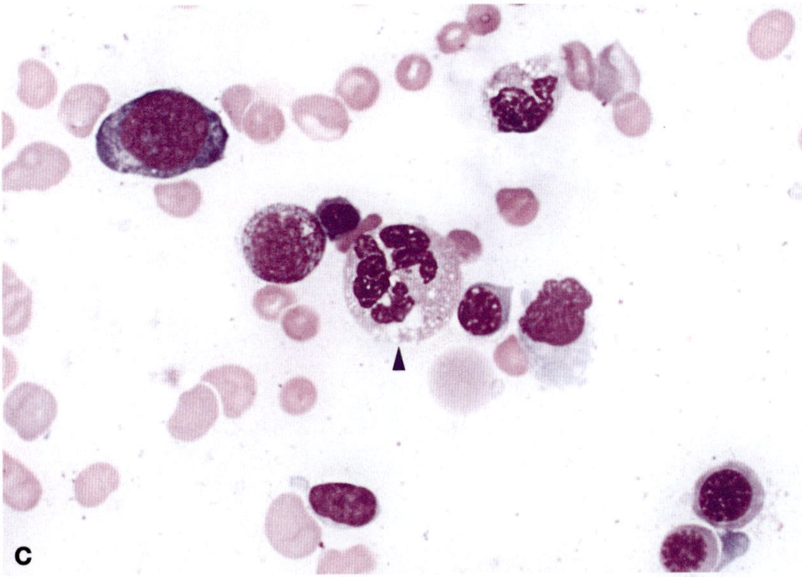

FIGURE 5.5 ***(continued)*** C, This aspirate shows an abnormally hypersegmented neutrophil with cytoplasmic vacuoles (arrowhead).

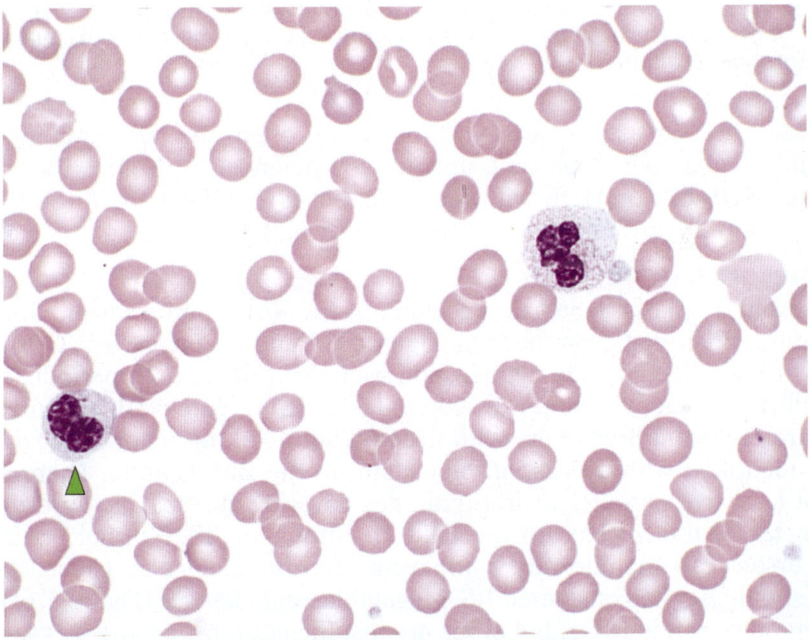

FIGURE 5.6 **The two dysplastic neutrophils in this peripheral blood are both hypogranular, one with relatively homogeneous pale bluish-purple cytoplasm (arrowhead) and the other with only partial cytoplasmic granulation.**

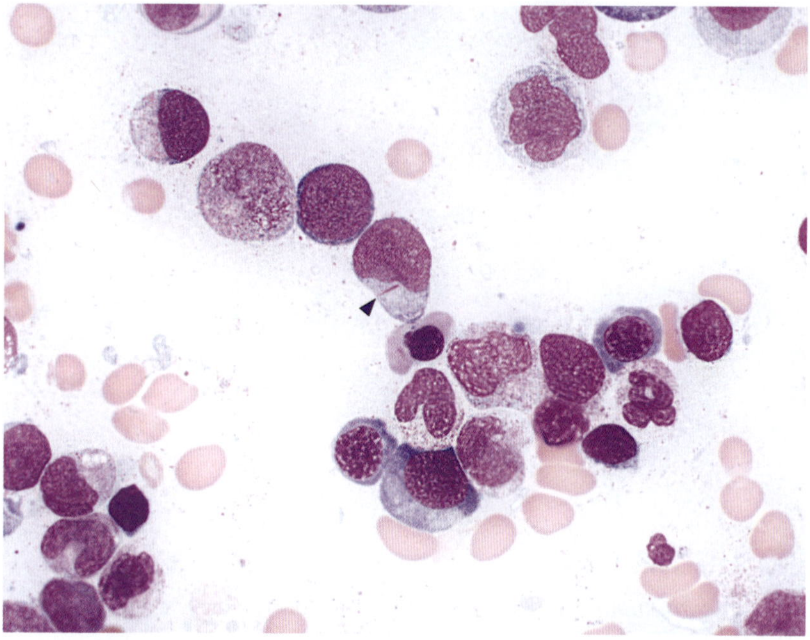

FIGURE 5.7 An Auer rod (arrowhead) present in a blast in a patient with myelodysplastic syndrome with myelodysplastic syndrome with excess blasts. There were too few blasts in the aspirate to make a diagnosis of acute myeloid leukemia based on morphology alone.

are seen in dysplastic neutrophils, but more often, the dysgranulopoiesis is subtle. Auer rods, if present, upgrade the diagnosis to MDS with excess blasts (MDS-EB; or MDS with increased blasts 2 [MDS-IB2] in the WHO 5th Edition) regardless of blast count (Figure 5.7).

Erythroid Dysplasia

Erythroid dysplasia is best appreciated on the BM aspirate smear. Nuclear budding and bridging may be seen (Figure 5.8A and B; eFigure 5.2). Cytoplasmic irregularities include cytoplasmic vacuoles (Figure 5.9), periodic acid-Schiff (PAS) reactivity, and ring sideroblasts (RS) (Figure 5.10; eFigure 5.3). RS are erythroid precursors with accumulations of mitochondrial ferritin, best identified with a Prussian blue stain on the BM aspirate. There must be at least five perinuclear iron granules covering at least one-third of the diameter of the nucleus to meet the definition of RS. Normal erythroid precursors can include rare cytoplasmic ferritin molecules (sideroblasts) and should not be considered RS. Megaloblastoid changes (Figure 5.11) are commonly seen in MDS, but alone are insufficient for the diagnosis as they may be seen in other, non-neoplastic settings.

Megakaryocytic Dysplasia

Megakaryocytic dysplasia is best appreciated on the BM core biopsy because many megakaryocytes can be evaluated at once (Figure 5.12). Identifying dysplastic megakaryocytes can be subjective, and care should be

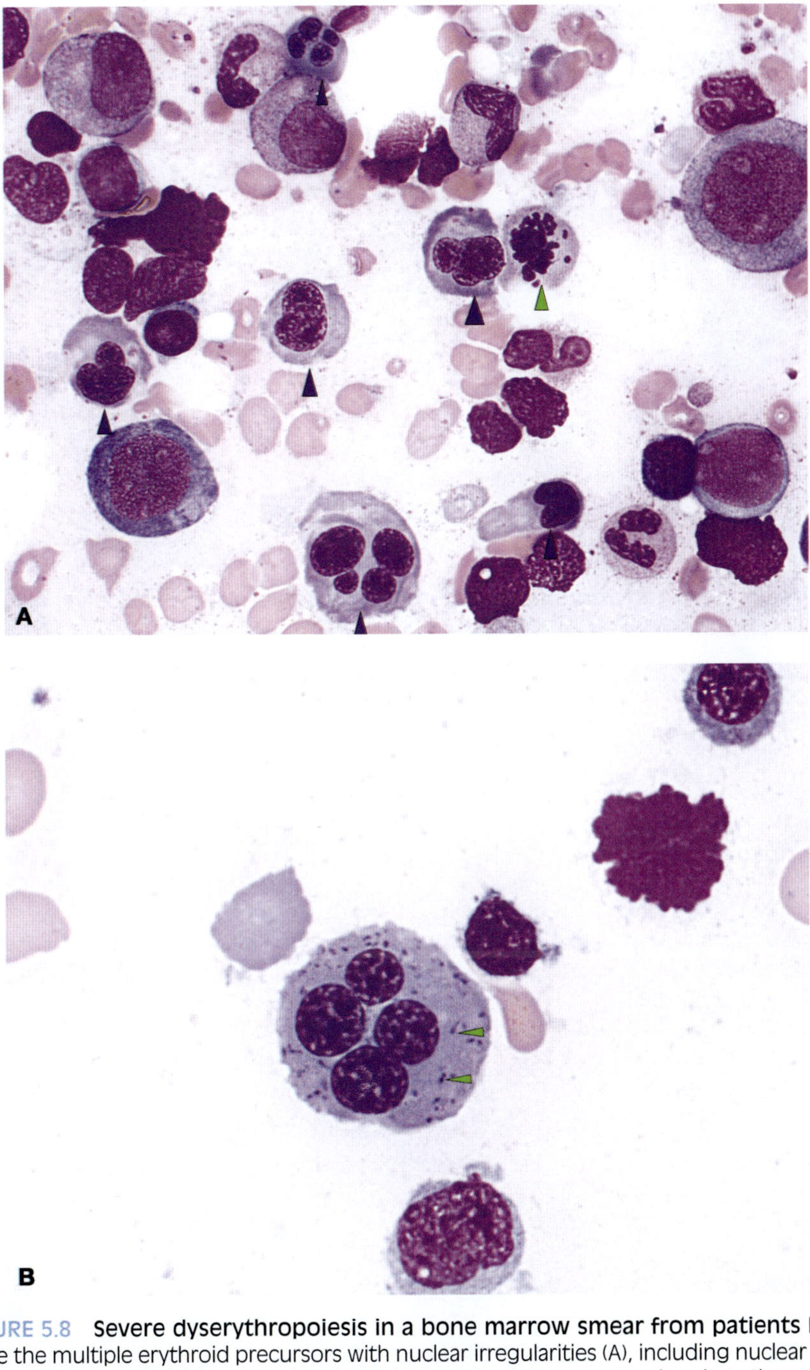

FIGURE 5.8 **Severe dyserythropoiesis in a bone marrow smear from patients MDS.** Note the multiple erythroid precursors with nuclear irregularities (A), including nuclear budding or blebbing (dark blue arrowheads) and karyorrhexis (green arrowhead). In the second aspirate (B), in addition to nuclear abnormalities, this erythroid precursor shows prominent cytoplasmic basophilic stippling (arrowheads).

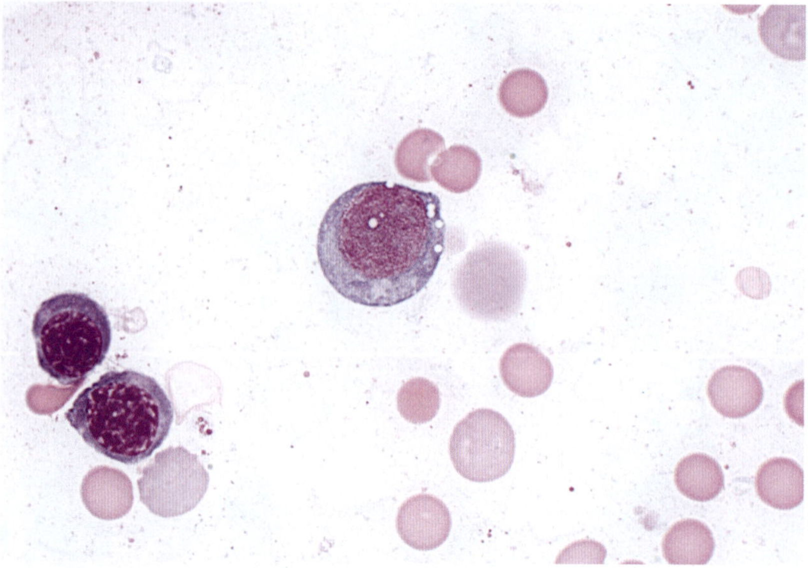

FIGURE 5.9 **This early erythroid precursor shows cytoplasmic vacuoles.** Although common in myelodysplastic syndrome, this finding is not specific.

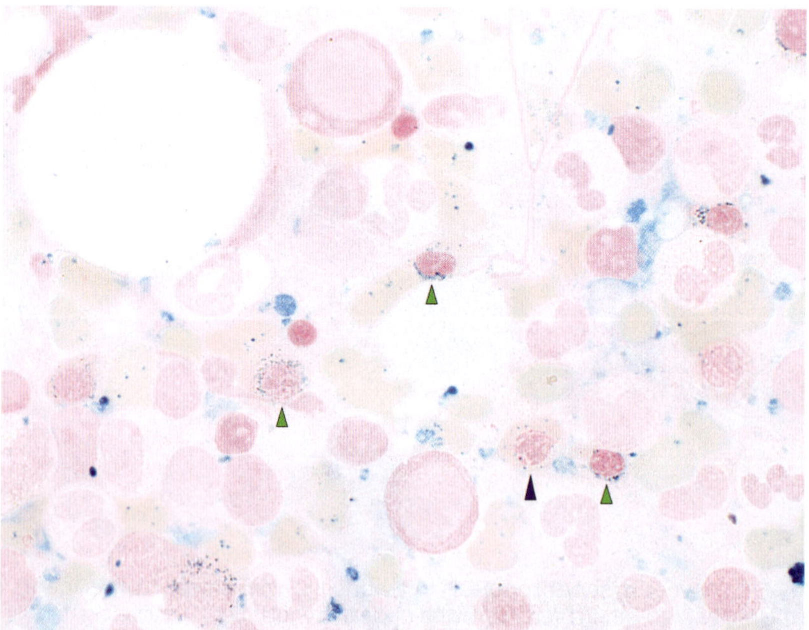

FIGURE 5.10 **An iron stain performed on this aspirate smear reveals abundant ring sideroblasts (green arrowheads), in addition to normal sideroblasts (dark blue arrowheads).** This patient was diagnosed with myelodysplastic syndrome with mutated *SF3B1*.

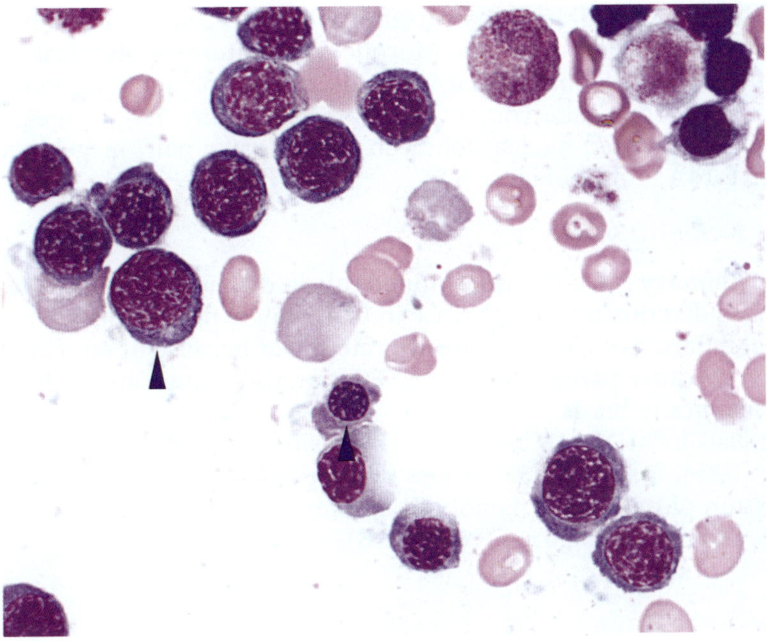

FIGURE 5.11 **Megaloblastic changes seen in an aspirate smear in a patient with MDS.** The nuclear chromatin is similar in both the immature erythroid precursor, left, and the more mature erythroid precursor, center (dark blue arrowheads), indicating a nuclear:cytoplasmic maturation asynchrony.

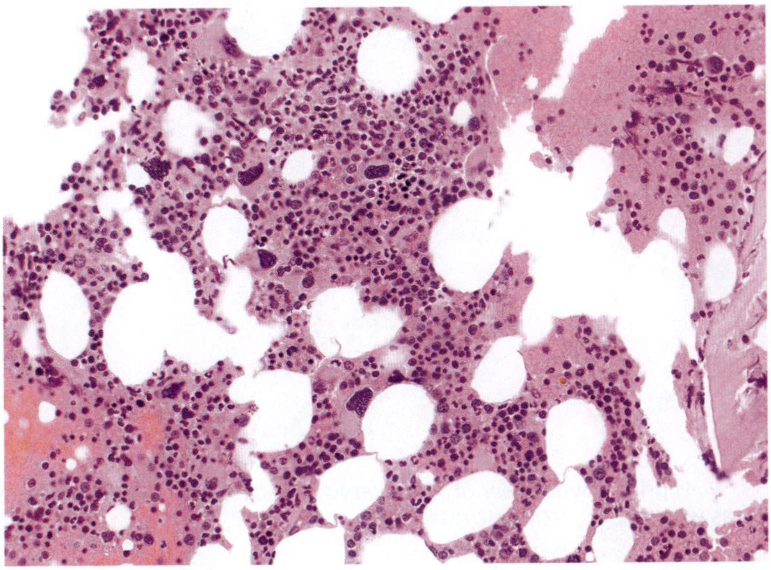

FIGURE 5.12 **This low-power core biopsy shows numerous dysplastic megakaryocytes, characterized by small size, and hypolobated and hyperchromatic nuclei.**

taken when making an initial diagnosis of MDS based only on unilineage megakaryocytic dysplasia. Morphologic features of dysplastic megakaryocytes include smaller than normal or monolobated megakaryocytes including micromegakaryocytes (Figure 5.13; eFigure 5.4), or megakaryocytes with separated nuclear lobes, so-called "pawn ball" megakaryocytes (Figure 5.14A and B; eFigure 5.5).

Immunophenotype

Flow cytometry (FC): FC has a limited role in diagnosing MDS. FC may be helpful to demonstrate an increase in blasts but is not a replacement for a manual differential count on the aspirate smear because of possible hemodilution or other preanalytic issues. FC can also demonstrate phenotypic abnormalities in blasts.

Blasts in MDS are usually CD34 positive, and may show especially bright CD34, loss of CD38, or loss or gain of CD117, as well as aberrant expression of myeloid or lymphoid markers including CD7, CD10, CD5, CD56, and others (Figure 5.15A and B).

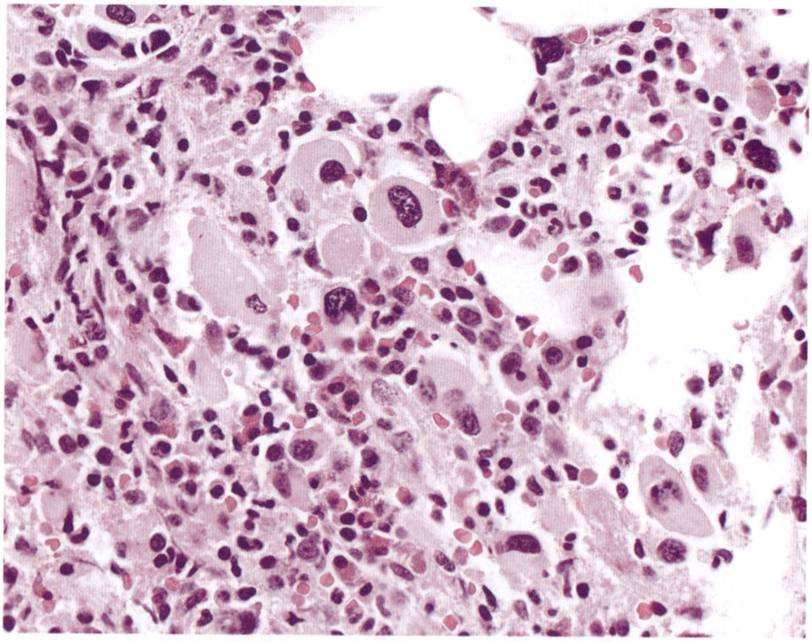

FIGURE 5.13 Higher power view of megakaryocytic dysplasia, including numerous small forms with hyperchromatic nuclei.

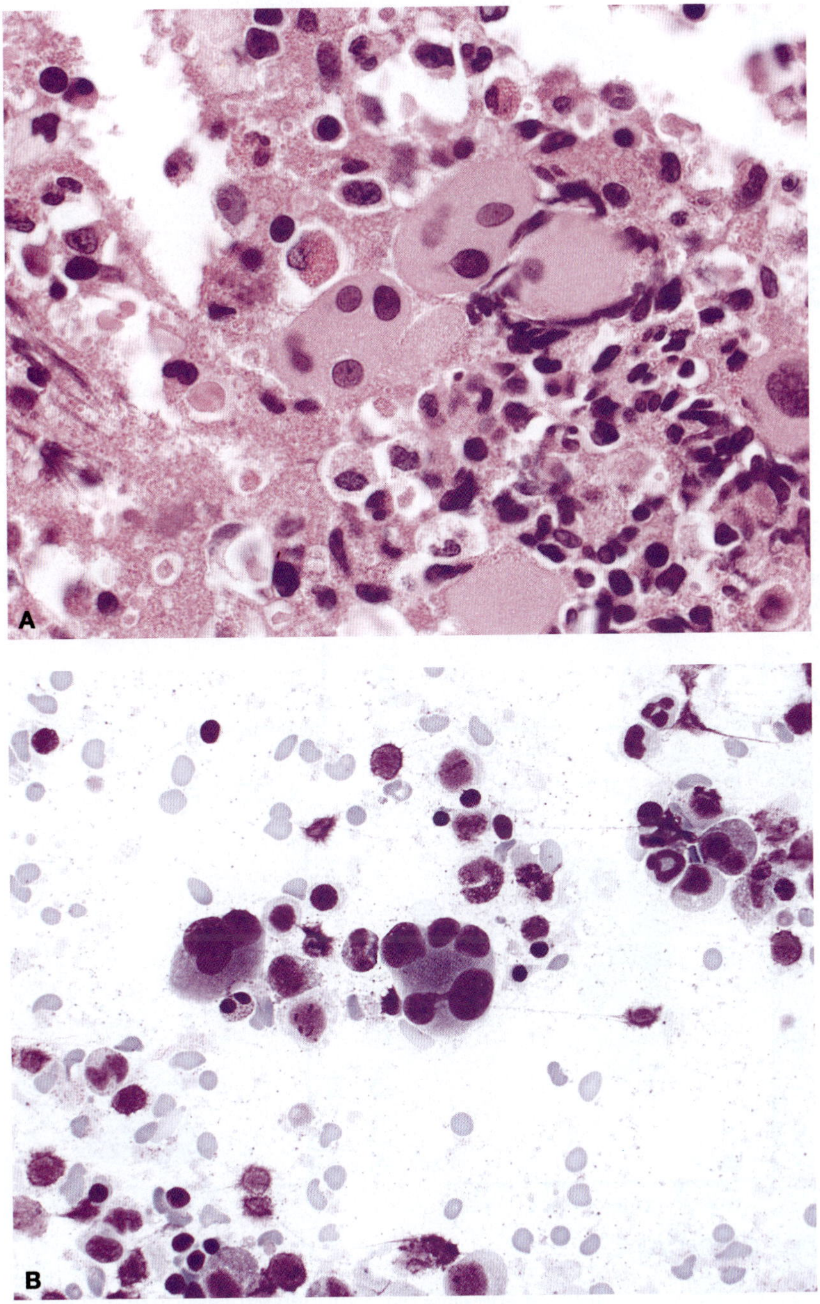

FIGURE 5.14 "Pawn ball" megakaryocytes have widely separated nuclear lobes, as seen on the core biopsy (A) and aspirate smear (B).

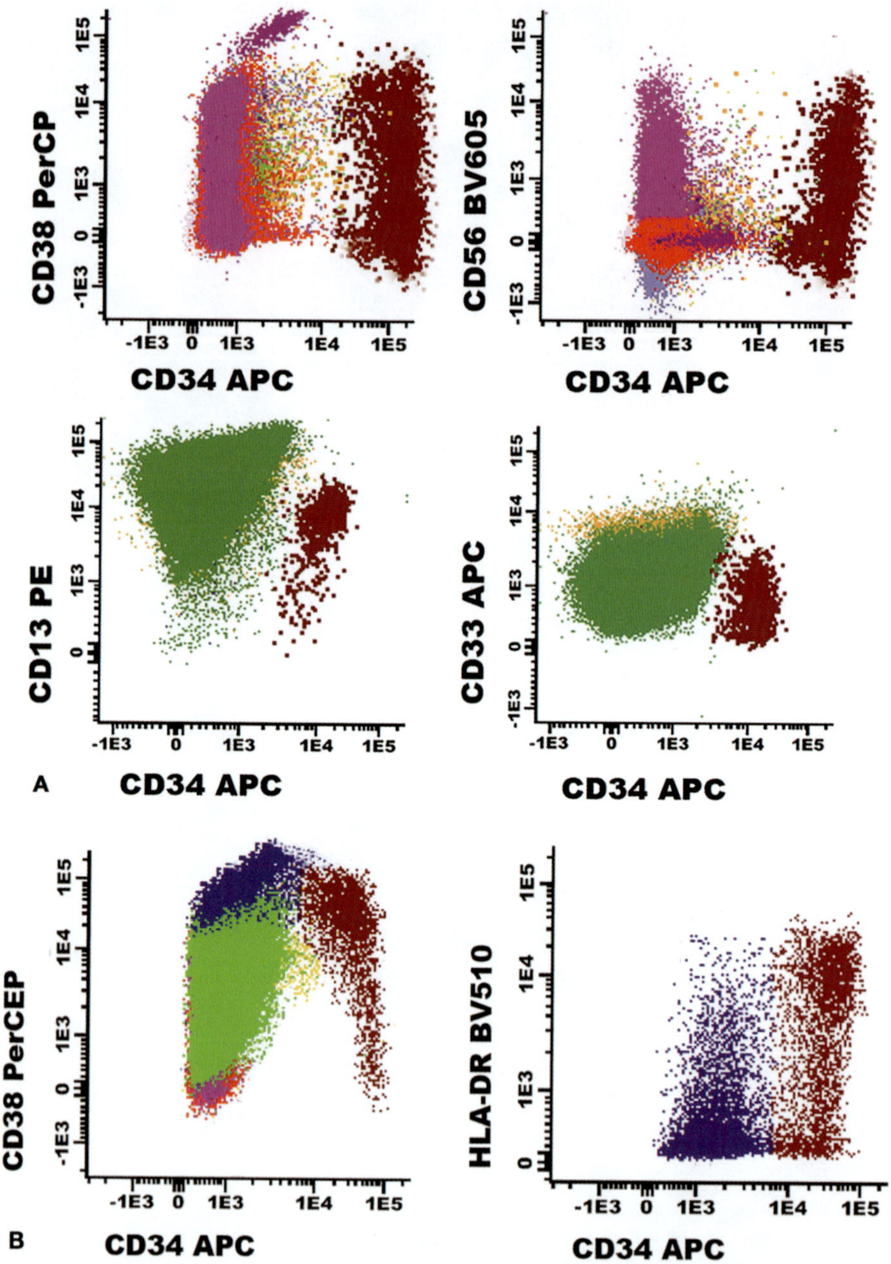

FIGURE 5.15 **Flow cytometry of aberrant blast antigen expression in myelodysplastic syndrome.** A, Abnormal blasts (brown population) express relatively bright CD34, show loss of CD38, and have aberrant expression of CD56 (top panels). The blasts also express relatively bright expression of CD13 relative to the much dimmer CD33 (bottom panels). B, Blasts (brown and blue population) have variable CD34 with a relatively more normal pattern of CD38 acquisition (left panel) but have significant loss of human leukocyte antigen-D related (HLA-DR; right panel).

FC is also useful to confirm the presence of abnormal myeloid maturation (Figure 5.16), the severity of which correlates with the degree of dysplasia. Asynchronous expression of CD10 and CD16 on myeloid cells is abnormal. Other myeloid markers, including CD13, CD11b, and CD16, have predictable patterns of expression with normal maturation, which may be disrupted in MDS. Care is needed not to overinterpret myeloid and monocytic marker expression because some reactive and regenerative conditions can be associated with abnormal levels of expression of markers such as CD14 and CD64 on granulocytes: CD64 is increased in sepsis. In addition, aberrant expression must be distinguished from quantitative abnormalities in maturation; loss of CD16 on granulocytes may simply represent a left shift. Finally, CD16 and CD14 are glycosylphosphatidylinositol (GPI)-linked proteins, and a lack of

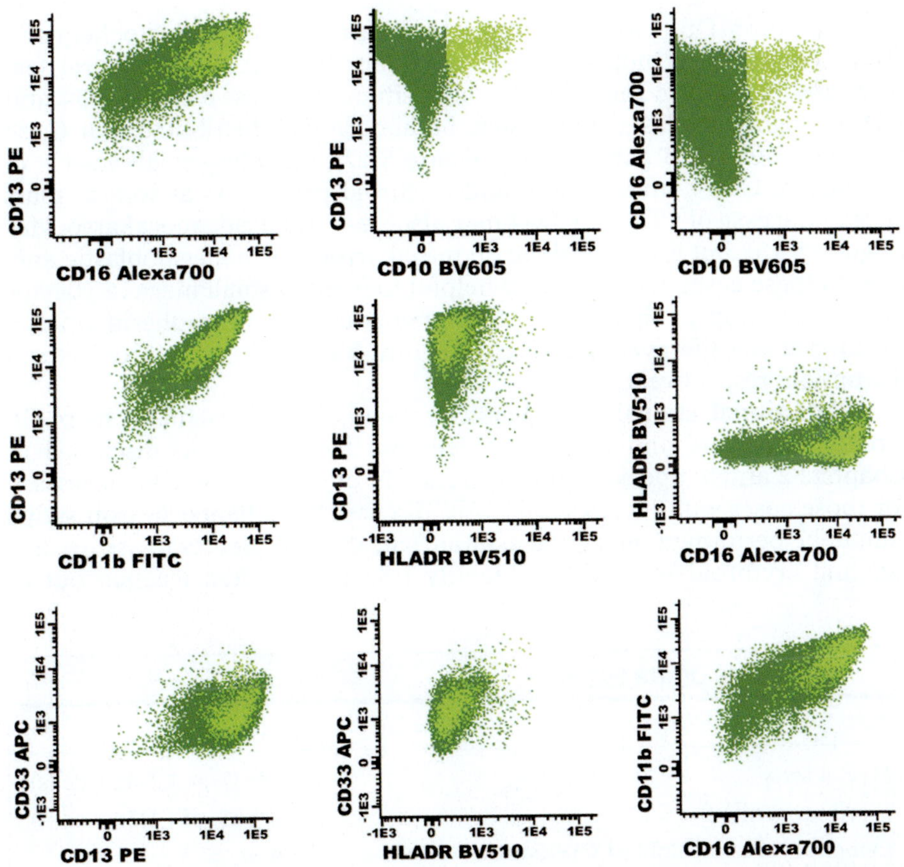

FIGURE 5.16 Abnormal myeloid maturation detected by flow cytometry, showing asynchronous expression of CD13, CD16, and CD11b on myeloid precursors (dark green), with few mature CD10+ neutrophils (light green).

expression may be seen in patients with paroxysmal nocturnal hemoglobinuria (PNH).

Other diagnostically useful information gleaned from FC includes (a) decreased light side scatter of neutrophils; (b) reduction or absence of normal B cell precursors in the BM; and (c) abnormal intensity of CD45 on blasts.[7] Quantitative thresholds for these three parameters, along with the number of CD34-positive blasts, have been combined to form a so-called "Ogata score,"[8] which is a simple screening method for MDS that has reasonable sensitivity and specificity (Table 5.4), although it is not considered diagnostic. If these types of abnormalities are noted, a more comprehensive workup may be recommended.

Patients with MDS may also have PNH clones, with loss of antigens bound to cell surface via GPI anchors. However, these patients typically have low-level PNH clones; large clones suggest actual PNH.

Immunohistochemistry

In cases of MDS with an inaspirable marrow, immunohistochemistry (IHC) on the core biopsy may be necessary to assess architectural features and to confirm the cellular composition and blast count. CD34 and CD117 highlight blasts, which may be abnormally distributed, but these also stain other BM components (Figure 5.17), including small vessels in the case of CD34, and myeloid and erythroid precursors as well as mast cells in the case of CD117. CD34 may also stain dysplastic megakaryocytes (Figure 5.18), but is also positive on megakaryocytes in megaloblastic anemia. In these cases, CD61 may be helpful to identify small megakaryocytes on the core biopsy (Figure 5.19). Myeloperoxidase and E-cadherin are useful to evaluate the overall BM architecture for ALIP or erythroid island disruption, respectively.

Additional stains: Cytochemical stains may be useful to help differentiate myeloid and monocytic cells on the aspirate, as discussed in Chapters 2 and 3. Special stains for reticulin or collagen may be necessary for those cases with increased fibrosis, discussed in Chapter 6. Iron stains should be performed on a good aspirate smear with spicules to assess storage and erythroid iron and to identify RS; iron is often leached out of

TABLE 5.4 The Ogata Score[a]

Feature	Cutoff value
Myeloblasts	>2% (% of CD45+ cells)
B cell progenitors	<5% (% of CD34+ cells)
Lymphocyte to myeloblast CD45 ratio	$\leq$4 or $\geq$7.5
Granulocyte to lymphocyte side scatter ratio	$\leq$6

[a]Score 1 point for each category. A sum of $\geq$2 points suggests myelodysplastic syndrome.

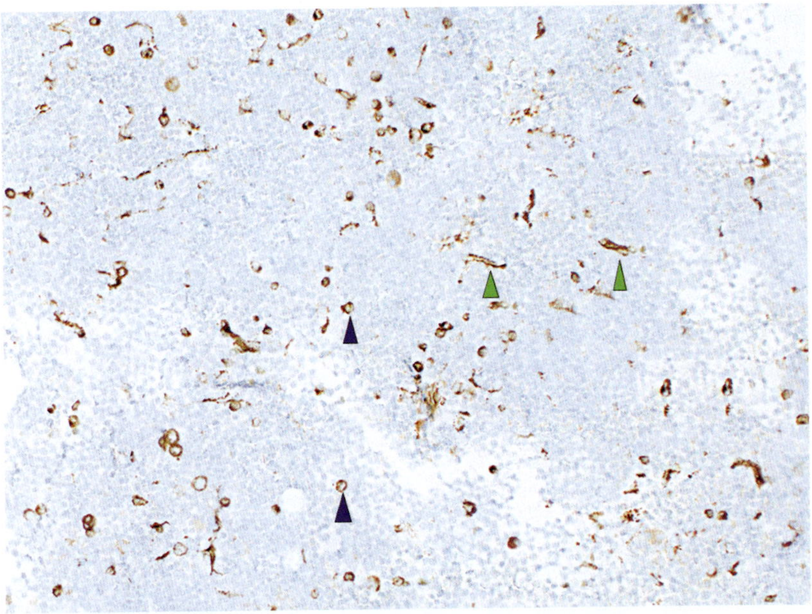

FIGURE 5.17 In this bone marrow core biopsy, CD34 highlights increased blasts (blue arrowheads) as well as small vessels (green arrowheads).

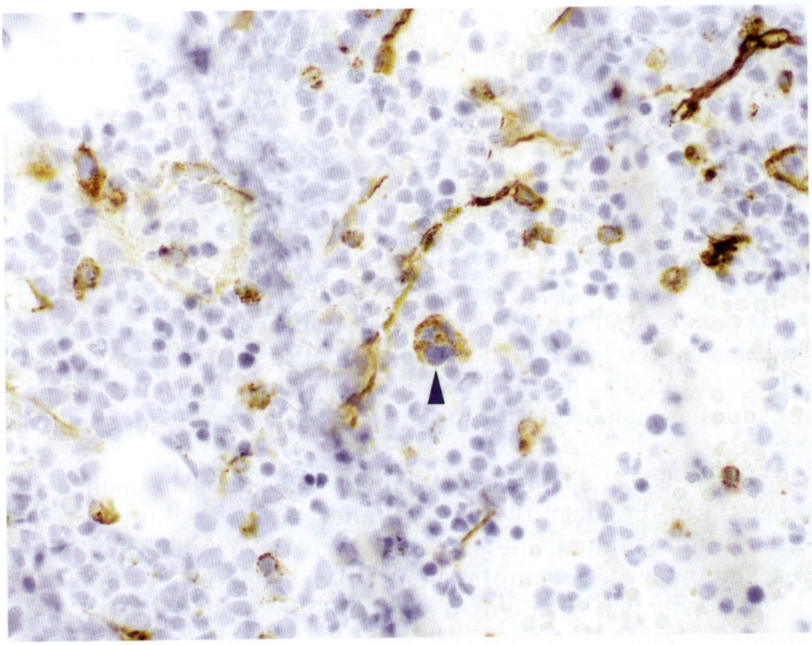

FIGURE 5.18 Abnormal megakaryocytes may express CD34 (arrowhead).

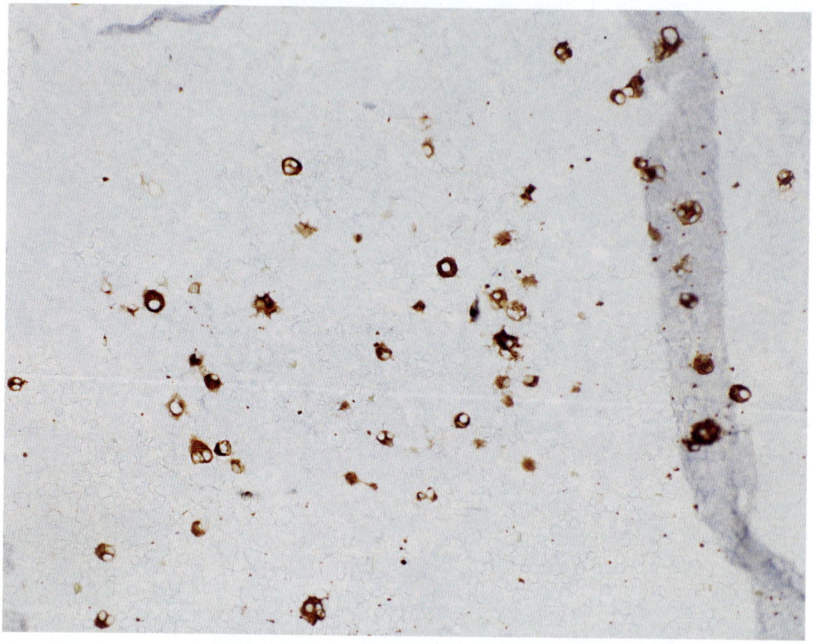

FIGURE 5.19 **Abnormal megakaryocytes and micromegakaryocytes are highlighted with CD61 on this core biopsy.**

marrow biopsies during the decalcification process, but iron stains can also be performed on particle/clot sections.

Genetics

It is well accepted that MDS is caused by mutations in hematopoietic stem cells; standard-of-care requires that both cytogenetic and molecular genetic studies be performed on all presumed MDS cases.

Conventional karyotypes and fluorescence in situ hybridization (FISH) panels are useful to detect chromosomal abnormalities and thus establish the presence of a clonal abnormality. With few exceptions, these are not used in the subclassification of MDS, but specific cytogenetic abnormalities are important for prognosis and factor into most clinical scoring systems.[9]

Molecular studies, in particular next-generation sequencing (NGS), are helpful in the diagnosis of MDS and are essential for recognition of certain entities. Somatic mutations are detected in about 90% of all MDS cases, and cytogenetic abnormalities are detected in up to 50% of cases. Certain genetic abnormalities are MDS defining, even in the absence of evidence of dysplasia (see later).[2]

Documentation of additional genetic abnormalities as they occur during the course of disease is important, as they may indicate progression to high-grade MDS and increased risk of transformation to AML.

TABLE 5.5 Morphologic Features Associated With Particular Genetic Abnormalities in MDS

Abnormality	Morphologic association
Loss of 17p	• Pseudo Pelger-Huet • Small vacuolated neutrophils
Isolated del(20q)	• Dysmegakaryopoiesis and low platelets
Inv(3)	• Abnormal megakaryocytes and thrombocytosis
Mutations in *SRSF2*, *RUNS1*, *TP53*, and *ASXL1*	• Granulocytic dysplasia
Del(5q)	• Small megakaryocytes
Mutations in *SF3B1*	• Ring sideroblasts

del, deletion; inv, inversion; MDS, myelodysplastic syndrome.

Interestingly, certain genetic and molecular abnormalities are associated with a certain phenotype or morphology (Table 5.5).

Differential Diagnosis

MDS may mimic other nonneoplastic disorders, and these must be excluded before a diagnosis of MDS is rendered (Table 5.6).

AA can mimic hypocellular MDS. Genetic testing may not be useful to differentiate between these disorders because AA may have trisomy 8, and up to one-third of AA cases have MDS-associated mutations.[10] Assessment of CD34-positive blasts is a better discriminator between the two: AA has a marked decrease in progenitors, whereas MDS has either normal levels or increased progenitors. AA can be effectively treated with immunosuppressive agents, and therefore, it is important to exclude this diagnosis before rendering a diagnosis of MDS.

MPNs may be difficult to differentiate from fibrotic MDS, particularly in the absence of a good-quality aspirate. Some characteristics that help rule out an MPN include (a) a lack of splenomegaly; (b) small megakaryocytes; (c) increased blasts; (d) no intrasinusoidal hematopoiesis.

Prognosis

MDS has variable prognoses and differs in the risk for AML transformation or death. These risks are determined by several factors, including patient age, cytopenias, blast count, karyotype, WHO (2016) subtype, multilineage dysplasia, and transfusion requirements. The most commonly utilized prognostic scores include (a) the International Prognostic Scoring System (IPSS), which assesses blast count, cytopenias, and karyotype; (b) the revised IPSS (IPSS-R), which assesses the same parameters in a more granular fashion;

TABLE 5.6 Nonneoplastic Mimics of MDS

Category	Nonneoplastic disorders causing dysplasia	Dysplasia
Nutritional	• Vitamin B_{12} deficiency • Folate deficiency • Copper deficiency	• Granulocytic hypersegmentation • Granulocytic hypersegmentation • Cytoplasmic vacuoles
Toxins	• Heavy metals (arsenic, lead, zinc) • Alcohol	• RS • RS, cytoplasmic vacuoles
Medications	• Isoniazid (in the absence of B6 supplement) • Antibiotics (Cotrimoxazole) • Immunosuppressants (tacrolimus, mycophenolate mofetil) • Chemotherapeutic agents • G-CSF	• RS • Granulocytic hyposegmentation • Granulocytic hyposegmentation • Dysplasia in all lineages • Granulocytic hyposegmentation, left shift, and hypergranulation
Infectious	• Parvovirus	• Giant erythroblasts with nuclear inclusions
Genetic	• Pelger-Huet anomaly (AD disorder resulting in mutations in lamin B receptor gene, *LBR*)	• Bisegmented neutrophils

AD, autosomal dominant; G-CSF, granulocyte colony-stimulating factor; MDS, myelodysplastic syndrome; RS, ring sideroblasts.

and (c) the WHO classification–based Prognostic Scoring System (WPSS), which evaluates karyotype and transfusion dependence in addition to the WHO (2016) subtype. Additionally, accumulated data so far have shown that the quantity and types of mutations may also affect prognosis and may be beneficial to include in the risk stratification system.

Precursors of MDS

Idiopathic Cytopenia of Undetermined Significance

Idiopathic cytopenia of undetermined significance (ICUS) represents those patients with cytopenia(s) but no evidence of dysplasia and no molecular or cytogenetic abnormalities (Table 5.7). In these cases, the clinician must exclude other causes of cytopenias. Such patients are typically assessed more comprehensively for other explanations of their cytopenias or followed with multiple BM examinations.

TABLE 5.7 Cytopenias and Potential Precursor Lesions to MDS

Disorder	Cytopenias	Clonal hematopoiesis	Dysplasia	Increased blasts
ICUS	+	–	–	–
CHIP	–	+	–	–
CCUS	+	+	–	–
Low-grade MDS[a]	+	+	+/–	–
High-grade MDS[b]	+	+	+/–	+

CCUS, clonal cytopenias of undetermined significance; CHIP, clonal hematopoiesis of indeterminate potential; ICUS, idiopathic cytopenia of undetermined significance; MDS, myelodysplastic syndrome.

[a]Low-grade MDS refers to MDS with *SF3B1*; MDS with del(5q); MDS, not otherwise specified without dysplasia; MDS with single lineage dysplasia; MDS with multilineage dysplasia.

[b]High-grade MDS refers to MDS with excess blasts (MDS-EB), MDS/acute myeloid leukemia (MDS/AML).

Clonal Hematopoiesis of Indeterminate Potential

Patients with certain abnormal genetic findings but no evidence of dysplasia or cytopenias are diagnosed with clonal hematopoiesis of indeterminate potential (CHIP). Although CHIP is increasingly common in otherwise healthy adults, such patients have an approximately 10-fold risk of developing MDS, at a rate of about 0.5% to 1% per year, and are commonly followed with additional BM examinations.

Clonal Cytopenia of Undetermined Significance

Clonal cytopenia of undetermined significance (CCUS) represents those patients with clonal hematopoiesis who also have cytopenia(s), but without morphologic changes sufficient to meet criteria for the diagnosis of MDS. Such patients nearly always progress to frank MDS. A newly recognized entity, called VEXAS syndrome (vacuoles, E1-enzyme, X-linked, autoinflammatory, somatic), is a multisystem form of clonal hematopoiesis associated with a somatic mutation in the *UBA1* gene; it may or may not be associated with definitive dysplastic changes and additional genetic abnormalities, but because of its unique clinical features is considered separately.

MDS Subtypes

The ICC and most clinicians formally divide MDS into low-grade and high-grade subtypes (Tables 5.8 and 5.9).

Low-Grade MDS

Subtypes without excess blasts all have in common a BM blast count <5% and a PB blast count of <2% (or 1% found only on one occasion); these have a low risk of transformation to AML. They differ mainly in the number of dysplastic cell lines and the presence or absence of specific mutations or cytogenetic abnormalities.

TABLE 5.8 Low-Grade MDS Subtypes

Category	Cytopenia	Dysplasia	Blasts	Genetics[a]
MDS with *SF3B1*	+	+	<5% BM <2% PB	• Must have *SF3B1* (VAF 10%) • Must exclude isolated del(5q); −7/del(7q); abn(3q26); complex karyotype
MDS with del(5q)	+[b]	+/−	<5% BM <2% PB	• Must have del(5q) (+/− one additional cytogenetic abnormality) • Must exclude −7/ del(7q)
MDS-NOS without dysplasia	+	−	<5% BM <2% PB	• Must have −7/del(7q) or complex karyotype • Must exclude *SF3B1*
MDS-NOS with SLD	+	+	<5% BM <2% PB	• Any • Must exclude *SF3B1* and del(5q)
MDS-NOS with MLD	+	+	<5% BM <2% PB	• Any • Must exclude *SF3B1* and del(5q)

abn, abnormal; BM, bone marrow; MDS, myelodysplastic syndrome; MLD, multilineage dysplasia; NOS, not otherwise specified; PB, peripheral blood; SLD, single lineage dysplasia; VAF, variant allele frequency.

[a]Must exclude multihit *TP53*.

[b]May have thrombocytosis.

TABLE 5.9 High-Grade MDS Subtypes

Category	Blasts	Genetics
MDS-EB	5%-9% BM 2%-9% PB	• Any • Must exclude multihit *TP53*
MDS/AML	10%-19% BM and PB	• Any • Must exclude AML-defining abnormalities • Must exclude *TP53* mutation
MDS with biallelic *TP53*	<20%	• Must have multihit *TP53* mutation

AML, acute myeloid leukemia; BM, bone marrow; EB, excess blasts; MDS, myelodysplastic syndrome; PB, peripheral blood.

MDS with *SF3B1* mutation is a low-grade lesion typically associated with RS, although neither RS nor other manifestations of dysplasia are required for diagnosis (Figure 5.20A and B; eFigure 5.6).

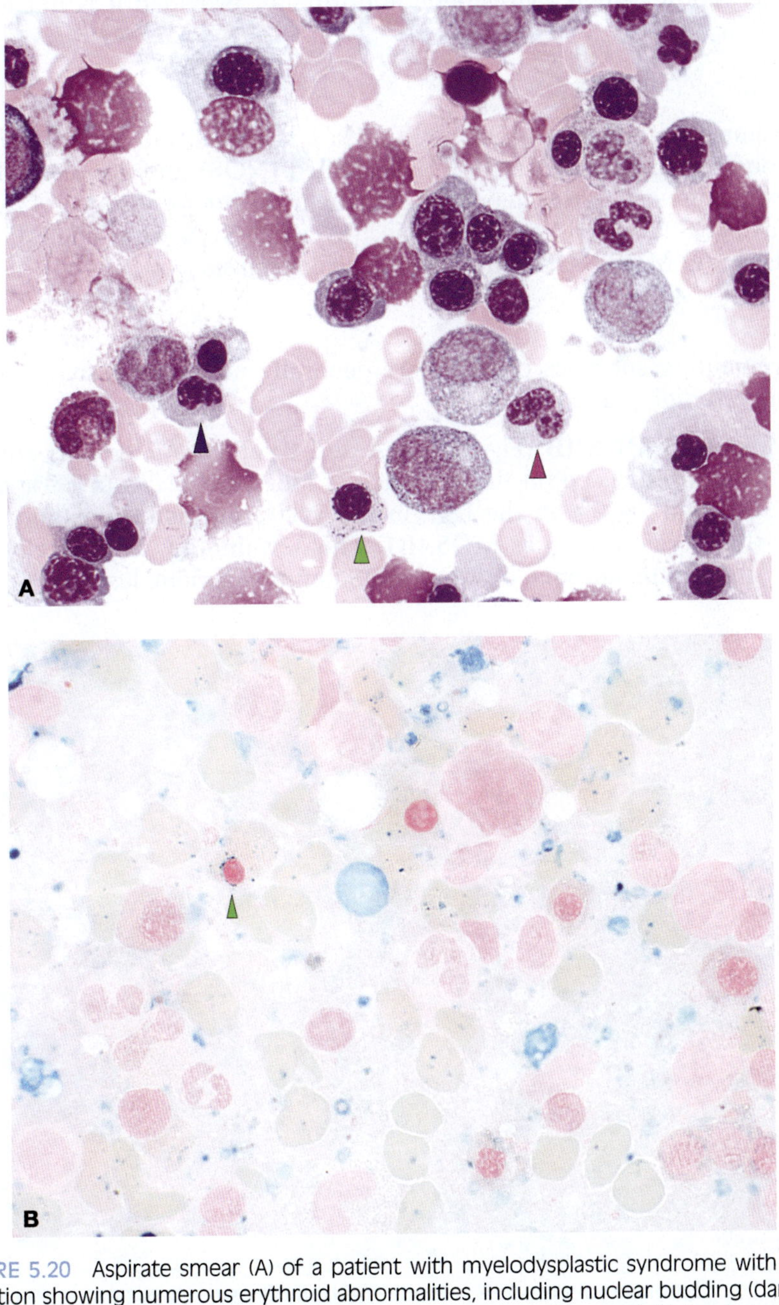

FIGURE 5.20 Aspirate smear (A) of a patient with myelodysplastic syndrome with *SF3B1* mutation showing numerous erythroid abnormalities, including nuclear budding (dark blue arrowhead) and basophilic stippling (green arrowhead), as well as myeloid dysplasia, including hypogranulation (pink arrowhead). An iron stain performed on the aspirate (B) showed abundant ring sideroblasts (arrowhead).

MDS with del(5q) is a low-grade lesion notable for characteristic changes in megakaryocytes (Figure 5.21; eFigure 5.7); it is most common in middle-aged females and is often accompanied by thrombocytosis. There may be another single cytogenetic abnormality, provided it is not monosomy 7 or del(7q).

MDS Not Otherwise Specified

The remaining cases of MDS with <5% BM blasts and <2% PB blasts are considered MDS not otherwise specified (NOS) and are divided into three separate categories depending on the presence or absence of dysplasia: (a) MDS-NOS without dysplasia; (b) MDS-NOS with single lineage dysplasia; (c) MDS-NOS with multilineage dysplasia.

High-Grade MDS

The remaining subtypes of MDS are generally more aggressive, and are considered high-grade.

MDS-EB/MDS-IB (Figure 5.22A and B; eFigure 5.8): This entity is diagnosed based on the presence of increased blasts (5%-9% in the BM and 2%-9% in the PB); in the WHO 5th edition classification this is referred to as MDS-IB1. This terminology is generally only used in the absence of other MDS-defining genetic lesions.

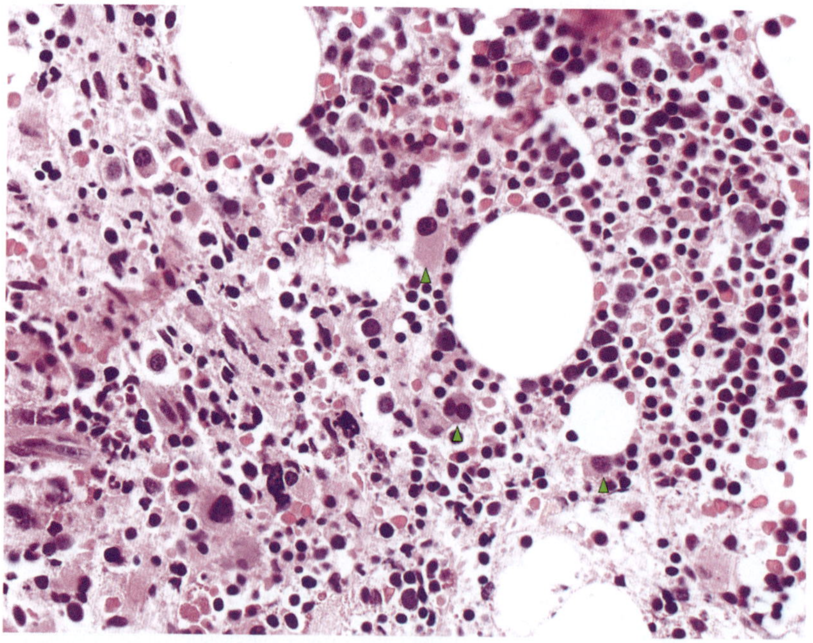

FIGURE 5.21 Megakaryocytes in this bone marrow biopsy of a patient with myelodysplastic syndrome with del(5q) are small and typically have round, unilobed, or sometimes bilobed nuclei (arrowheads).

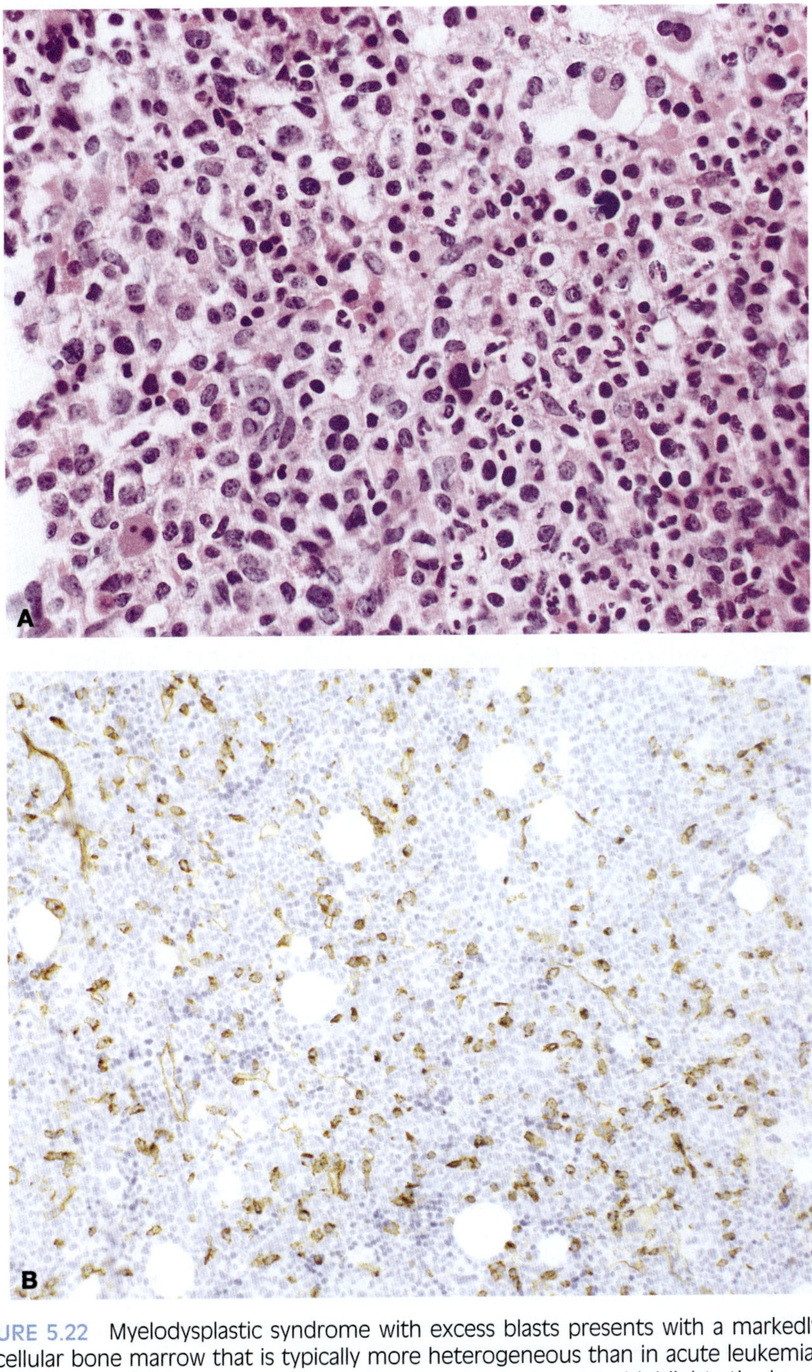

FIGURE 5.22 Myelodysplastic syndrome with excess blasts presents with a markedly hypercellular bone marrow that is typically more heterogeneous than in acute leukemia, but with increased blasts (A). An immunohistochemical stain for CD34 highlights the increased blasts (B).

MDS/AML: Cases of MDS with 10% to 19% blasts are classified as MDS-IB2 in the WHO 5th edition and are now referred to as MDS/AML in the ICC to emphasize the overlap with AML. The diagnosis requires detection of 10% to 19% blasts in the PB or BM, and a lack of AML-defining cytogenetic abnormalities and lack of mutations in *NPM1*, *bZIP*, *CEBPA*, or *TP53*. Cases meeting blast criteria for MDS/AML with *TP53* mutations are specifically classified as MDS/AML with mutated *TP53*.

MDS with mutated *TP53*: MDS with <10% blasts and multihit *TP53* mutations (or with a monoallelic mutation and a complex karyotype or loss of heterozygosity at 17p) is now considered a distinct category of MDS even if blasts are not increased or one of the other favorable genetic abnormalities is present, because of its very aggressive course.

MYELOID NEOPLASM (MDS/MPN) OVERLAP SYNDROMES

As the name suggests, these neoplasms display features of both MDS and MPNs,[1] with evidence of concurrent myeloproliferation and ineffective hematopoiesis.

The neoplasms in this category comprise CMML, atypical chronic myeloid leukemia (aCML), MDS/MPN with thrombocytosis and *SF3B1* mutations, MDS/MPN with RS and thrombocytosis, not otherwise specified (MDS-RS-T, NOS), and MDS/MPN, NOS (Table 5.10). Juvenile myelomonocytic leukemia (JMML), which was formally included in this category, is now subclassified as a germline mutation–associated disorder by the ICC and is beyond the scope of this chapter.

TABLE 5.10 MDS/MPN Categories

Disease	Cytosis	Cytopenia	Dysplasia
CMML	Monocytosis	Anemia	Dysplastic monocytes Dysplastic neutrophils
aCML[a]	Neutrophilia	Anemia	Dysplastic neutrophils
MDS/MPN-T-*SF3B1*	Thrombocytosis	Anemia	Ring sideroblasts
MDS/MPN-RS-T, NOS	Thrombocytosis	Anemia	≥15% ring sideroblasts
MDS/MPN-NOS	Any	Any	Any

aCML, atypical chronic myeloid leukemia; CMML, chronic myelomonocytic leukemia; MDS, myelodysplastic syndrome; MDS/MPN-T-*SF3B1*, MDS/MPN with thrombocytosis and *SF3B1* mutation; MDS/MPN-RS-T, NOS, MDS/MPN with ring sideroblasts and thrombocytosis, not otherwise specified; MPN, myeloproliferative neoplasm.

[a]aCML is replaced by the term "MPN with neutrophilia" in the WHO 5th edition classification.

Clinical

These disorders have numerous similarities with other primary BM disorders, and therefore, the correct diagnosis requires integration of clinical, morphologic, and genetic information. This includes knowledge of the patient's history including current and prior complete blood count (CBC) records, because some diagnoses rely on persistence of blood count abnormalities; moreover, some diseases have morphologic overlap in the marrow and are best distinguished by blood findings. Physical findings are also useful, particularly knowledge of splenomegaly, which suggests extramedullary hematopoiesis.

Evaluation of the PB typically shows cytoses in some lineages and cytopenias in others. Commonly, patients present with an elevated WBC count and anemia. Platelet counts are variable and may be normal, decreased, or increased, depending on the specific MDS/MPN subcategory.

Monocytosis is a key distinguishing feature in many disorders, and its presence rules out others. Monocytic and neutrophilic dysplasia is common in the PB, and these dysplastic changes may make differentiating between the two cell types difficult. Blasts may be slightly increased, but must be <20% of total cellularity in the PB and BM.

Morphology

Morphologic evaluation of the BM often shows a hypercellular marrow for age with hyperplasia of one or more lineages and progressive maturation of the myeloid and erythroid precursors. The proliferative lineage depends on the disorder: In cases of CMML, the myeloid component is elevated. In MDS/MPN with thrombocytosis and *SF3B1* mutations and MDS/MPN-RS-T, NOS, the erythroid and megakaryocytic lineages are increased. Megakaryocytes are often dysplastic appearing, resembling the megakaryocytes of MDS, with the exception of MDS/MPN with thrombocytosis (with or without *SF3B1* mutations), in which the megakaryocytes have an MPN-like appearance.

Immunophenotype

FC can confirm the increased monocytic cells, but cannot take the place of morphologic evaluation. Although monocytic markers are helpful to identify the lineage involved, monocyte quantitation by FC is not accurate and there is little specific correlation between monocyte phenotype and disease; in particular, an MPN with monocytosis may be difficult to distinguish from acute leukemia with monocytic differentiation. Likewise, FC can identify increased blasts, but should not be a replacement for morphologic blast assessment and enumeration.

Some cases have inadequate or poor BM aspirate smears, which precludes accurate morphologic assessment or blast enumeration. In those cases, IHC may be performed on the core biopsy to help assess blast count, although this is typically challenging because there is no phenotypic definition of a monoblast.

Genetics

A conventional karyotype is recommended for all cases of suspected MDS/MPNs. Although there are no defining cytogenetic abnormalities, an abnormal karyotype helps confirm the clonal nature of the disorder. FISH panels are helpful to detect the abnormalities commonly observed in MDS, including abnormalities of chromosomes 5, 7, and 17.

Molecular tests, including NGS panels, detect mutations commonly seen in MDS/MPNs and are useful to document clonality. Different entities generally have different mutational patterns although there is some overlap.

Chronic Myelomonocytic Leukemia

CMML is a clonal neoplasm that presents as a sustained monocytosis in the PB. To make this diagnosis, all reactive causes must be excluded, and certain criteria must be met (Table 5.11), including sustained monocytosis (>500/µL with at least 10% monocytes) of >3 months duration and dysplasia in at least one cell lineage, increased blasts, or cytogenetic or specific molecular abnormalities.

CMML is often further subclassified as "proliferative" or "dysplastic"[11,12] depending on the WBC count (Table 5.12) as these subtypes have different prognoses. As the name suggests, dysplastic CMML shows dysplastic features, with abnormal monocytes and hypogranular neutrophils in the PB, and dysplastic megakaryocytes in the BM. In addition to proliferative and dysplastic features, CMML is further subdivided based on the percentage of blasts in the PB or BM (Table 5.13).[13] Those cases with <10% blasts in the BM and <5% in the PB are considered CMML-1; those with 10% to 19% blasts in the BM or 5% to 19% blasts in the PB (or the presence of Auer rods) are considered CMML-2. If blasts are 20% or greater, the diagnosis is AML. CMML-0, which was previously designated as cases with <5% blasts in the BM and <1% in the PB, is no longer a recognized subtype.

TABLE 5.11 **Diagnostic Criteria for CMML**
Persistent monocytosis (>500/µL; ≥10% of WBC)
Exclusion of other disorders
Blasts <20%
Dysplasia of ≥1 lineage
OR genetic abnormality
OR ≥3 months monocytosis and no reactive causes

CMML, chronic myelomonocytic leukemia; WBC, white blood cell.

TABLE 5.12 Proliferative CMML Versus Dysplastic CMML

Myeloproliferative CMML	Myelodysplastic CMML
WBC >13 g/dL	WBC <13 g/dL
+/− Splenomegaly	−/+ Splenomegaly
−/+ Dysplasia	+ Dysplasia
Dysplasia-associated mutations in RAS pathway genes (*NRAS*, *KRAS*, *CBL*)	Dysplasia-associated mutations in *SRSF2*, *TET2*, and/or *ASXL1* (etc.)
Proliferative-associated mutations in *JAK2* and *SETBP1*	
Worse prognosis	Better prognosis

CMML, chronic myelomonocytic leukemia; g, grams; dL, deciliters; WBC, white blood cells.

TABLE 5.13 CMML Subgroups

Disease	PB blasts	BM blasts
CMML-1	<5%	5%-10%
CMML-2	5%-19%	10%-19%

BM, bone marrow; CMML, chronic myelomonocytic leukemia; PB, peripheral blood.

Clinical

This is a rare neoplasm, affecting 0.4/100,000 people, most often occurring in the elderly population. The median age at diagnosis is 65 to 75 years.

Patients present with symptoms based on the primary manifestation of the disease, that is, proliferative CMML often presents with constitutional symptoms, like fever, weight loss, and night sweats, whereas dysplastic CMML often presents with fatigue and increased infections, reflecting the sequelae of ineffective hematopoiesis. Although more common in proliferative CMML, both proliferative and dysplastic CMML may present with splenomegaly.

Morphologic

Monocytosis is invariably present (>500/µL; >10% of the WBC differential) and is part of the diagnostic criteria for both proliferative and dysplastic CMML. The monocytes are mature, but may have abnormal morphology, including abnormal nuclear chromatin, and are referred to as abnormal monocytes (Figure 5.23A-D; eFigure 5.9). Abnormal monocytes must be distinguished from promonocytes and monoblasts, which are considered blast equivalents.

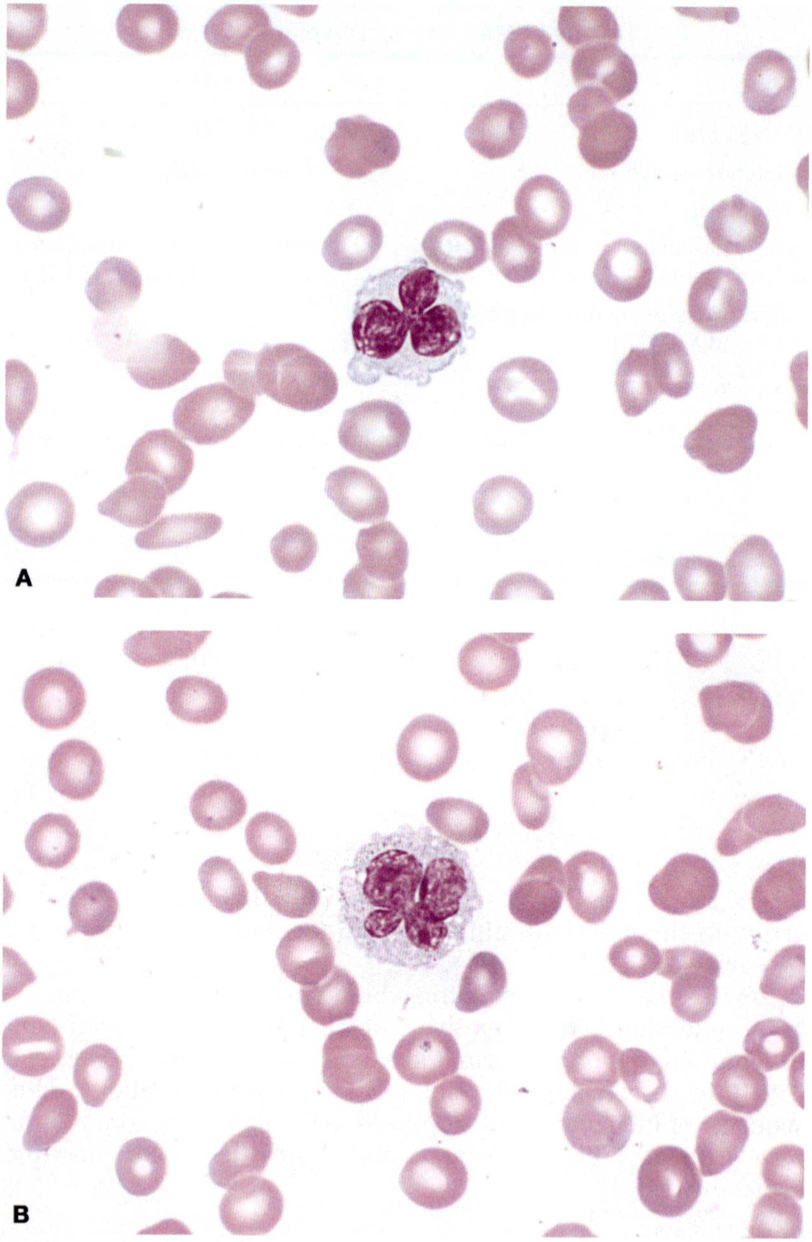

A

B

FIGURE 5.23 **Peripheral blood (PB) and bone marrow (BM) from a patient with chronic myelomonocytic leukemia.** Abnormal monocytes are identified in the PB (A and B), and a myeloid left shift with monocytosis is present in the BM aspirate (C and D).

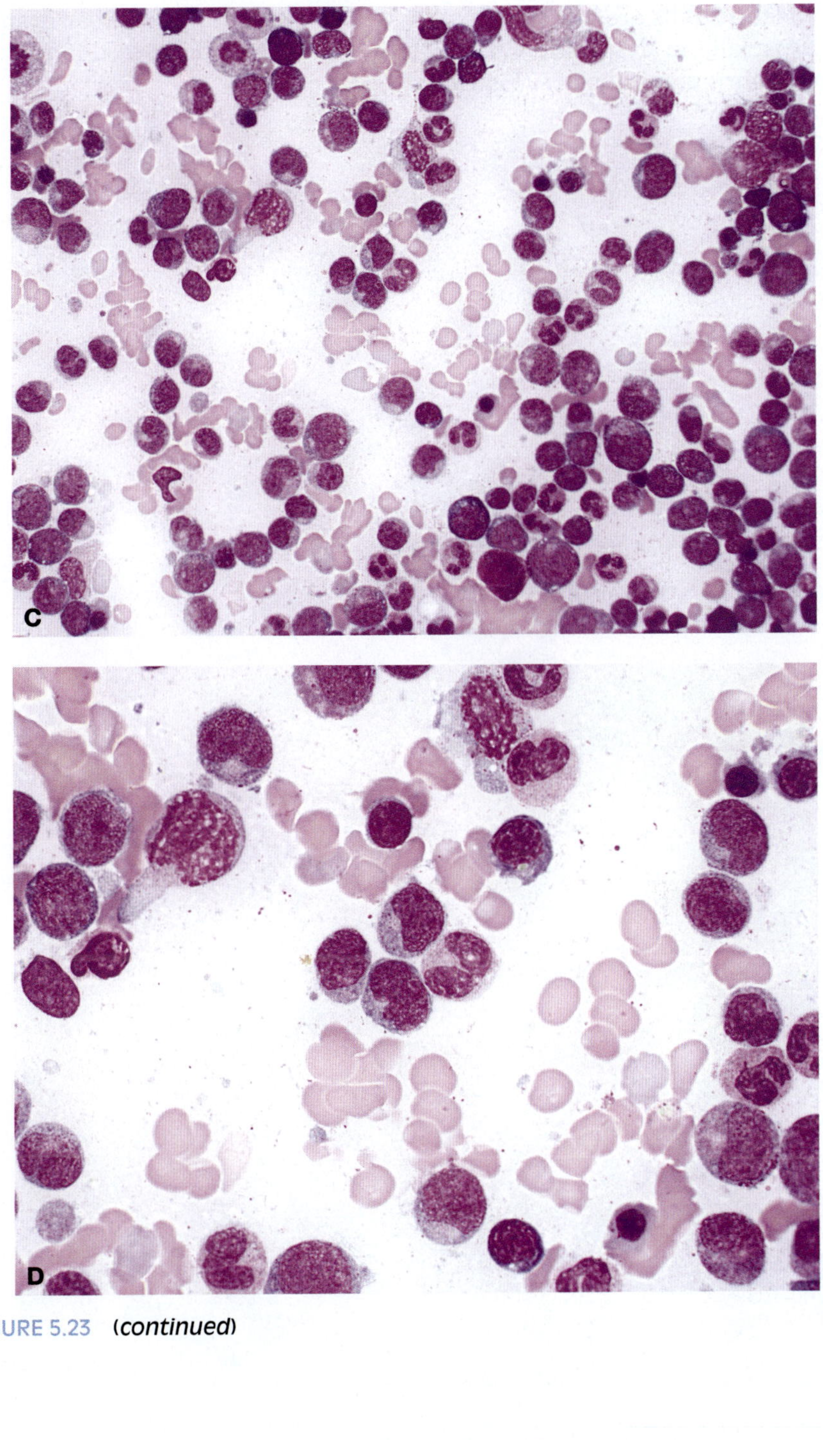

FIGURE 5.23 *(continued)*

Neutrophils are not significantly left-shifted, but may appear dysplastic, especially in dysplastic CMML, and are often difficult to differentiate from abnormal monocytes (Figure 5.24A-C).

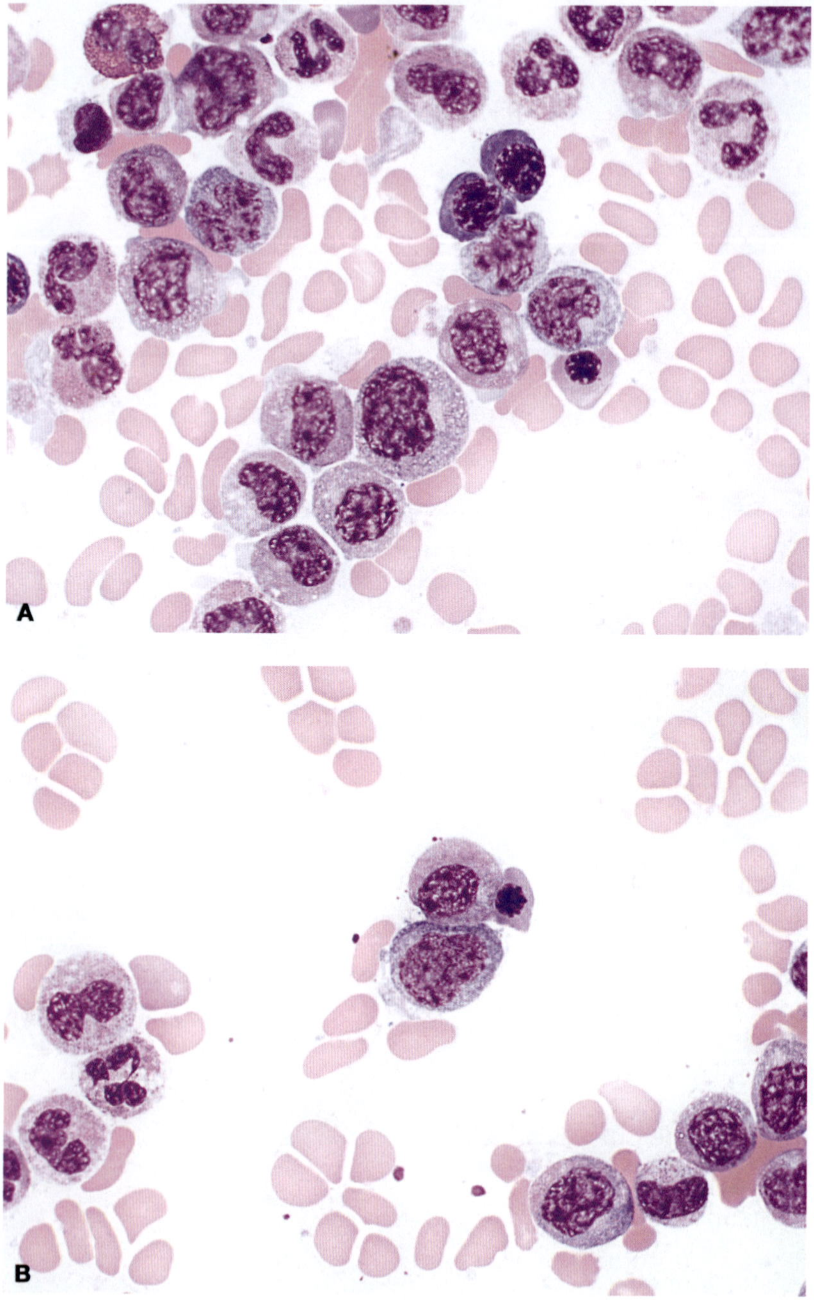

FIGURE 5.24 Neutrophils are often dysplastic in chronic myelomonocytic leukemia and may be difficult to differentiate from abnormal monocytes as seen in these bone marrow aspirates (A,B).

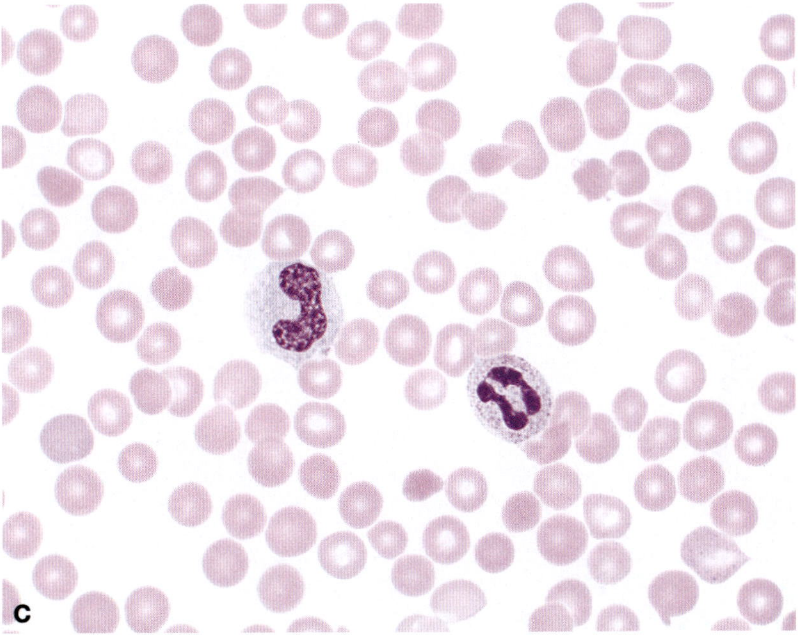

FIGURE 5.24 *(continued)* In Figure C, the peripheral blood in this patient with CMML shows abnormal myeloid cells. The cell on the left has morphologic features between a neutrophil and a monocyte.

Evaluation of the BM most often reveals a hypercellular for age marrow with a myelomonocytic hyperplasia. The monocytic component, plainly evident in the PB, may be difficult to appreciate on the BM core and even on the aspirate smear, which may simply resemble a marrow with a myeloid left shift (Figure 5.25A and B); IHC or cytochemical stains may be required to help highlight the monocytes. Megakaryocytes can appear small and hypolobated (in up to 80% of cases), and erythroid precursors, although typically relatively reduced, may display some dysplastic features.

Nodules of plasmacytoid dendritic cells (PDCs) are identified in the BM of 20% of patients with CMML and can be found at extramedullary sites. PDCs have round nuclei, fine chromatin, and eosinophilic cytoplasm. These nodules of PDCs in CMML are neoplastic and related to the CMML clone.[14,15] They express CD123, CD4, CD43, and only rarely express CD56. These nodules must be differentiated from blastic PDC neoplasms (BPDCN), which are aggressive and described further in Chapter 7.

Phenotype

FC simultaneously evaluates multiple monocytic markers on the population to detect aberrant features.[16] Decreased CD14 often only indicates monocytic immaturity, but an aberrant pattern of expression with human leukocyte antigen-D related (HLA-DR) can be a marker of aberrant

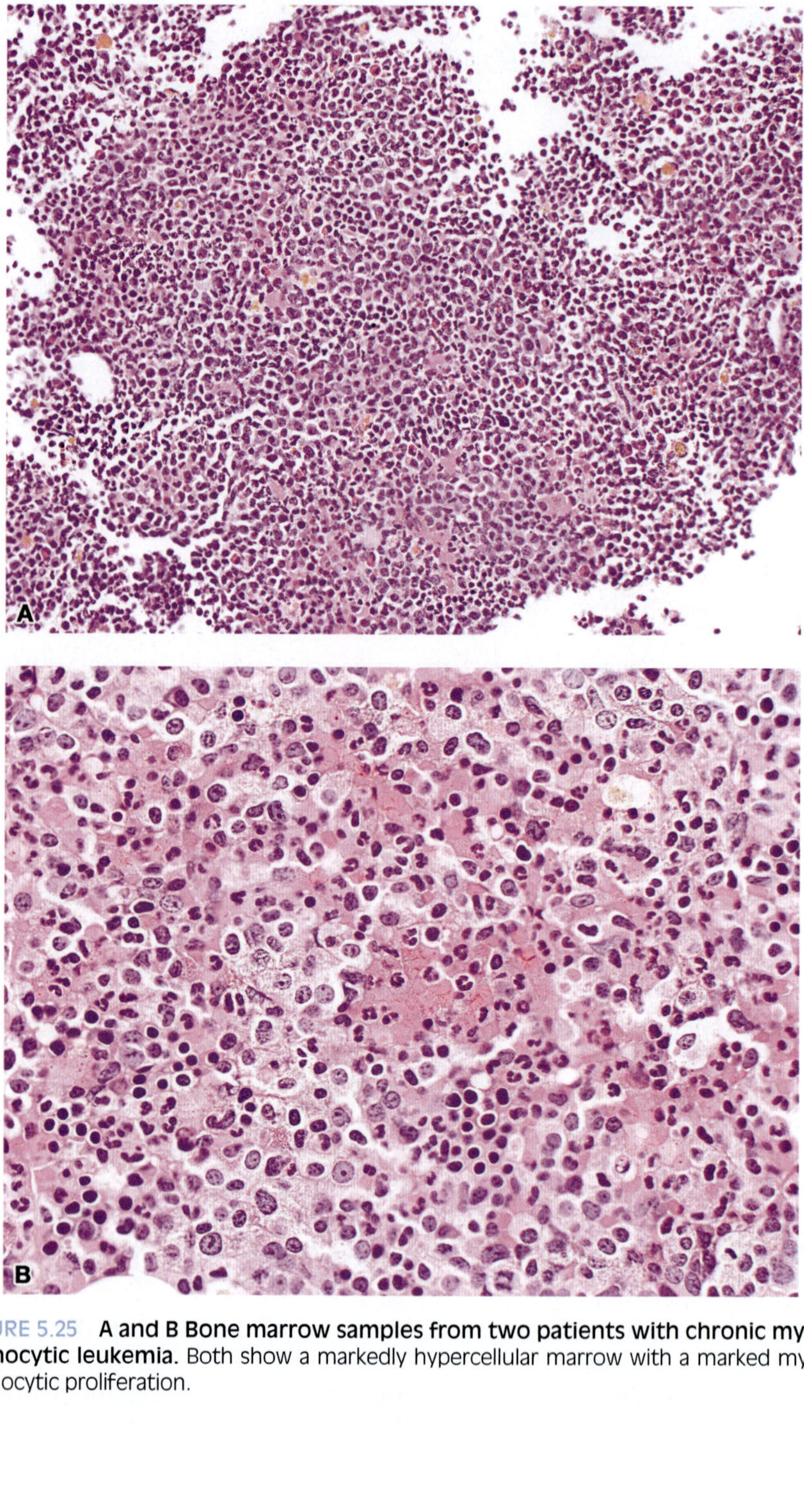

FIGURE 5.25 **A and B Bone marrow samples from two patients with chronic myelomonocytic leukemia.** Both show a markedly hypercellular marrow with a marked myelomonocytic proliferation.

expression. Increased classical monocytes (CD64 positive, CD14 positive, CD16 negative) may be used as a method to distinguish CMML from reactive monocytosis (Figure 5.26A and B).[17-19] CD56 expression on monocytes, although not specific, is more prevalent in CMML than in nonneoplastic diseases and may persist in the PB (Figure 5.27).[20]

Special stains for neuron-specific enolase (NSE) alone or in combination with chloroacetate ester (CAE) may be helpful to distinguish immature monocytes from mature monocytes and from dysplastic neutrophils.

Immunohistochemical monocytic markers are useful in cases with a dry tap aspirate. CD33, lysozyme, and CD68 highlight monocytic cells of all maturation stages and are typically much dimmer or negative for CD15 and myeloperoxidase. Mature monocytes express bright CD14 and CD163.

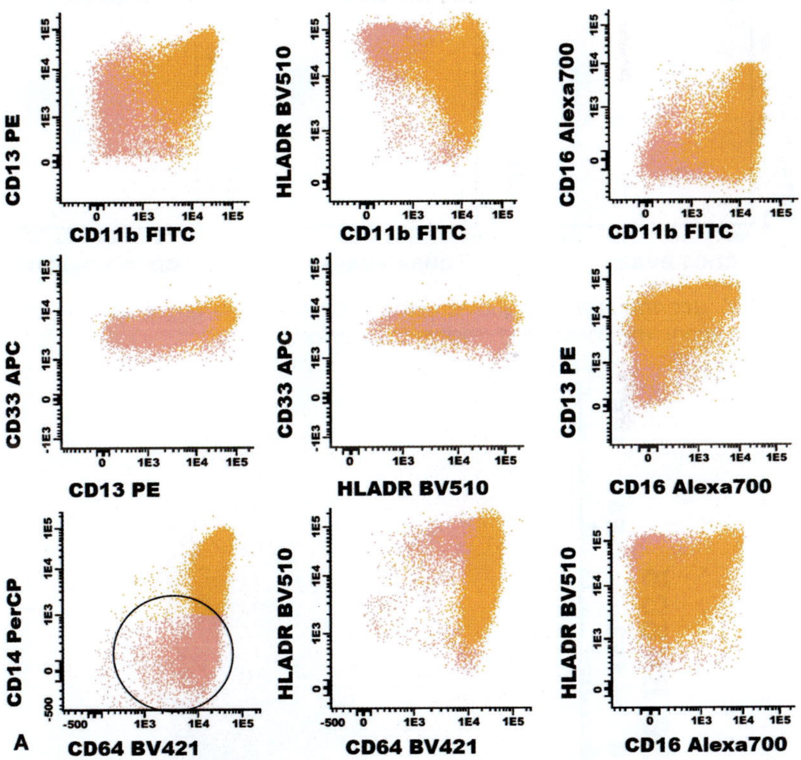

FIGURE 5.26 **Flow cytometry of two patients with monocytosis.** A, The monocytes in this patient's case show a much higher proportion of CD14-negative and CD64 dim immature monocytes (circled light pink population); this patient was diagnosed with chronic myelomonocytic leukemia.

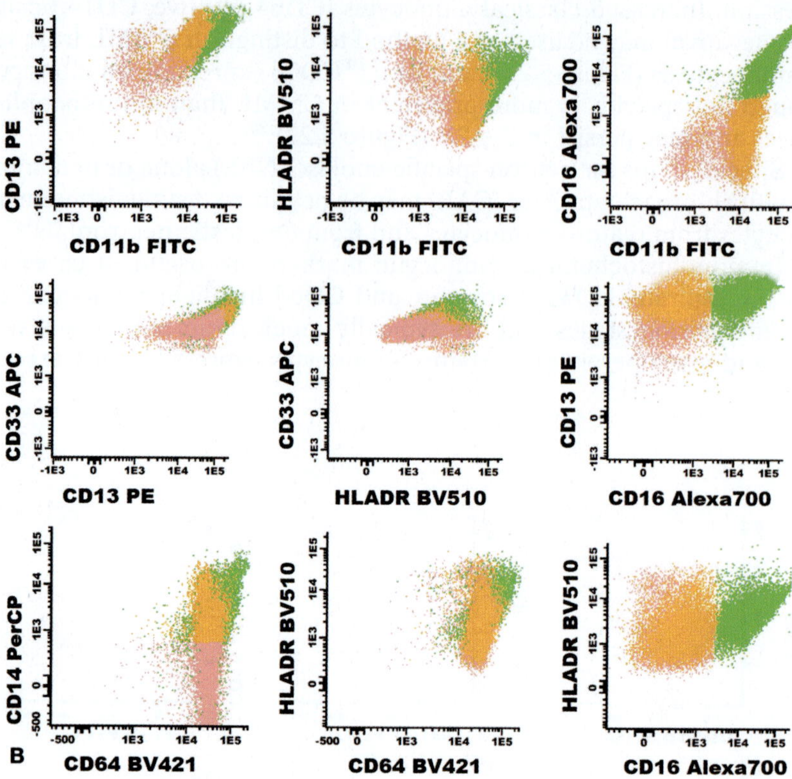

FIGURE 5.26 (*continued*) B, A subset of monocytes express bright CD16 in this case (green population). This patient had reactive monocytosis.

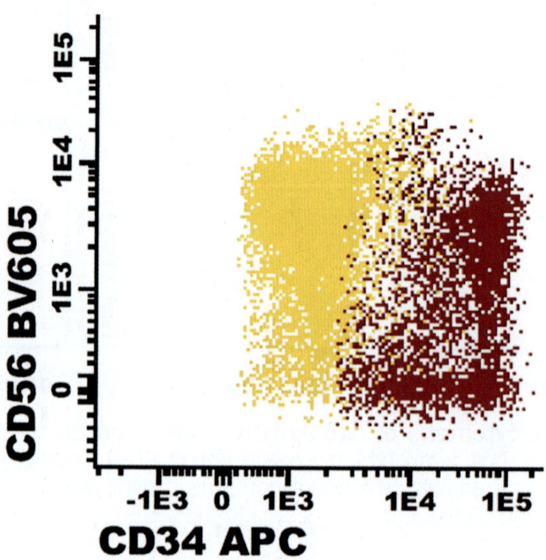

FIGURE 5.27 This flow cytometry example shows CD56 expression on monocytes (yellow population) as well as the blasts (brown population).

Genetics

A conventional karyotype is recommended for all cases of suspected CMML. Although there is no specific genetic alteration, the presence of any abnormality supports the diagnosis, as up to half of all cases have cytogenetic abnormalities. The most common cytogenetic abnormalities include trisomy 8, monosomy 7, and del(7q). Abnormalities of 11q23 are not commonly seen and suggests an alternate diagnosis of AML.

Most cases of CMML have somatic mutations including *ASXL1*, *TET2*, and *SRSF2* most commonly. *RUNX1*, *CBL*, *EZH2*, and *NRAS* are also seen. *NPM1* is not commonly seen in CMML and, if identified, may suggest either *de novo* AML or progression to AML. Even if AML cannot be documented, cases of CMML with *NPM1* mutations are clinically more aggressive.

Differential Diagnosis

The differential is broad and requires the exclusion of reactive and other neoplastic conditions. Reactive monocytosis is common in patients with infections, notably tuberculosis. Acute myelomonocytic leukemia or acute monocytic leukemia must be excluded. A definitive diagnosis of CMML should not be made based on blood findings without a marrow examination because in some cases of acute monocytic leukemia, monocytes may appear more mature in the PB (Figure 5.28A-D).

In more than half of all cases, the PB shows a neutrophilia in addition to the monocytosis. In these cases, it is critical to rule out *BCR::ABL1*-positive CML, as the p190 isoform of CML may present with increased monocytes, mimicking CMML. The proliferative form of CMML may have *JAK2* mutations and thus may be confused with other *BCR::ABL1*-negative MPNs, although other morphologic and laboratory findings can help exclude these. Neoplasms associated with eosinophilia and rearrangements of tyrosine kinase genes (see Chapter 6) may have significant monocytosis in addition to eosinophilia; especially in cases in which eosinophilia is not striking, these must also be ruled out as the therapy is very different.

CMML is commonly the associated neoplasm in cases of mastocytosis with associated myeloid neoplasm (SM-AMN), so that evidence of concomitant mastocytosis should be searched for in cases with increased mast cells or clinical findings.

CMML should also be distinguished from the newly recognized **clonal monocytosis of undetermined significance (CMUS)**.[2] This entity is defined as a persistent monocytosis in the absence of reactive causes, with the presence of one or more myeloid neoplasm–associated mutation(s), but lacking significant dysplasia or blasts in blood or marrow, and typically lacking a myeloid-predominant hypercellular marrow.

Prognosis

The prognosis varies, but the average survival for patients is 2 to 4 years.[21] Approximately 15% to 30% of patients progress to AML. Acquired mutations in *RUNX1* have been associated with progression to AML.

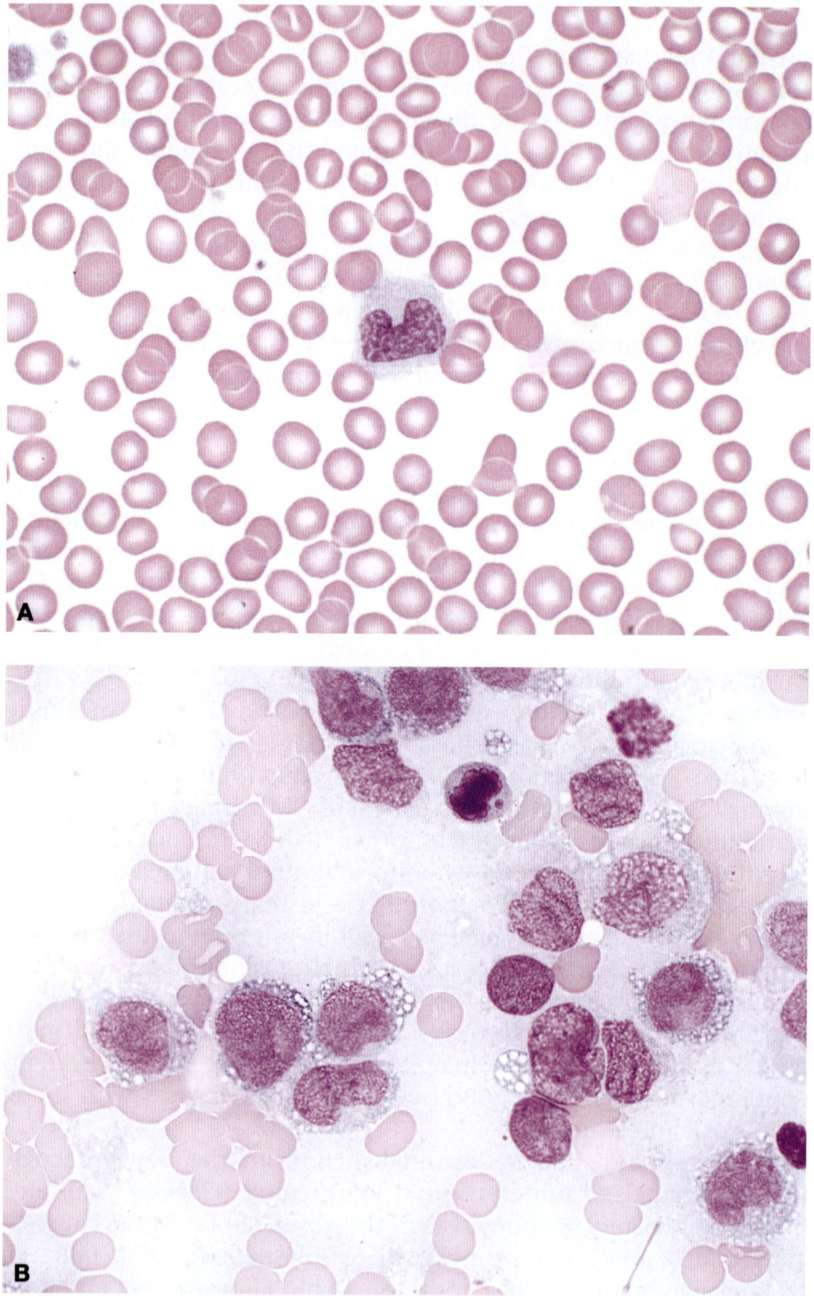

FIGURE 5.28 Mature-appearing monocytes (A) may be present in the peripheral blood (PB) of a patient with acute monoblastic leukemia in the bone marrow (BM) (B) and may be indistinguishable from the PB monocytes (C) in a patient with a BM showing chronic myelomonocytic leukemia (D).

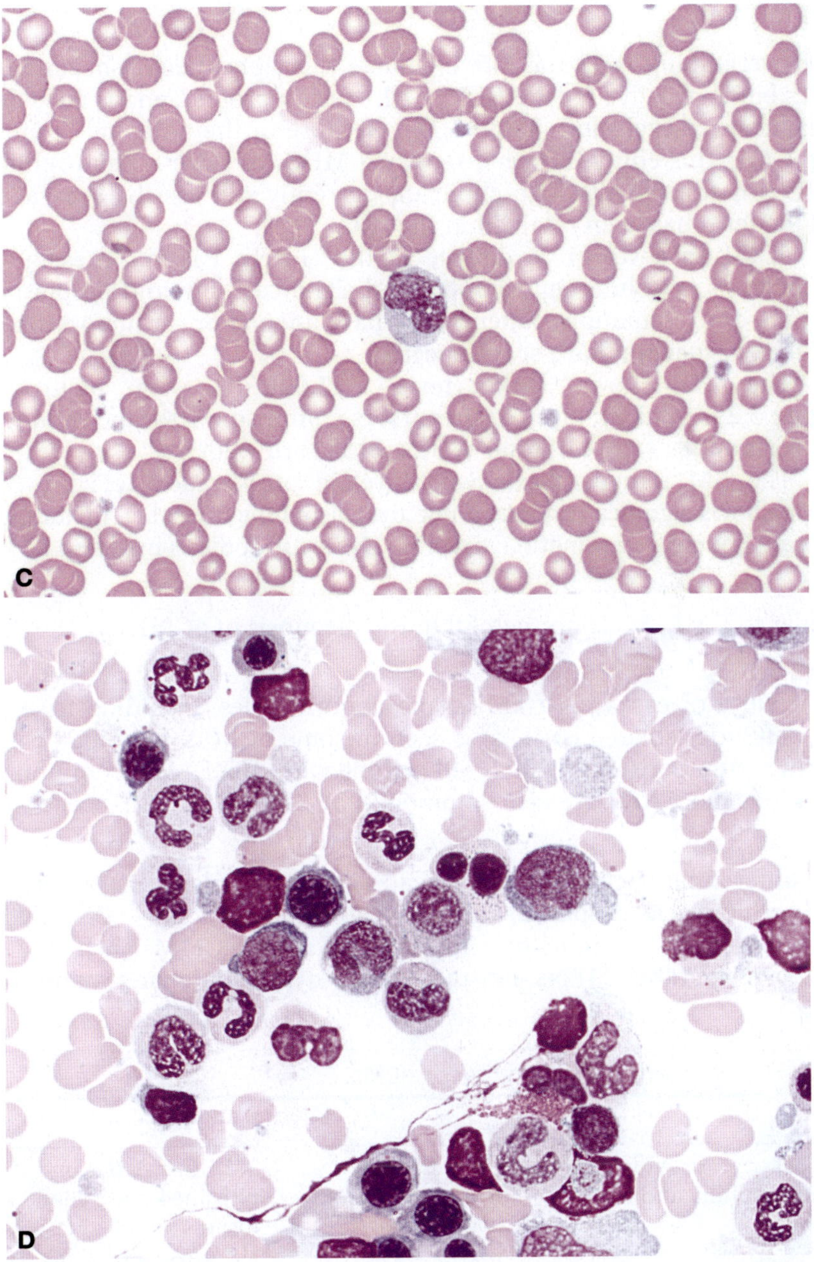

FIGURE 5.28 (*continued*)

Atypical CML

With overlapping MDS and MPN features, this clonal neoplasm can mimic CML, but is negative for the *BCR::ABL1* fusion protein, and is considered a diagnosis of exclusion (Table 5.14). Because of the potential confusion with CML, this entity has been renamed MDS/MPN with neutrophilia in WHO 5th edition, although clinicians currently still use the term aCML, and the term has been retained in the ICC.

aCML is a very rare disease of the elderly. Patients present with leukocytosis, absolute neutrophilia, and significant myeloid dysplasia. At the time of presentation, patients may have anemia or thrombocytopenia, and may or may not have splenomegaly.

The PB shows leukocytosis ≥13,000/µL with neutrophilia (Figure 5.29A and B); myeloid precursors comprise >10% and monocytes and eosinophils <10% of total WBCs. Blasts are <20%.

The BM is hyperplastic with myeloid proliferation (eFigure 5.10). aCML shows significant neutrophilic dysplasia (eFigure 5.11), including exaggerated nuclear chromatin clumping. Dyserythropoiesis may also be seen.

Immunophenotype

Similar to CML, FC is not helpful in the diagnosis of aCML.

Genetics

Up to 80% of cases have karyotypic abnormalities, including trisomy 8 and del(20q). Isolated iso(17q) is seen in some aCMLs, although it is not specific. Mutations in *SETBP1*, often along with *ASXL1*, are common, and mutations in *ETNK1* are also common in aCML.[22-24]

Differential

The differential includes reactive causes and neoplastic disorders, like CML, which lacks dysplasia; chronic neutrophilic leukemia (CNL), which lacks dysplasia and immature myeloid cells; and CMML, which has a monocytosis; other MPNs can rarely have dysplastic changes and might

TABLE 5.14 Diagnostic Criteria for aCML

PB	BM	Genetics
• Leukocytosis with neutrophilia and left shift • Cytopenias • No eosinophilia • No monocytosis • Blasts <20%	• Hypercellular BM with myeloid hyperplasia • Blasts <20%	• No *BCR::ABL1* or tyrosine kinase gene fusions • No MPN driver mutations • Mutations in *SETBP* in association with *ASXL1* supports diagnosis

aCML, atypical chronic myeloid leukemia; BM, bone marrow; MPN, myeloproliferative neoplasm; PB, peripheral blood.

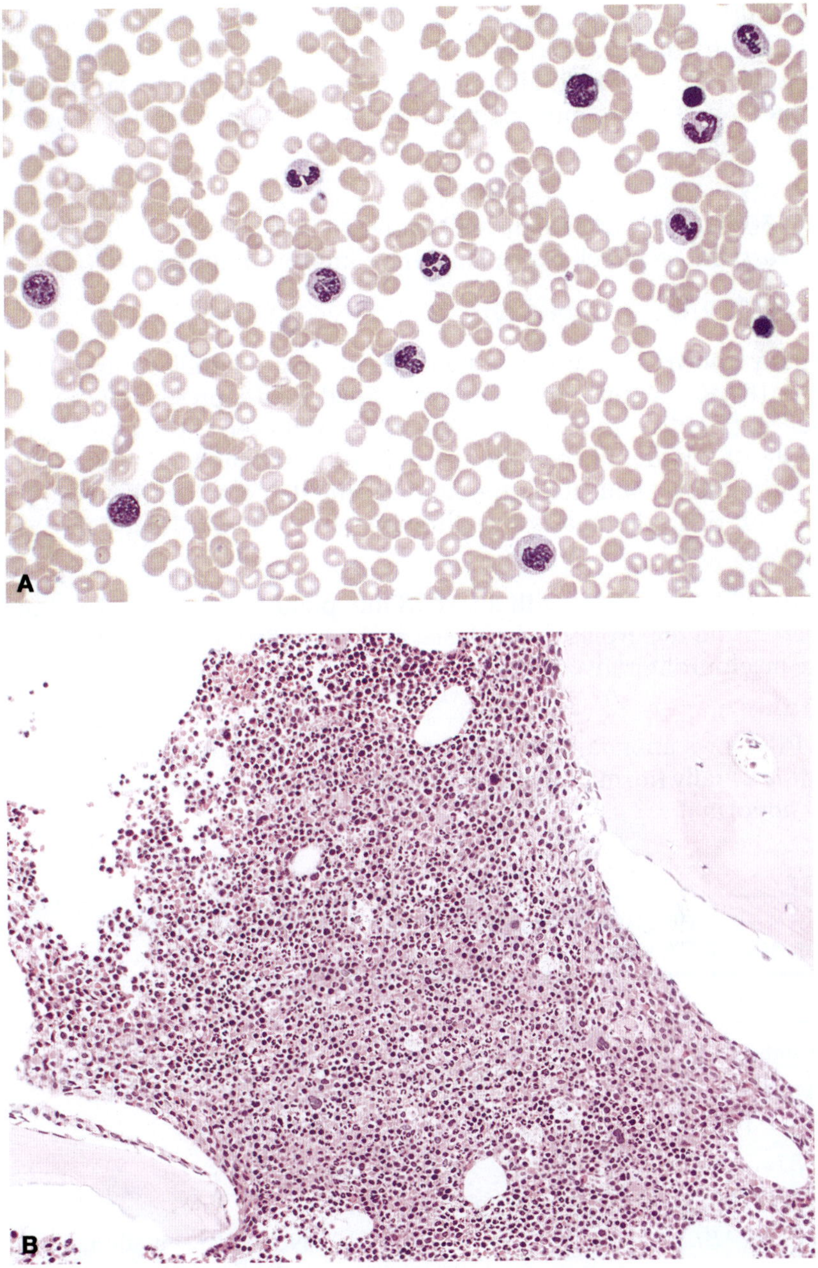

FIGURE 5.29 **Atypical chronic myeloid leukemia.** A, Neutrophilia in the peripheral blood, with some dysplastic-appearing neutrophils. The core biopsy (B) shows a markedly hypercellular marrow with a myeloid hyperplasia.

be considered. Genetic testing is useful to differentiate among these: *BCR::ABL1* would be seen in CML, whereas *JAK2*, *CALR*, or *MPL* would suggest an MPN. *CSF3R*, although rarely seen in aCML, is far more common in CNL, so care must be taken before making an aCML diagnosis if this is present.

Prognosis

About 30% to 40% of patients will evolve to AML. The overall survival is 2 to 3 years, but stem cell transplants have improved outcomes.[25]

MDS/MPN With Thrombocytosis and *SF3B1* Mutation

Formerly known as "refractory anemia with ring sideroblasts and thrombocytosis (RARS-T)" this entity is now defined by the presence of an *SF3B1* mutation (>10% variant allele frequency [VAF]) even if RS are not present. If >15% RS are identified in the absence of the mutation, but with characteristic morphologic and laboratory findings, the ICC employs the term "MDS/MPN with ring sideroblasts and thrombocytosis, NOS" (Table 5.15).

Clinical

This neoplasm presents with an MDS-like picture, with refractory anemia and erythroid hyperplasia, dysplasia, and typically with RS, but also shows some myeloproliferative features.

Morphologic

The PB shows anemia with anisocytosis and dimorphic RBCs. The WBC count is usually normal. Platelets are elevated and can appear morphologically abnormal.

TABLE 5.15 Diagnostic Criteria for MDS/MPN-T-*SF3B1* Versus MDS/MPN-RS-T, NOS

MDS/MPN-T-*SF3B1*	MDS/MPN-RS-T, NOS
Thrombocytosis	Thrombocytosis
Anemia +/− RS	Anemia + ≥15% RS
Blasts <1%	Blasts <1%
SF3B1 mutation	Clonality
JAK2, CALR, MPL mutation support dx	
No *BCR::ABL1*	No *SF3B1* mutation; no *BCR::ABL1*
Exclude reactive causes	Exclude reactive causes
Exclude other MDS/MPN	Exclude other MDS/MPN

dx, diagnosis; MDS, myelodysplastic syndrome; MPN, myeloproliferative neoplasm; NOS, not otherwise specified; RS, ring sideroblasts; T, thrombocytosis.

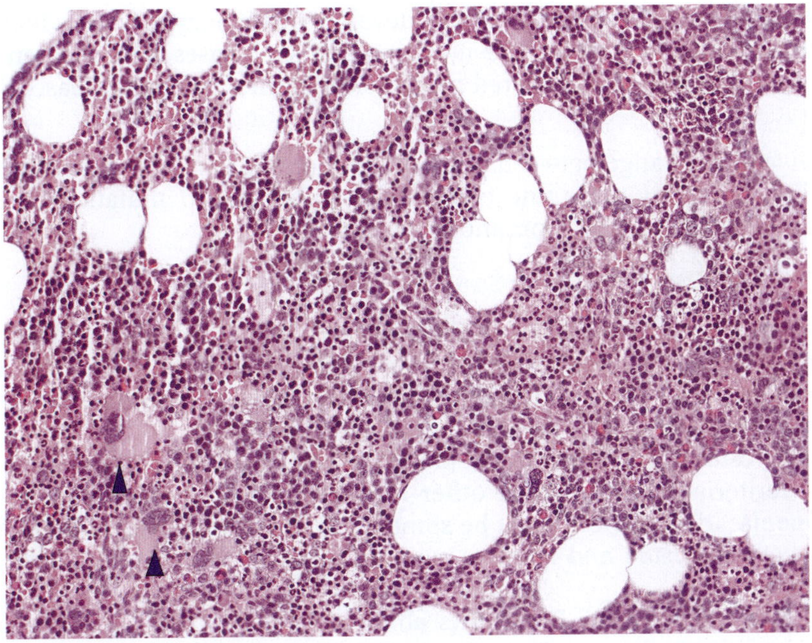

FIGURE 5.30 The core biopsy of this patient with myelodysplastic syndrome (MDS)-T-*SF3B1* shows an erythroid hyperplasia and increased atypical large megakaryocytes with morphologic features more typical of those seen in myeloproliferative neoplasm than MDS (arrowheads).

The BM shows erythroid hyperplasia and increased atypical megakaryocytes, similar to those seen in MPNs (Figure 5.30). Multilineage dysplasia may be seen. An iron stain performed on the aspirate smear often reveals increased RS.

Immunophenotype

FC plays no role in establishing this diagnosis, but may be used to characterize blasts for the purpose of disease monitoring when they are increased.

Genetics

In addition to the *SF3B1* mutation, 60% of cases also have the canonical *JAK2* mutation seen in MPNs, whereas <10% have *MPL* or *CALR* mutations.

Differential

Differential diagnostic considerations include MDS with del(5q), which presents with many similar findings (refractory anemia with increased megakaryocytes). However, the megakaryocytes in del(5q) are small and hypolobated, unlike the large atypical megakaryocytes of MDS/MPN-T-SF3B1. MDS with t(3;3)/inv(3) must also be ruled out, as these present with abnormal megakaryocytes and may have thrombocytosis. Cases of

MDS with *SF3B1* mutations may develop thrombocytosis late in their course from an acquired *JAK2* mutation and such cases are not given this diagnosis but rather considered progression of their original disease.

Prognosis

Survival times range between 76 and 128 months. Part of the justification behind separating these into two entities is that *SF3B1* mutations are associated with a favorable prognosis.

MDS/MPN, Not Otherwise Specified (MDS/MPN-NOS)

This entity is a diagnosis of exclusion, reserved for those MDS/MPN overlap cases that cannot be further subtyped (Table 5.16). The true incidence of this disorder is unknown, as they have been grouped together with other MPNs in the past.

To establish this diagnosis, blood counts of some lineage must meet MPN criteria, whereas some other lineage must meet MDS criteria for cytopenia. Ideally, there must be some marker of clonality, but if the findings have persisted and reactive causes excluded, this diagnosis can still be made.

Evaluation of the BM shows abnormal small MDS-like megakaryocytes in half of all cases. The other half must have a mixture of MDS- and MPN-like megakaryocytes.

Genetics

There is a similar cytogenetic and molecular profile to other MDS/MPNs, but nothing specific.

Differential

These cases may be difficult to differentiate from reactive causes. This diagnosis should not be rendered in a patient with cytotoxic or growth factor therapy. Additionally, this diagnosis should not be made in a patient with a known MPN who develops dysplastic features.

TABLE 5.16 Diagnostic Criteria for MDS/MPN, NOS

PB	BM	Genetics
• Cytoses • Cytopenia • <20% blasts	• MPN and MDS features, without meeting criteria for other MDS/MPNs • <20% blasts	• No *BCR::ABL1* or other tyrosine kinase fusions • Lacking t(3;3) or inv(3) • Lacking del(5q)

BM, bone marrow; del, deletion; inv, inversion; MDS, myelodysplastic syndrome; MPN, myeloproliferative neoplasm; NOS, not otherwise specified; PB, peripheral blood; t, translocation.

Cytogenetic/molecular studies should be performed to rule out CML, myeloid/lymphoid neoplasms with eosinophilia, del(5q), and t(3;3)/inv(3). Finding a high VAF MPN-associated mutation would more likely suggest evolution of an underlying MPN rather than MDS/MPN, NOS.

Recently, a provisional subtype of MDS/MPN-unclassifiable with isolated isochromosome (17q) has been proposed. Although it is not clear if it is simply a variant of aCML with a distinct cytogenetic abnormality, it shows similar clinical and laboratory features to aCML including frequent *SETBP1* mutations.

REFERENCES

1. Arber DA, Orazi A, Hasserjian R, et al. The 2016 revision to the World Health Organization classification of myeloid neoplasms and acute leukemia. *Blood.* 2016;127(20):2391-2405.
2. Arber DA, Orazi A, Hasserjian RP, et al. International consensus classification of myeloid neoplasms and acute leukemia: integrating morphological, clinical, and genomic data. *Blood.* 2022;140(11):1200-1228.
3. Khoury JD, Solary E, Abla O, et al. The 5th edition of the World Health Organization classification of haematolymphoid tumours: myeloid and histiocytic/dendritic neoplasms. *Leukemia.* 2022;36(7):1703-1719.
4. Ma X. Epidemiology of myelodysplastic syndromes. *Am J Med.* 2012;125(7 Suppl):S2-S5.
5. Amin HM, Yang Y, Shen Y, et al. Having a higher blast percentage in circulation than bone marrow: clinical implications in myelodysplastic syndrome and acute lymphoid and myeloid leukemias. *Leukemia.* 2005;19(9):1567-1572.
6. Jain AG, Zhang L, Bennett JM, Komrokji R. Myelodysplastic syndromes with bone marrow fibrosis: an update. *Ann Lab Med.* 2022;42(3):299-305.
7. Westers TM, Cremers EM, Oelschlaegel U, et al. Immunophenotypic analysis of erythroid dysplasia in myelodysplastic syndromes. A report from the IMDS flow working group. *Haematologica.* 2017;102(2):308-319.
8. Satoh C, Dan K, Yamashita T, Jo R, Tamura H, Ogata K. Flow cytometric parameters with little interexaminer variability for diagnosing low-grade myelodysplastic syndromes. *Leuk Res.* 2008;32(5):699-707.
9. Greenberg PL, Tuechler H, Schanz J, et al. Revised International Prognostic Scoring System for myelodysplastic syndromes. *Blood.* 2012;120(12):2454-2465.
10. Wilkins BS, Erber WN, Bareford D, et al. Bone marrow pathology in essential thrombocythemia: interobserver reliability and utility for identifying disease subtypes. *Blood.* 2008;111(1):60-70.
11. Cervera N, Itzykson R, Coppin E, et al. Gene mutations differently impact the prognosis of the myelodysplastic and myeloproliferative classes of chronic myelomonocytic leukemia. *Am J Hematol.* 2014;89(6):604-609.
12. Ricci C, Fermo E, Corti S, et al. RAS mutations contribute to evolution of chronic myelomonocytic leukemia to the proliferative variant. *Clin Cancer Res.* 2010;16(8):2246-2256.
13. Schuler E, Schroeder M, Neukirchen J, et al. Refined medullary blast and white blood cell count based classification of chronic myelomonocytic leukemias. *Leuk Res.* 2014;38(12):1413-1419.
14. Facchetti F, Cigognetti M, Fisogni S, Rossi G, Lonardi S, Vermi W. Neoplasms derived from plasmacytoid dendritic cells. *Mod Pathol.* 2016;29(2):98-111.

15. Lucas N, Duchmann M, Rameau P, et al. Biology and prognostic impact of clonal plasmacytoid dendritic cells in chronic myelomonocytic leukemia. *Leukemia.* 2019;33(10):2466-2480.
16. Xu Y, McKenna RW, Karandikar NJ, Pildain AJ, Kroft SH. Flow cytometric analysis of monocytes as a tool for distinguishing chronic myelomonocytic leukemia from reactive monocytosis. *Am J Clin Pathol.* 2005;124(5):799-806.
17. Hwang SM, Ahn H, Jeon S, Park J, Chang Y, Kim H. Monocyte subsets to differentiate chronic myelomonocytic leukemia from reactive monocytosis. *J Clin Lab Anal.* 2021;35(1):e23576.
18. Picot T, Aanei CM, Flandrin Gresta P, et al. Evaluation by flow cytometry of mature monocyte subpopulations for the diagnosis and follow-up of chronic myelomonocytic leukemia. *Front Oncol.* 2018;8:109.
19. Selimoglu-Buet D, Wagner-Ballon O, Saada V, et al. Characteristic repartition of monocyte subsets as a diagnostic signature of chronic myelomonocytic leukemia. *Blood.* 2015;125(23):3618-3626.
20. Lacronique-Gazaille C, Chaury MP, Le Guyader A, Faucher JL, Bordessoule D, Feuillard J. A simple method for detection of major phenotypic abnormalities in myelodysplastic syndromes: expression of CD56 in CMML. *Haematologica.* 2007;92(6): 859-860.
21. Such E, Germing U, Malcovati L, et al. Development and validation of a prognostic scoring system for patients with chronic myelomonocytic leukemia. *Blood.* 2013;121(15):3005-3015.
22. Gambacorti-Passerini CB, Donadoni C, Parmiani A, et al. Recurrent ETNK1 mutations in atypical chronic myeloid leukemia. *Blood.* 2015;125(3):499-503.
23. Meggendorfer M, Bacher U, Alpermann T, et al. SETBP1 mutations occur in 9% of MDS/MPN and in 4% of MPN cases and are strongly associated with atypical CML, monosomy 7, isochromosome i(17)(q10), ASXL1 and CBL mutations. *Leukemia.* 2013;27(9):1852-1860.
24. Piazza R, Valletta S, Winkelmann N, et al. Recurrent SETBP1 mutations in atypical chronic myeloid leukemia. *Nat Genet.* 2013;45(1):18-24.
25. Koldehoff M, Beelen DW, Trenschel R, et al. Outcome of hematopoietic stem cell transplantation in patients with atypical chronic myeloid leukemia. *Bone Marrow Transplant.* 2004;34(12):1047-1050.

6

MYELOPROLIFERATIVE NEOPLASMS (MPNS), NEOPLASMS ASSOCIATED WITH EOSINOPHILIA AND GENE REARRANGEMENTS, AND MASTOCYTOSIS

Myeloproliferative neoplasms (MPNs) encompass a broad category of clonal disorders that result in the uncontrolled proliferation of one or more hematopoietic lineage cells, namely, myeloid cells, erythroid cells, and/or megakaryocytes.[1] Unlike acute myeloid leukemias (AMLs), MPNs undergo complete maturation with no block in cellular development; unlike myelodysplastic syndrome (MDS), these neoplasms result in the accumulation of generally functional cells in the peripheral blood (PB) and bone marrow (BM), often significantly skewing the normal distribution of hematopoiesis. Until late stages, granulocytic function tends to be maintained so that infections are not common at presentation, but abnormalities in platelet function or consequences of increased red cell mass can produce symptoms. Although these disorders have an increased risk of transformation to acute leukemia, the risk varies greatly among them.

The MPNs comprise chronic myeloid leukemia (CML), polycythemia vera (PV), primary myelofibrosis (PMF), essential thrombocythemia (ET), chronic neutrophilic leukemia (CNL), and chronic eosinophilic leukemia (CEL); in some cases, precise classification is not possible, and a diagnosis of myeloproliferative disorder, unclassifiable may be used (Table 6.1).[2] In this chapter, we also briefly review neoplasms associated with eosinophilia and tyrosine kinase (TK) gene fusions and mastocytosis.

Although the pathophysiology differs for each MPN subcategory, in general, these disorders arise from dysregulation of protein kinases in a stem cell, via either point mutations or translocations, which leads to activation of intracellular signaling pathways.

It may be difficult to distinguish MPNs from reactive conditions, especially in the early phases of the disease.[3] Therefore, an accurate diagnosis requires integrating clinical, morphologic, and genetic information. Obtaining an accurate and complete patient history and both current and

TABLE 6.1 **MPN Categories**

Disease	PB	BM	Genetics
Chronic myeloid leukemia	• Leukocytosis with neutrophilia • Left-shifted myeloid cells but no increase in blasts • Basophilia	• Hypercellular marrow • Myeloid hyperplasia • Increased small megakaryocytes	• *BCR::ABL1* translocation
Polycythemia vera	• Erythrocytosis (Hgb >16 g/dL women; >16.5 g/dL men) • RBCs with anisopoikilocytosis	• Hypercellular marrow • Panmyelosis • Increased pleomorphic megakaryocytes	• *BCR::ABL1* negative • *JAK2* mutation
Primary myelofibrosis	<u>Prefibrotic:</u> • Leukocytosis and often anemia <u>Fibrotic:</u> • Leukoerythroblastosis	<u>Prefibrotic:</u> • Hypercellular marrow • Myeloid hyperplasia • Increased clusters of megakaryocytes with "cloud-like" nuclei; sinusoidal megakaryocytes <u>Fibrotic:</u> BM fibrosis grade 2-3	• *BCR::ABL1* negative • *JAK2, CALR or MPL* mutation
Essential thrombocythemia	• Thrombocytosis (platelets)	• Hypercellular or normocellular marrow • Increased atypical megakaryocytes with "staghorn"-like nuclei; no significant megakaryocytic clustering	• *BCR::ABL1* negative • *JAK2*, *CALR*, or *MPL* mutation

Chronic neutrophilic leukemia	• Leukocytosis (WBC ≥13,000/μL) with neutrophilia • Segmented and band neutrophils comprise >80% of WBC. • No monocytosis • No increase in blasts • Lacks features of other well-defined MPNs	• Hypercellular marrow • Myeloid hyperplasia • No granulocytic dysplasia • No increase in blasts	• *BCR::ABL1* negative • *CSF3R* or other activating mutation supports dx
Chronic eosinophilic leukemia	• Hypereosinophilia (eosinophils ≥1500/μL) • Blasts <20% • Lacks features of other well-defined MPNs	• Hypercellular marrow • Eosinophilic infiltrate, often with increased fibrosis (or increased blasts in PB/BM) • Increased atypical megakaryocytes (+/− dysplasia in other lineages) • Blasts <20%	• *BCR::ABL1* negative • No tyrosine kinase gene fusion • Demonstration of a clonal cytogenetic abnormality or mutation supports dx
Myeloproliferative neoplasm, unclassified	• Features of an MPN (cytoses) • Lacks features of other well-defined MPNs	• Features of an MPN (hypercellular BM) • Lacks features of other well-defined MPNs	• *BCR::ABL1* negative • *JAK2*, *CALR*, or *MPL* mutation or other clonal markers

BM, bone marrow; dL, deciliters; dx, diagnosis; g, grams; Hgb, hemoglobin; MPN, myeloproliferative neoplasm; PB, peripheral blood; RBC, red blood cells; μL, microliters; WBC, white blood cells.

prior levels of complete blood count (CBC) parameters can help distinguish an MPN from primary BM disorders, especially MDS or MDS/MPN, as discussed in Chapter 5. Physical examination can also help because organomegaly is common in MPNs and less common in reactive conditions or MDS.

CLINICAL

MPNs are rare, affecting approximately 6 to 10 per 100,000 people.[4,5] These disorders occur in middle-aged to elderly patients and are rarely seen in younger patients. Patients may or may not be symptomatic at presentation. The most common symptoms include fatigue, clotting disorders, and/or abdominal fullness from hepatosplenomegaly. Some patients are asymptomatic, and the disorder is detected incidentally on a routine exam.

The most common laboratory abnormality in MPNs is an abnormal CBC, with cytoses of one or more cell lineages (Figure 6.1), which helps differentiate among diagnostic categories. Variable eosinophilia, basophilia, or increased mast cells may be seen, depending on the specific MPN, but at initial presentation, blasts are not increased.

In later phases of disease, anemia and thrombocytopenia are more common; leukoerythroblastosis may be seen in the PB as a consequence of marrow fibrosis, which results in circulating marrow precursors of all lineages and numerous teardrop-shaped red blood cells (RBCs; Figure 6.2; eFigure 6.1). All MPNs have a risk of transformation to acute leukemia, typically referred to as blast phase (BP), although the risk varies greatly among different MPNs.

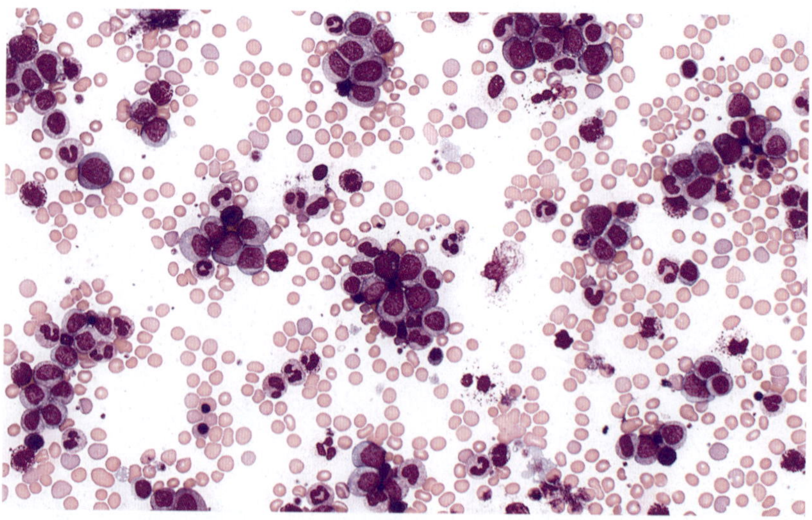

FIGURE 6.1 This peripheral blood shows a marked leukocytosis comprised of predominantly myeloid cells at all stages of maturation in this patient with chronic myeloid leukemia in chronic phase.

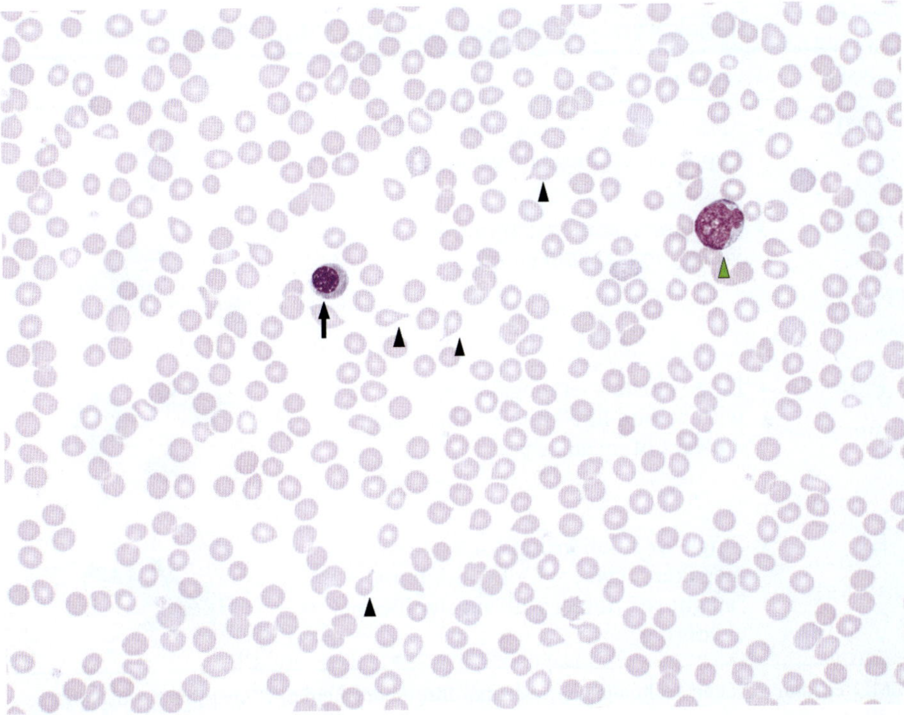

FIGURE 6.2 **Patients with significant fibrosis in the bone marrow will show a characteristic PB picture, as shown here.** Leukoerythroblastosis typically shows nucleated red blood cells (RBCs; black arrow), blasts (green arrowhead), or other immature myeloid cells, as well as teardrop-shaped RBCs (black arrowheads).

MORPHOLOGIC FEATURES

BM evaluation is necessary in the workup of MPNs. A core biopsy and aspirate smear are critical to assess cellularity, morphology, fibrosis, and percent blasts. It is also important to document the phase of disease, as many of these neoplasms are naturally biphasic or triphasic. In the proliferative phases of most MPNs, the BM is hypercellular for age, often with a panmyelosis, but with varying hyperplasia of different cell lineages in the different diseases. Fibrosis may be seen in all MPNs, although for some this will only occur at late stages.

Megakaryocytic atypia is characteristic of MPNs, and each disease entity shows slightly different morphologic features (Table 6.2). Significant dysplasia in the other lineages is not present.

Cellular maturation is complete, and in chronic phase (CP), blasts are not increased. Increased blasts up to 10%-19% of cells in the PB or BM indicate an accelerated phase (AP) of disease, although this term is not used in all types of MPNs. BP is diagnosed when blasts are ≥20% of cells in the PB or BM.

TABLE 6.2 Megakaryocytic Atypia in Myeloproliferative Neoplasms

Disease	Description	Morphology
CML	• "Dwarf" megakaryocytes: small, hypolobated megakaryocytes	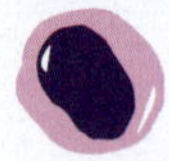
PV	• Pleomorphic megakaryocytes; variety in size and shape	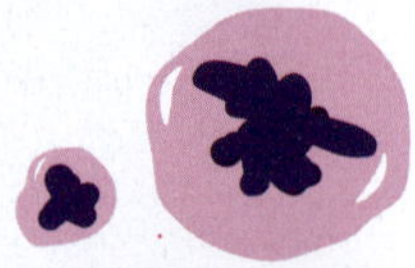
PMF	• Large clusters of megakaryocytes with "cloud-like" nuclei; sinusoidal clusters of megakaryocytes	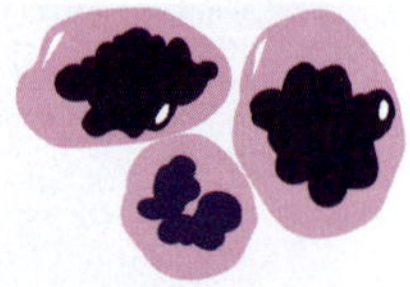
ET	• Single or small groups of megakaryocytes with hyperlobated "staghorn" nuclei with no significant clustering	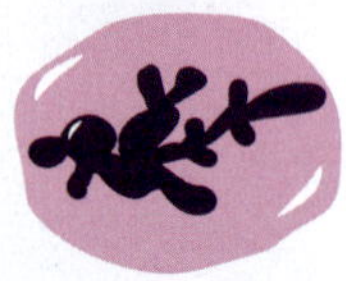

CML, chronic myeloid leukemia; ET, essential thrombocythemia; PMF, primary myelofibrosis; PV, polycythemia vera.

IMMUNOPHENOTYPE

Flow cytometric (FC) immunophenotyping of blood is not indicated in the CP of MPNs, although detecting an aberrant blast immunophenotype may be useful to identify that a patient has a marrow stem cell disorder. When blasts are increased, as in AP or BP, FC is useful to characterize the blasts. Because of the accompanying fibrosis seen in many MPNs, a BM aspirate may result in a "dry tap," so that neither morphology nor FC can be used to assess blast percentage; immunohistochemical (IHC) stains on the core biopsy may be a better way to document the percentage of blasts.

CD34 is the most useful marker because it highlights blasts in nearly all cases of MPNs. It is also positive on endothelial cells so that CD34 is useful to document the presence of neoangiogenesis and/or the presence of dilated sinuses that are prevalent in MPNs. CD61, CD42b, and Factor VIII may help identify atypical megakaryocytes. However, megakaryocytes are typically large in MPNs so that most of these are readily identifiable on hematoxylin and eosin (H&E).[6,7]

The grade of BM fibrosis is important to document, and special stains for reticulin and collagen should be performed in cases of suspected MPN (Figures 6.3A-D and 6.4A-D; eFigures 6.2 and 6.3),[8] as increased fibrosis may indicate advanced disease or, if present at diagnosis, inferior prognosis (Table 6.3A and B).[9]

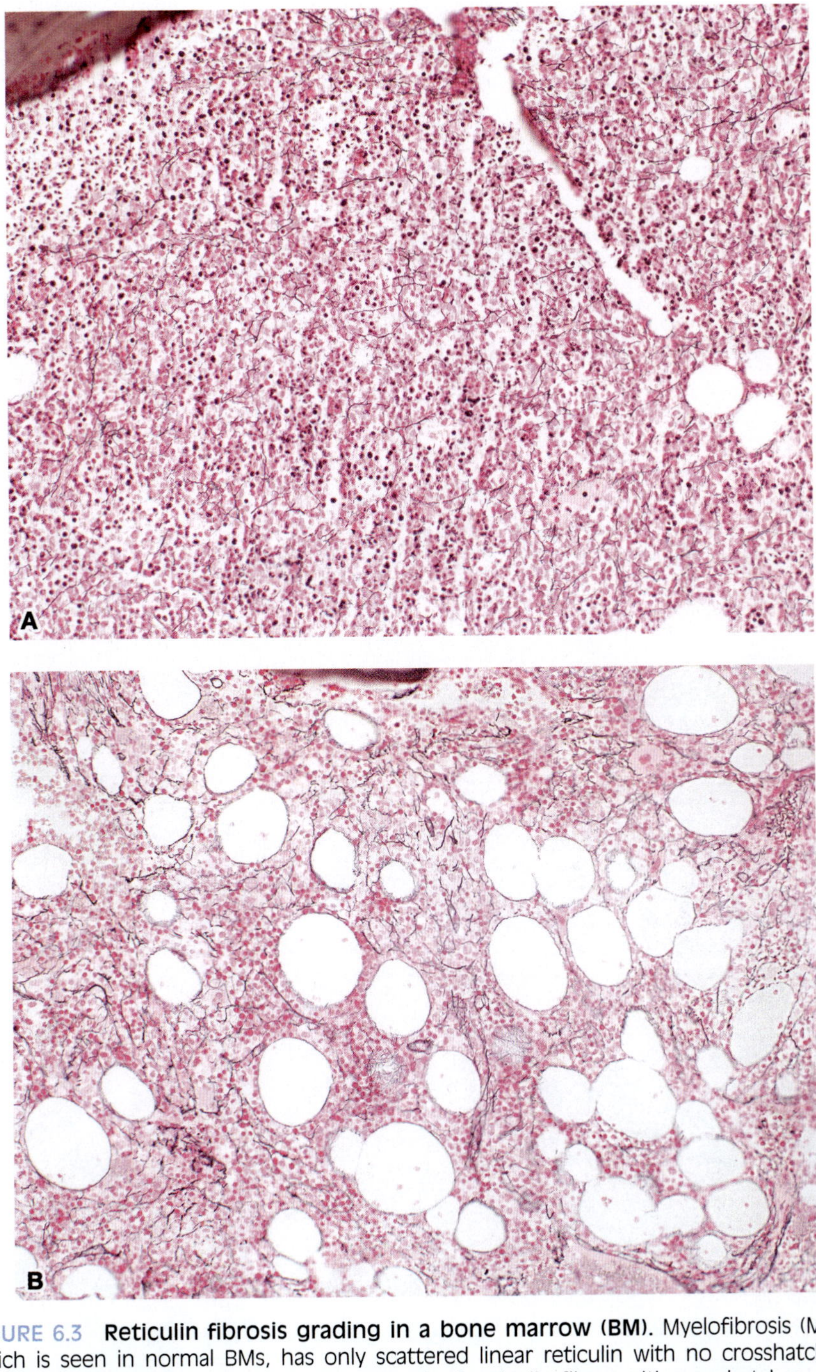

FIGURE 6.3 **Reticulin fibrosis grading in a bone marrow (BM).** Myelofibrosis (MF) 0, which is seen in normal BMs, has only scattered linear reticulin with no crosshatching/intersections (A). MF 1 shows a loose network of reticulin fibers with crosshatches, most prevalent in perivascular areas (B). MF 2 shows diffuse, dense reticulin with abundant crosshatching/intersections and focal thick bundles (C). MF 3 shows diffuse reticulin and coarse thick bundles, representing collagen fibrosis (D).

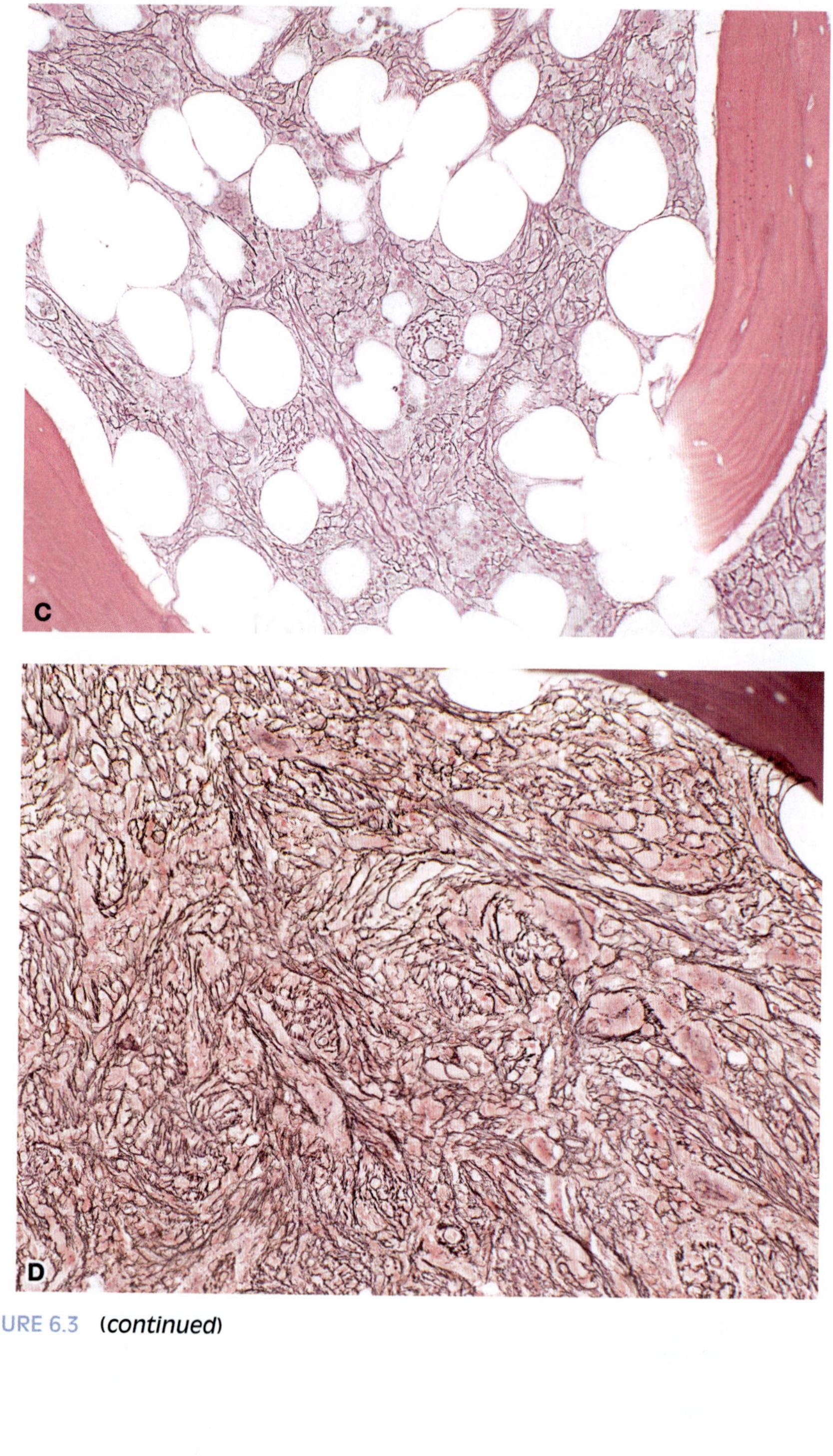

FIGURE 6.3 (*continued*)

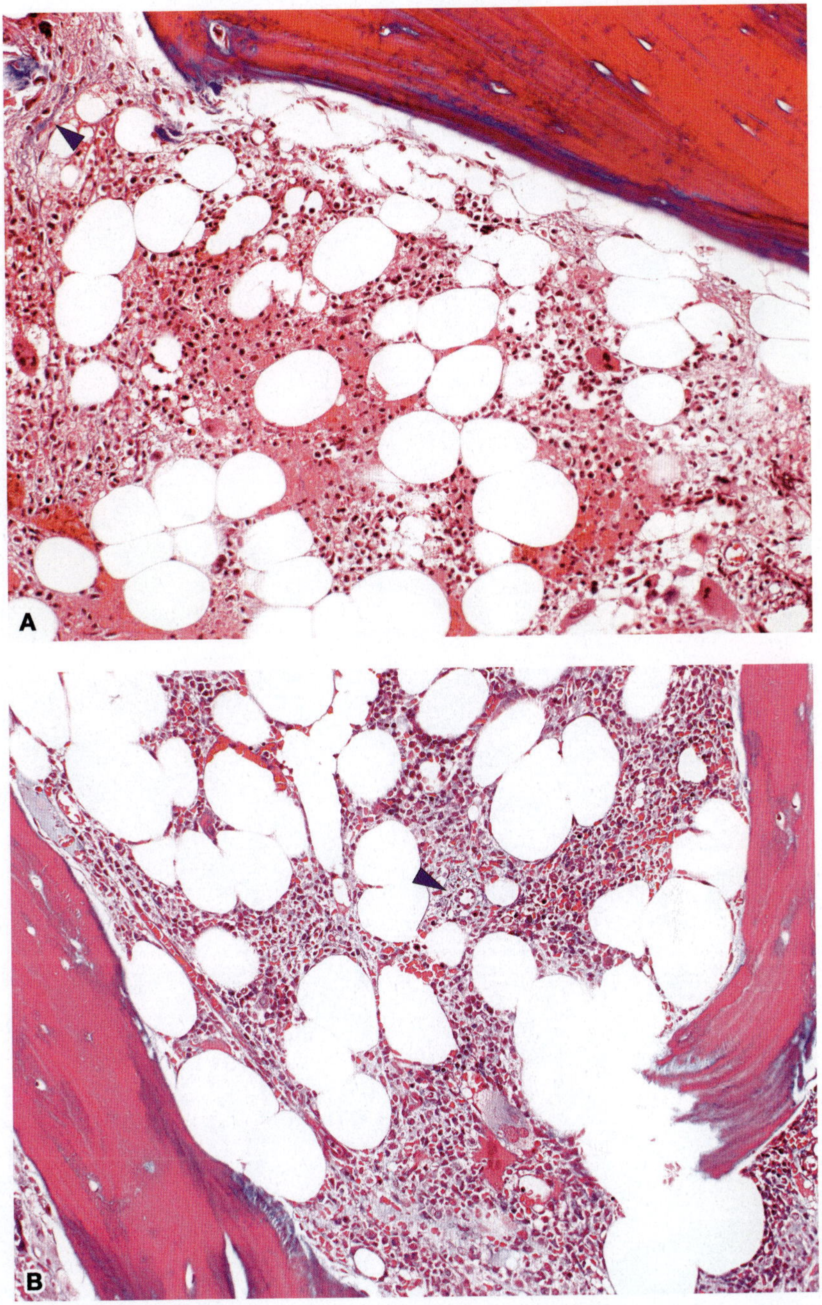

FIGURE 6.4 **Collagen fibrosis grading in a bone marrow (BM).** Grade 0, seen in normal BMs, shows only perivascular collagen or rare wisps of collagen (arrowhead), stained blue in this Masson trichrome stain (A). Grade 1 shows focal paratrabecular blue collagen and perivascular collagen (arrowhead), without connecting meshworks (B). Grade 2 shows focally connecting meshworks of collagen (C). Grade 3 shows complete diffuse collagen meshwork connections (D).

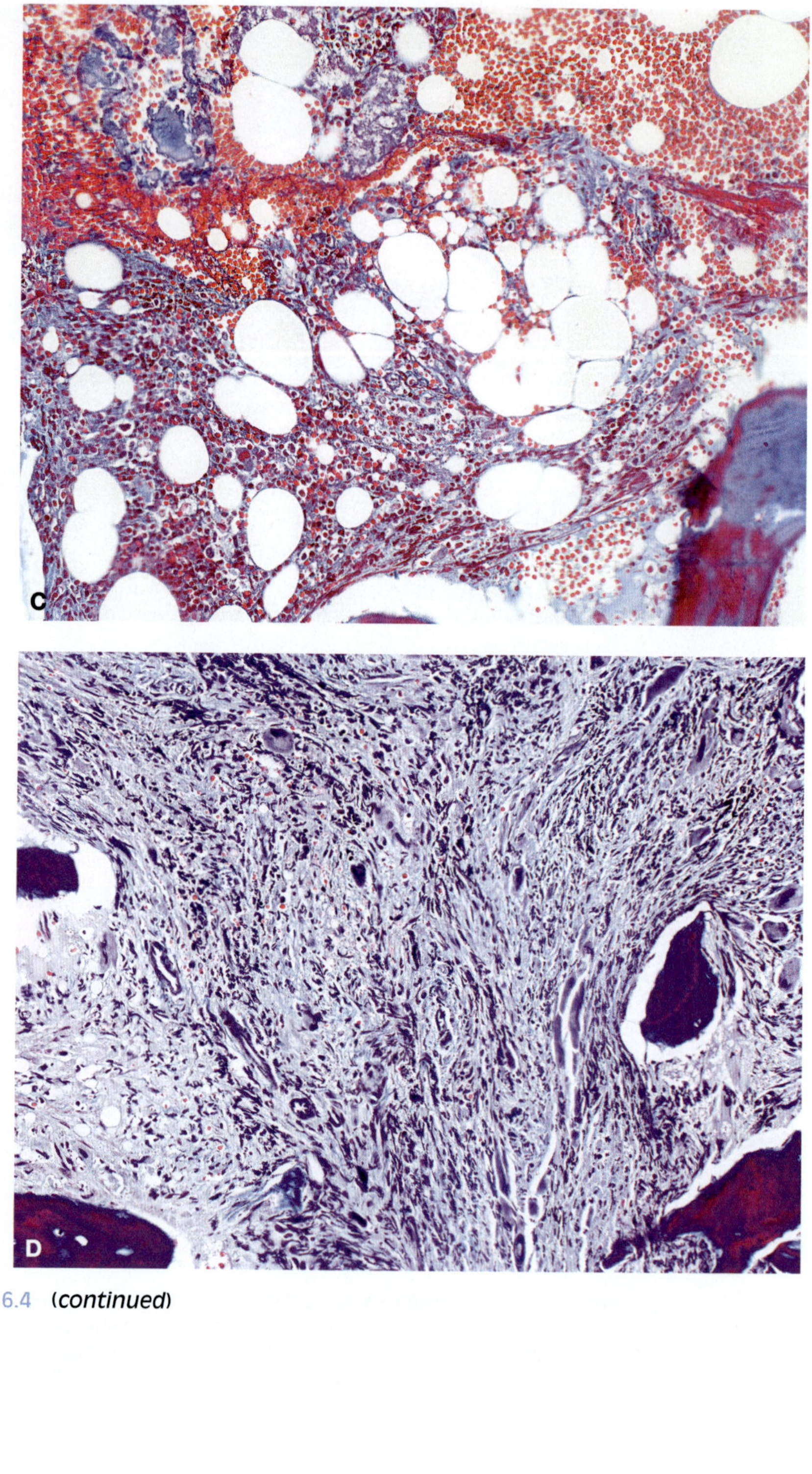

FIGURE 6.4 (*continued*)

TABLE 6.3A Bone Marrow Reticulin Fibrosis Grading

Features	MF 0	MF 1	MF 2	MF 3
Reticulin fibers	• Scattered linear reticulin with no crosshatching/ intersections	• A loose network of reticulin fibers with many crosshatches, most prevalent in perivascular areas	• Diffuse, dense reticulin with abundant crosshatching/ intersections and focal thick bundles	• Diffuse reticulin and coarse thick bundles, representing collagen fibrosis

MF, myelofibrosis.

TABLE 6.3B Bone Marrow Collagen Fibrosis Grading

Features	Grade 0	Grade 1	Grade 2	Grade 3
Collagen fibers	• Only focal perivascular collagen	• Focal paratrabecular blue collagen, without connecting meshworks	• Focally connecting meshworks of collagen	• Complete diffuse collagen meshwork connections

GENETICS

Genetic testing is essential to diagnose and classify an MPN. Most MPNs are associated with genetic and/or molecular abnormalities that result in the formation of an activated TK or involve other oncogenic signal transduction pathways, leading to unregulated cellular proliferation. The detection of these abnormalities is useful to help differentiate MPNs from each other, as well as from benign or reactive proliferations.

Conventional cytogenetic (karyotype) testing is useful to perform at diagnosis for all presumptive MPNs. An abnormal karyotype not only helps define the disorder as a clonal process, but also helps subclassify and/or definitively diagnose the disease. Additional BM biopsies performed over time can detect further abnormalities, which may herald progression to an AP or BP of the disease.

Florescence in situ hybridization (FISH) and reverse transcriptase (RT)-polymerase chain reaction (PCR) can detect chromosomal translocations that are not identified on the karyotype, because of either cryptic translocations or complex abnormalities. Quantitative PCR (qPCR) is especially useful for monitoring patients with CML, although it is generally not used in other MPNs.

Genetic sequencing, either with focused panels or by **next-generation sequencing (NGS),** is the most important tool in the diagnosis and classification of MPNs and related disorders because of the consistent finding of mutations in genes in signaling pathways, most commonly *JAK2*, *MPL*, *CALR*, *KIT*, and *CSF3R*, among others.

PROGNOSIS

The prognosis of patients varies with the disease subtype, as well as the phase of disease and the patient response to treatment. Patients who progress or show genetic evolution have worse outcomes.[1] BM failure may ultimately occur because of fibrosis, ineffective hematopoiesis (leading to infections or bleeding), or progression to a BP.

CHRONIC MYELOID LEUKEMIA, *BCR::ABL1*-POSITIVE

CML is the most common MPN. This neoplasm results from a progenitor hematopoietic cell with t(9;22)(q34;q11.2), resulting in the formation of *BCR::ABL1*, a novel fusion protein that acts as a constitutively active TK receptor. This leads to uncontrolled proliferation of myeloid cells, a hypercellular BM, and PB myeloid leukocytosis.

Clinical

CML has an annual incidence of 1 to 2 cases/100,000 people and represents 15% to 20% of leukemia cases in adults. The median age of diagnosis is 50 years. Nearly half of all patients are asymptomatic at the time of presentation, and the disease is detected incidentally. Symptomatic patients may present with fatigue, malaise, weight loss, excessive sweating, abdominal fullness, and bleeding episodes because of platelet dysfunction. On physical examination, patients typically have splenomegaly and may have hepatomegaly, although adenopathy is rare.

Morphologic

The CBC shows a marked myeloid proliferation (Figure 6.5; eFigure 6.4) with basophilia and occasional eosinophilia. Because basophilia is rare in reactive states, this finding should raise suspicions of CML (Figure 6.6; eFigure 6.5). A range of myeloid progenitors is present, especially myelocytes, resulting in a "myeloid bulge" appreciated on the PB smear (Figure 6.7; eFigure 6.6); blasts may be present but are not increased. Rarely, patients may present with only thrombocytosis, mimicking other MPNs. Monocytes are typically <3% of cellularity, except in rare cases of CML with the p190 isoform (discussed later), which resemble chronic myelomonocytic leukemia (CMML).

The BM biopsy reveals a hypercellular marrow with a markedly increased myeloid to erythroid (M:E) ratio (Figure 6.8A-C). Myeloid lineage cells are left-shifted but maturation is always complete (eFigure 6.7). Normally in the BM, immature myeloid cells are located

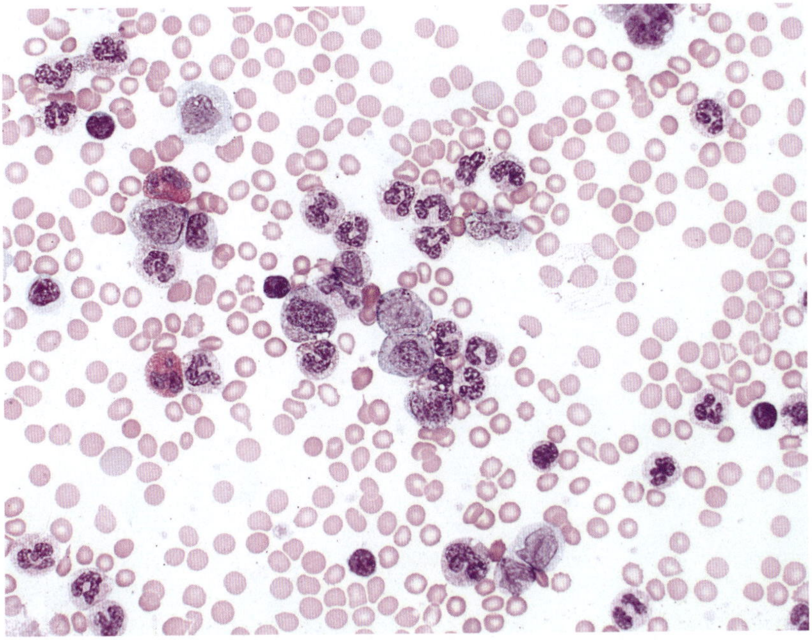

FIGURE 6.5 The typical peripheral blood smear in chronic myeloid leukemia shows a marked granulocytic leukocytosis with a left shift as seen here.

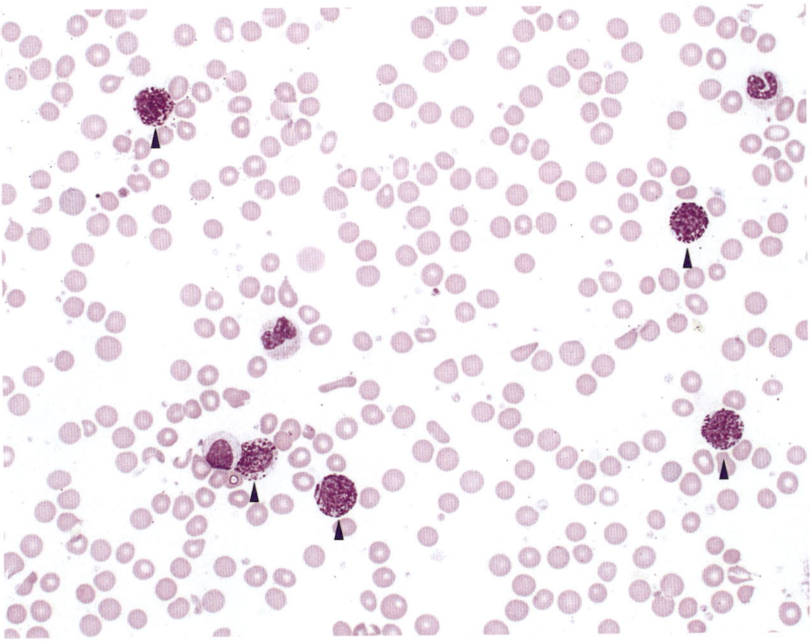

FIGURE 6.6 Chronic myeloid leukemia is invariably associated with basophilia (arrowheads).

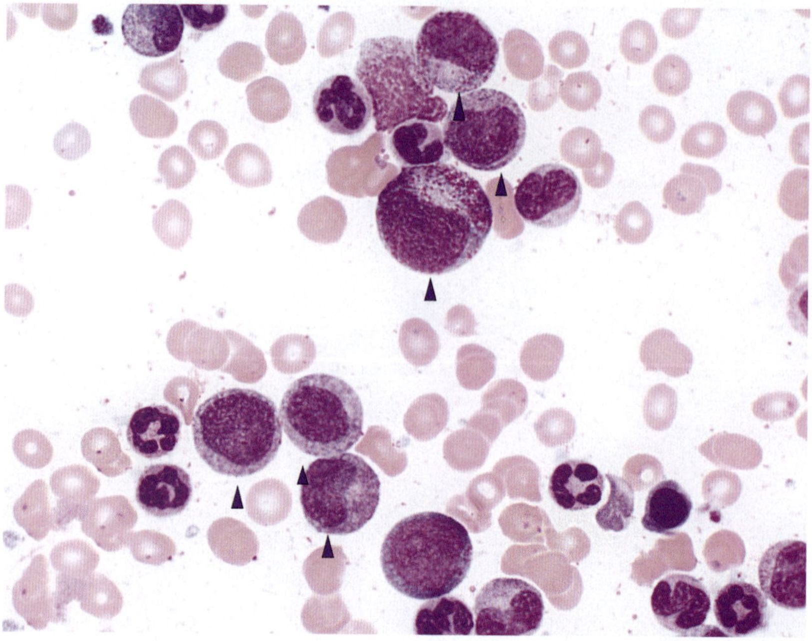

FIGURE 6.7 A peripheral blood smear in a patient with CML shows a significant increase in myelocytes and metamyelocytes (arrowheads) and is known as a "myeloid bulge."

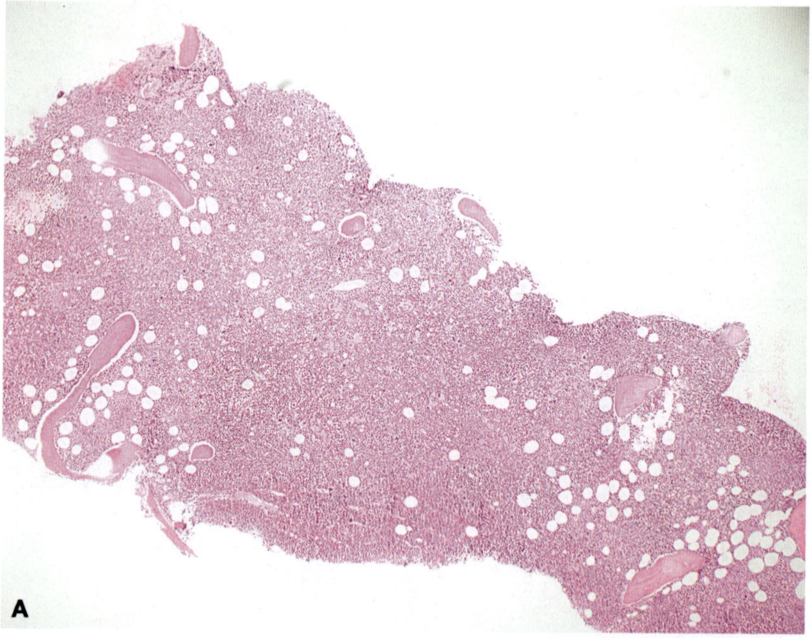

FIGURE 6.8 A bone marrow biopsy in chronic myeloid leukemia is characteristically markedly hypercellular, frequently approaching 100% (A). The marrow is overwhelmingly myeloid, typically with myeloid to erythroid ratios >10:1 (B). At high power (C), there are typically numerous neutrophils, but cells at all stages of maturation can be seen.

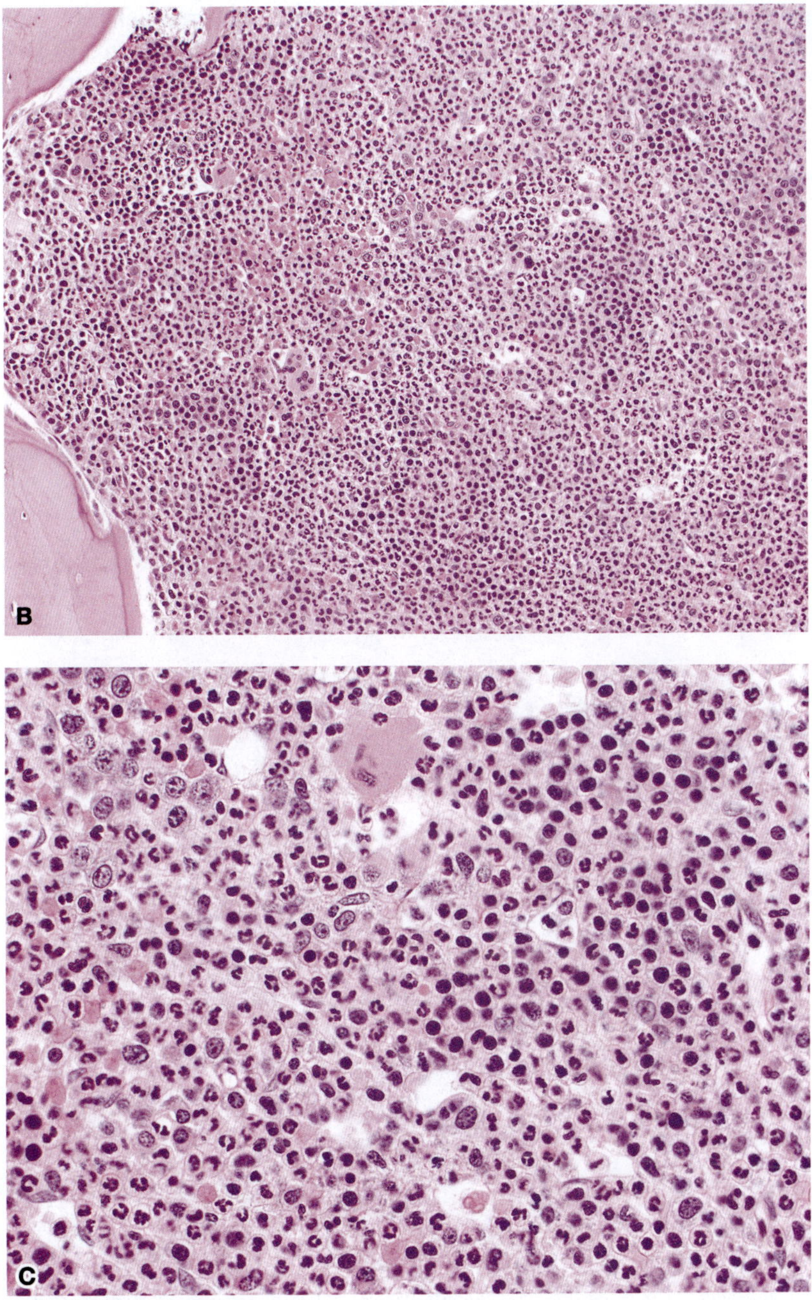

FIGURE 6.8 *(continued)*

adjacent to paratrabecular bone in layers of two to three cells. In patients with CML, however, the layers of immature cells are increased to 5 to 10 cells, and immature cells may be present scattered throughout the interstitium, a pattern referred to as "abnormal location of immature precursors" (ALIP).

Other morphologic features to note in the marrow are uniformly small hypolobated megakaryocytes (Figure 6.9A and B; eFigure 6.8), which may

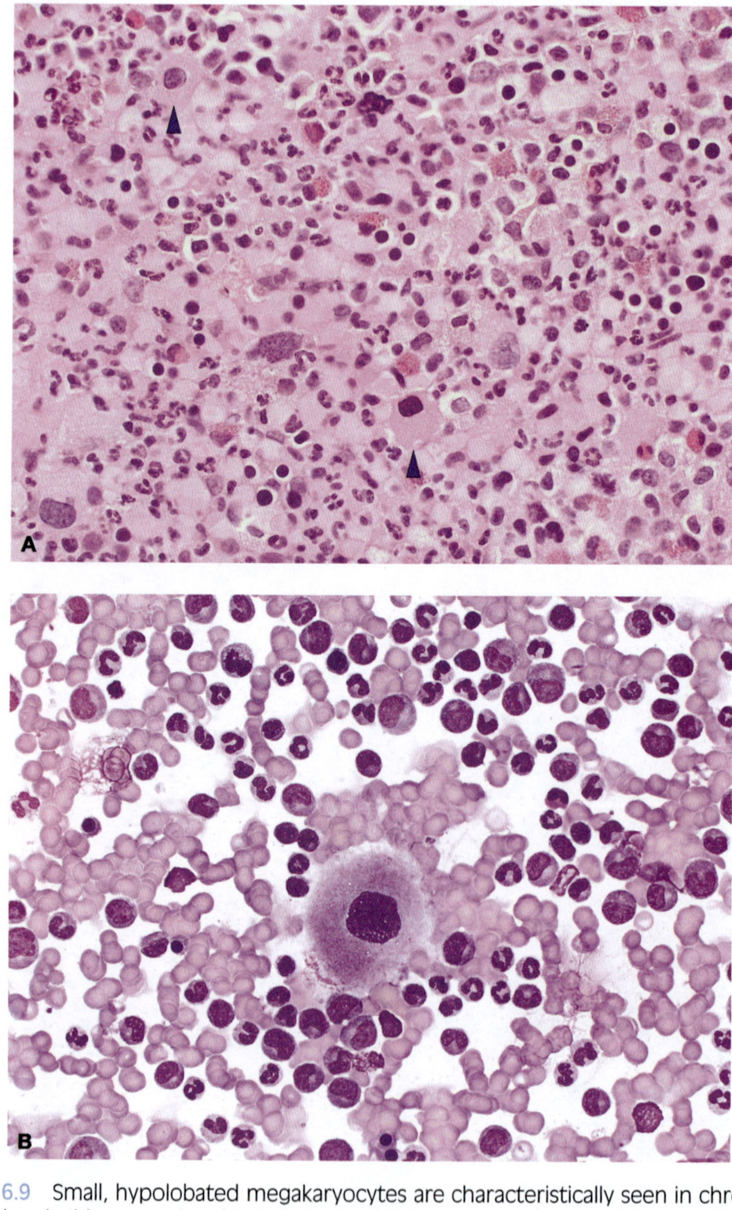

FIGURE 6.9 Small, hypolobated megakaryocytes are characteristically seen in chronic myeloid leukemia (blue arrowheads) and may be hard to see on the core biopsy at low power (A). A characteristic hypolobated megakaryocyte on an aspirate smear (B).

be markedly increased in up to half of all cases. There is no significant morphologic dysplasia in other lineages.[10] Pseudo-Gaucher cells and sea-blue histiocytes (Figure 6.10; eFigures 6.9 and 6.10) are identifiable on the aspirate smear in approximately 40% of all cases. These large histiocytic cells with abundant blue cytoplasm are phagocytosing cellular debris because of high cell turnover. At presentation, only about 30% of cases have significant fibrosis, but if present, it may indicate more aggressive disease.[9]

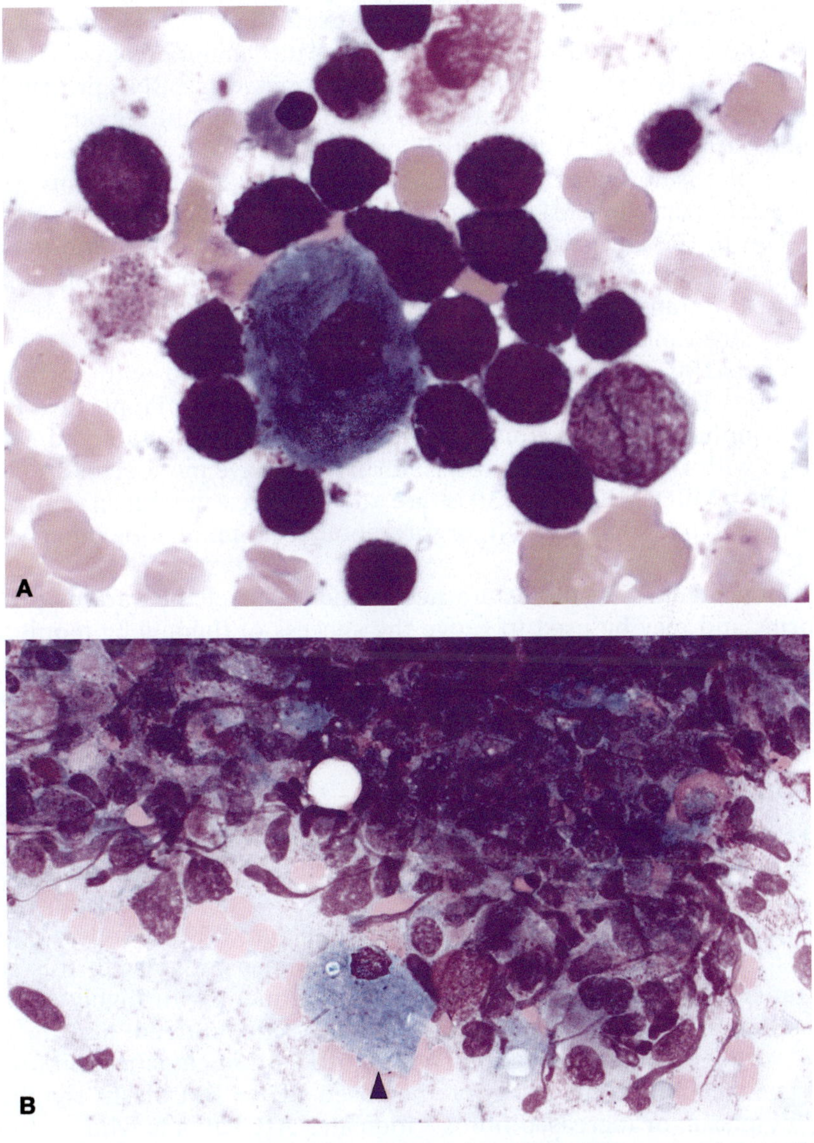

FIGURE 6.10 Because of the high cellular turnover, there may be scattered pseudo-Gaucher cells (A) and/or sea-blue histiocytes (B; arrowhead), as seen here.

Genetics

The *sine qua non* of CML is the *BCR::ABL1* translocation between the *BCR* gene on chromosome 22 and the *ABL1* gene on chromosome 9. The resultant diminutive chromosome 22, the "Philadelphia chromosome (Ph)," positions the native *BCR* next to the *ABL1* oncogene. The translocation t(9;22) is usually detected on a conventional karyotype, but approximately 5% to 10% of cases will require FISH or molecular analysis to detect cryptic or complex translocations involving chromosomes 9 and 22.[11]

The *ABL1* breakpoint is consistently present at exon 2 (a2), whereas the *BCR* breakpoint is variable, usually at exon 13 or 14 (e13 and e14, otherwise known as b2 and b3). This is known as the "major breakpoint cluster region" (M-BCR), which results in a chimeric messenger RNA protein with a molecular weight of 210 kDa (p210). Other breakpoint regions on *BCR* include exons 1-2 and exons 17-20, known as the m-BCR and μ-BCR, which result in the isoforms p190 and p230, respectively. All three forms (p210, p190, p230) occur in CML and are associated with different phenotypes.

The p210: This is the most common isoform in CML and patients present with typical CML morphology. In addition, small amounts of p230 and/or p190 transcripts are seen in most patients with p210 CML because of alternative splicing.[12]

The p190: CML with p190 is rare and associated with an inferior outcome.[13] This isoform is more often found in cases of Ph-positive B cell acute lymphoblastic leukemia/lymphoma (Ph+ B-ALL). As noted earlier, patients with CML with the p190 isoform often have monocytosis.

The p230: CML with p230 is rare and may present with either neutrophilic features resembling CNL or thrombocytosis, mimicking other MPNs like ET.[14]

Molecular PCR studies are necessary to detect the various protein isoforms and may be used to gauge the success of therapy by monitoring the transcript levels.

CML phases (Table 6.4): In the absence of therapy, patients with CML inexorably progress from a CP to BP, either abruptly or, more commonly, via an AP.

1. **Chronic phase (CP):** Most cases (95%) are diagnosed at this stage. Patients present with leukocytosis, increased absolute neutrophil count (ANC), and variable thrombocytosis. Blasts are not increased at this stage.
2. **Accelerated phase (AP)** (Figure 6.11; eFigure 6.11)**:** Rarely, a patient is first diagnosed in this stage. Patients may progress to this stage after a CP, although with the rise of treatment with highly effective TK inhibitors (TKIs), this stage is rarely encountered, and the new World Health Organization (WHO) 5th edition classification no longer recognizes this category. Increased PB or BM blasts, significant dysplasia, or increased fibrosis indicates AP. Patients who no longer respond to first-line TKIs may be treated with second-line TKIs. As in CP, the prognosis of patients in AP depends on response to therapy.

TABLE 6.4 Criteria for Chronic, Accelerated, and Blast Phase CML

Phase	PB	BM	Genetics
Chronic phase	<1% blasts	<5% blasts	*BCR::ABL1* translocation
Accelerated phase	10%-19% blasts Basophilia ≥20%	10%-19% blasts	*BCR::ABL1* + additional clonal cytogenetic abnormalities (in Ph+ cells)
Blast phase	Blasts ≥20%	Blasts ≥20% (or myeloid sarcoma) Lymphoblasts >5%	*BCR::ABL1* + additional clonal cytogenetic abnormalities (in Ph+ cells)

BM, bone marrow; CML, chronic myeloid leukemia; PB, peripheral blood; Ph, Philadelphia chromosome.

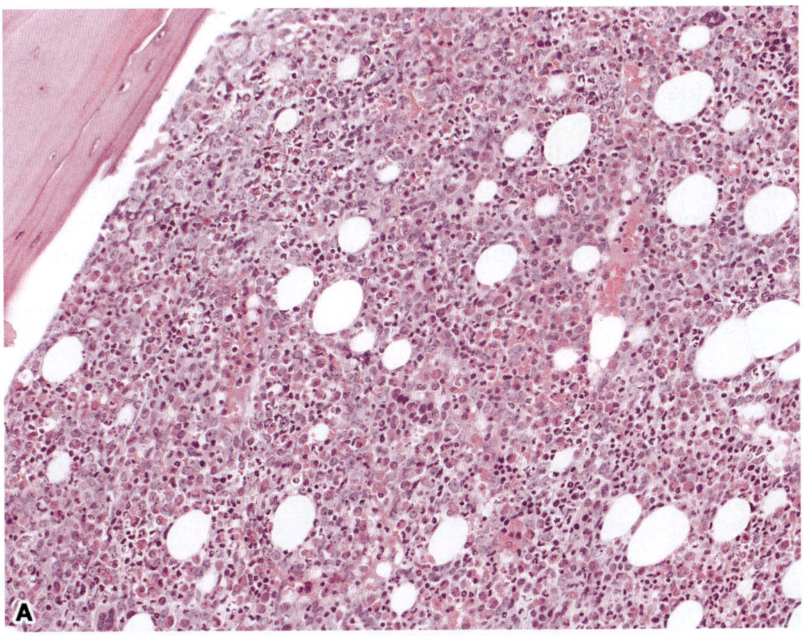

FIGURE 6.11 Bone marrow (BM) biopsy in a patient with accelerated phase chronic myeloid leukemia (CML) (A). There are fewer mature neutrophils and many more immature forms than in the typical chronic phase case. This case also shows an eosinophilia, which may sometimes be seen. However, BM biopsy morphology by itself cannot be used to diagnose accelerated phase because it may be difficult to tell increased blasts from just a left shift. B, Peripheral blood smear from a different case of accelerated phase CML showing many more blasts than would be expected in chronic phase, but not enough to be considered blast phase.

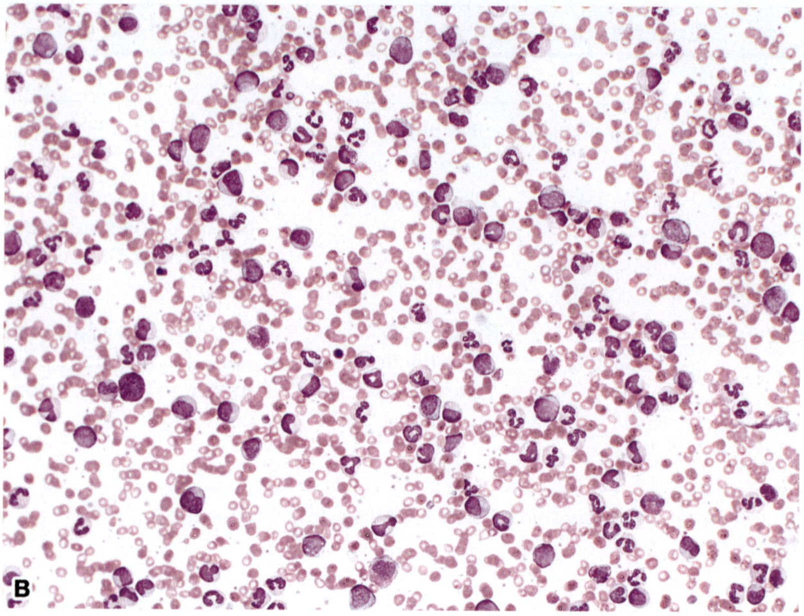

FIGURE 6.11 (*continued*)

3. **Blast phase (BP):** This is the final phase of the disease, defined as ≥20% blasts in the PB or BM or the presence of a myeloid sarcoma (Figure 6.12; eFigure 6.12). BP may be heralded by loss of response to therapy and/or additional genetic abnormalities. The majority of BPs present with increased myeloid blasts (70% of cases), whereas most of the remaining patients present with lymphoid blasts (Figure 6.13; eFigure 6.13), most often B lymphoblasts. Rare patients transform to

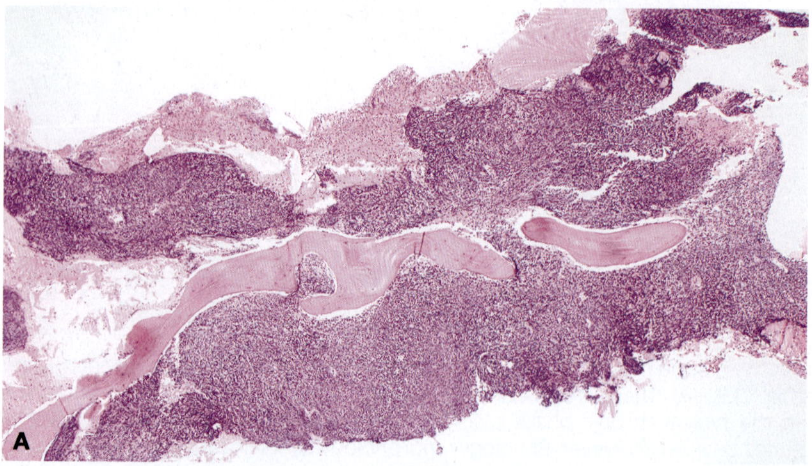

FIGURE 6.12 A bone marrow biopsy in blast phase chronic myeloid leukemia, as shown here, is markedly hypercellular (A) with sheets of blasts identified at higher power (B). These cases are usually morphologically indistinguishable from *de novo* acute myeloid leukemia.

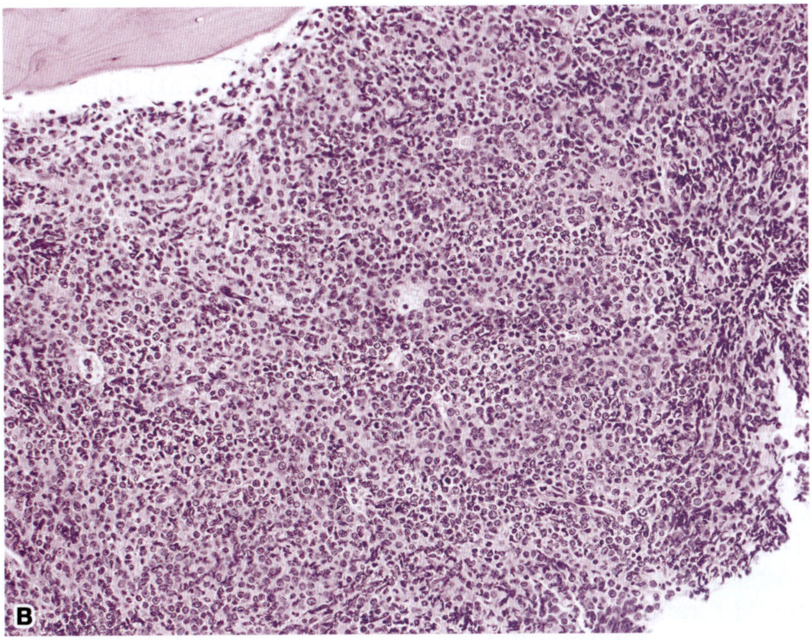

FIGURE 6.12 (*continued*)

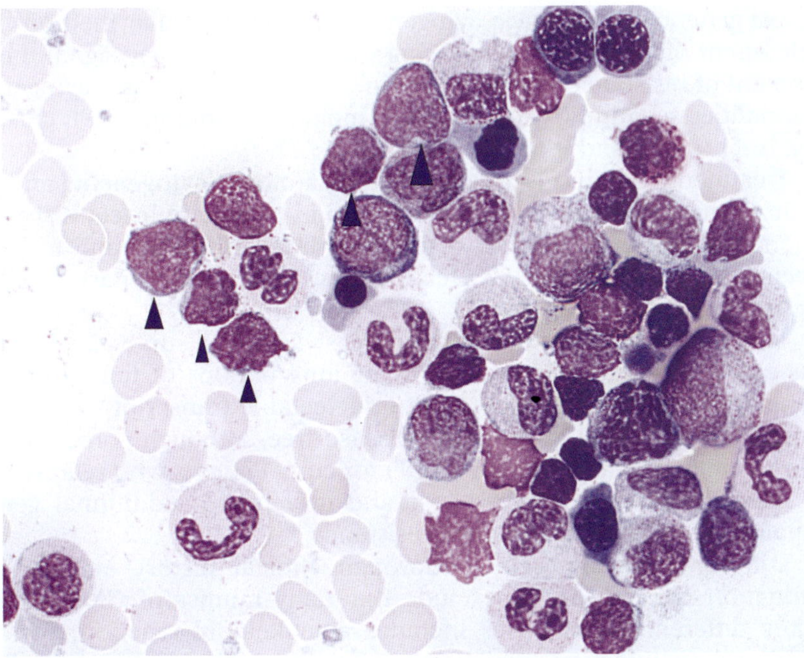

FIGURE 6.13 **Lymphoid blast phase of chronic myeloid leukemia (CML), with numerous lymphoblasts (arrowheads) displaying more compact chromatin and less cytoplasm than myeloid blasts.** Up to 30% of blast phase CMLs are lymphoid and are virtually always B cell acute lymphoblastic leukemia.

a T lymphoid BP and some patients to a mixed phenotype BP, virtually always B/myeloid. Classification of BP typically requires FC. Just as CML in myeloid BP is not classified as AML, CML in mixed BP is not considered mixed phenotype acute leukemia (MPAL). In general, the prognosis of BP is poor and not as treatable as *de novo* acute leukemia; patients ultimately succumb to bleeding or infections because of ineffective hematopoiesis.

TKI therapy in CML: *BCR::ABL1* acts as a constitutively active TK. It binds adenosine triphosphate (ATP) and transfers a phosphate to the tyrosine residue on its substrate, which leads to excess proliferation of myeloid cells. TKIs such as imatinib, the first-generation TKI, compete with ATP, block its binding site, and inhibit its action.[15] Up to 5% of CML patients are resistant to imatinib initially because of a mutation (T315I), and other patients may develop resistance with treatment over time. Patients who develop resistance may progress to AP or BP CML. Numerous second- and third-generation TKIs have been developed that can be used in cases of resistance and in some circumstances are even preferred as front-line therapy.

After TKI treatment, the BM may show normalization of cellularity and the M:E ratio, and a possible reversal of reticulin fibrosis.[16-18]

Disease monitoring: BM biopsies are recommended at certain time intervals to assess for disease progression. Clinicians monitor disease progression via several methods: *BCR::ABL1* transcript burden via PCR, evidence of genetic evolution via cytogenetic and/or molecular methods, and development of TKI resistance. Rising transcript levels may signal the development of resistance. The most common (or "major route") cytogenetic abnormalities seen in 80% of AP or BP include an additional Ph chromosome, iso(17q) +8 and +10.

Treatment response is assessed by hematologic, cytogenetic, and molecular parameters. A three $\log_{10}$ reduction in transcript levels is the goal of therapy. A major molecular response (MMR) is <0.1% and a deeper molecular response is <0.01%. Occasionally, a patient may have complete disappearance of the transcript.

TKI therapy has dramatically increased patient survival. Many patients can be maintained on therapy for long periods of time and some patients in long-term remission with undetectable transcript can even be removed from therapy and remain disease free, although some will still require stem cell transplantation (SCT) for cure. Patients who relapse post-SCT have a more aggressive course and may harbor additional genetic anomalies that give rise to therapy resistance.[19]

Differential diagnosis: A thorough clinical history and physical examination is necessary to exclude the many mimics of CML. One of the key differential diagnoses includes a leukemoid reaction, typically in response to infection, which can often be excluded by clinical history and other laboratory studies, although molecular studies are sometimes needed. In leukemoid reactions, WBCs rarely exceed 50,000/μL and often show toxic features, which are absent in CML. Additionally, basophilia is rare in leukemoid reactions. Historically, leukocyte alkaline phosphatase (LAP) scores were utilized to differentiate between CML and leukemoid reactions. This test is not often performed today because of the sensitivity, ease of use, and quick turnaround time of molecular tests.

The differential diagnosis also includes other neoplastic conditions like CMML, which is a diagnostic consideration in those cases of CML with p190 and monocytosis. CNL and atypical CML (aCML) are also in the differential diagnosis, but these lack *BCR::ABL1*. It is important to remember that *BCR::ABL1* is present in all cases of CML, but is not pathognomonic for CML, as it also occurs in B-ALL and in some cases of *de novo* AML.

Prognosis

With the advent of treatment with TKIs, patients with CML can expect nearly normal life spans. Prognosis depends on a patient's response to treatment, monitored using the methods indicated earlier. Approximately 70% to 90% of patients have a complete response, and there is a 90% progression-free survival/overall survival rate.

BCR::ABL1-NEGATIVE MPNs

Excluding *BCR::ABL1* CML is necessary in all suspected MPNs, as CML may present atypically, as described earlier. The so-called major "*BCR::ABL1*-negative MPNs," including PV, PMF, and ET, are clonal disorders that display an overtly proliferative phase and may progress to a fibrotic and cytopenic phase, most often in PMF and PV and only rarely in ET. Without treatment, these diseases may also progress to a BP indistinguishable from acute leukemia, although there are no formal criteria for AP with these MPNs. Like fibrosis, BP of ET is rare.

Genetic and molecular testing are essential for establishing a diagnosis of a *BCR::ABL1*-negative MPN, but in general, does not clearly distinguish among them. The majority have mutations in the pseudo-kinase domain of the *JAK2* gene at 9p24 in hematopoietic cells, which results in the constitutive activation of nuclear signaling pathways, leading to uncontrolled cellular proliferation.[20-23] The *JAK2* V617F mutation is found in 96% of PV cases, 65% of PMF cases, and 55% of ET cases and is considered a major criterion for the diagnosis of these neoplasms.[24-26] However, this mutation not specific to these diseases and can occur in other MDS/MPNs and rarely in primary AML or MDS. It can also rarely be seen with other more specific abnormalities, including *BCR::ABL1*.

Of those cases of PV that lack *JAK2* V617F mutations, most show mutations of *JAK2* exons 12 to 15.[27,28] Of those PMF and ET cases that lack *JAK2* mutations, other mutations have been detected in the thrombopoietin receptor gene, *MPL* and the calreticulin gene, *CALR*. *MPL* mutations cause the abnormal thrombopoietin receptors to phosphorylate Janus kinase (JAK) in the absence of its ligand, thrombopoietin, leading to uncontrolled proliferation via the JAK-signal transducer and activator of transcription (STAT) pathway.[29,30] *CALR* normally produces calreticulin, a calcium-binding protein involved in the regulation of protein expression.[31,32] Mutations truncate the calcium-binding domain and create a new novel peptide that activates JAK-STAT signaling and favors expansion of the megakaryocytic lineage.[33] *CALR* mutations are mutually exclusive with *JAK2* and *MPL* mutations.[31,32,34] A few patients with *BCR::ABL1*-negative MPNs lack any of the above mutations and are termed "triple-negative" MPNs; NGS studies will typically show other mutations. These patients have a worse prognosis.

Although demonstration of one of these molecular abnormalities can establish a BM proliferative process as neoplastic, subclassification relies on assessment of history and physical findings, especially on BM and PB findings.

POLYCYTHEMIA VERA

PV leads to an increase in RBC production independent from normal homeostatic regulation. It is rare, affecting approximately 0.8/100,000 patients per year.[35]

PV is considered a biphasic disease, with both a proliferative phase and a spent phase. There is also often a "pre-polycythemic stage," manifested by slightly elevated RBC parameters. PV is difficult to diagnose in this phase and is usually detected incidentally. Decreased serum erythropoietin (EPO) levels and *JAK2* mutations confirm the diagnosis at this stage (Table 6.5).[36,37]

TABLE 6.5 PV Diagnostic Criteria

	Major criteria		Minor criteria
Phase	**PB/BM**	**Genetics**	**Additional features**
PV[a]	• Increased Hgb (>16.5 g/dL men; >16.0 women) or Hct or RBC mass • Hypercellular BM with panmyelosis	• *JAK2* V617F or other *JAK2* exon 12-15 mutation	• Low serum EPO
Post-PV fibrosis[b]	• BM fibrosis (MF grade 2-3)		• Anemia • Splenomegaly • B symptoms[c] • Leukoerythroblastosis

BM, bone marrow; dL, deciliter; EPO, erythropoietin; g, grams; Hct, hematocrit; Hgb hemoglobin; MF, myelofibrosis; PB, peripheral blood; PV, polycythemia vera; RBC, red blood cell.
[a]Must fulfill all major criteria OR erythrocytosis and *JAK2* mutation with low serum EPO.
[b]Must have an established diagnosis of PV with fibrosis and at least two additional features.
[c]Weight loss, night sweats, fever.

THE PROLIFERATIVE POLYCYTHEMIC STAGE

Patients are most often diagnosed in this stage and may experience symptoms such as headache, dizziness, pruritus, paresthesia, and plethora (reddening of the skin of the palms of the hands or face). Splenomegaly is very common (70%), and hepatomegaly is also detected in a subset of patients (40%). The increased RBC mass leads to increased blood viscosity, and patients often suffer from hypertension and vascular abnormalities, including thrombosis: Up to 20% of patients present with arterial or venous thrombosis as the first manifestation of their disease. Approximately 40% of patients with idiopathic splanchnic vein thrombosis (SVT) harbor the *JAK2* mutation.[38,39] Detection of mesenteric thrombosis or manifestations of Budd-Chiari syndrome should always prompt a workup for potential PV.

A CBC reveals erythrocytosis with increased hemoglobin (Hgb) and hematocrit (Hct). Occasionally, a patient may also present with an associated increased ANC or thrombocytosis. Because of the unregulated erythroid production, patients may become functionally iron deficient and may have normal or even decreased red cell parameters, and present instead with pronounced thrombocytosis.

The BM is hypercellular for age with panmyelosis, or hyperplasia of all three hematopoietic lineages, although erythroid and megakaryocytic hyperplasia are most evident (Figure 6.14; eFigure 6.14). Although this is considered a major criterion for the diagnosis of PV, a marrow biopsy may

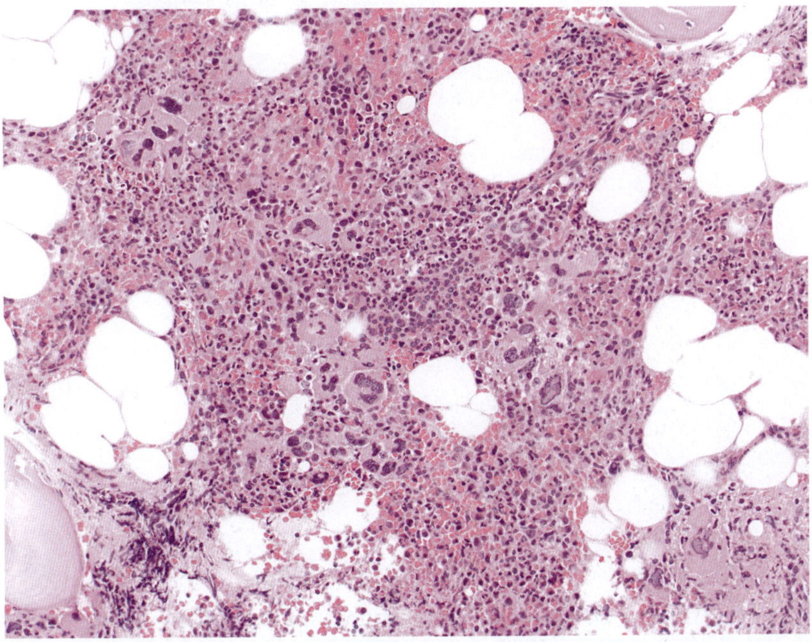

FIGURE 6.14 **This figure shows a bone marrow from a patient with polycythemia vera (PV), showing panmyelosis rather than erythroid predominance; erythroid activity can be depressed because patients may become iron deficient.** The highly pleomorphic megakaryocytes seen here are common in PV.

not be needed in patients with a *JAK2* mutation and sustained significant erythrocytosis (Hct > 55.5% men, >49.5% women).

Megakaryocytes appear very pleomorphic, with a variety of sizes and shapes, but there is no significant dysplasia in the other lineages. Up to 20% of patients have some degree of BM fibrosis at presentation.

Post-PV MF ("spent phase"): Over time, PV may progress to an overtly fibrotic or even osteosclerotic stage (Figure 6.15; eFigure 6.15), and clinical history is key to making the diagnosis at this point. A diagnosis

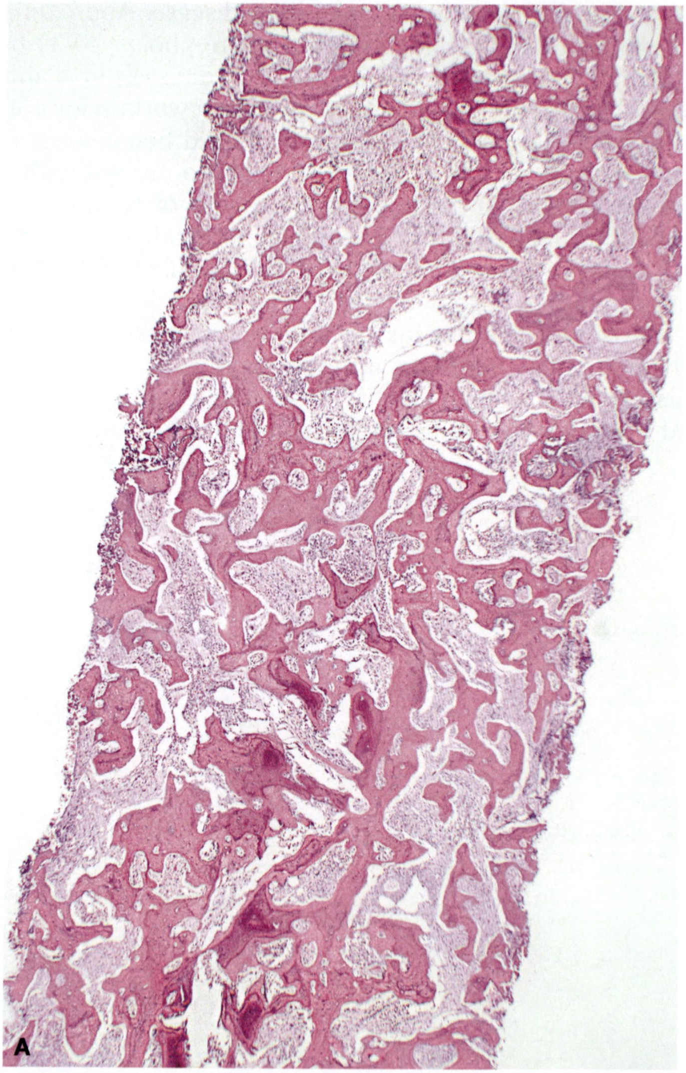

FIGURE 6.15 This low-power view (A) of a bone marrow biopsy shows marrow fibrosis and marked osteosclerosis in a patient with a long-standing history of polycythemia vera, a finding referred to as post–polycythemic myelofibrosis. Figure B shows the same biopsy at higher power.

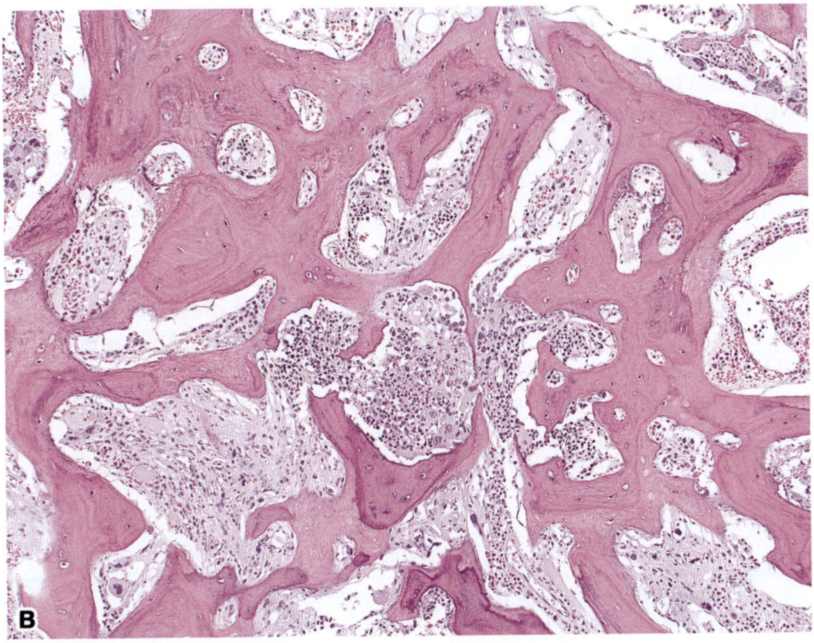

FIGURE 6.15 (*continued*)

of spent phase PV requires (a) definitive history of PV; (b) BM fibrosis of grade 2 or 3; and (c) at least two of the following features: increase in or new development of palpable splenomegaly, anemia, leukoerythroblastosis, weight loss, night sweats, and/or fever. Over time, patients develop ineffective hematopoiesis and become cytopenic. Splenomegaly may become massive because of an extramedullary hematopoiesis.

Genetics

Approximately 96% of PV cases have a *JAK2* V617F mutation and the other 4% have *JAK* exon 12 to 15 mutations. *MPL* and *CALR* mutations are not reported in PV.[31]

Approximately 20% of PV cases have cytogenetic abnormalities detected at diagnosis, most often +8, +9, del(20q), del(13q), and del(9p), whereas 80% of spent phase cases have cytogenetic abnormalities.

Differential Diagnosis

The differential diagnosis includes other causes for erythrocytosis, including secondary or reactive causes[26]:

Congenital: High O_2 affinity hemoglobinopathies; methemoglobinemia; EPO receptor mutations; familial erythrocytosis

Secondary: Reaction to hypoxia or excess production of EPO; other MPNs

Prognosis: Survival is good, with a median life expectancy of 10 years. The 15-year survival is 65%.[41] Adverse findings include increased leukocytosis and abnormal karyotypes.[42] Disease progression is rare in PV, with an incidence of only 5% to 15% of patients likely to progress to MDS/AML.[43] The cause of death for most patients is either a secondary malignancy or a thrombotic event (50%).[44]

PRIMARY MYELOFIBROSIS

This neoplasm is characterized by granulocytic and megakaryocytic proliferation with progressive BM fibrosis. PMF is a rare clonal neoplasm, affecting 0.5/100,000 people per year.

Like PV, this is a biphasic neoplasm with invariable disease progression from a prefibrotic phase, with myeloid and megakaryocytic hyperplasia in the BM, to an overtly fibrotic phase, with variable cellularity, abnormal megakaryocytes, increased fibrotic connective tissue, and extramedullary hematopoiesis (Table 6.6).

TABLE 6.6 PMF Diagnostic Criteria

	Major criteria		Minor criteria
Phase	**PB/BM**	**Genetics**	**Additional features**
Pre-PMF[a]	• Hypercellular BM with myeloid hyperplasia and atypical megakaryocytes • Lacks diagnostic criteria for other MPN	• No *BCR::ABL1* translocation • *JAK2, CALR,* or *MPL* mutation (or other clonal marker or absence of reactive fibrosis)	• Leukocytosis (WBC ≥11,000/µL) • Anemia • Elevated LDH • Splenomegaly
Overt PMF[a]	• BM biopsy with increased atypical megakaryocytes and associated fibrosis (MF grade 2-3) • Lacks diagnostic criteria for other MPN	• No *BCR::ABL1* translocation • *JAK2, CALR,* or *MPL* mutation (or other clonal marker or absence of reactive fibrosis)	• Leukocytosis (WBC ≥11,000/µL) • Anemia • Elevated LDH • Splenomegaly • Leukoerythroblastosis

BM, bone marrow; LDH, lactase dehydrogenase; MF, myelofibrosis; MPN, myeloproliferative neoplasm; PB, peripheral blood; PMF, primary myelofibrosis; WBC, white blood cell; µL, microliter.
[a]Diagnosis requires all major criteria and at least one minor criteria.

Prefibrotic phase: Unlike PV, only about 30% of cases are diagnosed in the prefibrotic phase, and it may be difficult to differentiate from ET at this stage (eFigure 6.16). Over half of patients are symptomatic at presentation and display fatigue, fever, night sweats, or other constitutional symptoms. A CBC reveals variable cytoses, including neutrophilia and/or thrombocytosis, confirmed by PB examination. In the prefibrotic phase, the BM is hypercellular for age, with myeloid and megakaryocytic hyperplasia.

Overtly fibrotic phase: In this phase, patients will have variable cytopenias, especially anemia, and the PB often shows leukoerythroblastosis.

BM examination in the overtly fibrotic stage reveals characteristic findings. The BM aspirate is often inaspirable ("dry tap"), and the core biopsy shows a variably hypocellular marrow with increased fibrosis (Figure 6.16A and B; eFigure 6.17). The degree of reticulin fibrosis and collagen fibrosis is assessed and graded using a reticulin stain and a trichrome stain, respectively. As discussed earlier, sequential grading of reticulin and collagen fibrosis is important to track disease progression.

Abundant abnormal megakaryocytes are observed in this stage. The megakaryocytes have a characteristic morphology and location, which can help differentiate pre-PMF from ET. Megakaryocytes are more pleomorphic than in other MPNs and often show "cloud-like," round, condensed nuclei (Figure 6.17; eFigure 6.18). They often form large clusters of cells located near bony trabecula or within expanded sinuses within which hematopoiesis may also be identified (Figure 6.18; eFigure 6.19). The

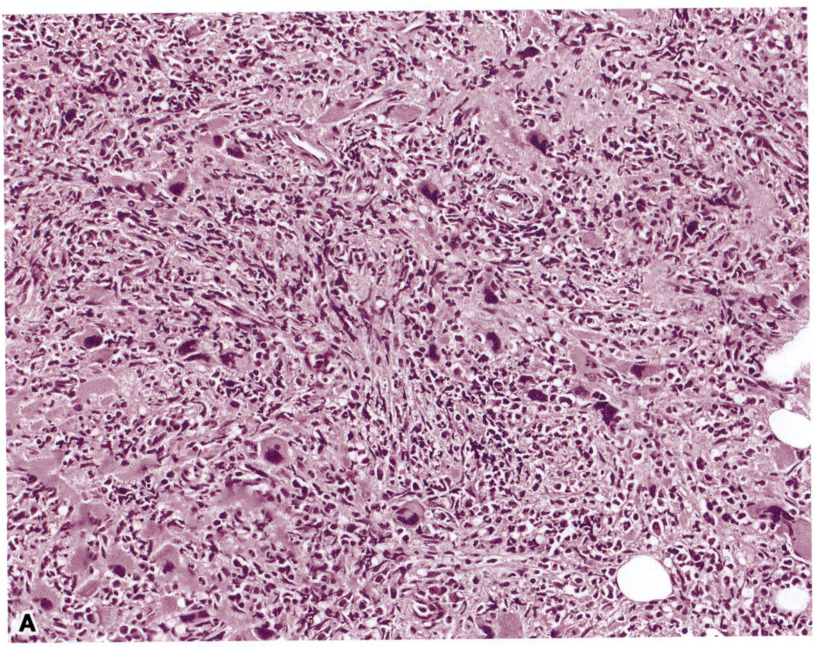

FIGURE 6.16 The marrow in a case of primary myelofibrosis is hypercellular with atypical megakaryocytes and marrow fibrosis apparent as a streaming effect (A). The fibrosis is highlighted by a reticulin stain (B).

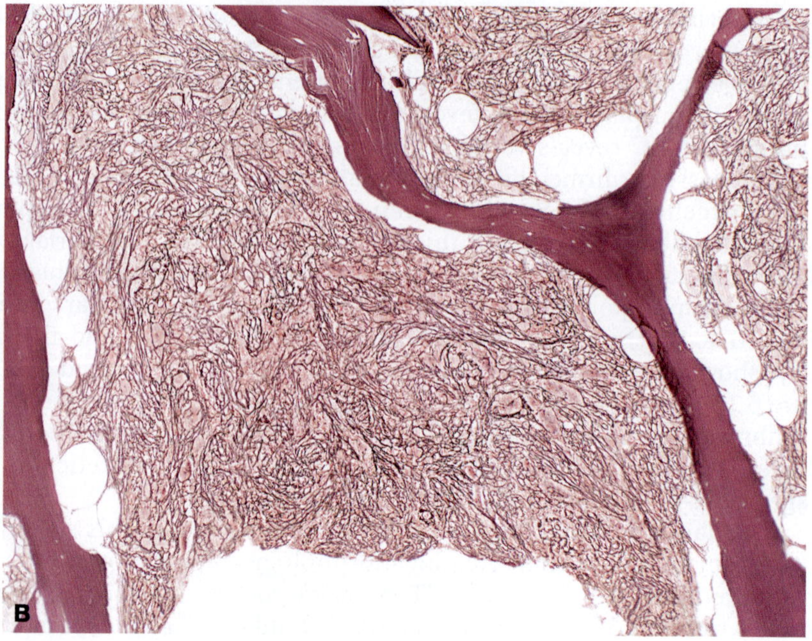

FIGURE 6.16 (*continued*)

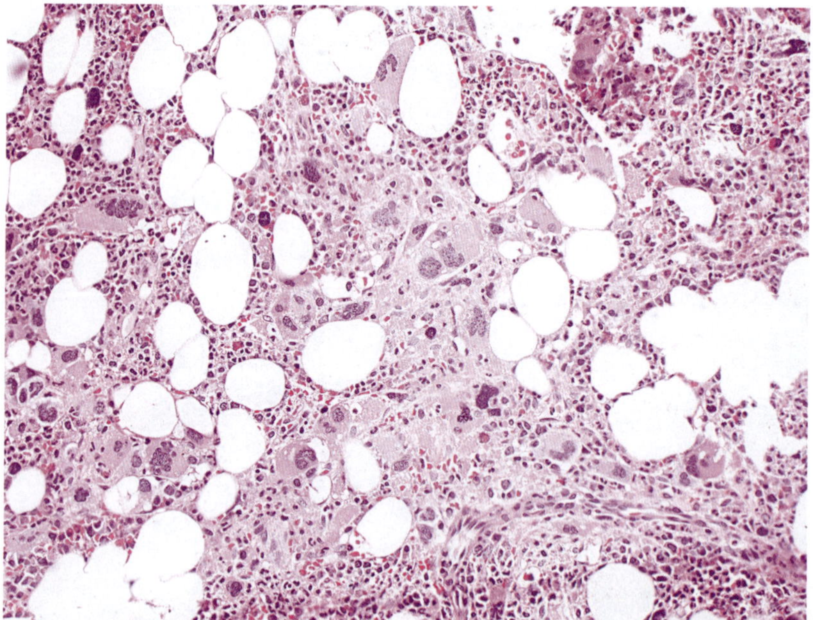

FIGURE 6.17 Primary myelofibrosis megakaryocytes have nuclei that have been described as "cloud-like" or globoid, with condensed chromatin, as shown here.

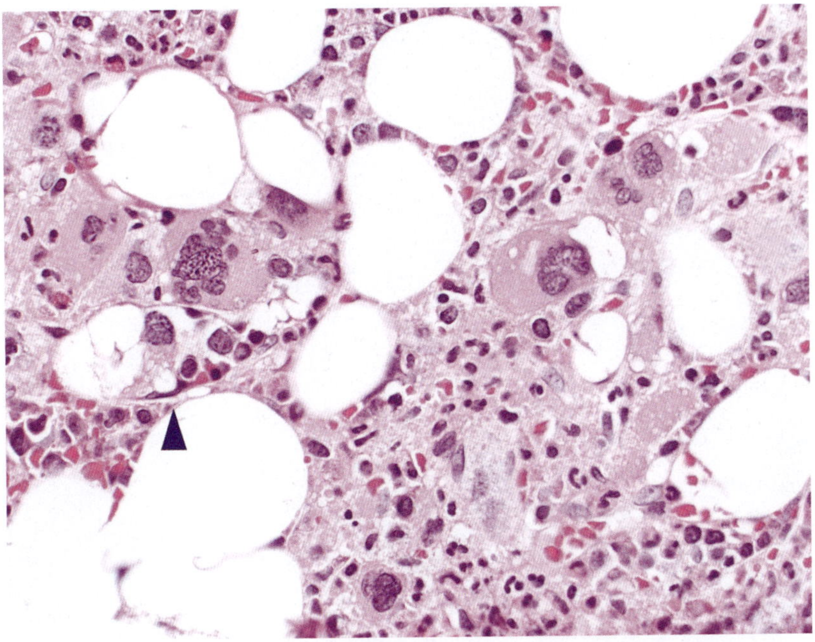

FIGURE 6.18 In primary myelofibrosis, the bone marrow often shows dilated sinuses that contain hematopoietic elements (arrowhead), including megakaryocytes.

number of blasts should be assessed, but this may prove difficult because of the lack of an adequate aspirate smear. In these cases, IHC stains for CD34 are useful to detect increased blasts on the core biopsy. CD34 also highlights increased vessels, which correlates with the degree of fibrosis, and may be prognostically relevant.[45] This stage may also show abundant osteosclerosis (Figure 6.19).

Genetics

There is no specific genetic defect, but 65% have *JAK2* V617F mutations, 8% have *MPL* mutations, and 24% have *CALR* mutations; the rest are negative for all three mutations ("triple negative").

Differential Diagnosis

The differential diagnosis includes any insult to the BM that results in fibrosis. Radiation, viruses, toxins, and other factors can cause a marked fibrosis nearly indistinguishable from PMF. Gray platelet syndrome can show a resemblance to early fibrotic phase PMF in the BM, but these usually show hypogranulated platelets in the PB, a finding not seen in PMF. Autoimmune disorders may mimic PMF in the BM, but these typically present with cytopenias in the PB.[46,47]

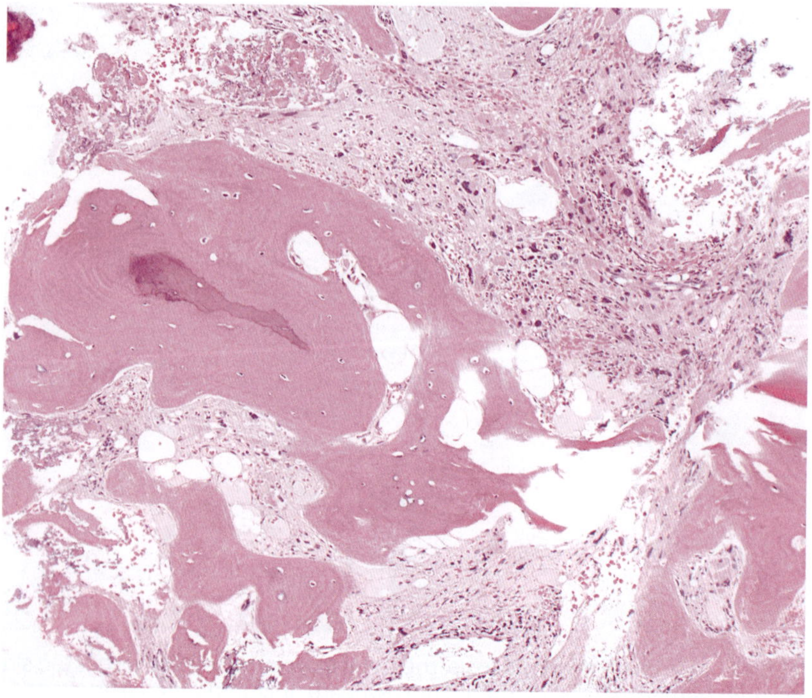

FIGURE 6.19 Late-stage primary myelofibrosis with abundant osteosclerosis and fibrotic marrow with atypical megakaryocytes, often compressed by surrounding fibrosis.

Prognosis

The prognosis depends on the phase of disease and risk status: prefibrotic PMF has a 10-year survival of 72% and a 15-year survival of 59%; overt PMF has 3- to 7-year overall survival, but treatment with interferon or JAK1/JAK2 inhibitors may delay or reverse fibrosis. Progression to BP is more common than in PV and has been reported in 5% to 30% of patients in different studies. *CALR*-mutated patients have a better prognosis and a longer overall survival than those with *JAK2* and *MPL* mutations.[32]

ESSENTIAL THROMBOCYTHEMIA

ET is a clonal disorder that results in the proliferation of abnormal megakaryocytes in the BM, thrombocytosis in the PB, and increased risk of thrombosis and/or hemorrhage (Table 6.7). This affects approximately 1/100,000 people per year, mostly people in their 50s-60s, although there is a second peak seen in patients in their 30s. Unlike PV and PMF, ET does not show significant BM fibrosis at diagnosis.

TABLE 6.7 ET Diagnostic Criteria

	Major criteria		Minor criteria
Phase	**PB/BM**	**Genetics**	**Additional features**
ET[a]	• Thrombocytosis (platelets ≥ 450,000/µL) • Increased atypical megakaryocytes with "staghorn" nuclei in BM • Lacks diagnostic criteria for other MPN	• No *BCR::ABL1* translocation • *JAK2*, *CALR*, or *MPL* mutation	• Presence of clonal marker or absence of evidence of reactive thrombocytosis
Post-ET fibrosis[b]	BM fibrosis (MF grade 2-3)		• Anemia • Elevated LDH • Splenomegaly • B symptoms[c] • Leukoerythroblastosis

BM, bone marrow; ET, essential thrombocythemia; LDH, lactase dehydrogenase; MF, myelofibrosis; PB, peripheral blood.

[a]Must fulfill all major criteria OR thrombocytosis, increased atypical megakaryocytes, and absence of *BCR:ABL1* in addition to the presence of a clonal marker (or absence of evidence of reactive thrombocytosis).

[b]Must have an established diagnosis of ET with fibrosis and at least two additional features.

[c]Weight loss, night sweats, fever.

Clinical

Most patients (>50%) are asymptomatic at presentation. Those patients with symptoms may show bleeding in the mucosa, gastrointestinal (GI) tract, or elsewhere. Patients may also have the propensity to clot, causing paresthesias and transient ischemic attacks (TIAs).

A CBC shows a markedly elevated platelet count and relatively normal WBC and Hgb. Morphologic review of the PB smear confirms thrombocytosis and reveals platelets with marked anisocytosis (Figure 6.20) as well as occasional circulating megakaryocytic nuclei and micromegakaryocytes. Platelet granulation abnormalities, however, are not seen.

Morphology

The BM is often normocellular for age and shows large, "staghorn" megakaryocytes with hyperlobulated hyperchromatic nuclei (Figure 6.21A and B; eFigure 6.20). Although there are some interobserver discrepancies,[48]

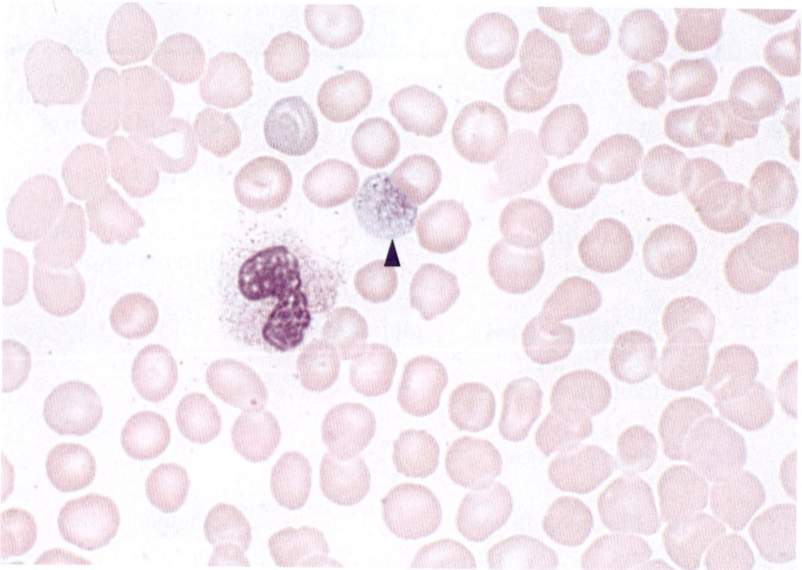

FIGURE 6.20 This is a peripheral blood smear in a patient with essential thrombocythemia showing a giant platelet (arrowhead).

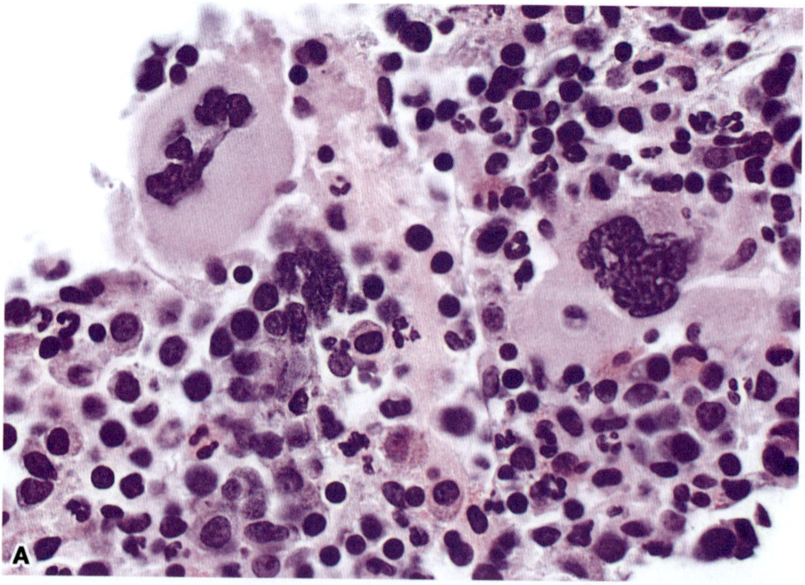

FIGURE 6.21 This bone marrow in a patient with essential thrombocythemia shows megakaryocytes with "staghorn" nuclei on the core biopsy (A). There is no significant fibrosis. The aspirate smear also reveals a giant megakaryocyte with a hyperlobated nucleus (B).

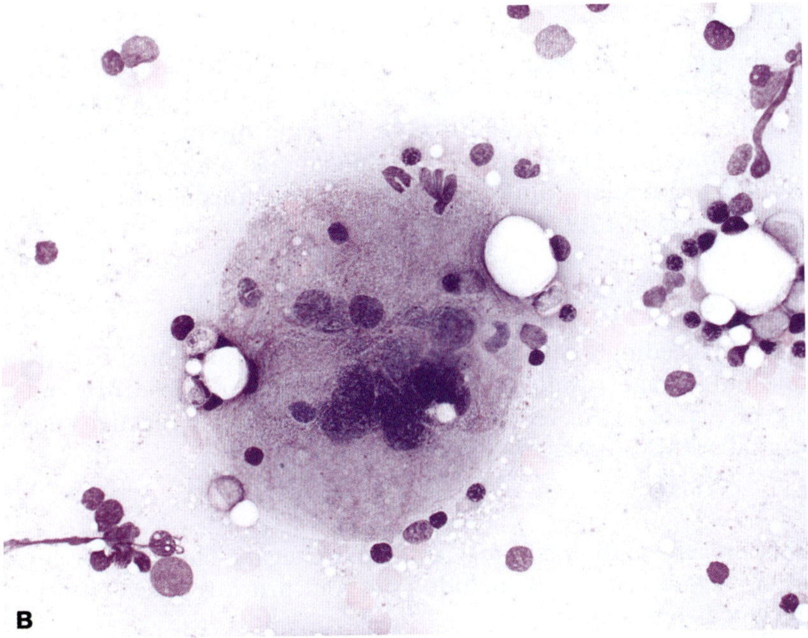

FIGURE 6.21 *(continued)*

they are generally easy to distinguish from megakaryocytes in other MPN subtypes. These megakaryocytes are the largest of all MPNs. Megakaryocyte clusters of three cells or more are infrequent, and very large clusters should suggest prefibrotic PMF as an alternate diagnosis. Fibrosis is rare at diagnosis (10%) and never above grade 1, although more significant fibrosis is found in post-ET MF.

Genetics

Approximately 55% of cases show *JAK2* V617F mutations, typically at a lower variant allele frequency than either PV or PMF. *JAK2* exon 12 mutations are not seen. The remaining cases have mutations in *MPL* (3%) or in *CALR* (30%). Patients with *CALR*-mutated ET tend to be younger and have higher platelet count and lower Hgb than those with *JAK2*-mutated ET.[34]

Differential Diagnosis

The differential diagnosis is broad and includes MDS/MPN with ring sideroblasts and thrombocytosis, prefibrotic PMF, MDS with del(5q) inv(3) AML/MDS, and CML; of these, only the first two will have mutations in *JAK2*, *MPL*, or *CALR*. Reactive thrombocytosis also needs to be excluded: Iron deficiency is a common confounder, especially in those patients with only mild thrombocytosis.

Prognosis

Approximately <5% of ET cases accelerate, generally via progression to post-ET MF; transformation to AML is rare, and life expectancy is near normal. It is important to differentiate ET from prefibrotic PMF because the latter have different disease complications and poorer survival.[49] *CALR*-mutated patients appear to have a better thrombosis-free survival than those without *CALR*.[33]

CHRONIC NEUTROPHILIC LEUKEMIA

This is an exceedingly rare MPN that presents with a clonal expansion of the myeloid lineage, resulting in a high ANC. CNL mimics CML, but there is no evidence of *BCR::ABL1*. As there are many other reactive causes for neutrophilia, this is a diagnosis of exclusion.

Clinical

Patients present with splenomegaly, hepatomegaly, bleeding, or bruising. Other signs and symptoms include gout and pruritus, elevated uric acid, and elevated serum vitamin B_{12}.

Morphologic

The PB shows absolute neutrophilia; historically, the WBC threshold was 25,000/µL, although this has recently been lowered to 13,000/µL. At least 80% of cells are granulocytes at the band or neutrophil stage, and there are usually <5% immature myeloid forms, and rare-to-no blasts; the marrow is markedly hypercellular and myeloid dominant but contains cells of all stages of maturation (Figure 6.22; eFigure 6.21). Toxic granulations and Döhle bodies may be seen, but these are not specific, as they are also seen in reactive neutrophilia. Significant eosinophilia, basophilia, or monocytosis should suggest other diagnoses.

Patients have a hypercellular BM with granulocytic hyperplasia. Often, increased macrophages may be identified phagocytosing granulocytes. Fibrosis is rare, and significant dysplasia should be absent and should instead suggest aCML.

Occasionally, underlying plasma cell dyscrasias are associated with CNL, so that patients with CNL should be evaluated for these disorders. It is postulated that in a subset of cases, this association may be due to granulocyte colony-stimulating factor (G-CSF)-secreting plasma cells, whereas other cases have both clonal neutrophils and plasma cells.[50]

Genetics

CNL is cytogenetically normal in 90% of cases. Mutations in *CSF3R* are strongly associated with CNL, often together with mutations of *SETBP1*, *SRSF1*, or *ASXL1*. MPN-associated driver mutations (*JAK2*, *MPL*, and *CALR*) are usually absent.

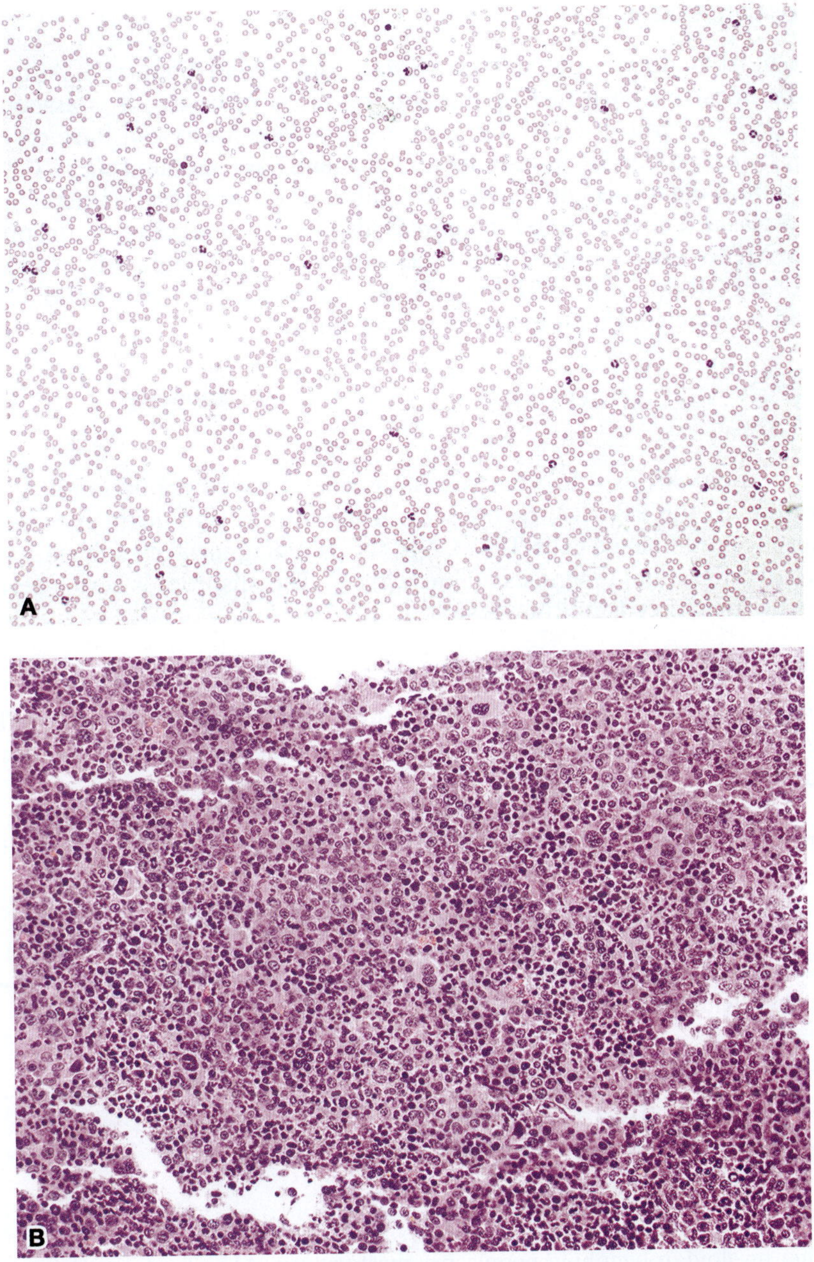

FIGURE 6.22 Chronic neutrophilic leukemia (CNL), as shown in this peripheral blood (A), presents with neutrophilia; unlike chronic myeloid leukemia (CML) immature myeloid cells and basophils are absent, although this diagnosis should not be made without excluding a *BCR::ABL1* translocation (B). As in CML, a core biopsy in CNL is markedly hypercellular and overwhelmingly myeloid and, in contrast to the blood, contains a range of maturing myeloid cells.

Differential Diagnosis

CNL must be differentiated from aCML, discussed in Chapter 5. Although aCML does not have *CSF3R* mutations (<10% of cases), it is associated with *SETBP1* and/or *ETNK1* mutations (one-third of cases). Rare cases of CNL can lack *CSF3R* mutations and if these have mutated *SETBP1*, the differential diagnosis can be very difficult and usually rests on assessment of dysplasia. The differential diagnosis also includes reactive neutrophilia; other MPNs are less often confused with CNL, although it is critical to perform PCR for *BCR::ABL1* to rule out the neutrophilic variant of CML, which is associated with the variant isoform p230.

CHRONIC EOSINOPHILIC LEUKEMIA, NOT OTHERWISE SPECIFIED

CEL is a clonal disorder that results in uncontrolled proliferation of eosinophils in the PB, BM, or other tissues, with no significant increase in other myeloid lineage cells. Like CNL, this is a diagnosis of exclusion, with a broad differential diagnosis (Table 6.8).[51-54] This disorder is very rare, and the true incidence is unknown.

Clinical

Patients may present with the signs and symptoms of hypereosinophilia. Organ damage to the heart, lung, GI tract, and skin is due to eosinophilic degranulation.

CBC findings include hypereosinophilia (>1500 K/µL) present for >6 months. Eosinophils are mature, but may show some dysplasia, including

TABLE 6.8 The Differential Diagnosis of Chronic Eosinophilic Leukemia

Myeloid/lymphoid neoplasms with eosinophilia and tyrosine kinase gene fusions
Other MPNs with *JAK2, CALR, MPL* and increased eosinophils
CML with *BCR::ABL1* with eosinophilia
CMML with eosinophilia
aCML with eosinophilia
Lymphocytic variant of HES
Other myeloid or lymphoid neoplasms: mastocytosis, ALL, T cell lymphoma, CHL, etc.
Reactive causes: Parasites, allergies, pulmonary disease, angiolymphoid hyperplasia, collagen vascular disease, Kimura disease, *etc.*

[a]CML, atypical CML; ALL, acute lymphoblastic leukemia; CHL, classic Hodgkin lymphoma; CML, chronic myeloid leukemia; CMML, chronic myelomonocytic leukemia; HES, hypereosinophilic syndrome; MPN, myeloproliferative neoplasm.

hyper- or hypogranulation, and/or hypo- or hypersegmentation. Dysplasia does not exclude reactive causes, however, as reactive eosinophils may also be morphologically atypical.[55] Immature eosinophilic forms are not prominent.

Morphologic

BM findings include a hypercellular marrow with a marked eosinophilic proliferation (Figure 6.23A; eFigure 6.22). As in the PB, eosinophils may show some dysplasia, and there may be dysplastic megakaryocytes, but there should be no significant dysplasia of erythroid or neutrophilic lineages. There may be a concomitant myeloid proliferation, as well as mildly increased myeloid blasts, but blasts must constitute <20% of total cells. The BM often shows fibrosis because of eosinophilic degranulation. Charcot-Leyden crystals may be seen in the BM or in other tissue biopsies (Figure 6.23B; eFigure 6.23).

Immunohistochemical stains, including mast cell tryptase or CD117, should be performed to rule out systemic mastocytosis (SM), which can show similar morphologic findings in the BM (see below).

Genetics

CEL is not associated with any characteristic genetic abnormalities, but molecular studies are useful to rule out other disorders associated with eosinophilia. Reactive eosinophils may be seen in other MPNs; these are not part of the clone, but are reacting to increased levels of interleukin (IL)-2, IL-3, IL-5, or granulocyte-macrophage CSF.

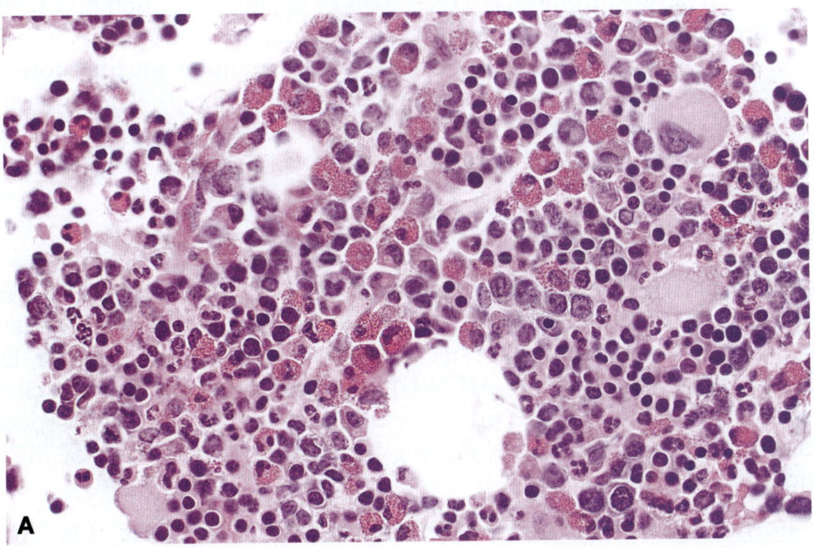

FIGURE 6.23 Chronic eosinophilic leukemia (CEL) presents with eosinophilia in the peripheral blood and bone marrow (BM) (A), although the diagnosis is one of exclusion. Charcot-Leyden crystals (arrowhead) may be seen in the BM or in tissue biopsies in CEL (B).

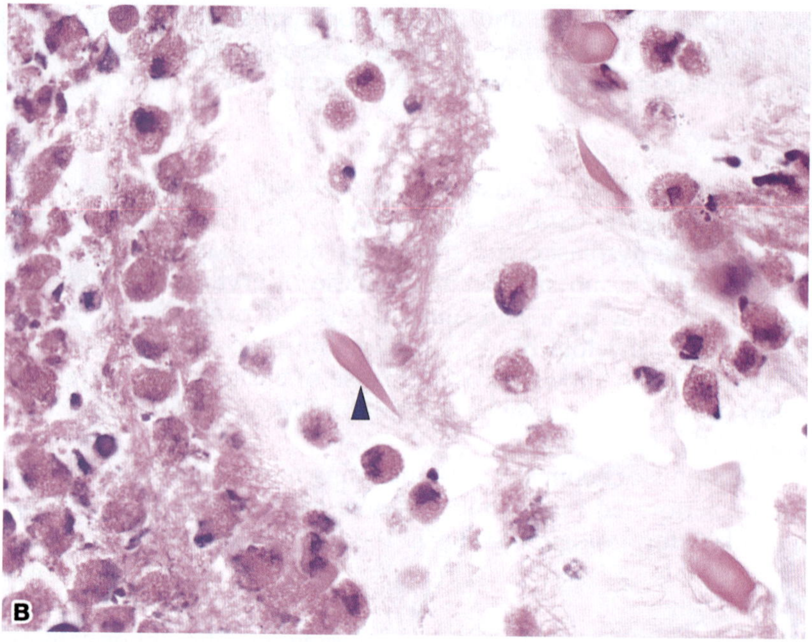

FIGURE 6.23 *(continued)*

IDIOPATHIC HYPEREOSINOPHILIA/IDIOPATHIC HYPEREOSINOPHILIC SYNDROME

Idiopathic hypereosinophilia is a diagnosis of exclusion, which may be diagnosed in certain cases where eosinophilic clonality cannot be established. Idiopathic hypereosinophilic syndrome (HES) includes all the aforementioned criteria, with associated tissue damage (Table 6.9). The differential diagnosis includes infection, inflammation, toxins, growth factors, cytokines, immunosuppressives, and malignancies like cancer or lymphoma.

MYELOPROLIFERATIVE NEOPLASM, UNCLASSIFIABLE

This group of neoplasms represents approximately 10% of all MPNs and is reserved for those clonal MPNs that cannot be further subtyped, either because of overlapping features or because of a lack of specific criteria. Diagnosis of MPN, unclassifiable (MPN-U) requires that there be both clinical features of an MPN and the presence of a characteristic MPN-associated mutation. The most common reasons for making a diagnosis of MPN-U include:

1. Early stage of an MPN: At the earliest stages of disease, it is difficult and sometimes impossible to tell the difference between MPNs.
2. Late stage of an MPN: Similarly, it is difficult to determine the specific disorder at the very latest stages of a disorder when fibrosis obscures morphologic features.

TABLE 6.9 iHES Diagnostic Criteria

PB	BM	Genetics	Other
• Hypereosinophilia (eosinophils ≥1500/μL)	• Normal BM with exception of increased eosinophils	• No genetic abnormalities other than CHIP	• Organ damage • Exclusion of autoimmune or neoplastic condition • Exclusion of lymphocyte variant HES

BM, bone marrow; CHIP, clonal hematopoiesis of indeterminate potential; HES, hypereosinophilic syndrome; iHES, idiopathic HES; PB, peripheral blood.

3. Coexisting neoplasm that obscures the MPN: Occasionally, the patient may have a secondary malignancy that occupies the marrow space, precluding accurate morphologic assessment of the MPN.

It is recommended to note on the report the differential diagnosis and reasons for the ambiguity. However, a diagnosis of MPN-U should not be made on the basis of an inadequate sample or incomplete clinical information; rather, the report should be descriptive and raise MPN as a diagnostic consideration, indicating the factors precluding diagnosis. In addition, other diagnostic considerations should be carefully considered in patients with prior toxic therapy.

Differential Diagnosis

The differential diagnosis includes MDS with fibrosis or MDS/MPN. Significant dysplasia, cytopenias, or monocytosis favors the latter. Other reactive causes must be excluded.

MYELOID/LYMPHOID NEOPLASMS WITH EOSINOPHILIA AND TK GENE FUSIONS

This separate category of neoplasms is now comprised of fusions involving six different TK genes, each with a most common fusion partner, but also including variants that produce similar, although often not identical, diseases. All of these occur because of the formation of an aberrant TK, either through mutation or through gene rearrangement. The detection of these genetic abnormalities is sufficient for diagnosis regardless of morphology. They may present as myeloid or lymphoid neoplasms and are often, but not always, associated with eosinophilia. It is important to recognize and diagnose these disorders, as some, most notably those with platelet-derived growth factor receptor (PDGFR)α/β, are effectively treated with commonly used TKIs, whereas others respond to specific kinase inhibitors.

1. **Neoplasms with *PDGFRa* rearrangements:** The most common rearrangement, *FIPIL1::PDGFRa*, occurs because of a deletion at 4q12 involving the *CHIC2* gene. This is a cryptic deletion, which requires detection by FISH, as it cannot be identified by normal karyotype. Patients present with morphologic findings consistent with CEL, but may also present with AML or T cell ALL (T-ALL)-like morphology. Variant translocations occur, and the features of the disease often depend on the fusion partner.
2. **Neoplasms with *PDGFRB* rearrangements:** These rearrangements, most often t(15;12)(q32;p13.2) *ETV6::PDGFRB*, present with morphologic features of CMML with eosinophilia (Figure 6.24; eFigure 6.24). There are >30 partner genes that produce variant translocations.
3. **Neoplasms with *FGFR1* rearrangements:** This disorder often presents as T-ALL with eosinophilia and less commonly as CEL, B-ALL, AML, or MPAL. It does not respond to the usual TKIs but responds to fibroblast growth factor receptor (FGFR) inhibition.
4. **Neoplasms with *PCM1::JAK2*:** This results from t(8;9)(p22;p24.1), and patients typically present either with an MPN with eosinophilia or with myeloblastic or B-lymphoblastic transformations. *ETV6* and *BCR* have been described as alternate partners.
5. **Neoplasms with *ETV6::FLT3*:** This may present as T-ALL/lymphoblastic lymphoma (LBL) or myeloid sarcoma with MPN-like BM features.
6. **Neoplasms with *ETV6::ABL1*:** These have similarities to *BCR::ABL1*-positive CML with eosinophilia in CP or in myeloid or lymphoid BP; they are typically responsive to second-generation TKIs.

MASTOCYTOSIS

Mastocytosis is considered a separate, unique group of disorders resulting in a clonal proliferation of mast cells forming aggregates in different organs. Severe cases may lead to organ failure.

The various subtypes are categorized based on pathologic features, anatomic location, and clinical findings. Most cases involve the skin, and up to 30% of systemic mastocytosis (SM) have an associated myeloid neoplasm (AMN); such cases are referred to as SM-AMN.

Normal mast cells are oval cells with round-to-oval nuclei and abundant cytoplasm with metachromatic granules (Figure 6.25A), although this may not be appreciated on H&E as tissue processing may leach the granules. Neoplastic mast cells are typically spindle-shaped (Figure 6.25B; eFigure 6.25) and may be hypogranular. Abnormal mast cells may aggregate in clusters or may be diffusely interspersed. In SM, BM biopsies often show aggregates of mast cells associated with lymphocytes and eosinophils (Figure 6.26A-D; eFigure 6.26). There may be associated fibrosis and bony trabeculae may be thickened or sclerotic.

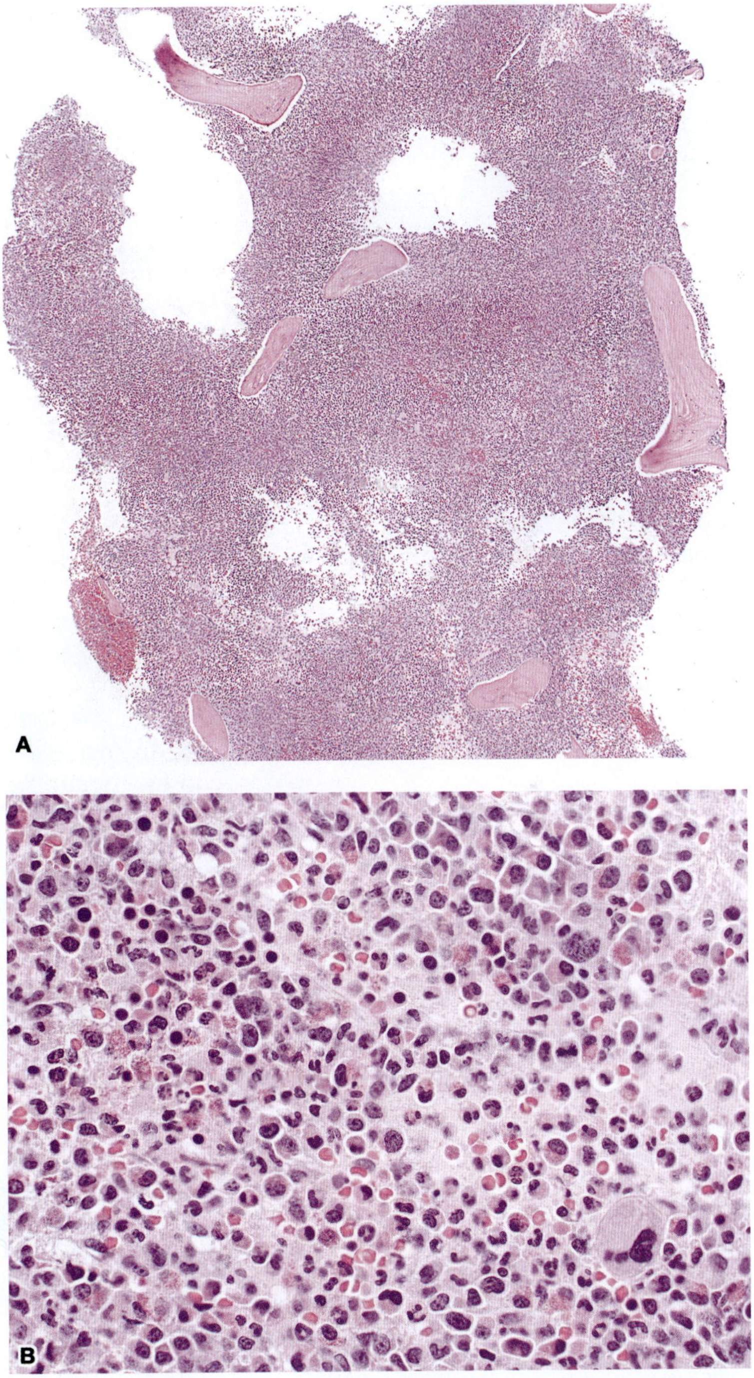

FIGURE 6.24 **This patient had a myeloid neoplasm with eosinophilia and a tyrosine kinase gene fusion, in this case a rearrangement of *PDGFRB*.** The bone marrow core biopsy at low power (A) and at high power (B) shows a myeloid hyperplasia and increased eosinophils, although the morphologic features are not specific and diagnosis requires demonstration of the specific gene fusion.

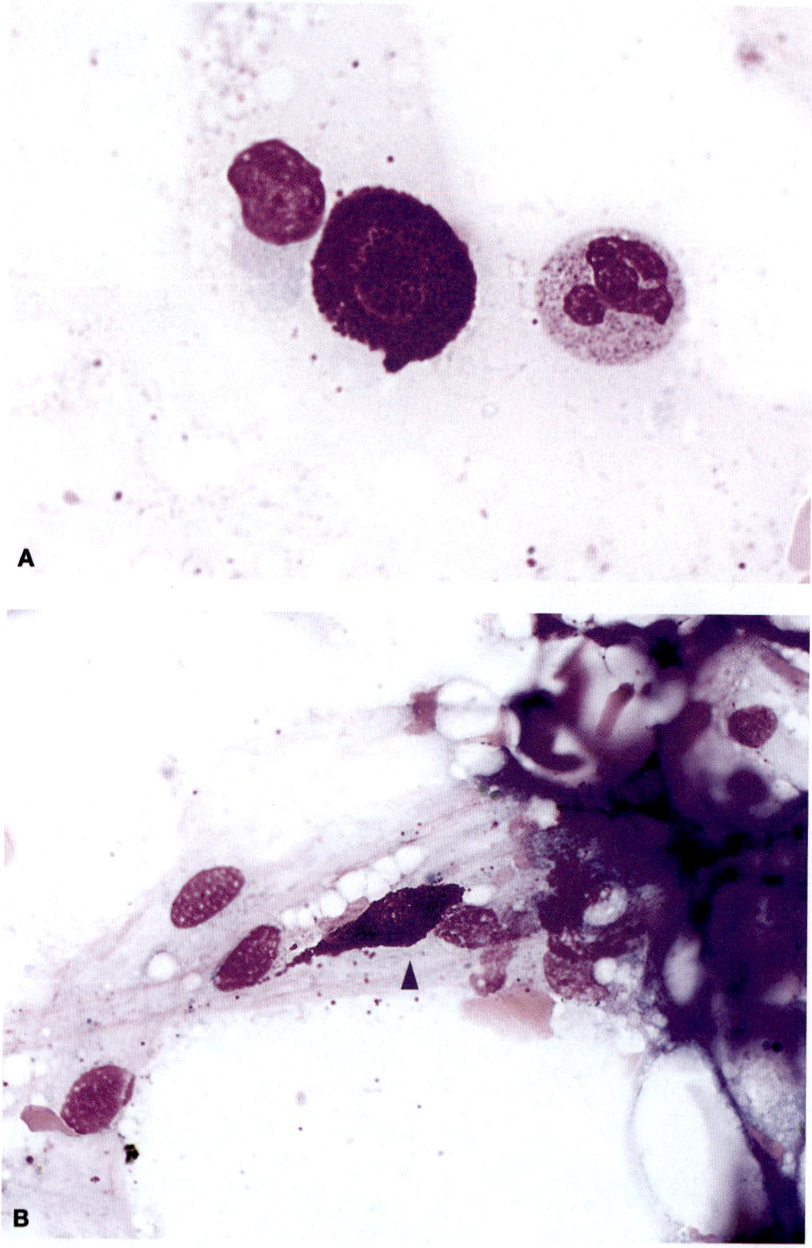

FIGURE 6.25 Normal mast cells are oval with round-to-oval nuclei and metachromatic cytoplasmic granules (A), as seen in this aspirate smear. Abnormal mast cells are more often spindle-shaped (B, arrowhead) or hypogranular.

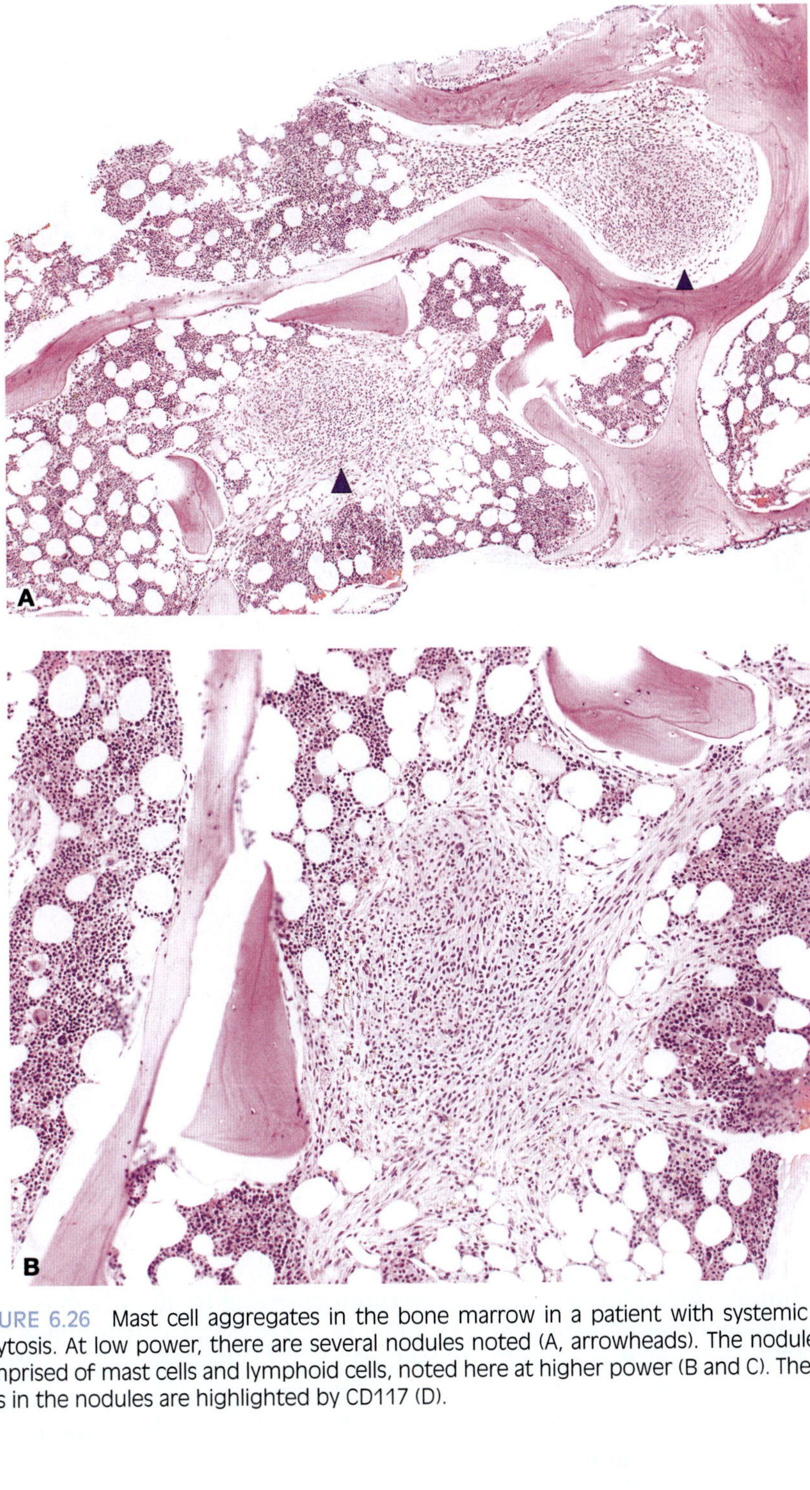

FIGURE 6.26 Mast cell aggregates in the bone marrow in a patient with systemic mastocytosis. At low power, there are several nodules noted (A, arrowheads). The nodules are comprised of mast cells and lymphoid cells, noted here at higher power (B and C). The mast cells in the nodules are highlighted by CD117 (D).

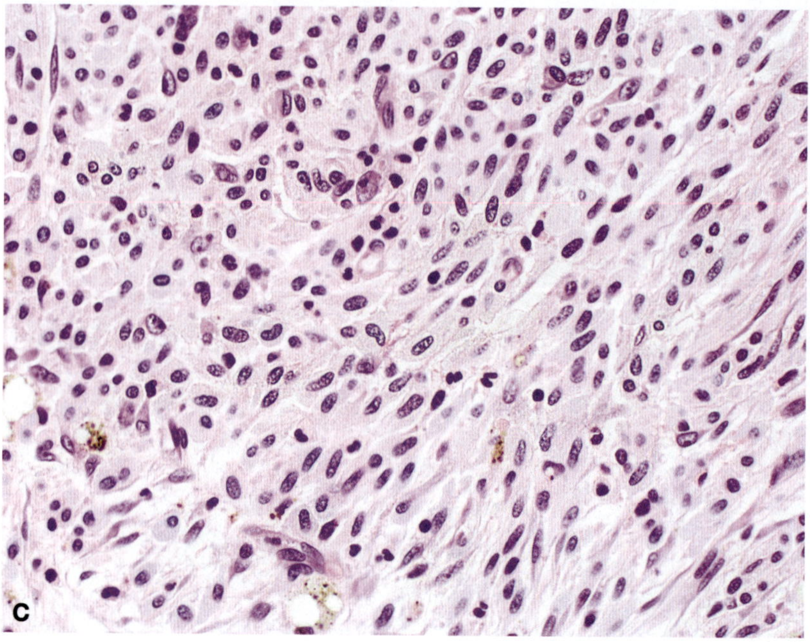

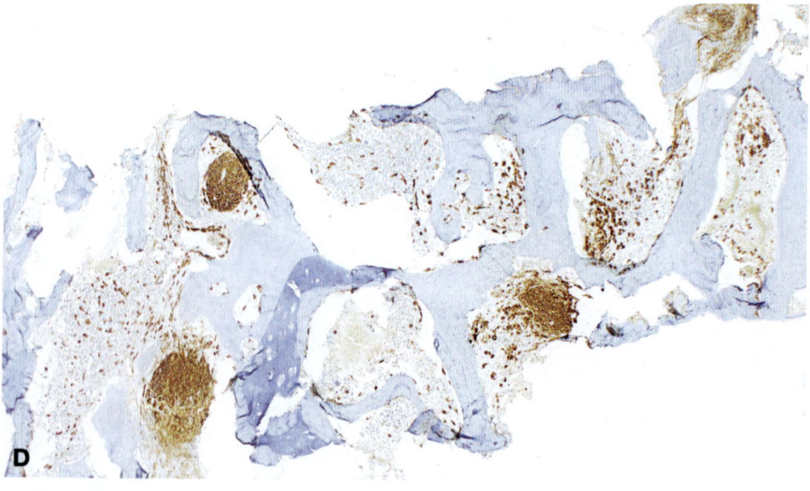

FIGURE 6.26 *(continued)*

Immunohistochemical stains are often essential to identify mast cells on tissue sections (Figure 6.27A-D; eFigure 6.27): Mast cell tryptase and CD117 highlight all mast cells. Neoplastic mast cells also express CD25 and to a lesser degree CD2 or CD30.[56-58] CD30 is particularly important to recognize cases in which mast cells lack the characteristic spindle cell morphology important for diagnosis.

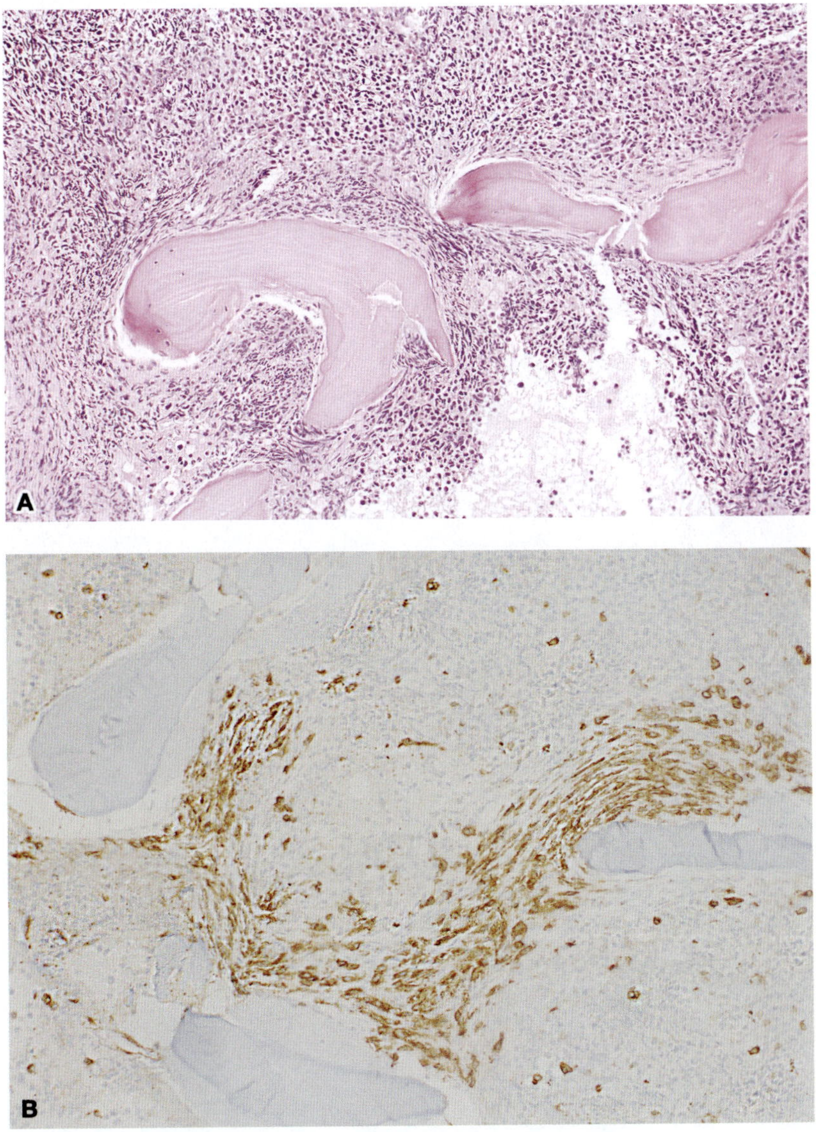

FIGURE 6.27 This mast cell infiltrate noted on hematoxylin and eosin (A) is also highlighted by immunohistochemical stains for CD117 (B), mast cell tryptase (MCT) (C), and CD25 (D). The hypercellular myeloid-predominant background suggests additional involvement by an systemic mastocytosis (SM)-associated myeloid neoplasm (AMN). The most common AMN to co-occur with systemic mastocytosis is chronic myelomonocytic leukemia.

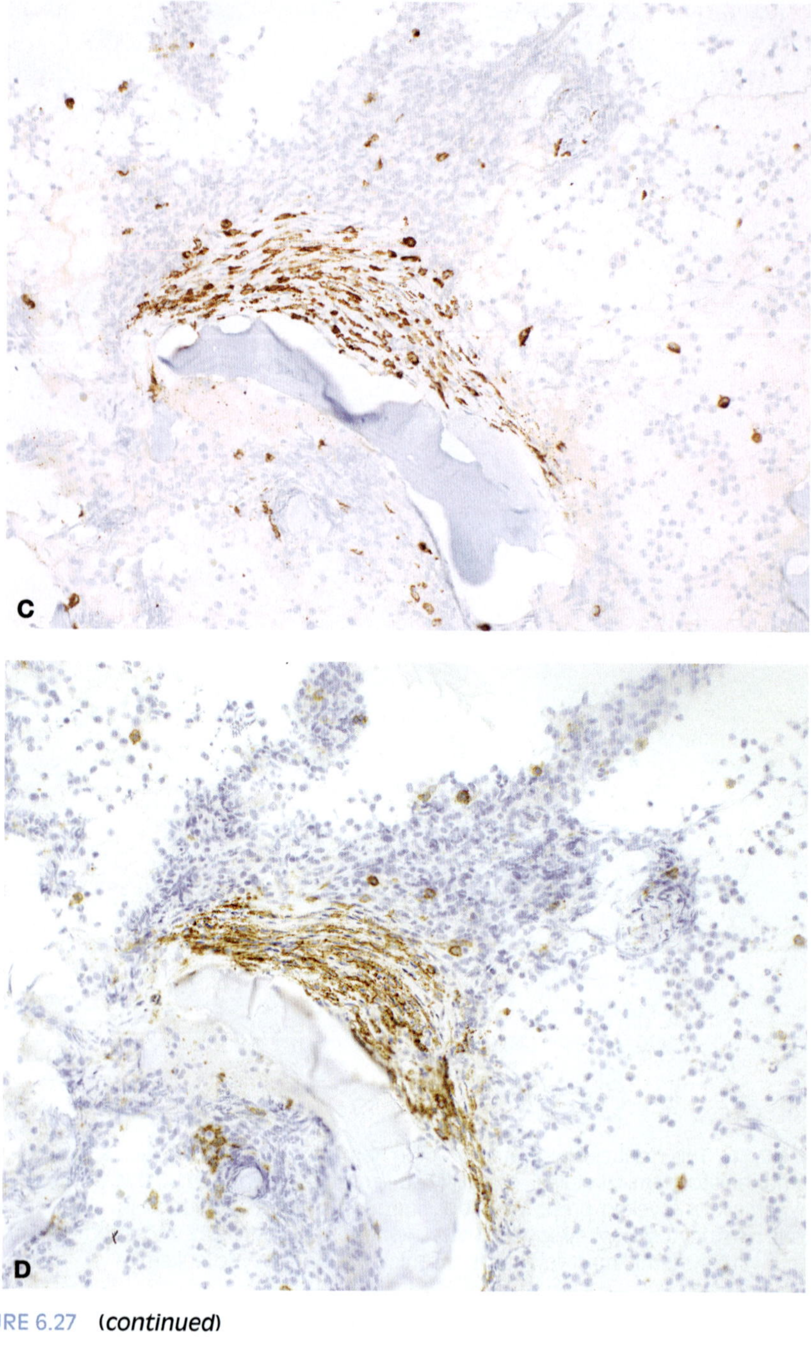

FIGURE 6.27 (*continued*)

1. **Cutaneous Mastocytosis:** This disorder usually presents in childhood. The three subvariants include: (a) maculopapular rash; (b) diffuse cutaneous; and (c) mastocytoma. All three subvariants display urticaria pigmentosa. Stroking the skin causes a wheal to form (urticaria/Darier sign); melanin pigment is identified (pigmentosum).
2. **Systemic Mastocytosis:** This more often presents in middle-age patients. A diagnosis of SM requires one extracutaneous site of disease and almost always involves the BM. The major and minor criteria are listed in Table 6.10. Mastocytosis is further subtyped based on the manifestation of symptoms (B and C findings; Table 6.11); the five

TABLE 6.10 SM Diagnostic Criteria

Criteria[a]	Features
Major	• Multiple clusters of mast cells (>15 cells per cluster) in BM or other noncutaneous organ
Minor	• >25% of mast cells are spindled or immature
	• Mast cells express CD25, CD2, or CD30
	• *KIT* D816V mutation or other activating *KIT* mutation
	• Elevated serum tryptase >20 ng/mL

BM, bone marrow; SM, systemic mastocytosis.
[a]In the absence of the major criteria, at least three out of four minor criteria must be met.

TABLE 6.11 B and C Findings in SM

Category	Features
B	• MC aggregates comprise >30% of BM cellularity on biopsy.
	• Serum tryptase >200 ng/mL
	• Cytopenias (excluding C findings) or cytoses
	• Exclude reactive causes.
	• Criteria for other myeloid neoplasms are not met
	• Hepatomegaly without impairment of liver function, or splenomegaly without features of hypersplenism
C	• BM dysfunction caused by neoplastic MC infiltration (≥1 cytopenia)
	• Hepatomegaly with impaired liver function
	• Splenomegaly with hypersplenism
	• Skeletal involvement with osteolytic lesions
	• Malabsorption/weight loss because of GI MCs

BM, bone marrow; GI, gastrointestinal; MC, mast cell; SM, systemic mastocytosis.

subtypes are listed below. Patients typically present with organomegaly, anemia, neutropenia, thrombocytopenia, and an elevated eosinophil count. There may be other cytoses depending on the presence of an AMN.

- Indolent Mastocytosis: 1 B finding; low mast cell burden; may or may not involve skin. The WHO 5th edition describes a provisional entity of indolent mastocytosis involving the BM only, without skin lesions,[59] known as bone marrow mastocytosis (BMM). Studies have shown that in these cases, the *KIT* mutations are limited to the BM mast cells; they often involve elderly males, are more clinically indolent, and have lower serum tryptase levels. In half of these patients, mast cell mediator release is triggered exclusively by insects.[60]
- Smoldering Mastocytosis: >1 B finding, more than one organ involved; may progress.
- Aggressive Mastocytosis: 1 C finding, mast cells comprise <20% of nucleated cells in BM; skin involvement may be absent or present.
- Mastocytosis with AMN: The symptoms, course, and prognosis depend on *both* malignancies, and both must be listed as separate entities on the diagnostic line. *KIT* mutations are often found in both neoplastic entities. CMML is very common and aCML is also often seen; both have *KIT* mutations. Lymphoid neoplasms are rare and do not share *KIT* mutations.[61-63]
- Mast Cell Leukemia (MCL): Mast cells comprise >20% of cells in BM aspirate. Typical MCL has >10% in PB, but the more common aleukemic variant has <10% mast cells in PB. The survival is poor, with <1 year survival. *KIT* mutations are detected in many lineages.

3. **Mast cell sarcoma:** This represents an accumulation of mast cells in an extracutaneous site.

Genetics

Mast cells express C-KIT (CD117) receptors on their surface. The KIT ligand, stem cell factor (SCF), normally binds to the receptor and causes proliferation of mast cells and mediator release. Molecular mutations in *KIT* (D816V) are found in >90% of patients with mastocytosis and comprise part of the diagnostic criteria.[64-66] The mutation is a gain of function mutation that causes uncontrolled proliferation of mast cells.

Differential Diagnosis

The differential diagnosis includes mast cell hyperplasia and mast cell activation. These are accumulations of reactive, nonclonal mast cells and are not considered mastocytosis. Mast cell activation syndrome (MCAS) occurs in both SM and in other non-mastocytosis settings. Occasionally,

MCAS may involve clonal mast cells, but the other findings are not sufficient to make a diagnosis of mastocytosis. This situation, known as monoclonal MCAS, should be followed closely.

REFERENCES

1. Arber DA, Orazi A, Hasserjian R, et al. The 2016 revision to the World Health Organization classification of myeloid neoplasms and acute leukemia. *Blood.* 2016;127(20):2391-2405.
2. Arber DA, Orazi A, Hasserjian RP, et al. International consensus classification of myeloid neoplasms and acute leukemia: integrating morphological, clinical, and genomic data. *Blood.* 2022;140(11):1200-1228.
3. Gianelli U, Iurlo A, Vener C, et al. The significance of bone marrow biopsy and JAK2V617F mutation in the differential diagnosis between the "Early" prepolycythemic phase of polycythemia vera and essential thrombocythemia. *Am J Clin Pathol.* 2008;130(3):336-342.
4. Johansson P. Epidemiology of the myeloproliferative disorders polycythemia vera and essential thrombocythemia. *Semin Thromb Hemost.* 2006;32(3):171-173.
5. Rollison DE, Howlader N, Smith MT, et al. Epidemiology of myelodysplastic syndromes and chronic myeloproliferative disorders in the United States, 2001–2004, using data from the NAACCR and SEER programs. *Blood.* 2008;112(1):45-52.
6. Gianelli U, Vener C, Raviele PR, et al. VEGF expression correlates with microvessel density in Philadelphia chromosome-negative chronic myeloproliferative disorders. *Am J Clin Pathol.* 2007;128(6):966-973.
7. Boveri E, Passamonti F, Rumi E, et al. Bone marrow microvessel density in chronic myeloproliferative disorders: a study of 115 patients with clinicopathological and molecular correlations. *Br J Haematol.* 2008;140(2):162-168.
8. Thiele J, Kvasnicka HM, Facchetti F, Franco V, van der Walt J, Orazi A. European consensus on grading bone marrow fibrosis and assessment of cellularity. *Haematologica.* 2005;90(8):1128-1132.
9. Hidalgo-López JE, Kanagal-Shamanna R, Quesada AE, et al. Bone marrow core biopsy in 508 consecutive patients with chronic myeloid leukemia: assessment of potential value. *Cancer.* 2018;124(19):3849-3855.
10. Xu Y, Dolan MM, Nguyen PL. Diagnostic significance of detecting dysgranulopoiesis in chronic myeloid leukemia. *Am J Clin Pathol.* 2003;120(5):778-784.
11. Foucar K, Reichard K, Czuchlewski D. *Bone Marrow Pathology*. 3rd ed. ASCP Press; 2010.
12. van Rhee F, Hochhaus A, Lin F, Melo JV, Goldman JM, Cross NC. p190 BCR-ABL mRNA is expressed at low levels in p210-positive chronic myeloid and acute lymphoblastic leukemias. *Blood.* 1996;87(12):5213-5217.
13. Verma D, Kantarjian HM, Jones D, et al. Chronic myeloid leukemia (CML) with P190 BCR-ABL: analysis of characteristics, outcomes, and prognostic significance. *Blood.* 2009;114(11):2232-2235.
14. Melo JV. The molecular biology of chronic myeloid leukaemia. *Leukemia.* 1996;10(5):751-756.
15. Druker BJ, Tamura S, Buchdunger E, et al. Effects of a selective inhibitor of the Abl tyrosine kinase on the growth of Bcr-Abl positive cells. *Nat Med.* 1996;2(5):561-566.
16. Frater JL, Tallman MS, Variakojis D, et al. Chronic myeloid leukemia following therapy with imatinib mesylate (Gleevec). Bone marrow histopathology and correlation with genetic status. *Am J Clin Pathol.* 2003;119(6):833-841.
17. Hasserjian RP, Boecklin F, Parker S, et al. ST1571 (imatinib mesylate) reduces bone marrow cellularity and normalizes morphologic features irrespective of cytogenetic response. *Am J Clin Pathol.* 2002;117(3):360-367.

18. Buesche G, Ganser A, Schlegelberger B, et al. Marrow fibrosis and its relevance during imatinib treatment of chronic myeloid leukemia. *Leukemia*. 2007;21(12):2420-2427.
19. Huang Q, Wu Y, Snyder DS, et al. Clinical and pathologic analysis of 16 cases of relapsed chronic myeloid leukemia after stem cell transplantation. *Am J Clin Pathol*. 2007;128(4):565-570.
20. Baxter EJ, Scott LM, Campbell PJ, et al. Acquired mutation of the tyrosine kinase JAK2 in human myeloproliferative disorders. *Lancet (London, England)*. 2005;365 (9464):1054-1061.
21. James C, Ugo V, Le Couédic JP, et al. A unique clonal JAK2 mutation leading to constitutive signalling causes polycythaemia vera. *Nature*. 2005;434(7037):1144-1148.
22. Kralovics R, Passamonti F, Buser AS, et al. A gain-of-function mutation of JAK2 in myeloproliferative disorders. *N Engl J Med*. 2005;352(17):1779-1790.
23. Levine RL, Wadleigh M, Cools J, et al. Activating mutation in the tyrosine kinase JAK2 in polycythemia vera, essential thrombocythemia, and myeloid metaplasia with myelofibrosis. *Cancer Cell*. 2005;7(4):387-397.
24. Tefferi A, Vardiman JW. Classification and diagnosis of myeloproliferative neoplasms: the 2008 World Health Organization criteria and point-of-care diagnostic algorithms. *Leukemia*. 2008;22(1):14-22.
25. Tefferi A. Essential thrombocythemia, polycythemia vera, and myelofibrosis: current management and the prospect of targeted therapy. *Am J Hematol*. 2008;83(6):491-497.
26. Patnaik MM, Tefferi A. The complete evaluation of erythrocytosis: congenital and acquired. *Leukemia*. 2009;23(5):834-844.
27. Butcher CM, Hahn U, To LB, et al. Two novel JAK2 exon 12 mutations in JAK2V617F-negative polycythaemia vera patients. *Leukemia*. 2008;22(4):870-873.
28. Kouroupi E, Zoi K, Parquet N, et al. Mutations in exon 12 of JAK2 are mainly found in JAK2 V617F-negative polycythaemia vera patients. *Br J Haematol*. 2008;142(4):676-679.
29. Abdel-Wahab OI, Levine RL. Primary myelofibrosis: update on definition, pathogenesis, and treatment. *Ann Rev Med*. 2009;60:233-245.
30. Pikman Y, Lee BH, Mercher T, et al. MPLW515L is a novel somatic activating mutation in myelofibrosis with myeloid metaplasia. *PLoS Med*. 2006;3(7):e270.
31. Nangalia J, Massie CE, Baxter EJ, et al. Somatic CALR mutations in myeloproliferative neoplasms with nonmutated JAK2. *N Engl J Med*. 2013;369(25):2391-2405.
32. Klampfl T, Gisslinger H, Harutyunyan AS, et al. Somatic mutations of calreticulin in myeloproliferative neoplasms. *N Engl J Med*. 2013;369(25):2379-2390.
33. Rotunno G, Mannarelli C, Guglielmelli P, et al. Impact of calreticulin mutations on clinical and hematological phenotype and outcome in essential thrombocythemia. *Blood*. 2014;123(10):1552-1555.
34. Rumi E, Pietra D, Ferretti V, et al. JAK2 or CALR mutation status defines subtypes of essential thrombocythemia with substantially different clinical course and outcomes. *Blood*. 2014;123(10):1544-1551.
35. Ma X, Vanasse G, Cartmel B, Wang Y, Selinger HA. Prevalence of polycythemia vera and essential thrombocythemia. *Am J Hematol*. 2008;83(5):359-362.
36. Kvasnicka HM, Thiele J. Prodromal myeloproliferative neoplasms: the 2008 WHO classification. *Am J Hematol*. 2010;85(1):62-69.
37. Tagariello G, Di Gaetano R, Sartori R, et al. The JAK2(V617F) tyrosine kinase mutation in blood donors with upper-limit haematocrit levels. *Blood Transfus*. 2009;7(2):111-116.
38. Barbui T, Carobbio A, Rambaldi A, Finazzi G. Perspectives on thrombosis in essential thrombocythemia and polycythemia vera: is leukocytosis a causative factor? *Blood*. 2009;114(4):759-763.
39. De Stefano V, Za T, Rossi E, et al. Recurrent thrombosis in patients with polycythemia vera and essential thrombocythemia: incidence, risk factors, and effect of treatments. *Haematologica*. 2008;93(3):372-380.

40. Reilly JT. Pathogenetic insight and prognostic information from standard and molecular cytogenetic studies in the BCR-ABL-negative myeloproliferative neoplasms (MPNs). *Leukemia*. 2008;22(10):1818-1827.
41. Passamonti F, Rumi E, Pungolino E, et al. Life expectancy and prognostic factors for survival in patients with polycythemia vera and essential thrombocythemia. *Am J Med*. 2004;117(10):755-761.
42. Gangat N, Strand J, Li CY, Wu W, Pardanani A, Tefferi A. Leucocytosis in polycythaemia vera predicts both inferior survival and leukaemic transformation. *Br J Haematol*. 2007;138(3):354-358.
43. Finazzi G, Caruso V, Marchioli R, et al. Acute leukemia in polycythemia vera: an analysis of 1638 patients enrolled in a prospective observational study. *Blood*. 2005;105(7):2664-2670.
44. Gruppo Italiano Studio Policitemia. Polycythemia vera: the natural history of 1213 patients followed for 20 years. *Ann Intern Med*. 1995;123(9):656-664.
45. Ponzoni M, Savage DG, Ferreri AJ, et al. Chronic idiopathic myelofibrosis: independent prognostic importance of bone marrow microvascular density evaluated by CD105 (endoglin) immunostaining. *Mod Pathol*. 2004;17(12):1513-1520.
46. Pullarkat V, Bass RD, Gong JZ, Feinstein DI, Brynes RK. Primary autoimmune myelofibrosis: definition of a distinct clinicopathologic syndrome. *Am J Hematol*. 2003; 72(1):8-12.
47. Piatek CI, Vergara-Lluri ME, Pullarkat V, et al. Autoimmune myelofibrosis: clinical features, course, and outcome. *Acta Haematol*. 2017;138(3):129-137.
48. Wilkins BS, Erber WN, Bareford D, et al. Bone marrow pathology in essential thrombocythemia: interobserver reliability and utility for identifying disease subtypes. *Blood*. 2008;111(1):60-70.
49. Gangat N, Wolanskyj AP, McClure RF, et al. Risk stratification for survival and leukemic transformation in essential thrombocythemia: a single institutional study of 605 patients. *Leukemia*. 2007;21(2):270-276.
50. Dinçol G, Nalçaci M, Doğan O, et al. Coexistence of chronic neutrophilic leukemia with multiple myeloma. *Leuk Lymphoma*. 2002;43(3):649-651.
51. Bain B. The idiopathic hypereosinophilic syndrome and eosinophilic leukemias. *Haematologica*. 2004;89(2):133-137.
52. Bain BJ, Fletcher SH. Chronic eosinophilic leukemias and the myeloproliferative variant of the hypereosinophilic syndrome. *Immunol. Allergy Clin. North Am*. 2007;27(3):377-388.
53. Gotlib J. Eosinophilic myeloid disorders: new classification and novel therapeutic strategies. *Curr Opin Hematol*. 2010;17(2):117-124.
54. Tefferi A, Gotlib J, Pardanani A. Hypereosinophilic syndrome and clonal eosinophilia: point-of-care diagnostic algorithm and treatment update. *Mayo Clin Proc*. 2010; 85(2):158-164.
55. Fletcher S, Bain B. Eosinophilic leukaemia. *Br Med Bull*. 2007;81-82:115-127.
56. Horny HP. Mastocytosis: an unusual clonal disorder of bone marrow-derived hematopoietic progenitor cells. *Am J Clin Pathol*. 2009;132(3):438-447.
57. Hahn HP, Hornick JL. Immunoreactivity for CD25 in gastrointestinal mucosal mast cells is specific for systemic mastocytosis. *Am J Surg Pathol*. 2007;31(11):1669-1676.
58. Horny HP, Sotlar K, Valent P, Hartmann K. Mastocytosis: a disease of the hematopoietic stem cell. *Dtsch Arztebl Int*. 2008;105(40):686-692.
59. Zanotti R, Bonifacio M, Lucchini G, et al. Refined diagnostic criteria for bone marrow mastocytosis: a proposal of the European competence network on mastocytosis. *Leukemia*. 2022;36(2):516-524.
60. Alvarez-Twose I, Zanotti R, González-de-Olano D, et al. Nonaggressive systemic mastocytosis (SM) without skin lesions associated with insect-induced anaphylaxis shows unique features versus other indolent SM. *J Allergy Clin Immunol*. 2014;133(2):520-528.

61. Bernd HW, Sotlar K, Lorenzen J, et al. Acute myeloid leukaemia with t(8;21) associated with "occult" mastocytosis. Report of an unusual case and review of the literature. *J Clin Pathol.* 2004;57(3):324-328.

62. Nagai S, Ichikawa M, Takahashi T, et al. The origin of neoplastic mast cells in systemic mastocytosis with AML1/ETO-positive acute myeloid leukemia. *Exp Hematol.* 2007;35(11):1747-1752.

63. Pullarkat V, Bedell V, Kim Y, et al. Neoplastic mast cells in systemic mastocytosis associated with t(8;21) acute myeloid leukemia are derived from the leukemic clone. *Leuk Res.* 2007;31(2):261-265.

64. Metcalfe DD. Mast cells and mastocytosis. *Blood.* 2008;112(4):946-956.

65. Chatterjee A, Ghosh J, Kapur R. Mastocytosis: a mutated KIT receptor induced myeloproliferative disorder. *Oncotarget.* 2015;6(21):18250-18264.

66. Akin C. Molecular diagnosis of mast cell disorders: a paper from the 2005 William Beaumont Hospital symposium on molecular pathology. *J Mol Diagn: JMD.* 2006;8(4):412-419.

7

ACUTE LYMPHOBLASTIC LEUKEMIA/LYMPHOMA (ALL) AND OTHER ACUTE LEUKEMIAS

Acute lymphoblastic leukemias (ALLs) are clonal neoplasms of immature lymphoid precursors involving the peripheral blood (PB) and/or bone marrow (BM). Lymphoblastic lymphomas (LBLs) involve tissues without PB or BM involvement; when disease involves both PB and tissue, the distinction is arbitrary. In this chapter, we focus on ALL involving the BM.

ALL is broadly divided into B- and T-ALL, with the former more common than the latter. Extensive studies of ALL, which afflicts children more than adults, have established diagnostic strategies, optimal risk stratification, and effective treatment protocols.

In Chapter 4, we previously discussed acute myeloid leukemias (AMLs); in this chapter, we also briefly touch on other acute leukemias that are less common than either AML or ALL.

In general, patients with ALL present with similar morphologic findings. Moreover, blasts that characterize this disease are not always morphologically distinguishable from those of other acute leukemias, including some AMLs. Thus, immunophenotyping plays a crucial role in the diagnosis and classification of ALL. As with AML, there are numerous distinct genetic entities within ALL, although, with one rare exception discussed later, there are no morphologic clues to recognize these. Detailed discussion of all these different entities is outside the scope of this chapter, although some of the more common or more clinically relevant ones will be covered.

B-ACUTE LYMPHOBLASTIC LEUKEMIA

Epidemiology

B-ALL is more common in the pediatric population than in the adult population (>75% are children <6 years of age). There are approximately 1 to 5 cases per 100 000 patients and 6000 new cases per year. Although the exact etiology is unknown, patients with certain genetic disorders are at an increased risk, as discussed later.

Presentation

B-ALL involves the BM and usually the PB, although occasionally, aleukemic cases occur. It also involves the liver, spleen, lymph nodes (LNs), and sanctuary sites like the central nervous system (CNS).

Patients often present with lethargy and fatigue because of anemia or may show bruising and bleeding because of thrombocytopenia. The white blood cell (WBC) count is variable; some genetic subtypes of B-ALL are associated with very high WBC counts, whereas others show modest elevations or even low WBC counts. Unlike AML, which requires at least 20% blasts for a diagnosis (or certain genetic abnormalities), there is no lower blast limit for diagnosing ALL, although in practice oligoblastic ALL is rare. In patients with primary tissue-based presentations, a threshold of 25% blasts is conventionally used for distinguishing ALL from LBL, although this is only important for protocol purposes.

Morphology

Lymphoblasts are small- to medium-sized cells with fine chromatin and variably visible nucleoli (Figure 7.1A and B; eFigure 7.1). The cytoplasm is typically scant, but may be more abundant, and although vacuoles are typically associated with Burkitt lymphoma/leukemia, they may be seen in cases of ALL as well (Figure 7.2A). When a lymphoblast's cytoplasm protrudes at one end, they are referred to as "hand mirror cells" (Figure 7.2B), although this has no clinical significance. Lymphoblasts may also have coarse azurophilic cytoplasmic granules; occasionally, such cells may be seen in up to 10% of cases of B-ALL and rarely can they be so numerous as to be confused with AML (Figure 7.2C; eFigure 7.2).

In the BM, lymphoblasts can be confused with normal B cell precursors (hematogones) (Figure 7.3; eFigure 7.3). Most hematogones are smaller than blasts and have very high N:C ratios with the barest rim of cytoplasm, lack nucleoli, and have homogeneous chromatin. However, they sometimes may be indistinguishable from lymphoblasts on morphologic grounds alone, especially in less-than-optimal smear preparations.

Immunophenotype

Distinguishing B-lymphoblasts from blasts of other acute leukemias and from hematogones requires immunophenotyping via flow cytometry (FC) or immunohistochemistry (IHC).

Flow Cytometry

FC is especially useful in diagnosing B-ALL because of the quick turnaround time and high sensitivity for minimal residual disease (MRD) testing. To recognize B-ALL, it is necessary to distinguish it from more mature B cell neoplasms on the one hand, and from normal B precursors on the other. Because there is wide variability in phenotype among cases of ALL, no single marker will be diagnostic in any particular case so that panels of antibodies need to be used (Table 7.1).

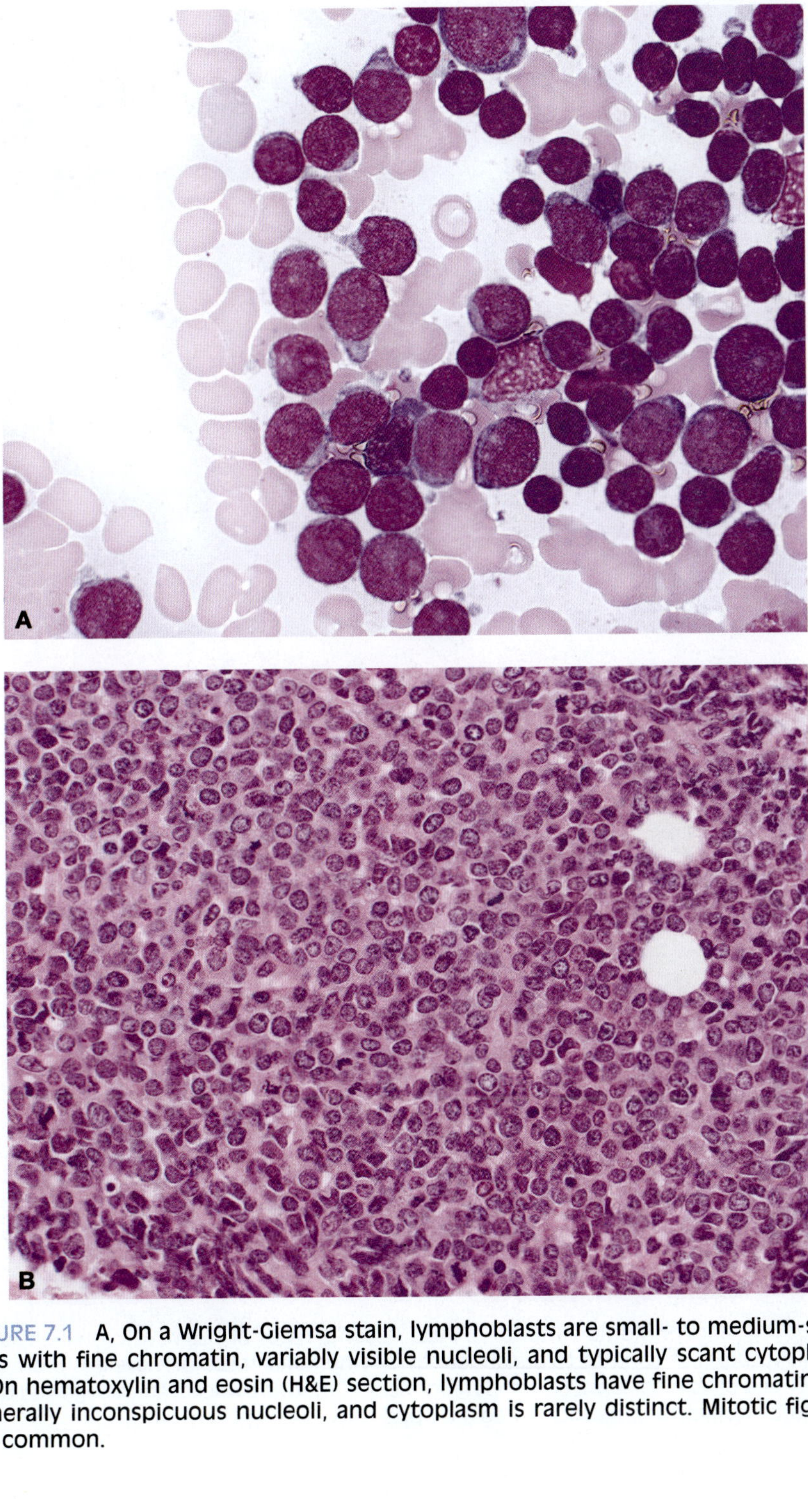

FIGURE 7.1 A, On a Wright-Giemsa stain, lymphoblasts are small- to medium-sized cells with fine chromatin, variably visible nucleoli, and typically scant cytoplasm. B, On hematoxylin and eosin (H&E) section, lymphoblasts have fine chromatin and generally inconspicuous nucleoli, and cytoplasm is rarely distinct. Mitotic figures are common.

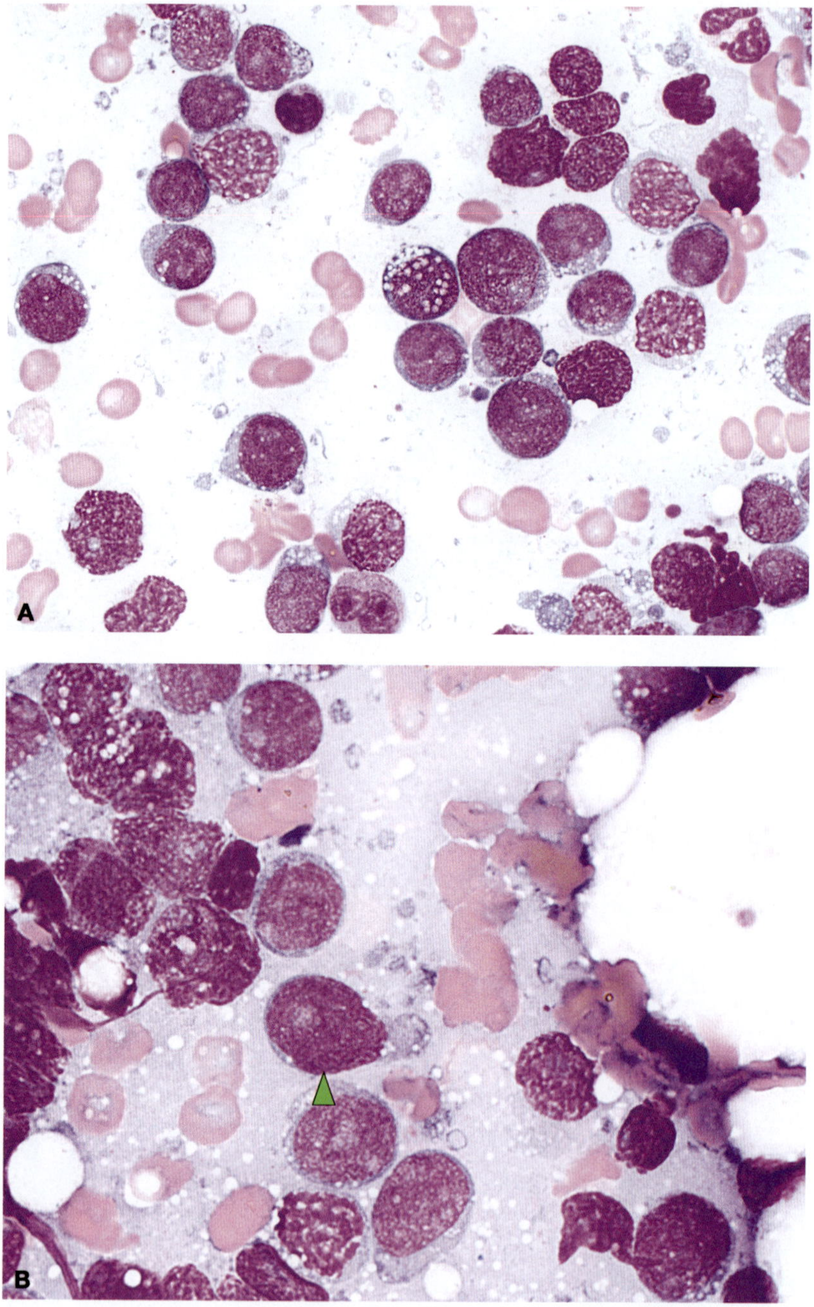

FIGURE 7.2 **Morphologic variants of ALL.** A, Some cases of ALL have prominent cytoplasmic vacuoles. In contrast to Burkitt leukemia/lymphoma, these will have less prominent nucleoli and paler cytoplasm. B, "Hand mirror cells" (green arrowhead) are recognized by an eccentric cytoplasmic projection called a uropod.

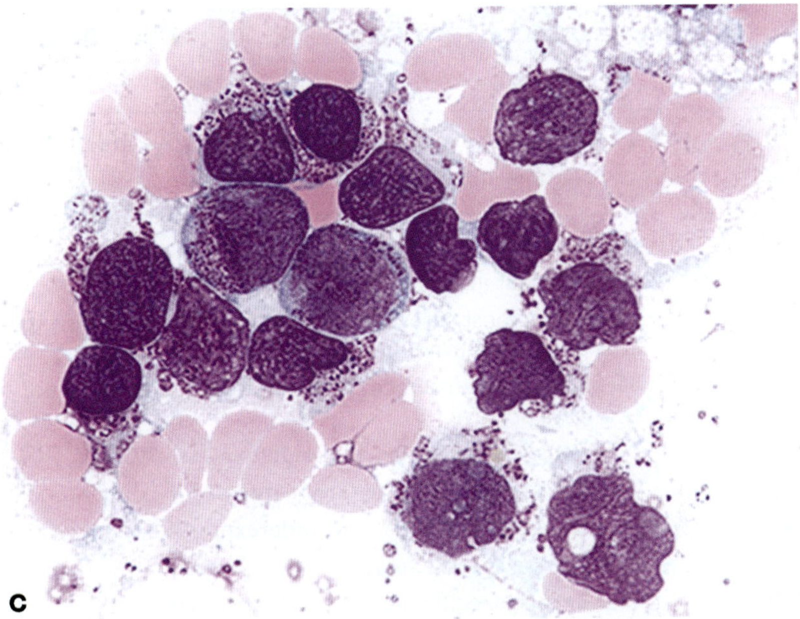

C

FIGURE 7.2 (*continued*) C, Granular lymphoblasts have coarse eosinophilic granules; although these resemble myeloid or even promyelocytic granules, they are myeloperoxidase negative. ALL, acute lymphoblastic leukemia.

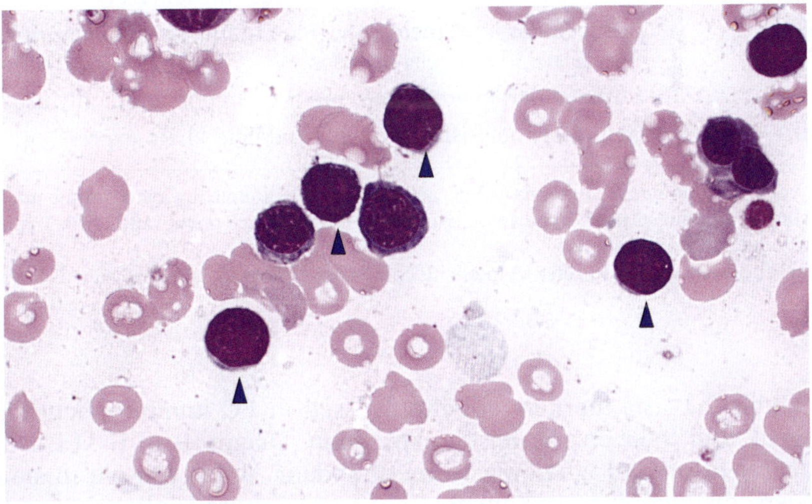

FIGURE 7.3 **Normal B cell precursors (hematogones) (arrowheads) have homogeneous compact chromatin and a very thin rim of cytoplasm, often only at one side of a cell.**

TABLE 7.1 Markers Useful in Flow Cytometric Analysis of B-ALL

Marker	Comment
CD19	Highly sensitive and lineage specific; positive in rare AMLs
CD20	Lineage specific, but often negative
CD22	Sensitive but expressed at low levels and may be dim; also on basophils
CD24	Sensitive but also present on granulocytes
CD10	Positive in most cases; not lineage specific; helps distinguish B precursors from mature B cells
CD34	Definitive immature marker but not lineage specific; not always positive
CD38	Not lineage specific; usually underexpressed[a]
CD58	Not lineage specific; often overexpressed
CD45	Not lineage specific; usually underexpressed
CD123	Not lineage specific; may be overexpressed
CD304	Not lineage specific; may be overexpressed
CD73	Not lineage specific; often overexpressed
CD81	Not lineage specific; may be underexpressed
CD13,15,33	Often positive; also positive in AMLs; does not imply MPAL
CD9	Not lineage specific; often overexpressed
CD79a	Intracellular; moderately specific but on some T-ALL
TdT	Intracellular; not lineage specific but indicates immaturity; negative in 5%-10% of cases
cμ	Intracellular; expressed on pre-B cells; not commonly used
SmIg	Can rarely be positive, with clonal light chain expression

ALL, acute lymphoblastic leukemia; AML, acute myeloid leukemia; cμ, cytoplasmic mu heavy chain; MPAL, mixed phenotype acute leukemia; SmIg, surface membrane Ig; TdT, terminal deoxynucleotidyl transferase.

[a]Under- and overexpression refer to intensity compared to normal hematogones.

Table 7.1 lists markers commonly used in FC immunophenotyping of B-ALL and their characteristic expression. Diagnosis of B-ALL is typically straightforward when blasts are abundant. When present in smaller numbers, distinction from hematogones can be more challenging and depends on aberrant levels of expression of various markers; this is possible because hematogones have reproducible patterns of maturation, as well as a continuum of antigen expression, acquisition, and loss during differentiation (see Chapter 2). Any variation of this normal pattern is detectable by FC (Figure 7.4).

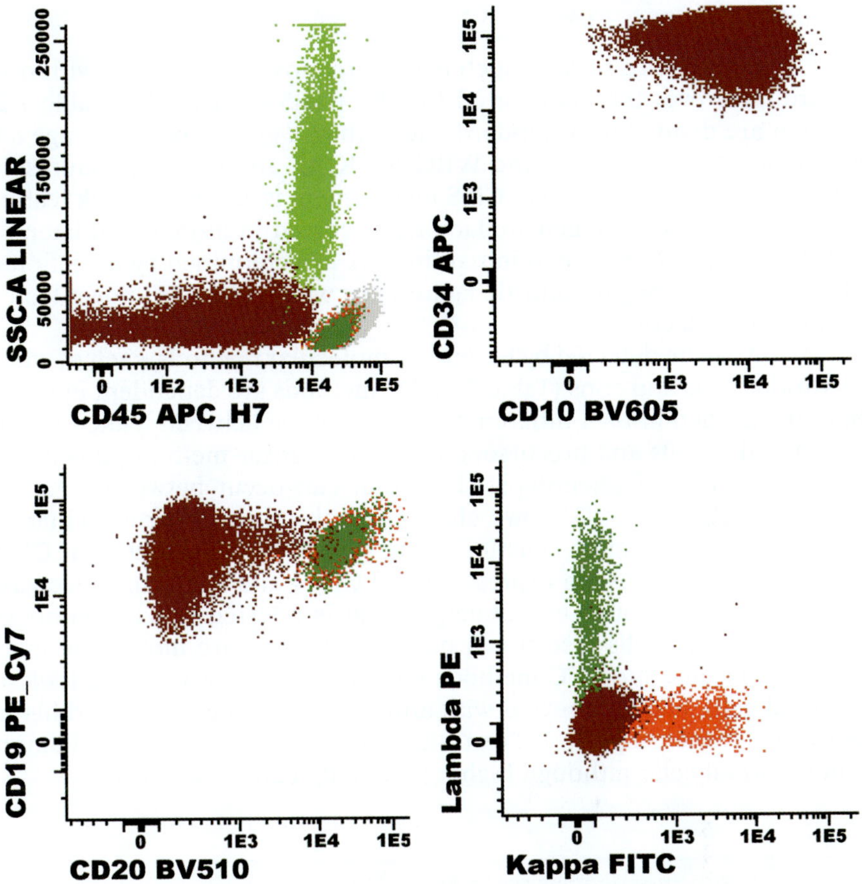

FIGURE 7.4 **The typical FC appearance of B-ALL.** Blasts (brown) have dim-to-negative CD45 with bright expression of CD19, CD10, and CD34. CD20 is often variable, as shown here, but is more often negative than strongly uniformly positive. Surface light chain is almost always negative. Also shown are normal myeloid cells (light green) and normal residual mature B cells (red and green). ALL, acute lymphoblastic leukemia; FC, flow cytometry.

Immunohistochemistry

In most circumstances, a combination of morphologic and FC findings can establish a diagnosis of B-ALL. However, in cases in which an adequate aspirate cannot be obtained, or in rare cases when ALL in the marrow presents with patchy disease, IHC can provide useful information. Many of the most common markers used in FC are not routinely available in IHC. However, PAX5 is a marker rarely used in FC that is highly sensitive and specific for B cell lineage. Distinguishing B-ALL from hematogones can be more challenging by IHC because small differences in intensity cannot be reliably detected, although the distribution of immature cells can be used to recognize relatively low levels of immature blasts.

Prognostic Factors in ALL

Children with B-ALL have a much better prognosis than adults, with overall cure rates over 90% compared to 60% to 85% for adults (Table 7.2). Children are divided into standard and high-risk groups based on age and WBC count (age >10 years and WBC >50K/µL are high-risk features; infants <1 year also fare poorly). CNS involvement is also a high-risk feature. Risk group and specific genetic factors, discussed in more detail later, determine therapy. Response to initial therapy, as determined by detection of MRD, is a very strong prognostic factor even when all other known factors are taken into account.[1]

MRD can be detected by FC and by molecular methods, each of which has various pros and cons (Table 7.3). FC methods are dependent upon the above-mentioned known differences in phenotype between leukemic cells and normal B cells and precursors. In applying these methods, it is important to be aware of phenotypic shifts that can occur between diagnosis and follow-up. Some well-known changes involve those that reflect maturation of residual leukemic cells following steroid therapy, such that CD20 and CD45 will increase in expression and CD34 and CD10 may decrease. Some genetic subgroups can undergo what is referred to as B-monocyte transition, where cells lose B cell markers and acquire monocytic markers.[2] Also, because most FC methods rely on gating with CD19 to look for abnormal cells, patients treated with anti-CD19 therapy require a different approach.[3] Done properly, FC can routinely detect 1 leukemic cell among 10,000 normal cells, although higher sensitivity can be obtained.[4]

TABLE 7.2 Prognostic Factors in ALL

Factor	Comment
Age	Adults worse than children; infants <1 and children >10 years old have adverse risk
White blood cell count	>50K/µL worse in children
Genetics	*ETV6::RUNX1* and high hyperdiploid are good risk in children
	Hypodiploid is poor risk
	Ph+ and Ph-like is poor risk
	Other genetic entities also associated with risk (see text)
Response to initial therapy	MRD after induction is the most important adverse factor

ALL, acute lymphoblastic leukemia; Ph, Philadelphia chromosome; MRD, minimal residual disease.

TABLE 7.3 Comparison of MRD detection methods

	Translocation PCR	Clone-specific PCR	Flow cytometry	NGS
Sensitivity	10^{-4}-10^{-6}	10^{-5}	10^{-4}-10^{-5}	10^{-6}
% of informative cases	<50	90	>95	>90
Turn-around time	1-2 days	Weeks	Hours	Days to weeks
Expense	Low	High	Moderate	Moderate
Need for pre-treatment sample	None	Essential	Desirable but not necessary	Essential

MRD, minimal residual disease; PCR, polymerase chain reaction; NGS, next generation sequencing.

Genetics

Molecular methods identify tumor-specific sequences of clonally rearranged IGH or TCR genes. This method relies on the detection of unique clonal sequences at diagnosis and the subsequent use of patient-specific primers to assess for MRD. Polymerase chain reaction (PCR) is extremely sensitive. This approach achieves sensitivity of up to 10^{-5} in >90% of cases and has been validated in numerous clinical trials. However, it is expensive and time consuming to synthesize and validate these primers, and the method is being replaced by next-generation sequencing (NGS) techniques that use multiplex PCR to identify tumor-specific abnormalities and to identify them in post-therapy samples. This technique can achieve sensitivities of better than 10^{-6} and has been well standardized; it is available in the United States as a Food and Drug Administration (FDA)–approved send-out test but is not generally available in individual labs. Real-time quantitative (q)PCR testing for specific fusion genes can be performed but is uncommonly used, except in the case of *BCR::ABL1* rearranged ALL, although as discussed later, this may not be reliable and is not recommended for MRD detection.

SUBCLASSIFICATION OF B-ALL

Historically, B-ALL was subtyped based on blast maturation stage as distinguished by phenotype and morphology. However, these categories, L1, L2, and L3 (L3 now recognized as Burkitt lymphoma/leukemia), show no independent clinical significance, and therefore, B-ALL is currently subtyped based on genetic features, which define clear-cut, non-overlapping biologic entities, often with distinct clinical behaviors and prognosis (Table 7.4).

TABLE 7.4 B-ALL With Recurrent Genetic Abnormalities

Subtype	Comment
B-ALL with t(9;22)(q34.1;q11.2)/ *BCR::ABL1*	Two types, lymphoid only vs multilineage
B-ALL with t(v;11q23.3)/*KMT2A* rearranged	Common in infants
B-ALL with t(12;21)(p13.2;q22.1)/ *ETV6::RUNX1*	Common in children, good prognosis
B-ALL, hypodiploid	Two types, low hypodiploid and near haploid
B-ALL with t(5;14)(q31.1;q32.3)/ *IL3::*IGH	Associated with eosinophilia
B-ALL with t(1;19)(q23.3;p13.3)/ *TCF3::PBX1*	
B-ALL, *BCR::ABL1*–like	Two types; ABL1 class translocations vs JAK-STAT activation
B-ALL with iAMP21	Only children, poor prognosis
B-ALL with *MYC* rearrangement	Distinct from Burkitt lymphoma
B-ALL with *DUX4* rearrangement	Good prognosis
B-ALL with *MEF2D* rearrangement	Poor prognosis
B-ALL with *ZNF384(362)* rearrangement	Often MPAL
B-ALL with *NUTM1* rearrangement	Rare, seen in infants
B-ALL with *HLF* rearrangement	Very rare, poor prognosis
B-ALL with *UBTF::ATXN7L3/ PAN3,CDX2 ("CDX2/UBTF")*	Very recently recognized
B-ALL with mutated *IKZF1* N159Y	Rare
B-ALL with mutated *PAX5* P80R	Rare, more common in adults

ALL, acute lymphoblastic leukemia; MPAL, mixed phenotype acute leukemia.

Cytogenetics, including karyotyping and fluorescence in situ hybridization (FISH), is commonly used to identify these subtypes, but recognition of all the known genetically distinct lesions of B-ALL requires sophisticated sequencing techniques including exome, transcriptome, and even whole-genome sequencing or gene expression profiling; with adoption of new techniques, a number of new entities have recently been added to the classification. Only one of these entities, the very rare ALL with t(5;14)(q31;q32)(IGH::*IL3*), can be suspected morphologically because of the marked eosinophilia that accompanies the overexpression of interleukin 3 (IL3) caused by the translocation. The more common clinically relevant lesions are discussed briefly later. In general, immunophenotyping cannot be used to identify these entities, although where noted there are some immunophenotypic correlates that can suggest them.

B-ALL With t(9;22) (q34;q11.2), *BCR::ABL1*

Epidemiology and Presentation

Philadelphia chromosome (Ph)-positive B-ALL is more common in adults than in children (25% of adults vs 2%-5% of children).

Phenotype

Characteristically, B-lymphoblasts express CD33 and CD13, although this is not specific; CD25 is relatively more specific but genetic studies are essential to identify these patients. Rarely, they may have a T cell phenotype.

Genetics

The *BCR::ABL1* translocation can be detected via karyotype, PCR, or FISH. Detecting this abnormality is important for prognosis and has treatment implications, namely the use of tyrosine kinase inhibitors (TKIs). Some patients with Ph+ ALL have a disease that is more similar in clinical behavior to chronic myeloid leukemia (CML) in lymphoid blast crisis. Although ALL more commonly uses the p190 isoform of the *BCR::ABL1* transcript, and CML uses the p210 isoform, this does not definitively distinguish these. Rather, in patients with CML-like disease, it is possible to detect the *BCR::ABL1* translocation in myeloid as well as lymphoid cells. This may be difficult to do at diagnosis when myeloid cells are rare and may require nonroutine sorting techniques. However, following therapy, these cases are often recognized because of persistent detection of *BCR::ABL1* by PCR when FC and IGH PCR is negative.

Prognosis

Historically, the prognosis of Ph+ B-ALL has been very poor, but TKI therapy has greatly improved the outcome, although it is still considered a relatively poor prognostic factor.

BCR::ABL1-Like B-ALL

Epidemiology and Presentation

This is an important but heterogeneous B-ALL subtype first recognized by gene expression profiling as a group of cases that clustered closely with Ph+ ALL but lacked *BCR::ABL1* translocation. It comprises 10% to 25% of all B-ALLs, and incidence increases with age. WBC counts are typically high at diagnosis.

Phenotype

In those cases with *CRLF2* rearrangements, upregulation of thymic stromal lymphopoietin receptor (TSLPR), the product of the *CRLF2* gene, can be detected by FC as it is present on the cell surface. Detection of the antigen correlates very closely with detection of the fusion by FISH, which is the reference method for diagnosis.

Genetics

There are many genetic lesions identified in this B-ALL subtype, including gene fusions and mutations. It can be divided broadly into classes, with one type characterized by rearrangements of tyrosine kinase genes and the other by Janus kinase (JAK) pathway activation. Among the former, the most important genes involved are those of the *ABL* class, including *ABL1/2*, *PDGFRA/B*, and *CSF1R*, whereas the most common of the latter is characterized by fusions of *CRLF2*. *JAK* mutations are common in the latter as well.

Prognosis

Many patients with *ABL* class rearrangements have a remarkable response to TKIs such as imatinib and dasatinib. Other kinase fusions, *CRLF2*-rearranged cases or *JAK*-mutated cases, have a poorer prognosis and to date no effective targeted therapies have been identified.

B-ALL With t(v;11q23.3), *KMT2A (MLL)* Rearranged

Epidemiology and Presentation

This B-ALL is often encountered in young infants <1 year old and has even been identified in fetuses in utero. The WBC count is very high at presentation, usually >100K/μL. CNS involvement is common.

Phenotype

The blasts have an immunophenotype consistent with a pro-B cell stage, positive for CD10 and CD15, and negative for CD20 and CD24.

Genetics

KMT2A (*MLL*) at 11q23 is an oncogene with numerous rearrangement partners, and different partners may give rise to T or myeloid leukemias. In B-ALL, the most common partner is *AFF1* (*AF4*).

Prognosis

This disease has a poor prognosis, especially in patients <6 months old.

B-ALL With t(12;21)(p13q22), *ETV6::RUNX (TEL::AML1)*

Epidemiology and Presentation

This leukemia is rare in adulthood but represents 25% of childhood B-ALL. In children, it is much more common in those with good risk clinical features (WBC count <50K/μL and 1-10 years of age). This translocation likely occurs in utero as an initial leukemogenic event, with subsequent lesions producing leukemic transformation.

Phenotype

These blasts have a unique phenotype: These express CD10 and CD19 and usually show complete absence of CD9, CD20, and CD66c. CD27 is typically positive and CD44 absent or low.[5] CD13 and/or other myeloid-associated markers may be expressed.

Genetics

FISH or molecular studies are necessary as the translocation may be cryptic.

Prognosis

This has a good overall prognosis although not quite as good in children with high-risk disease. Over 90% of patients are cured, although late relapses may occur; some of these may be new second leukemias arising from the original latent preleukemic clone.

Hyperdiploid B-ALL

Epidemiology and Presentation

This subtype represents 25% of all pediatric cases and <10% of adult cases. In children, it is much more common in those with good risk clinical features.

Phenotype

The phenotype is similar to other B-ALL cases, with the exception that CD45 is usually negative.

Genetics

The karyotype usually reveals between 50 and 60 chromosomes with no structural abnormalities. The hyperdiploidy is nonrandom: extra copies of chromosomes 21, X, 14, and 4 are the most common, whereas chromosomes 1, 2, and 3 are the least common. This subtype must be differentiated from hypodiploidy with endoreduplication (doubling of the apparent number of chromosomes).

Prognosis

The specific chromosomes that are duplicated, rather than the number of chromosomes, may have an impact on prognosis. Those patients with the best prognosis are those with gains of chromosomes 4, 10, and 17. In general, B-ALL with hyperdiploidy has a very favorable prognosis, with >95% cure rate in children.

Hypodiploid B-ALL

Epidemiology and Presentation

This subtype comprises <5% of overall cases of B-ALL.

Genetics

By definition, this subtype shows <46 chromosomes on the karyotype. There are two important subtypes that should be distinguished: near haploid (23-29 chromosomes) and low hypodiploid (33-39 chromosomes). The latter is frequently associated with p53 deletions, often constitutional. Hypodiploid ALL with 40-43 chromosomes is exceptionally rare; those with 44-45 chromosomes are biologically and clinically different and not typically considered part of this category.

Prognosis

These neoplasms have a very poor prognosis, with near haploid ALL even worse than low hypodiploid.

B-ALL With Intrachromosomal Amplification of Chromosome 21 (iAMP21)

Epidemiology and Presentation

This type of B-ALL occurs in children who present with a low WBC count and thus would otherwise be considered standard risk. It is almost never seen in adults. Up to 2% of cases are seen in patients with a Robertsonian translocation, t(15;21) (q10q10). The pathogenesis of this disease involves chromothripsis, with repeated breakage and reannealing of DNA; patients with the t(15;21) translocation are predisposed to chromothripsis and have a 3000-fold increase in developing this B-ALL.

Genetics

This abnormality is typically detected with a FISH probe for *RUNX1*, which reveals additional (>5) copies of the gene. About 20% of cases have this as the sole abnormality.

Prognosis

Patients who are treated with standard risk therapy fare poorly, but this can largely be overcome by treating them more aggressively.

OTHER SUBTYPES

Most of the newly recognized subtypes (see Table 7.4) are uncommon or very rare. Although there are not generally well-characterized standard assays for these, many can be recognized by FISH and most by either exome or transcriptome sequencing. Worth noting is the relatively more common (5%-10% of cases) *DUX4* rearranged subtype, which has an excellent prognosis. Although definitive recognition of this entity genetically requires complex analysis including whole-genome sequencing, expression of CD371 by FC has been shown to be an excellent surrogate marker.[6] *ZNF384* rearrangement is also not rare and, as discussed later, is also common in B/myeloid mixed phenotype acute leukemia (MPAL). Finally, B-ALL may sometimes have *MYC* rearrangements, and these may also be associated with *BCL2* or *BCL6* rearrangements and may be difficult to distinguish from high-grade B cell lymphomas, although they have a different mutational profile and also differ from the lymphomas by having unmutated IGH V region genes.[7] There are also a number of new provisional subtypes of B-ALL, currently generally recognized because they cluster together in gene expression profiling studies; genetic drivers are known for some but not all of these.

T-Acute Lymphoblastic Leukemia

In contrast with immature B cells that develop in the BM, early T cells migrate to the thymus to mature. T cells undergo phenotypic changes as they mature, progressing from the thymic cortex toward the medulla. Detecting the normal patterns of antigen acquisition during cellular maturation is instrumental in identifying abnormal populations.

Epidemiology and Presentation

T-ALL most commonly involves older children, adolescents, and young adults, comprising 15% of all childhood ALL cases, with a male predominance. T-ALL is also relatively more common in older adults.

In T-ALL, BM and PB are invariably both involved, unlike B-ALL, which can be aleukemic. Patients often have a high WBC. T-ALL also can involve LNs, tonsils, liver, spleen, testicles, CNS, and skin. An anterior mediastinal mass in a patient with leukemia is highly suggestive of T-ALL.

Morphology

Morphologically, T-lymphoblasts may look indistinguishable from other blasts; in adults, T-ALL may also resemble more mature lymphocytes so that immunophenotyping is critical for the diagnosis.

Immunophenotype

T-ALL is phenotypically heterogeneous, but phenotypes broadly reflect different stages of T cell maturation (Table 7.5). The most immature T cells

TABLE 7.5 Markers Used in Flow Cytometric Analysis of T-ALL

Marker	Comment
cCD3	Highly sensitive and specific; some cases may be dim
CD7	Highly sensitive but not specific; present on many AMLs
CD5	Expressed on most cases but dimmer than normal; negative or low on ETP ALL
CD2	Expressed on many cases
sCD3	Often negative; almost always dim when positive
CD4, CD8	May be coexpressed, or both absent, or one expressed but not the other; usually different intensity from normal T cells
CD1a	Often coexpressed with CD4 and CD8
CD10	Expressed on a significant subset of cases; can help identify abnormal population in marrow
CD34	Definitive immature marker but not lineage specific; uncommonly positive
CD117	Good marker of immaturity; often positive in ETP ALL
CD99	Good marker of immaturity; present on most cases but may be dim
CD38	Not lineage specific; may be overexpressed
CD45	Not lineage specific; may be as bright as normal lymphocytes
CD48	Underexpressed in most cases and a useful aberrant marker
CD56	Uncommonly positive
CD13,15,33	Often positive and does not imply MPAL
TdT	Intracellular; not lineage specific but indicates immaturity; negative in 10%-15% of cases

ALL, acute lymphoblastic leukemia; AML, acute myeloid leukemia; cCD3, cytoplasmic CD3; ETP, early T-precursor; MPAL, mixed phenotype acute leukemia; sCD3, surface CD3.

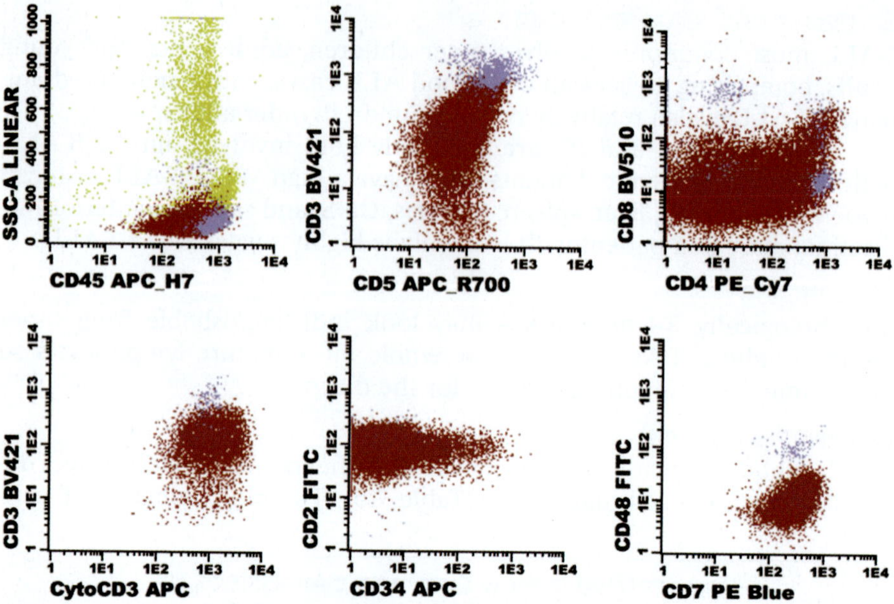

FIGURE 7.5 **T-ALL can show many phenotypic patterns by FC, but classically, the blasts (brown population) express CD7, bright cytoplasmic CD3 with dim or negative surface CD3, and dim CD5.** CD2, CD4, and CD8 are variably expressed and CD34 may be expressed, either uniformly or partially, as shown here. ALL, acute lymphoblastic leukemia; FC, flow cytometry.

express cytoplasmic, but not surface, CD3 and express bright CD7 but may lack other T cell markers (Figure 7.5). Very early T cell precursors will also express TdT, CD99, and CD34. As T cells mature, they will express CD5 and CD2 followed by coexpression of CD4 and CD8 along with CD1a. With further maturation, surface CD1a is lost and surface CD3 is expressed, and cells differentiate into separate $CD4^+$ and $CD8^+$ T cell subsets. In T-ALL, levels of expression of many of these antigens are different from that of normal T cells, but because T cell precursors are not normally found in the marrow, distinguishing normal and abnormal T precursors is not usually a problem. However, T-ALL may not always express TdT, and T cells with a more mature phenotype may be difficult. Although patterns of expression of markers can be used to subclassify T-ALL, with the exception of early T-precursor ALL, discussed later, these are not typically defined in clinical practice.

Genetics

The majority of cases of T-ALL have genetic alterations that initiate leukemogenesis by aberrantly activating transcription factors. These can be clustered into several entities based on gene expression profiling and different subgroups defined by the specific transcription factors involved, including

HOXA, LMO1, LMO2/LYL1, TLX1/3, TAL1/2, SPI1(PU.1), and *NKX1/2.* However, in contrast to most cases of B-ALL, there are a variety of different alterations that can produce the same pattern of transcription activation, so that these groups cannot be identified by routine diagnostic methods. Moreover, although some of these entities have prognostic associations, these factors have not been used in clinical trials to classify patients and are not used to direct therapy.

Prognosis

In contrast to B-ALL, age and WBC count are only weakly prognostic in T-ALL and do not determine therapy. As noted earlier, genetic prognostication is not done routinely. MRD is an important prognostic factor. However, patients with T-ALL respond more slowly to therapy, so that later time points and/or higher thresholds are used to identify patients in need of therapeutic intensification. If immature T cells are present in the marrow, recognition of MRD may be straightforward, but the same caveats about maturation-induced changes in phenotype apply to T-ALL, including loss of TdT expression. In addition, small numbers of natural killer (NK) cells express cytoplasmic but not surface CD3. Thus, detecting small numbers of T-ALL cells after therapy can be challenging.

Early T-Precursor ALL

Normal early T cell precursors (ETPs) retain some myeloid differentiation potential, and this leukemia also shares some myeloid-associated phenotypic and genetic features. It is defined by phenotype as a leukemia that has CD7 and cCD3; has one or more myeloid markers or immature markers including HLA-DR, CD34, or CD117; lacks CD1a and CD8; and is only dim-to-negative for CD5 (<75%) (Figure 7.6). They often have mutations in genes typically associated with myeloid leukemia, including those involving RAS, JAK, and FLT-3 signaling pathways, or epigenetic regulators. Recently, it has been found that about 30% of cases of ETP ALL are associated with a rearrangement of the *BCL11B* gene. Interestingly, about 30% of cases of T/myeloid MPAL and even some cases of myeloid or undifferentiated leukemia have this same rearrangement, and all of these cases cluster tightly together by gene expression profiling.[8]

The prognosis of ETP ALL in children was originally suggested to be very poor, but with appropriate intensive therapy, the outcome is not different from that of other children with ALL.

LEUKEMIAS OF AMBIGUOUS LINEAGES

These are clonal neoplasms composed of blasts with no discernable lineage. These neoplasms are rare, comprising <5% of all leukemias. Phenotyping is required, either by FC or IHC.

They comprise **MPAL** and **Acute Undifferentiated Leukemia.**

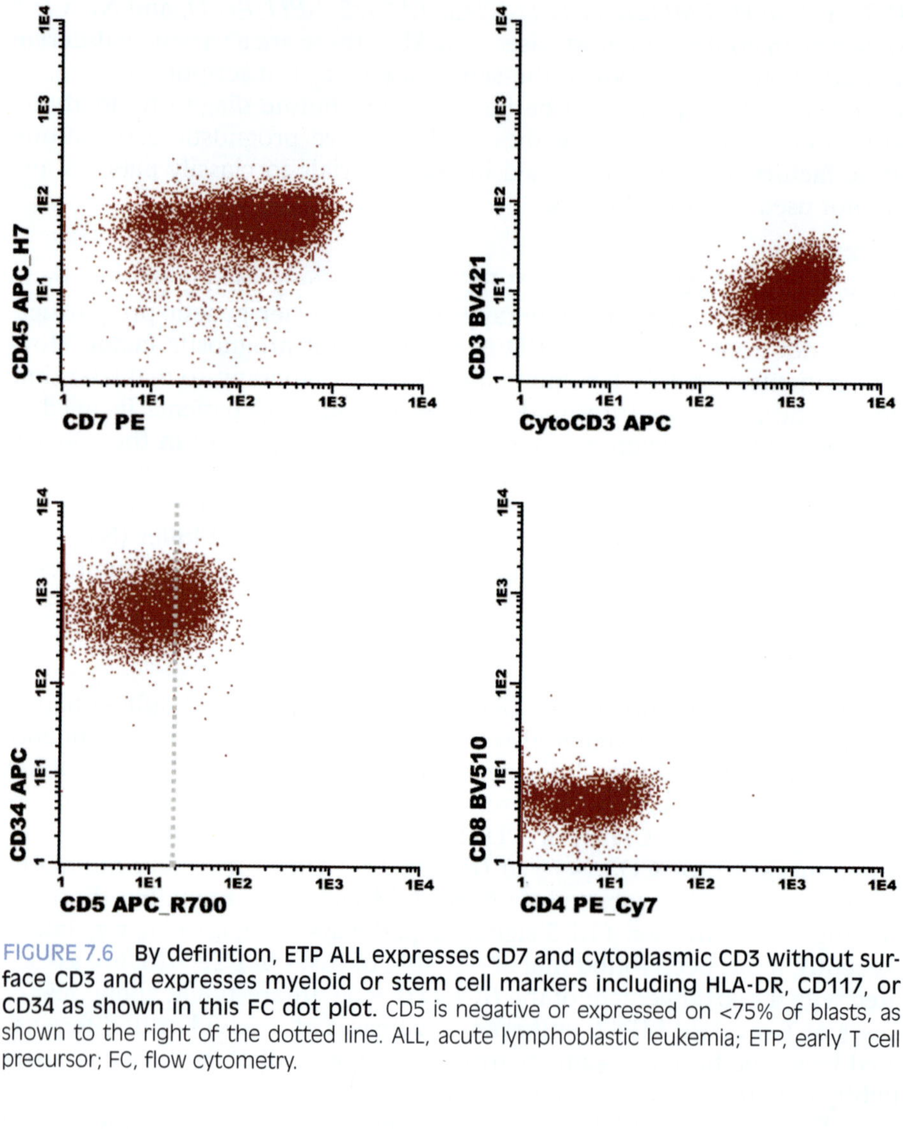

FIGURE 7.6 **By definition, ETP ALL expresses CD7 and cytoplasmic CD3 without surface CD3 and expresses myeloid or stem cell markers including HLA-DR, CD117, or CD34 as shown in this FC dot plot.** CD5 is negative or expressed on <75% of blasts, as shown to the right of the dotted line. ALL, acute lymphoblastic leukemia; ETP, early T cell precursor; FC, flow cytometry.

Mixed Phenotype Acute Leukemia

Blasts express antigens of one or more lineages. MPAL includes cases with leukemic blasts of different lineages or those with a single blast population of unclear lineage because of coexpression of antigens of multiple lineages (Figure 7.7A-D). These are not considered different entities because both populations may be present in a patient either simultaneously or over time. This category does not include leukemias that are clearly of one lineage with aberrant markers of another lineage.

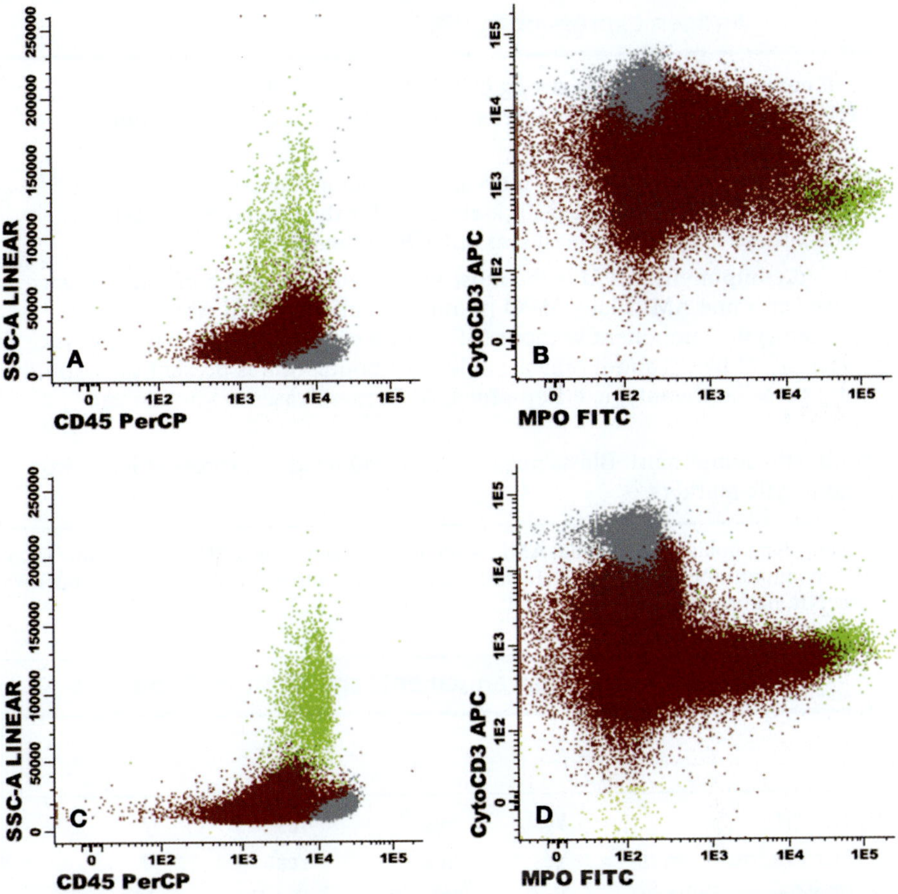

FIGURE 7.7 **FC dot plots of two cases of MPAL (T/myeloid).** A and B, So-called "biphenotypic pattern," where the majority of blasts show coexpression of cytoplasmic CD3 and myeloperoxidase. C and D, So-called "bilineal pattern," where the majority of blasts express cytoplasmic CD3 and myeloperoxidase separately. These are not considered different entities because the pattern seen in an individual may change over time (brown: leukemic blasts; gray: normal T cells; green: residual myeloid elements). FC, flow cytometry; MPAL, mixed phenotype acute leukemia.

Morphology

In cases of MPAL, a threshold of 20% blasts is needed for a diagnosis, but is not required for each distinct population.

In the BM, blasts look indistinguishable from other subtypes, although MPAL may be suspected if a dimorphic population of blasts is present, particularly if one is monocytic.

Immunophenotype

MPAL is divided into B/myeloid and T/myeloid MPAL based on the combination of antigens expressed (Table 7.6). Most cases of MPAL involve

TABLE 7.6 Antigen Expression in MPAL

T cell component: Requires strong cCD3 (at the level of normal T cells). IHC may cross-react with NK cells, which have cytoplasmic, but not surface, CD3.

B cell component: CD19 is the most specific, but at least one other B cell marker (CD79a, cCD22, CD10) is required for the diagnosis; if CD19 is weak, there should be at least two other B cell markers.

Myeloid component: MPO is the most specific marker of the myeloid lineage; however, some AMLs lack MPO (minimally differentiated AML) or have a monocytic component without MPO. Rare cases of B-ALL may express weak MPO by FC and if only a single blast population is present that would otherwise fit phenotypic criteria for B-ALL, these cases are not considered MPAL.

Monocytic component: Blasts negative for MPO need to express at least two monocytic markers.

ALL, acute lymphoblastic leukemia; AML, acute myeloid leukemia; cCD3, cytoplasmic CD3; IHC, immunohistochemistry; MPAL, mixed phenotype acute leukemia; MPO, myeloperoxidase; NK, natural killer.

TABLE 7.7 Chromosomal Rearrangements shared by MPAL and ALL

Entity	B-ALL	B/My MPAL	T-ALL	T/My MPAL
BCR::ABL1	Yes	Yes	Yes	?
KMT2A rearrangement	Yes	Yes	Yes	?
ZNF384 rearrangement	Yes	Yes	No	No
BCL11B rearrangement	No	No	Yes (ETP)	Yes

ALL, acute lymphoblastic leukemia; AML, acute myeloid leukemia; ETP, early T precursor; MPAL, mixed phenotype acute leukemia.

blasts with coexpression of myeloid antigens with lymphoid antigens. B/T or B/T/myeloid cases are exceedingly rare.

Genetics

Although there are a variety of nonrecurring cytogenetic abnormalities seen in MPAL, certain translocations can be seen in ALL and MPAL and/or AML; in some cases, patients with these lesions who present with ALL may recur as AML (Table 7.7).

MPAL with *BCR::ABL1* may be difficult to distinguish from CML in mixed blast crisis when there is no evidence of residual myeloid maturation in the latter. The karyotype may be complex, and patients have a poor prognosis, worse than other MPALs, although TKI therapy is effective.

MPAL with *KMT2A* rearrangements is relatively more common in young children or infants and prognosis is poor. The myeloid component is typically monocytic and easily recognized morphologically, although they can also appear undifferentiated. The lymphoid component is usually positive for CD19 although other B cell markers may be lacking, and is negative for CD10, but expresses CD15. The most common translocations are t(4;11), t(9;11), and t(11;19).

The differential diagnosis includes B-ALL with *KMT2A* translocations that express myeloid antigens and AML with *KMT2A* rearrangements.

B/myeloid MPAL with *ZNF384* rearrangements. This recently recognized subgroup of cases accounts for nearly half of B/myeloid MPAL[9] and has a virtually identical gene expression profile to cases of ALL with the same translocation. This translocation has not, to date, been seen in cases of AML, although cases of lineage switch from B-ALL to AML have been reported. Prognosis compared to ALL with the same translocation is unknown.

Acute Undifferentiated Leukemia

These leukemias lack all lineage-specific markers. AML with minimal differentiation, defined by its lack of myeloperoxidase (MPO) but expression of other markers of myeloid differentiation, must be ruled out.

Undifferentiated leukemias are positive for HLA-DR, CD34, CD38, and may express TdT or CD7, and lack other B cell, T cell or myeloid markers. Rare leukemias such as acute basophilic leukemia or dendritic cell leukemia must be ruled out. Occasionally, leukemias will express myeloid and lymphoid markers but not meet criteria for MPAL. These are best considered "unclassifiable acute leukemias," or "acute leukemias of ambiguous lineage, NOS."

BLASTIC PLASMACYTOID DENDRITIC CELL NEOPLASM

Normal plasmacytoid dendritic cells (PDCs) are monocytic-derived cells found in small quantities in primary and secondary lymphoid organs, as well as in the PB. These cells secrete interferon-α and can transform into antigen-presenting cells when activated. PDCs may accumulate in reactive conditions and neoplastic processes and rarely may transform into malignant neoplasms.[10]

PDCs are difficult to identify by the naked eye on a BM biopsy and are usually only visualized when they cluster and appear as bland-appearing monocytic cells. Clusters of these may be seen in conjunction with chronic myelomonocytic leukemia (CMML) (Figure 7.8A-E), or other myeloid neoplasms, but are not neoplastic themselves.

Blastic plasmacytoid dendritic cell neoplasms (BPDCN) are rare precursor hematopoietic neoplasms composed of immature PDCs. This is an aggressive disease, with an average survival time of <2 years. It is most

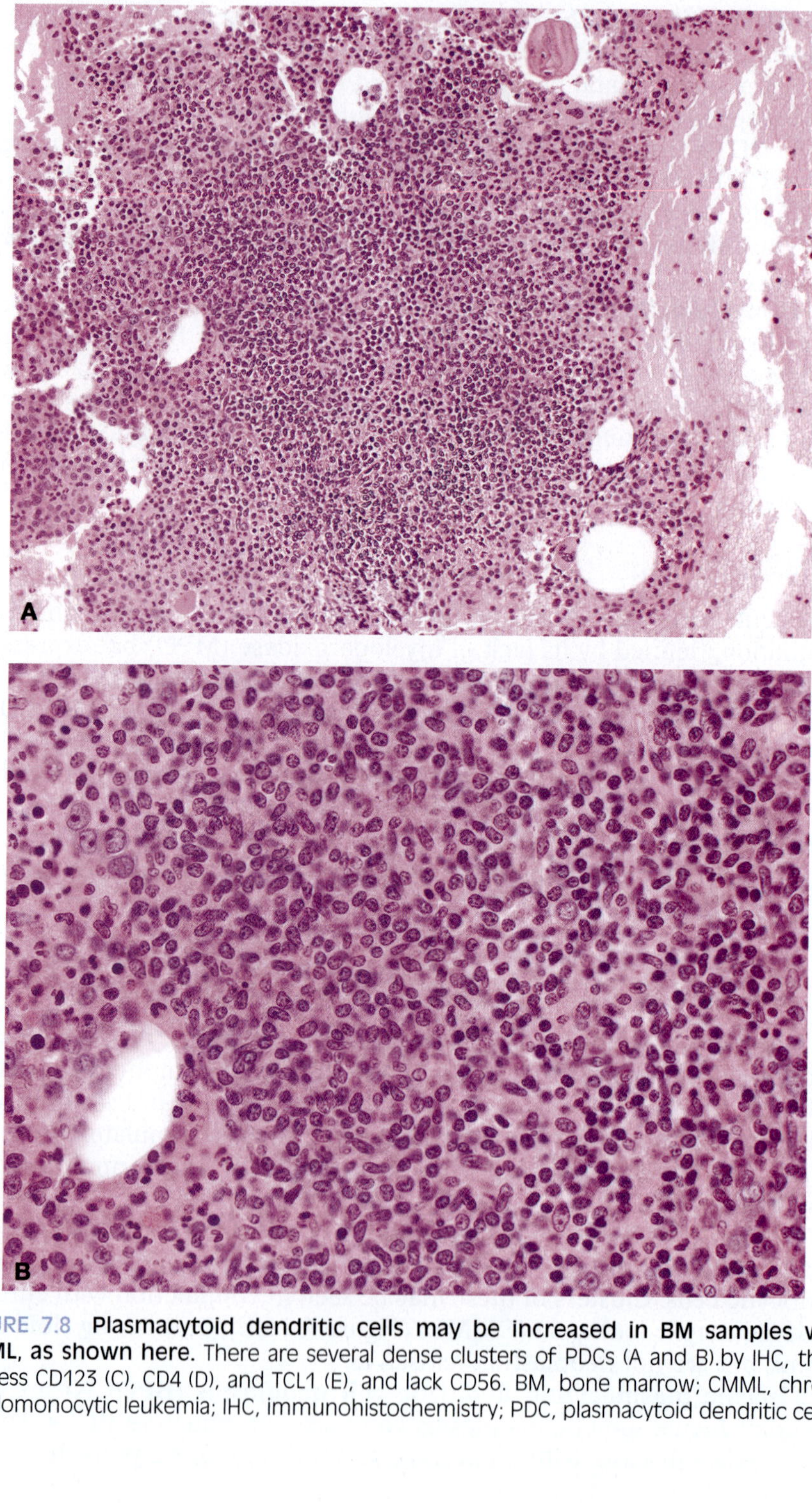

FIGURE 7.8 **Plasmacytoid dendritic cells may be increased in BM samples with CMML, as shown here.** There are several dense clusters of PDCs (A and B).by IHC, these express CD123 (C), CD4 (D), and TCL1 (E), and lack CD56. BM, bone marrow; CMML, chronic myelomonocytic leukemia; IHC, immunohistochemistry; PDC, plasmacytoid dendritic cell.

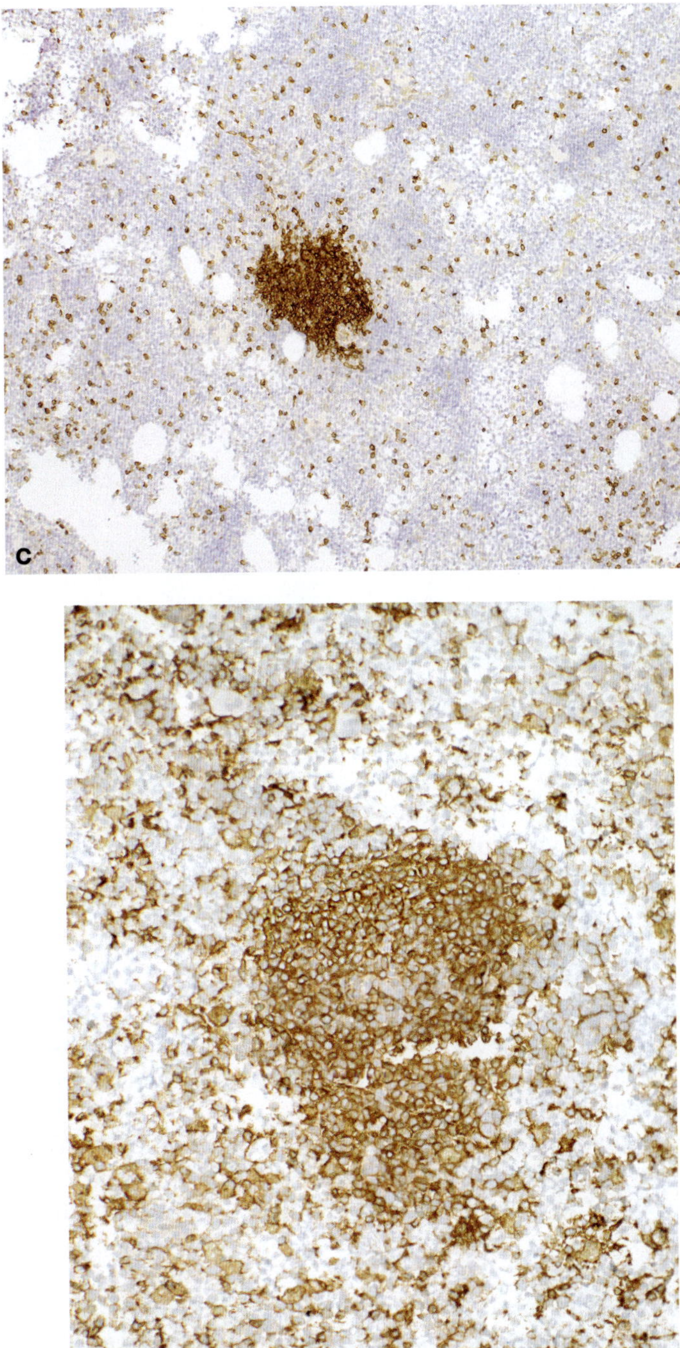

FIGURE 7.8 *(continued)*

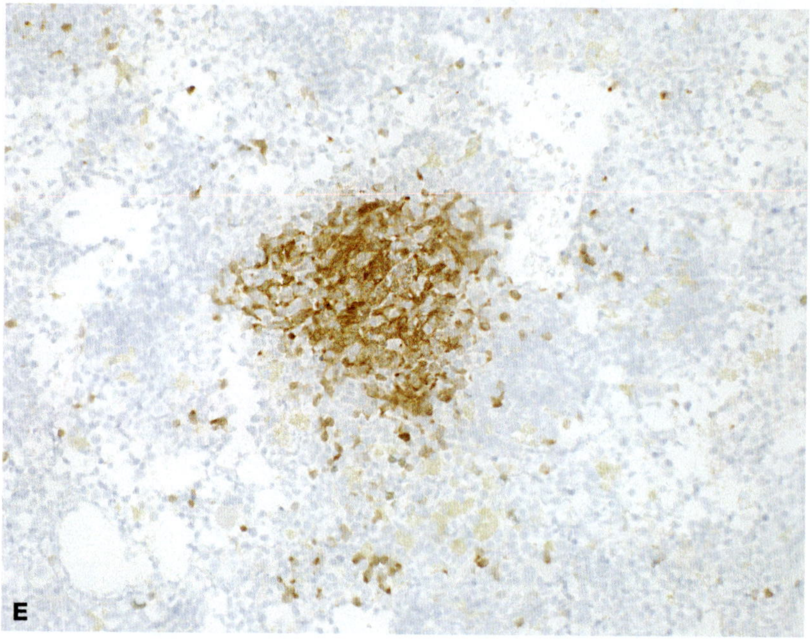

FIGURE 7.8 *(continued)*

commonly seen in elderly patients (60-70 years of age), but children can also rarely be affected. Approximately 10% to 20% are associated with, or develop into, CMML, MDS, or AML, although how these may be pathogenically related is unknown.

Epidemiology and Presentation

BPDCN usually presents as an asymptomatic cutaneous lesion, either a solitary purple nodule or a few bruise-like papules, to disseminated disease with multiple macules and papules, although it may present in the absence of cutaneous disease.

LNs are involved in up to 20% of patients at diagnosis. PB and BM are invariably involved as the disease progresses. Up to 60% to 90% of patients will have systemic involvement throughout the course of the disease.

Morphology

BM involvement can be subtle or diffuse. Microscopically, these neoplasms are composed of medium-sized blasts that resemble either myeloblasts or lymphoblasts, with irregular nuclei, fine chromatin, and one to two nucleoli (Figure 7.9A-E; eFigure 7.4).

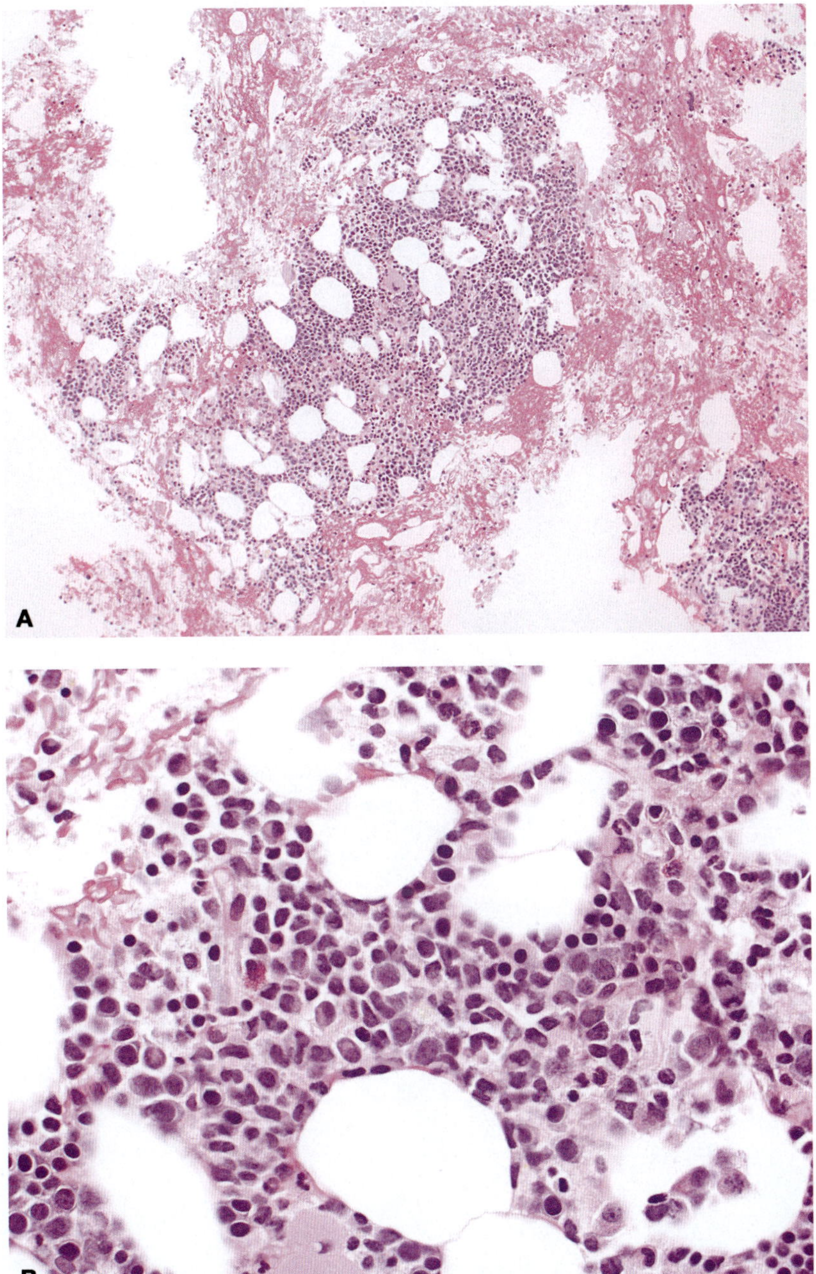

FIGURE 7.9 **BM involvement of BPDCN can be subtle or diffuse (A and B).** BPDCNs are medium-sized blasts that resemble either myeloblasts or lymphoblasts, with irregular nuclei, fine chromatin, and one to two nucleoli (C). BPDCN cells have no distinctive morphologic characteristics and must be defined by immunophenotype. They express CD4 (D) and CD56 (E). BM, bone marrow; BPDCN, blastic plasmacytoid dendritic cell neoplasm.

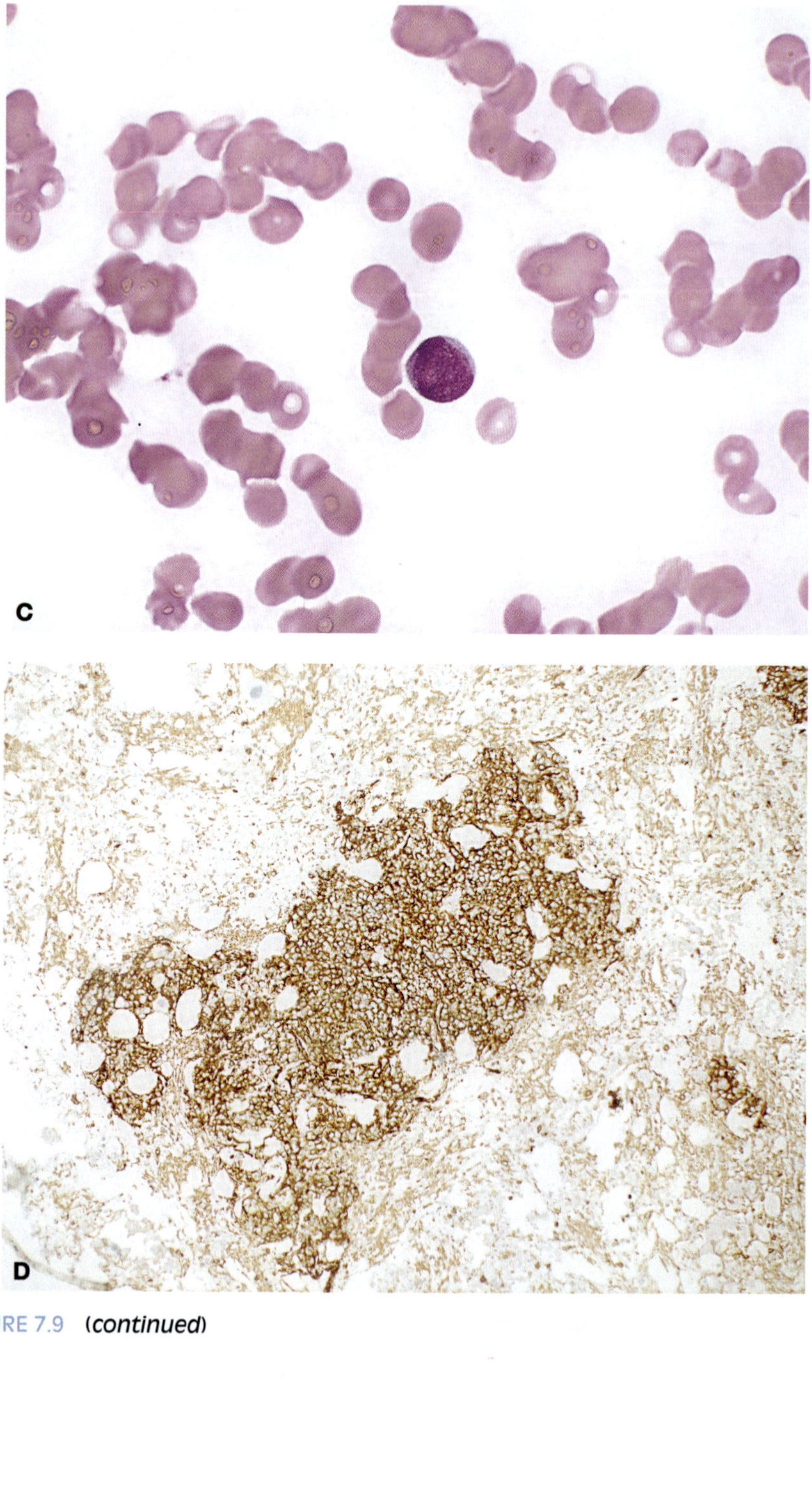

FIGURE 7.9 (*continued*)

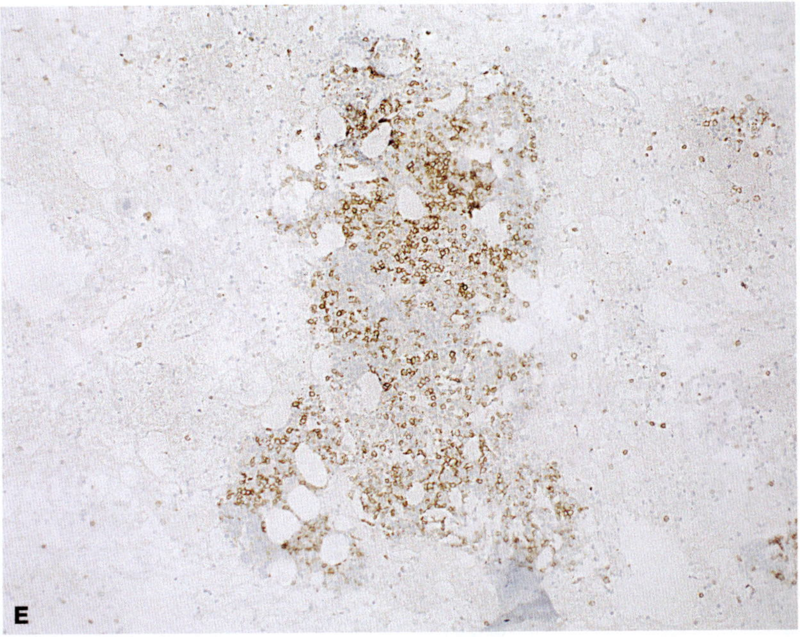

FIGURE 7.9 *(continued)*

Immunophenotype

By FC, normal PDCs can be found in the "blast pocket," but unlike myeloid blasts, they lack CD34 and express bright CD123. Expression of HLA-DR helps differentiate these cells from basophils (Figure 7.10).

Abnormal BPDCN cells also reside in the blast pocket, and like their benign mature counterparts, BPDCN cells are positive for CD123 and HLA-DR. They are also positive for CD4 and CD56 (Figure 7.11), as well as relatively more specific CD303, and TCL1A. Fewer than 10% are negative for CD4 or CD56, but this does not exclude the diagnosis. The differential diagnosis includes AML, which can express CD123, CD4, and CD56, although CD123 in particular is generally not as intense as in BPDCN; CD303 and TCL1A are more specific. BPDCNs may have variable expression of CD34 and CD117, depending on their stage of maturation.[11]

IHC can also help differentiate these cells (eFigure 7.5). BCL2, BCL6, and IRF4/MUM1 are positive in BPDCNs. S100 may be expressed in 25% to 30% of cases, especially in pediatric patients. Up to a third of cases are TdT-positive.

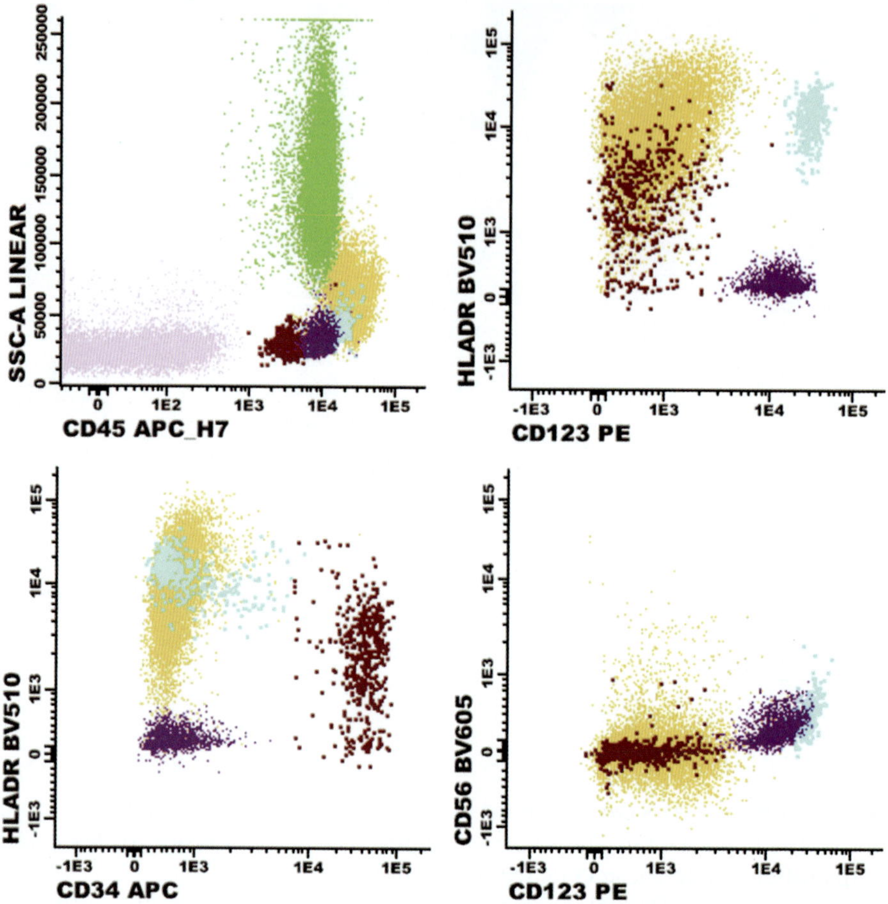

FIGURE 7.10 **By FC, normal PDCs (light blue) and basophils (purple) can both be found in the "blast pocket."** These both have bright CD123 but can be distinguished based on expression of HLA-DR. Normal PDCs lack CD56 (green: myeloid cells; orange: monocytes; pink: nucleated red cells; brown: myeloblasts). FC, flow cytometry; PDC, plasmacytoid dendritic cell.

Genetics

BPDCN cells do not have any associated mutations or specific rearrangements, but they often have complex karyotypes.

Prognosis

This is an aggressive disease. Most patients usually initially respond to chemotherapy, but almost always relapse and are rarely if ever cured without stem cell transplant.

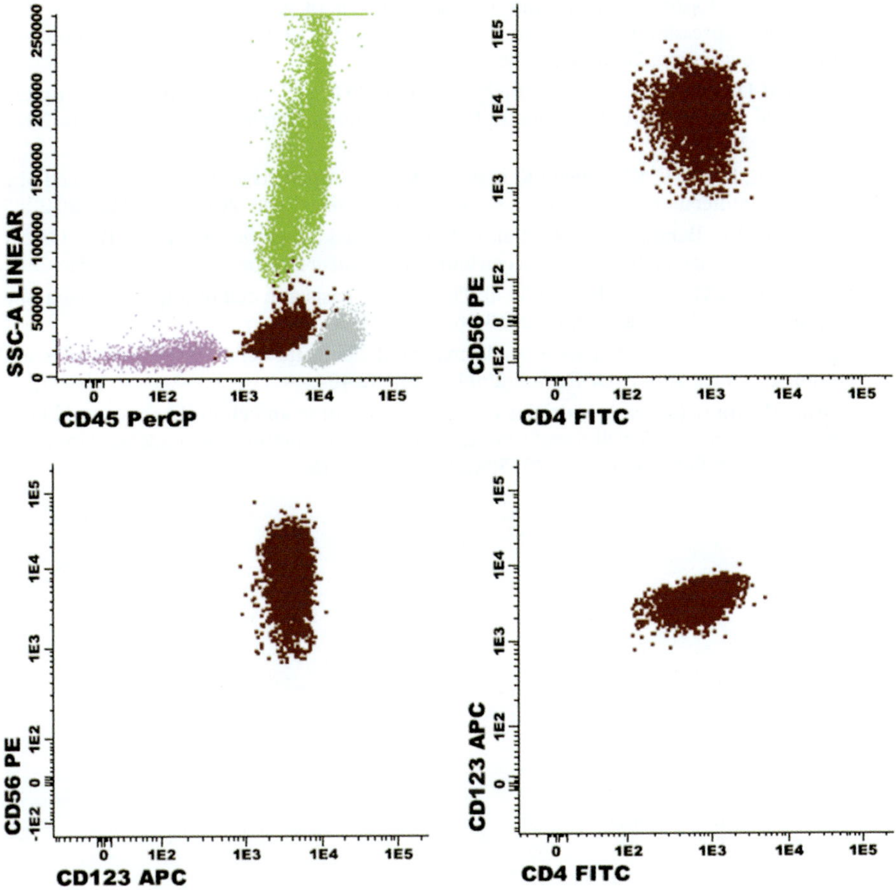

FIGURE 7.11 **By FC, BPDCNs (brown population) are positive for CD123, CD4, and CD56 (purple: NRBCs; gray: lymphocytes; green: myeloid cells).** FC, flow cytometry; BPDCN, blastic plasmacytoid dendritic cell neoplasm.

REFERENCES

1. Borowitz MJ, Devidas M, Hunger SP, et al. Clinical significance of minimal residual disease in childhood acute lymphoblastic leukemia and its relationship to other prognostic factors: a Children's Oncology Group study. *Blood*. 2008;111(12):5477-5485.
2. Novakova M, Zaliova M, Fiser K, et al. DUX4r, ZNF384r and PAX5-P80R mutated B-cell precursor acute lymphoblastic leukemia frequently undergo monocytic switch. *Haematologica*. 2021;106(8):2066-2075.
3. Cherian S, Miller V, McCullouch V, Dougherty K, Fromm JR, Wood BL. A novel flow cytometric assay for detection of residual disease in patients with B-lymphoblastic leukemia/lymphoma post anti-CD19 therapy. *Cytometry B Clin Cytom*. 2018;94(1):112-120.
4. Theunissen P, Mejstrikova E, Sedek L, et al. Standardized flow cytometry for highly sensitive MRD measurements in B-cell acute lymphoblastic leukemia. *Blood*. 2017;129(3):347-357.

5. Vaskova M, Mejstrikova E, Kalina T, et al. Transfer of genomics information to flow cytometry: expression of CD27 and CD44 discriminates subtypes of acute lymphoblastic leukemia. *Leukemia*. 2005;19(5):876-878.
6. Schinnerl D, Mejstrikova E, Schumich A, et al. CD371 cell surface expression: a unique feature of DUX4-rearranged acute lymphoblastic leukemia. *Haematologica*. 2019; 104(8):e352-e355.
7. Wagener R, López C, Kleinheinz K, et al. IG-MYC$^+$ neoplasms with precursor B-cell phenotype are molecularly distinct from Burkitt lymphomas. *Blood*. 2018;132(21):2280-2285.
8. Montefiori LE, Bendig S, Gu Z, et al. Enhancer hijacking drives oncogenic BCL11B expression in lineage-ambiguous stem cell leukemia. *Cancer Discov*. 2021;11(11):2846-2867.
9. Alexander TB, Gu Z, Iacobucci I, et al. The genetic basis and cell of origin of mixed phenotype acute leukaemia. *Nature*. 2018;562(7727):373-379.
10. Jegalian AG, Facchetti F, Jaffe ES. Plasmacytoid dendritic cells: physiologic roles and pathologic states. *Adv Anat Pathol*. 2009;16(6):392-404.
11. Martín-Martín L, López A, Vidriales B, et al. Classification and clinical behavior of blastic plasmacytoid dendritic cell neoplasms according to their maturation-associated immunophenotypic profile. *Oncotarget*. 2015;6(22):19204-19216.

8

MATURE LYMPHOID LEUKEMIAS/LYMPHOMAS

The term "lymphoma" usually denotes a lymphoid malignancy based primarily in lymph nodes (LNs) or tissue, whereas "leukemia" refers to disease that primarily involves the peripheral blood (PB) or bone marrow (BM). However, for many lymphoid malignancies, these terms are used somewhat interchangeably, especially in the absence of complete clinical or laboratory data, and strict definitions do not always apply. This chapter covers mature lymphoid malignancies and the reactive disorders that mimic them; acute leukemias and tumors of precursor cells are discussed in Chapter 7.

PRESENTATION

Lymphoid malignancies have predilections for involvement at certain anatomic sites: Some with frequent or primary involvement of the PB and BM, including hairy cell leukemia (HCL), splenic marginal zone lymphoma (SMZL) (both of which also involve the spleen), lymphoplasmacytic lymphoma (LPL) and T cell prolymphocytic leukemia (T-PLL). Others are more likely to be primarily tissue or LN based. Chronic lymphocytic leukemia/small lymphocytic lymphoma (CLL/SLL) typically involves LN, BM, and PB; others, including follicular lymphoma (FL), Burkitt lymphoma/leukemia (BL), and mantle cell lymphoma (MCL), can involve tissue, BM, and PB, although less often than CLL/SLL; whereas others such as diffuse large B cell lymphoma (DLBCL) uncommonly involve marrow and rarely circulate. Many, but not all, T cell malignancies can also involve marrow or blood, as discussed at the end of the chapter.

The presence or absence of disease at specific sites cannot be inferred based on the presence of disease at other locations. For instance, the presence of an abnormal lymphoid component in the BM does not necessarily imply PB or nodal involvement, and although uncommon, PB disease may not involve the BM.

Depending on the type and location of the leukemia or lymphoma, patients present with a variety of symptoms, including lymphadenopathy (LAD), hepatosplenomegaly (HSM), or other "B symptoms," specifically fevers, night sweats, or weight loss. Abnormalities of the complete blood count (CBC) are common, including leukocytosis with absolute lymphocytosis, sometimes associated with anemia or thrombocytopenia. Rarely, a patient may present with leukopenia, as in HCL. Other cytopenias are common, particularly when the marrow is extensively involved.

BM BIOPSY

Lymphoid cells can be identified as small round mature cells with mostly regular nuclei and condensed chromatin (eFigure 8.1). Although mature T cells usually outnumber mature B cells in a normal marrow, B cell neoplasms are far more common than T cell or natural killer (NK) cell neoplasms because B cells undergo somatic hypermutation during the normal course of maturation, providing an opportunity for generating deleterious mutations.

Lymphoid cells normally comprise <40% of total cellularity.[1] Increases in lymphocytes are abnormal, but do not necessarily imply the presence of a neoplasm.

Reactive: Occasionally, BM biopsies reveal a reactive lymphocytosis or lymphoid hyperplasia:

- **Diffuse lymphocytosis:** Rarely, patients with infection may present with diffuse lymphocytosis. Relative lymphocytosis may occur after chemotherapy.
- **Small lymphoid aggregates:** Occasionally, small aggregates of lymphoid cells are scattered throughout the interstitium, comprised of a mixture of B cells and T cells, with a predominance of the latter (Figure 8.1A-C; eFigure8.2). This is physiologically normal in elderly patients and does not indicate a lymphoproliferation disorder.

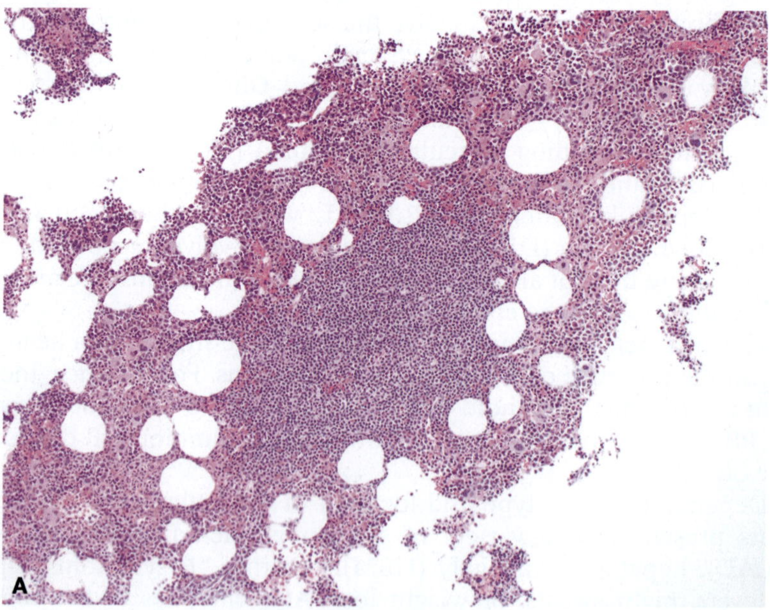

FIGURE 8.1 **Benign lymphoid aggregate.** A, A bone marrow clot section with a loose but well-defined aggregate of mostly small lymphoid cells, which are a mixture of B cells and T cells, as highlighted by CD20 (B) and CD3 (C).

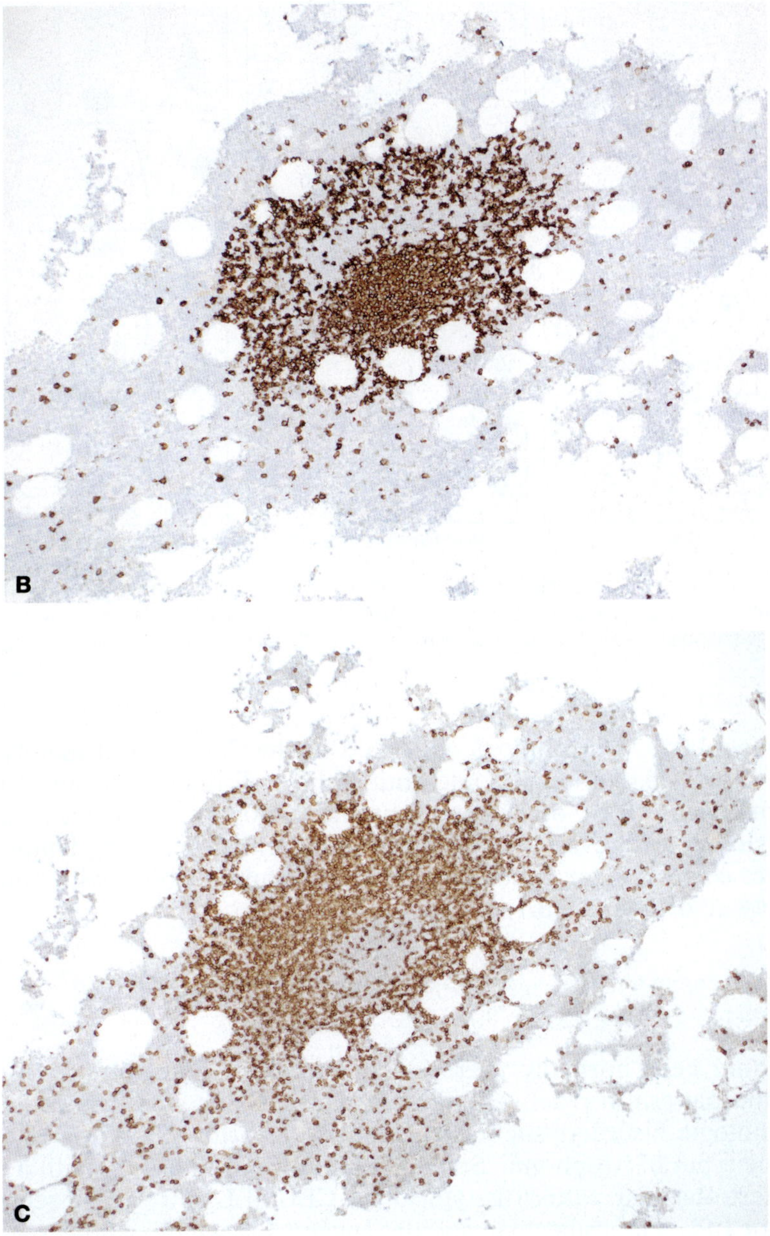

FIGURE 8.1 (*continued*)

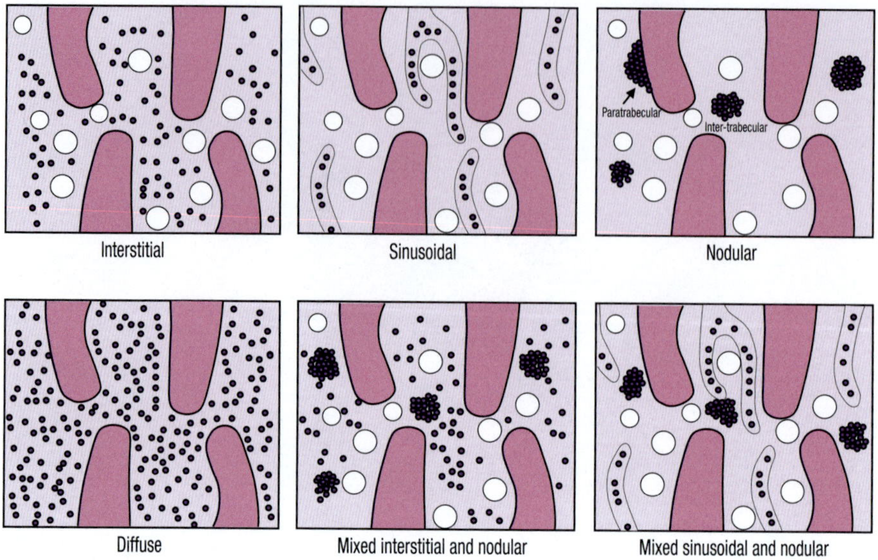

FIGURE 8.2 **Schematic of different patterns of bone marrow infiltration by mature leukemia/lymphoma.** Black dots represent lymphoid cells. White circles represent fat cells. Dark pink shapes represent trabecular bone. Black outlines represent sinuses.

Neoplastic: Morphologic clues aid in the diagnosis of mature lymphoid disorders. Although some entities have distinct infiltrative growth patterns (Figure 8.2),[2] other important morphologic clues include cell size and cytology. However, in most cases, differentiating among lymphomas requires correlating morphologic and architectural features with immunophenotypic data (Table 8.1).[3]

B CELL LYMPHOMAS WITH PREDOMINANTLY NODULAR PATTERNS OF INFILTRATION

Lymphoid cells normally aggregate in nodules, and although this is a common pattern in reactive infiltrates, particularly with advanced age or immunologic disorders such as rheumatoid arthritis (RA), it is also seen in some types of lymphoma. Small lymphoid cell infiltration with a nodular intertrabecular pattern is typical for CLL/SLL and can be seen with MZL or LPL. Paratrabecular nodules suggest FL, whereas MCL can have intertrabecular nodules or nodules near bone, but not paratrabecular. Cytologically, these lymphoid cells are small and mature appearing. Flow cytometry (FC) is instrumental in differentiating among neoplasms. Large cell lymphomas can also be distributed in a nodular pattern, although not as commonly; these will be discussed later in the chapter. FC also helps distinguish between B cell and T cell neoplasms. B cell neoplasms far outnumber T cell neoplasms; and these will be discussed first.

TABLE 8.1 Common Patterns of Bone Marrow Leukemic/Lymphomatous Infiltration

	Cell size	Neoplasm	Infiltration pattern				
			Interstitial or diffuse	Nodular[a]	Sinusoidal	Nodular and sinusoidal	Single cell
B cell	**Small**	**CLL**	+	+			
		MCL	+	+[a]			
		HCL	+				
		SMZL		+	+	+	
		LPL	+	+			
		MZL	+	+			
		FL		+[a]			
	Medium	**BL**	+				
	Large	**DLBCL**	+	+			
		TCHRLBCL					+
		CHL					+
T cell	**Medium-large**	**T-PLL**	+				
		HSTCL			+		+
		ATLL	+				
		T-LGL			+		
		AITL	+	+			
		PTCL-NOS	+				

AITL, angioimmunoblastic T cell lymphoma; ATLL, adult T cell leukemia/lymphoma; BL, Burkitt lymphoma; CHL, classic Hodgkin lymphoma; CLL, chronic lymphocytic leukemia; DLBCL, diffuse large B cell lymphoma; FL, follicular lymphoma; HCL, hairy cell leukemia; HSTCL, hepatosplenic T cell lymphoma; LGL, large granular lymphocytic leukemia; LPL, lymphoplasmacytic lymphoma; MCL, mantle cell lymphoma; MZL, marginal zone lymphoma; PTCL-NOS, peripheral T cell lymphoma, not otherwise specified; SMZL, splenic marginal zone lymphoma; TCHRLBCL, T cell histiocyte-rich large B cell lymphoma; T-PLL, T-prolymphocytic leukemia.

[a]The nodules seen with MCL and FL are characteristically, but not invariably, closely associated with bone, with FL right up against it and MCL somewhat removed. In leukemic phase, MCL and FL marrow infiltration can be interstitial or diffuse.

CLL/SLL AND MONOCLONAL B CELL LYMPHOCYTOSIS

CLL/SLL is B cell neoplasm composed of small mature B cells involving the BM, PB, LNs, spleen, and other tissues.[4] The term CLL refers to the leukemic form of the disease, which involves the PB and BM only. SLL refers to nonleukemic cases, involving LN or tissue only. However, CLL and SLL are genetically identical, and the terms are often used synonymously.

Epidemiology

CLL/SLL is the most common leukemia of adults in Western countries. This disease affects men more than women (M:F = 1.5-2:1) and is more prevalent in older adults. CLL/SLL has a high genetic predisposition: there is a 2 to 7 times increased risk of developing the disease in first-degree relatives of CLL/SLL patients, as well as an increased incidence of CLL/SLL phenotype monoclonal B cell lymphocytosis (MBL), discussed later.

Presentation

Patients may be asymptomatic or symptomatic. Asymptomatic patients are typically diagnosed with routine blood work, including a CBC with an elevated absolute lymphocyte count. Symptomatic patients may present with LAD or organomegaly and commonly have symptoms associated with cytopenias because of BM infiltration, splenic sequestration, or autoimmune hemolytic anemia, including fatigue, recurrent infections, and/or bleeding disorders. A small monoclonal immunoglobulin (Ig) paraprotein may be present in the blood.

To diagnose CLL, > 5000/µL (5×10^9/L) circulating clonal B cells with the appropriate morphology and immunophenotype must be present for at least 3 months.[5] Patients with lower counts but significant cytopenias and/or disease-related symptoms may also be diagnosed with CLL/SLL.

Morphology

Morphologic evaluation of the PB reveals leukocytosis with lymphocytosis. The abnormal CLL/SLL cells are small lymphoid cells with mature, clumped chromatin and scant cytoplasm (Figure 8.3; eFigure 8.3). CLL/SLL cells that are broken, also known as "smudge cells" or "basket cells" may be abundant. An albumin-treated slide may aid morphologic assessment because it prevents this phenomenon from occurring. In addition to anemia, red blood cells (RBCs) may show abnormal size and shape; microspherocytes in particular may suggest a diagnosis of autoimmune hemolytic anemia. Platelet counts may be decreased because of autoimmune thrombocytopenia or splenic sequestration but they are more typically normal, and can even be increased.

Large abnormal lymphoid cells with prominent nucleoli, known as "prolymphocytes," are present in some cases, but should represent <2% of

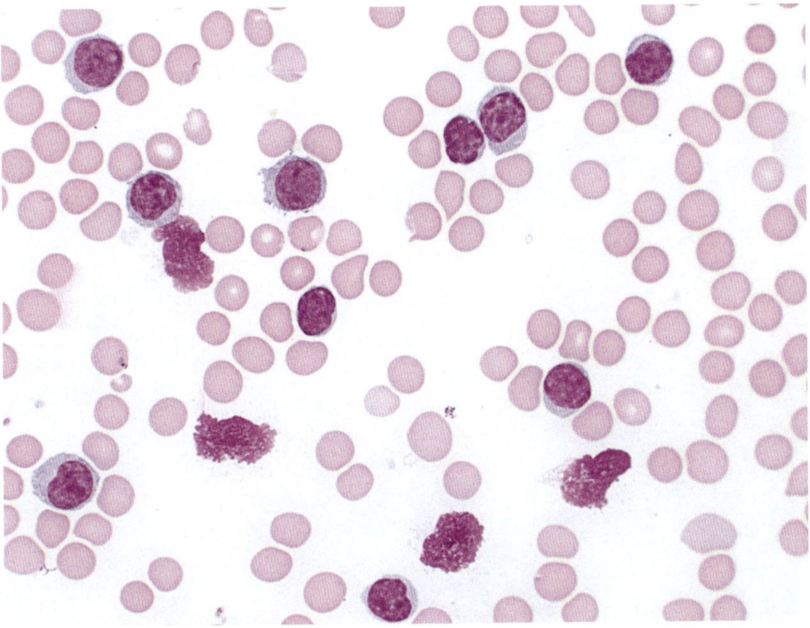

FIGURE 8.3 **Chronic lymphocytic leukemia/small lymphocytic lymphoma cells in the peripheral blood.** Lymphoid cells are small with clumped chromatin and scant and sometimes moderate amounts of cytoplasm. Small nucleoli may be seen (upper left). Smudge cells are common.

the total white blood cells (WBCs). Greater numbers of prolymphocytes may indicate a more aggressive disease course, especially if these represent an increase from prior levels. Historically, a diagnosis of B-PLL was made when prolymphocytes constitute ≥55% of lymphoid cells, although whether B-PLL even exists as an entity is controversial, and this is no longer a criterion.

Although not an official diagnosis, occasionally the term "atypical CLL/SLL" has been used for cases when cells exhibit greater nuclear irregularity and less condensed nuclear chromatin than usual CLL/SLL cells. These findings are more frequent in cases with trisomy 12; the immunophenotype also often differs from typical cases.

The BM typically reveals a diffuse interstitial lymphocytosis and occasionally nodules or nonparatrabecular aggregates of the atypical lymphoid cells (Figure 8.4A-C; eFigure 8.4). In the absence of other features, the BM lymphoid infiltrate must constitute at least 30% of total cellularity for a diagnosis of CLL/SLL.

Immunophenotype

FC and/or immunohistochemical (IHC) phenotyping is critical for the diagnosis. CLL/SLL cells are positive for dim CD20, CD19, CD5, CD23,

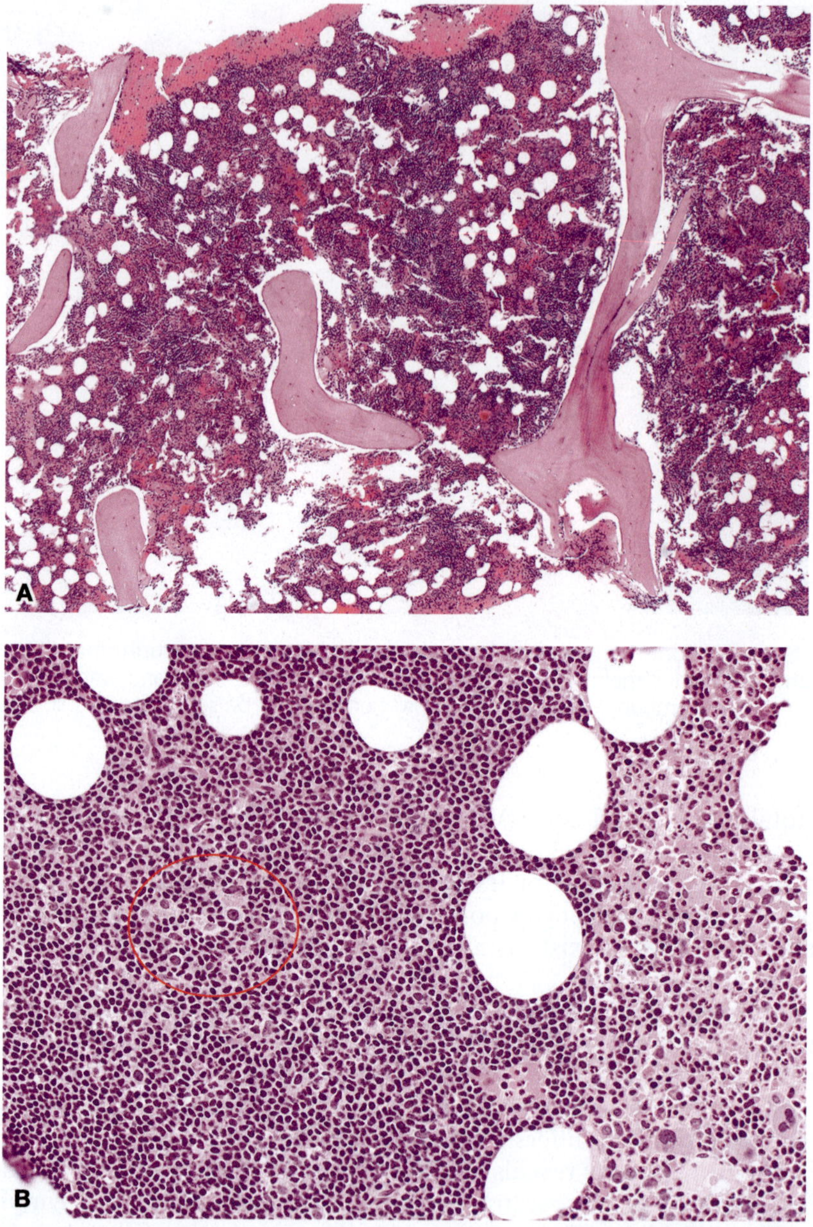

FIGURE 8.4 **A bone marrow biopsy in a patient with chronic lymphocytic leukemia/small lymphocytic lymphoma.** A, Low-power view showing a diffuse interstitial lymphocytosis and confluent nonparatrabecular aggregates. B, Higher power view of a large lymphoid aggregate comprised mostly of small lymphocytes with occasional larger cells (circled), suggesting a growth center. C, The bone marrow aspirate shows sheets of atypical mature lymphoid cells with round nuclei with slight size variability and varying degrees of chromatin clumping.

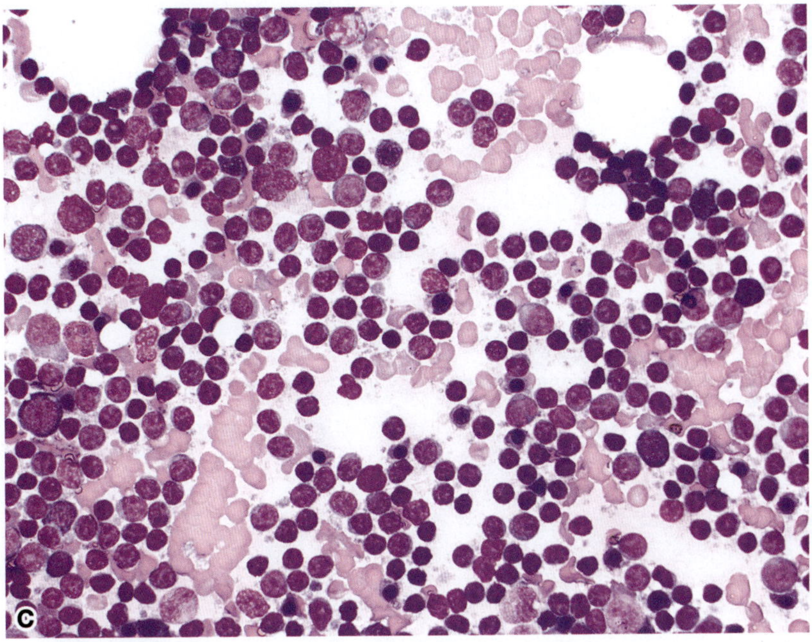

FIGURE 8.4 *(continued)*

weak CD11c, and CD200 (Figure 8.5) and have restricted light chains, which are typically dimly expressed. They are negative for CD10, CD38, and FMC7, the latter an epitope on the CD20 molecule. These FC findings are characteristic and helpful in differentiating CLL/SLL from MCL, which is another CD5-positive mature B cell neoplasm, but which lacks CD200 and has relatively bright CD20 (see later).

Genetics

Approximately 80% of CLL/SLL cases have cytogenetic abnormalities detected by fluorescent in situ hybridization (FISH). The most common include del(13q14.3) (50% of cases) and trisomy 12 (20% of cases). Less commonly detected are deletions of 11q22-23, 17p13, and 6q21. Del(13q) affects microRNA genes; Del(11q) affects ATM; and del(17p) affects p53. The distribution of these cytogenetic abnormalities varies based on mutational status of Immunoglobulin (IG) genes.

Up to 40% to 50% of CLL/SLL cases have unmutated IG genes, whereas 50% to 60% show somatic hypermutation of IG genes. These two subgroups, mutated and unmutated, differ in both biology and clinical features; unmutated CLL/SLL often expresses CD38 and ZAP70 by FC, although the correlation is imperfect.

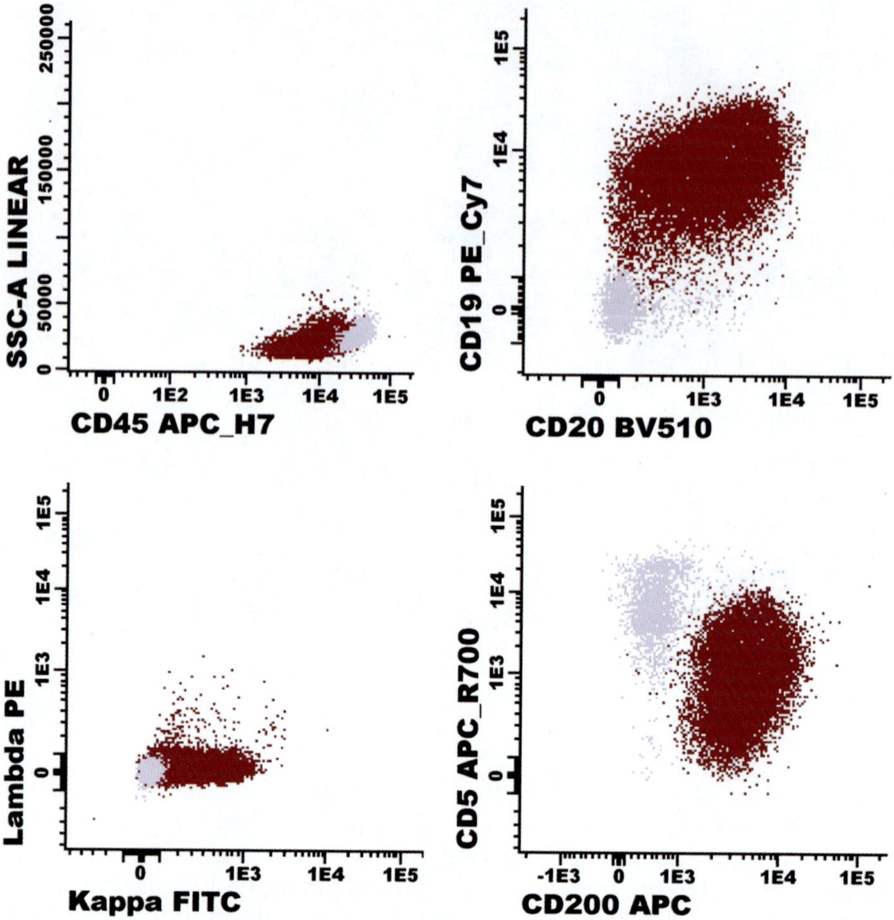

FIGURE 8.5 Flow cytometry of chronic lymphocytic leukemia cells (brown) with dimmer CD45 than background T cells (gray); dim variable expression of CD20 and relatively brighter CD19; dim clonal expression of kappa light chain; and coexpression of CD5 and CD200, the former dimmer than that seen in background T cells. SSC, side scatter.

Staging and Prognosis

CLL/SLL is clinically staged using the Rai and Binet system to define disease extent and prognosis. For patients at a low stage, those with mutated CLL/SLL have a better prognosis than those with unmutated CLL/SLL.

Patients with a worse prognosis have the following features: unmutated CLL (or its surrogate markers), del(11q), del(17p), and del(6q). Other poor predictors include a rapid cell doubling time in the PB (<1 year) and serum markers of high cell turnover, like lactate dehydrogenase (LDH). Some cases of CLL/SLL will progress to a more aggressive disease, with increasing numbers of prolymphocytes, sometimes referred to as prolymphocytic transformation. Richter transformation typically refers to progression of nodal disease with the histologic appearance of DLBCL, which occurs in 2% to 8% of cases. Less than 1% of cases will progress to classic Hodgkin lymphoma (CHL).

MONOCLONAL B CELL LYMPHOCYTOSIS

Cases that do not fulfill the quantitative criteria for CLL/SLL or other leukemia are known as MBL.[6] The WBC counts are lower than those of CLL/SLL ($<5 \times 10^9$ K/μL), although the absolute count should be noted, as it affects the likelihood of progression to CLL/SLL.

- High-count MBL: ($>0.5 \times 10^9$/L): progression to CLL = 1% to 2% per year
- Low-count MBL: ($<0.5 \times 10^9$/L): most likely clinically insignificant

MBL occurs in 3.5% of patients over the age of 40 and, similar to CLL/SLL, increases the risk of infections and other neoplasms.

MANTLE CELL LYMPHOMA/LEUKEMIA

MCL is a clonal neoplasm of mature B cells characterized in the great majority of cases by Cyclin D1 protein expression because of the IGH::*CCND1* translocation.[6] This lymphoid neoplasm has a myriad of clinical presentations, which correspond with disease course and prognosis, and range from aggressive to indolent.[7]

Epidemiology

MCL represents 3% to 10% of all non-Hodgkin lymphoma (NHL) and affects middle-aged to elderly patients with a male predominance.

Presentation

MCL classically affects the LN, spleen, BM, and/or PB. Other extranodal sites include the gastrointestinal (GI) tract, in the form of multiple lymphomatous polyposis. The central nervous system (CNS) may be involved, especially in relapsed disease. Most patients have widespread disease, or stage III/IV, at diagnosis and almost all have PB involvement, which presents as a marked lymphocytosis. There is also a leukemic non-nodal variant of the disease, with pure PB involvement and little-to-no LN involvement. In the PB, the abnormal cells are morphologically variable; some may resemble CLL and others may display irregular nuclei (Figure 8.6; eFigure 8.5). Many cases previously diagnosed as B-PLL are now recognized as leukemic MCL.

Morphology

The pattern of BM infiltration is typically diffuse, or diffuse and nodular (eFigure 6). The cells are small-to-medium and monomorphic with irregular nuclear borders, dispersed chromatin, and nonvisible nucleoli (Figure 8.7). There are several morphologic variants that may cause diagnostic confusion,

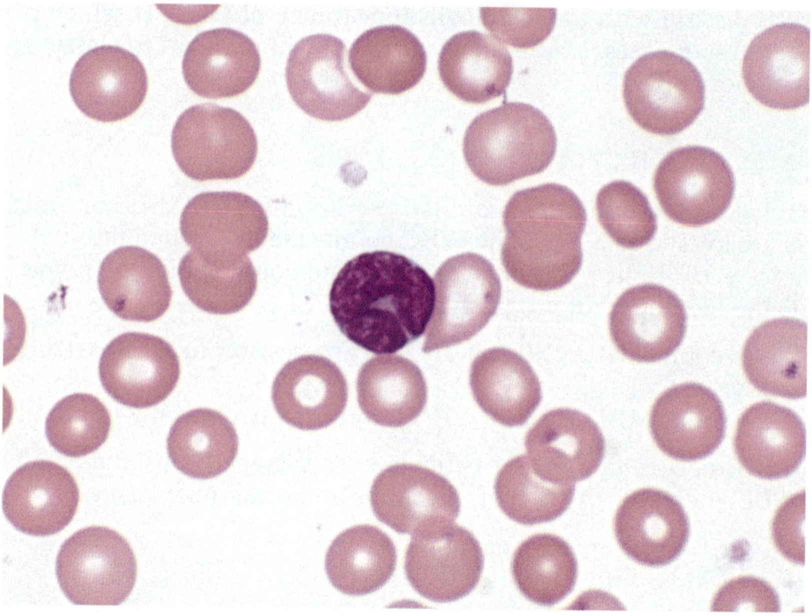

FIGURE 8.6 A circulating cell in mantle cell lymphoma with a highly irregular nuclear shape.

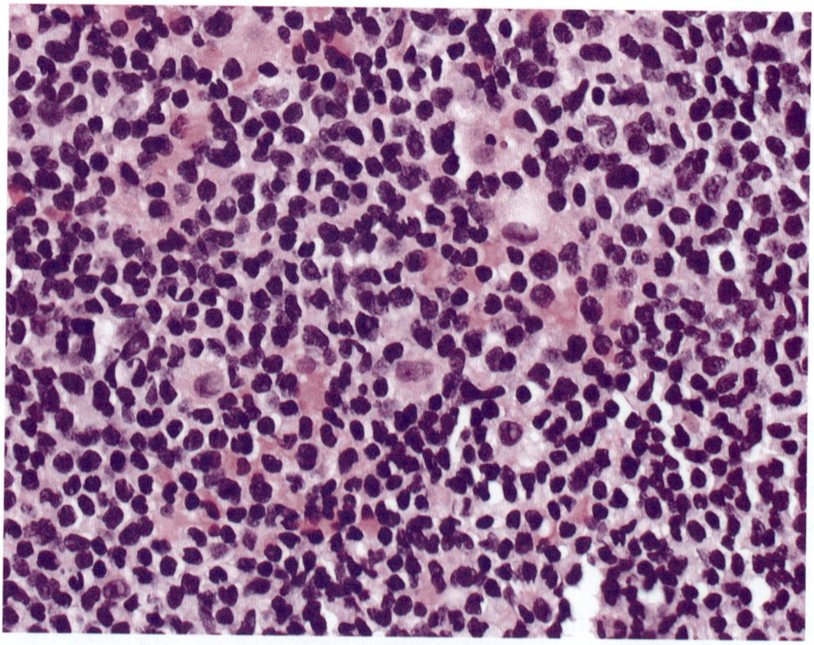

FIGURE 8.7 High-power view of mantle cell lymphoma in the bone marrow showing small mature atypical lymphoid cells with irregular nuclei.

including the blastoid, pleomorphic, small cell, and marginal zone lymphoma (MZL)-like variants. The small cell variant is often seen in leukemic, non-nodal disease.

Immunophenotype

In contrast to CLL/SLL, the abnormal B cells are positive for bright CD20, CD5, FMC7, and CD43, with dim-to-negative CD23 and negative CD200 (Figure 8.8; eFigure 8.7). Light chains are more brightly expressed than in CLL/SLL, and lambda light chain restriction is more prevalent than kappa. Cyclin D1 is positive in >95%, even in rare CD5-negative cases (Figure 8.9). SOX11, a specific and sensitive marker for MCL, is positive in >90% of cases, even in Cyclin D1–negative cases and in cases with blastoid morphology.

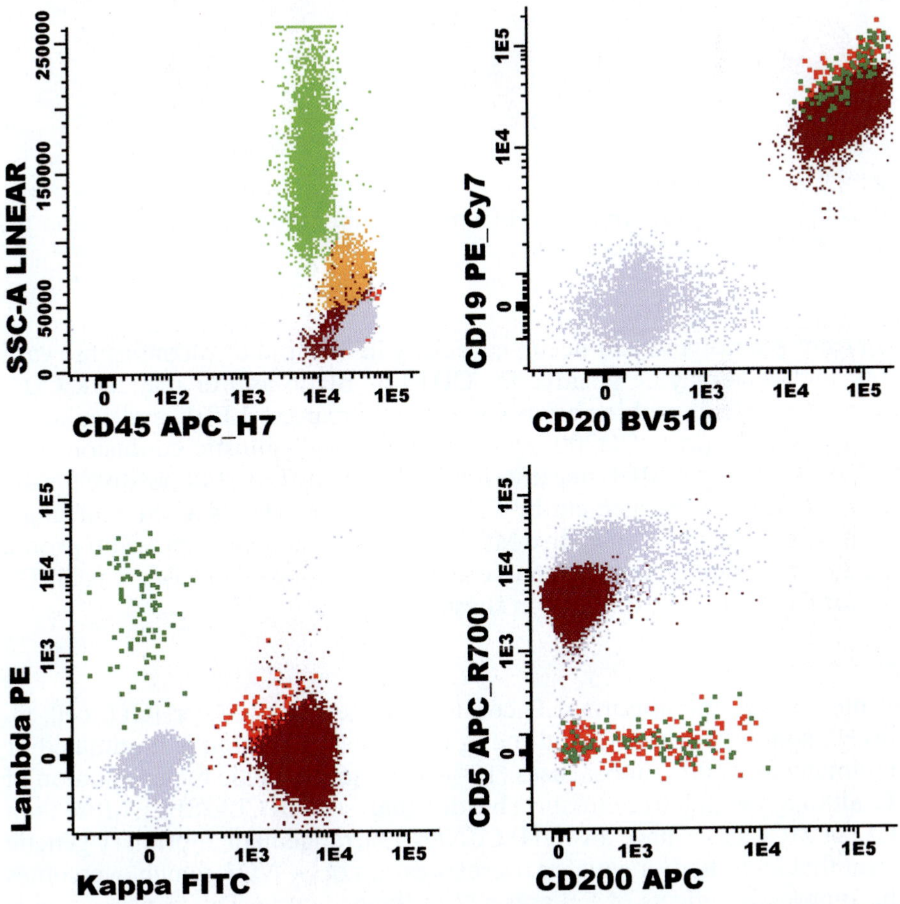

FIGURE 8.8 **Flow cytometry of leukemic phase mantle cell lymphoma (compare to chronic lymphocytic leukemia [CLL]).** Neoplastic cells (brown) have brighter CD45, CD19, and CD20 compared to CLL, are positive for CD5, and lack CD200 (light green: neutrophils; orange: monocytes; red and green: residual normal κ- and λ-positive B cells). SSC, side scatter.

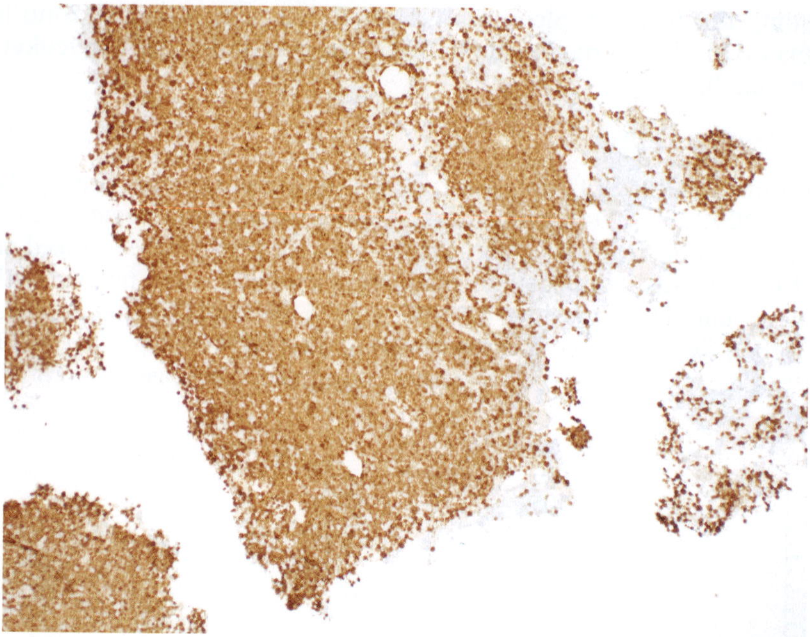

FIGURE 8.9 **Mantle cell lymphoma in a marrow clot section stained for Cyclin D1.** More than 95% of cases will be positive.

Aberrant phenotypes can occur, especially in blastoid or pleomorphic variants, and cells may be positive for CD10 or BCL6 and/or may lack CD5. Blastoid or pleomorphic variants may rarely express LEF1, and leukemic variants may express CD200, which may cause diagnostic confusion with CLL/SLL. Rarely is MCL negative for Cyclin D1 by IHC, but positive for the IGH::*CCND1* rearrangement by FISH. Rare cases also lack the rearrangement. These cyclin D1–negative MCL have a similar gene expression profile (GEP) and a similar clinical course as Cyclin D1–positive cases. Cyclin D2 and/or Cyclin D3 is expressed in these cases.

Genetics

In most cases, the abnormal B cell is a pre-germinal center (GC) cell, although some are post-GC, and the Ig variable (IgV) region is unmutated or minimally mutated in most cases (15%-40% show somatic hypermutation of IG, although with lower mutation burden than seen in CLL/SLL). More than 95% of MCL cases have an IGH::*CCND1* rearrangement, a primary genetic event that leads to dysregulated overexpression of *CCND1*, which overcomes the suppressive effects of *RB* and p27 in the cell cycle. The translocation is not sufficient in and of itself for the formation of this lymphoma, however; numerous nonrandom chromosomal abnormalities are also typically present, including gain of 3q, 7p, and 8q and loss of 1p, 6q, or 9p or copy-neutral loss of heterozygosity (LOH). Mutations are seen in *CCND1* (35%) and other genes, including *NOTCH2*, which has prognostic significance.

Prognosis

The prognostic impact is determined by morphologic subtype, *TP53* deletions/mutations, and the Ki67 proliferation index; patients with >30% Ki67-positive cells are considered to have a poor prognosis. The median survival for typical MCL is 3-5 years, and most patients are never cured of their disease. Although MCL does not transform to DLBCL, it can transform to a higher-grade lesion with blastoid features.

Leukemic MCL variant, which involves the PB, BM, and/or spleen, has a more indolent course than typical nodal-based MCL.[8] Morphologically, the cells are small and indistinguishable from other small cell leukemias, like CLL/SLL. These are SOX11-negative and may also be negative for CD5. Unlike typical MCL, they have few cytogenetic abnormalities other than the *CCND1* rearrangement. As mentioned earlier, the *CCND1* rearrangement is not sufficient for disease formation alone, as up to 7% of healthy individuals have PB cells with *CCND1* rearrangements.

This variant has a better prognosis than typical MCL, with longer survival times (79 months average). However, it may become aggressive with the addition of genetic abnormalities, including *TP53* mutations.

FOLLICULAR LYMPHOMA

FL is a systemic lymphoid neoplasm involving the LNs, BM, PB, spleen, and other tissues. The neoplastic cells are clonal B cells with a GC phenotype and a characteristic follicular growth pattern mimicking secondary lymphoid follicles. This neoplasm arises out of a combination of complex genetic abnormalities, most of which begin with translocation t(14;18) in a precursor B cell followed by additional genetic abnormalities, including copy number changes and gene mutations.[9]

Epidemiology

FL represents approximately 20% to 30% of all NHLs in the Western world. Patients are typically elderly (median 65 years), and young patients are rarely diagnosed. Patients with increased environmental exposure to pesticides or herbicides have a higher incidence of abnormal B cells with t(14;18) identified in their PB.

Presentation

FL is an indolent, chronic, and relapsing disease. Patients often present with LAD, which may be present for months to years and have widespread disease at diagnosis. The spleen may be involved, but other organs and/or non-nodal tissues are rarely involved. Less than 20% of all patients have B symptoms or increased LDH levels.

In some cases, a CBC may reveal leukocytosis with lymphocytosis comprised of atypical lymphoid cells. The cells in the PB are medium-to-large, with irregular, often cleaved, nuclei and relatively scant cytoplasm (Figure 8.10). There is often an accompanying anemia and occasionally thrombocytopenia.

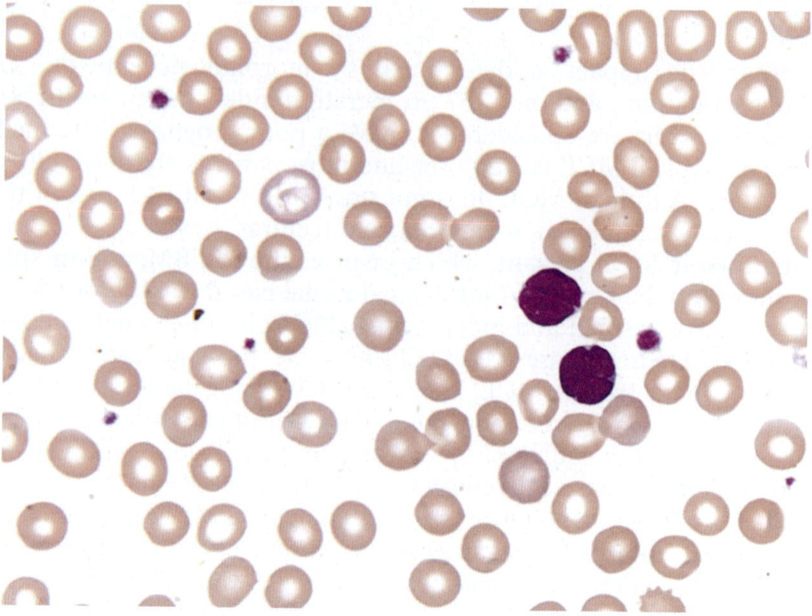

FIGURE 8.10 Follicular lymphoma cells in the peripheral blood are small-to-medium-sized cells with scant cytoplasm and irregular nuclei, typically with a deep cleft.

Morphology

Up to 70% of FL patients have BM involvement, including 30% to 40% of patients with low-grade FL in peripheral LNs. Characteristic morphologic findings in the BM biopsy include a paratrabecular nodular lymphoid infiltrate (Figure 8.11A and B; eFigure 8.8). A truly follicular pattern, like that seen in the LN, is rarely seen in the BM. However, as in the LN, the abnormal cells recapitulate GC cells, with centrocytes and varying numbers of centroblasts. Centrocytes are small-to-medium lymphoid cells with irregular or cleaved nuclei, condensed chromatin, and no visible nucleoli. Centroblasts are large, round lymphoid cells with large nuclei, vesicular chromatin, and one to three small, peripheralized nucleoli. Interestingly, up to 10% to 25% of patients with low-grade FL in the BM have a high-grade FL (grade 3) or DLBCL in other tissues. In fact, this low-grade component may be the only clue of underlying FL in a patient presenting with DLBCL elsewhere.

The core biopsy is the best specimen to examine, as involvement in the aspirate smear may be subtle or nonexistent. The paratrabecular lymphoid aggregates are not often aspirated, and this may lead to a false-negative result on the aspirate, as well as the FC.

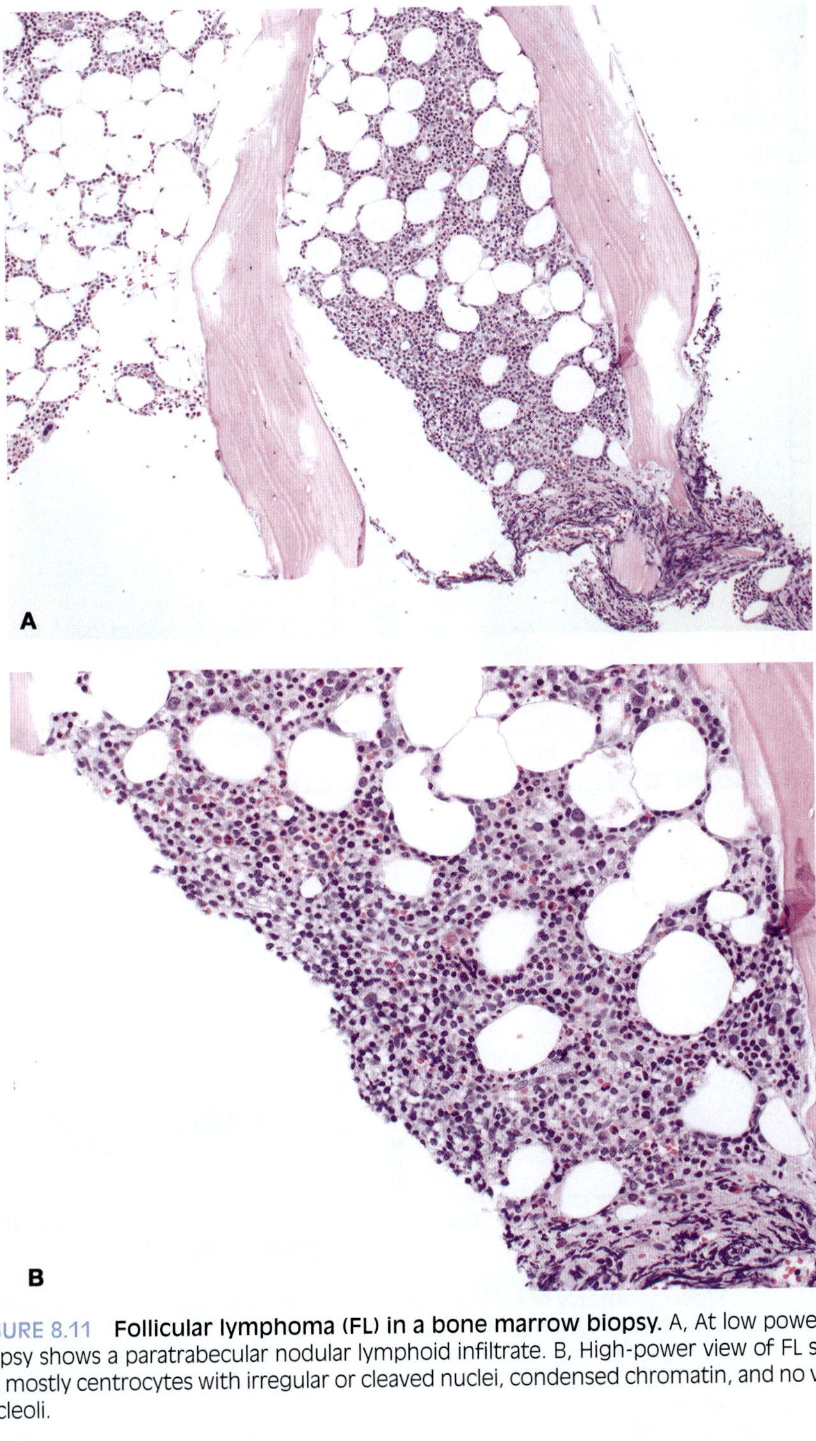

A

B

FIGURE 8.11 **Follicular lymphoma (FL) in a bone marrow biopsy.** A, At low power, the biopsy shows a paratrabecular nodular lymphoid infiltrate. B, High-power view of FL showing mostly centrocytes with irregular or cleaved nuclei, condensed chromatin, and no visible nucleoli.

Immunophenotype

The FC phenotype of FL is characteristic, although not absolutely specific (Figure 8.12). The hallmark of FL is expression of CD10, a GC marker. CD10 is also expressed on BL and DLBCL of GC B cell (GCB) type. Other mature B cell malignancies can express CD10, including MCL, HCL, and LPL, but this is rare. Immature B cells in B cell acute lymphoblastic leukemia (B-ALL) also express CD10; thus, the diagnosis of FL requires assessment for markers of maturity, including CD20 and surface Ig light chains.

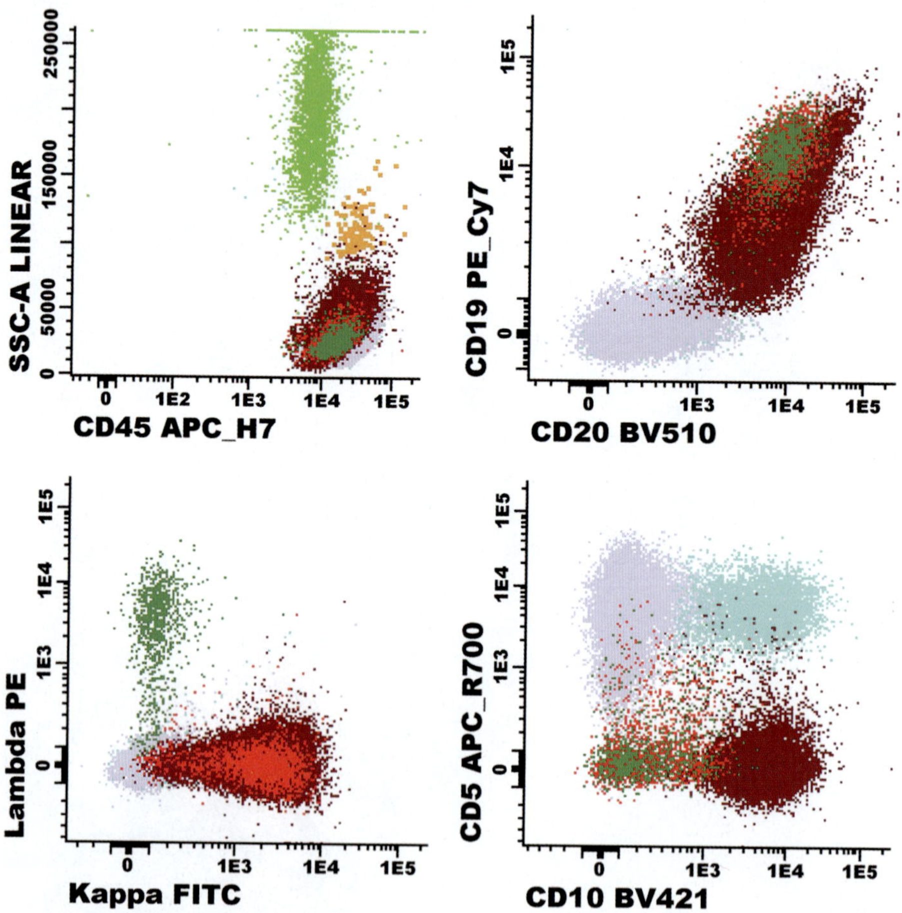

FIGURE 8.12 **Flow cytometry of follicular lymphoma (brown) shows relatively bright CD45 and CD20 with dim variable CD19.** Kappa light chain is relatively bright and CD10 is positive but CD5 negative. Note that in this case there are many CD10+ T follicular helper cells (light blue) in addition to other T cells (gray). There are some contaminating granulocytes (light green) and monocytes (orange) in this fine needle aspiration specimen, along with some background polyclonal CD10-negative B cells (red and green). SSC, side scatter.

CD10 is also positive on physiologically normal GCB, requiring demonstration of light chain restriction or other phenotypic aberrancy; CD38 in particular can be useful for distinguishing FL from reactive GC cells as CD38 intensity is decreased in FL.

However, as mentioned earlier, paratrabecular lymphoid nodules are often difficult to aspirate, so that FC diagnosis of FL may not be reliable on a BM specimen. IHC stains performed on a core biopsy are useful to demonstrate paratrabecular accentuation of CD20-positive B cells and to assess BCL6 and BCL2 expression (eFigure 8.9). Ki67 is also useful to assess the proliferation index. However, it can be very difficult to interpret both Ki67 and CD10 by IHC in the BM because of the high proliferative index of normal background hematopoietic cells and the abundance of neutrophils, which also express CD10.

Genetics

The IGH::*BCL2* rearrangement resulting from t(14;18) is identified in 80% to 85% of FL cases. This translocation occurs in precursor B cells in the BM during heavy chain rearrangement. These cells undergo additional alterations and eventually reach the GC with multiple genetic lesions. In the highly selective environment of the GC, the cells with t(14;18) have a survival advantage because of the overexpression of BCL2, a negative regulator of apoptosis.

The translocation t(14;18) is not definitional, however, as some *bona fide* FL do not have the translocation. Nor is it sufficient for lymphomagenesis alone, as it is found in 50% to 70% of normal healthy individuals. Cases of BCL2-negative FL have the same prognosis as BCL2-positive cases.

Other structural abnormalities are common in FL, including loss of 1p36, 6q, 17p and gains of 1q, 7, 8, 12q, 18q, and X. Abnormalities of 3q27/*BCL6* are found in 5% to 15% of FL cases. In general, high-grade FL has more genetic alternations than low-grade FL.

In addition to chromosomal abnormalities, there are often extensive mutations detected in FL cells. Mutations are detected in chromatin modifiers (histone methylators/methyltransferase), including *KMT2D* (89%), *CREBBP* (41%), and *EZH2* (7% of cases). Copy number changes, copy-neutral loss of heterozygosity (LOH), and abnormalities of *TNFRSF14*, located on 1p36, are the most common abnormalities seen in FL. *MYC* and *TP53* alterations are associated with FL transformation.

Next-generation sequencing (NGS) is useful to detect mutations in the common genes listed earlier, but the diagnosis usually depends on the morphology, phenotype, and/or FISH. FISH is a better diagnostic tool than polymerase chain reaction (PCR) because of variation of breakpoint regions in FL. The IgV undergoes extensive and ongoing somatic hypermutation. Although historically FL had a low rate of detection by PCR because of mutations in the complementarity-determining regions (CDRs), causing problems with primer binding, currently 90% to 100% of cases are detected via PCR because of better primer sets.

Prognosis

Patient prognosis is related to the extent of disease. Several prognostic models are used; the most common is a modification of the International Prognostic Index (IPI), known as Follicular lymphoma (FL) IPI. FLIPI uses five clinical predictors of survival. The Lugano Classification, a modification of the Ann Arbor staging classification, is used for clinical staging.

Like many low-grade lymphomas, FL is treatable, but ultimately incurable with conventional chemotherapy. Despite this, patients often have favorable outcomes. After the introduction of rituximab, up to 80% of patients have an overall survival (OS) of >10 years. The median survival for FL grades 1-3A is approximately 12 years.

The natural course of FL is frequent disease recurrence and subsequent progression from low grade to high grade. Histologic transformation occurs in approximately 30% to 40% of patients at a rate of about 3% each year. Many new treatments, including biologics, are available that permit long-term management of patients.

REVIEW OF THE DIFFERENTIAL DIAGNOSIS OF NODULAR LYMPHOID AGGREGATES OF SMALL MATURE LYMPHOID CELLS

- The main differential diagnosis includes CLL/SLL, MCL, MZL, and FL. CLL/SLL and MCL have an interstitial distribution and express CD5. FL has a paratrabecular distribution and expresses CD10 and BCL6. MZL may show interstitial aggregates with associated germinal centers. A subset of MZL can express CD5.
- Additional markers including CD23, LEF1, and CD200 may be helpful in differentiating CLL/SLL from MCL (Table 8.2). Intensity of expression of markers, especially of CD20 and light chains, is important. FMC7, which is not commonly used, tends to follow CD20 expression; it is dim on CLL/SLL and bright on MCL.
- CD5 may be positive on physiologic, naïve B cells, so that assessment of light chain restriction on any CD5-positive B cells is necessary.
- The differential diagnosis for CD10-positive mature B cell leukemias/lymphomas detected by FC includes FL, BL, and DLBCL (Table 8.3),

TABLE 8.2 CD5-Positive B Cell Neoplasms

CD5 positive	Size	CD23	CD200	CD20 intensity	sIg intensity
CLL	Small	+	+	Dim	Dim
MCL	Small	−/+	−	Moderate	Moderate
DLBCL	Large or small	Variable	Variable	Variable	Variable

CLL, chronic lymphocytic leukemia; DLBCL, diffuse large B cell lymphoma; MCL, mantle cell lymphoma; sIg, surface immunoglobulin.

TABLE 8.3 **CD10-Positive B Cell Neoplasms**

CD10 positive	Size	CD38	CD10 intensity	sIg
FL	Small-medium	+	Moderate	Variable
BL	Small-medium	+ Bright	Bright	Bright
DLBCL	Large or small	Variable	Variable	Variable

BL, Burkitt lymphoma; DLBCL, diffuse large B cell lymphoma; FL, follicular lymphoma; sIg, surface immunoglobulin.

among others (e.g. subset of LPL and HCL), and morphologic correlation is necessary.

- CD10 is present on physiologically normal GCB. Occasionally, these may appear to be light chain restricted by FC.[10]
- FC can occasionally lack surface light chains, but normal GCB can also lack surface light chains.

B CELL LYMPHOMAS WITH PREDOMINANTLY DIFFUSE OR INTERSTITIAL PATTERNS OF INFILTRATION

Some B cell neoplasms show lymphoid cells distributed throughout the interstitium without recognizable nodules. This may be patchy and often subtle involvement, or sheet-like growth. Although CLL/SLL can show this pattern, other examples of B cell neoplasms with this pattern of infiltration include HCL and BL.

HAIRY CELL LEUKEMIA

Epidemiology and Presentation

HCL is a rare mature B cell leukemia that involves the PB, BM, and spleen. Patients are typically elderly, have a male predominance, and present with splenomegaly and CBC abnormalities, including anemia, leukopenia, and monocytopenia.[11]

Morphology

The BM is variably cellular, but often overall hypocellular for age. HCL appears as a variably subtle interstitial and septal lymphoid infiltrate (Figure 8.13A and B; eFigure 8.10). The abnormal cells are medium-sized and have abundant cytoplasm, giving them a "fried egg" appearance on hematoxylin and eosin (H&E) (Figure 8.14A and B). The background marrow shows increased reticulin fibrosis, resulting in a "dry tap" BM aspirate (Figure 8.15; eFigure 8.11).

Atypical lymphoid cells are present in the PB, displaying abundant circumferential cytoplasmic projections, giving the cells a "hairy" appearance (Figure 8.16; eFigure 8.12).

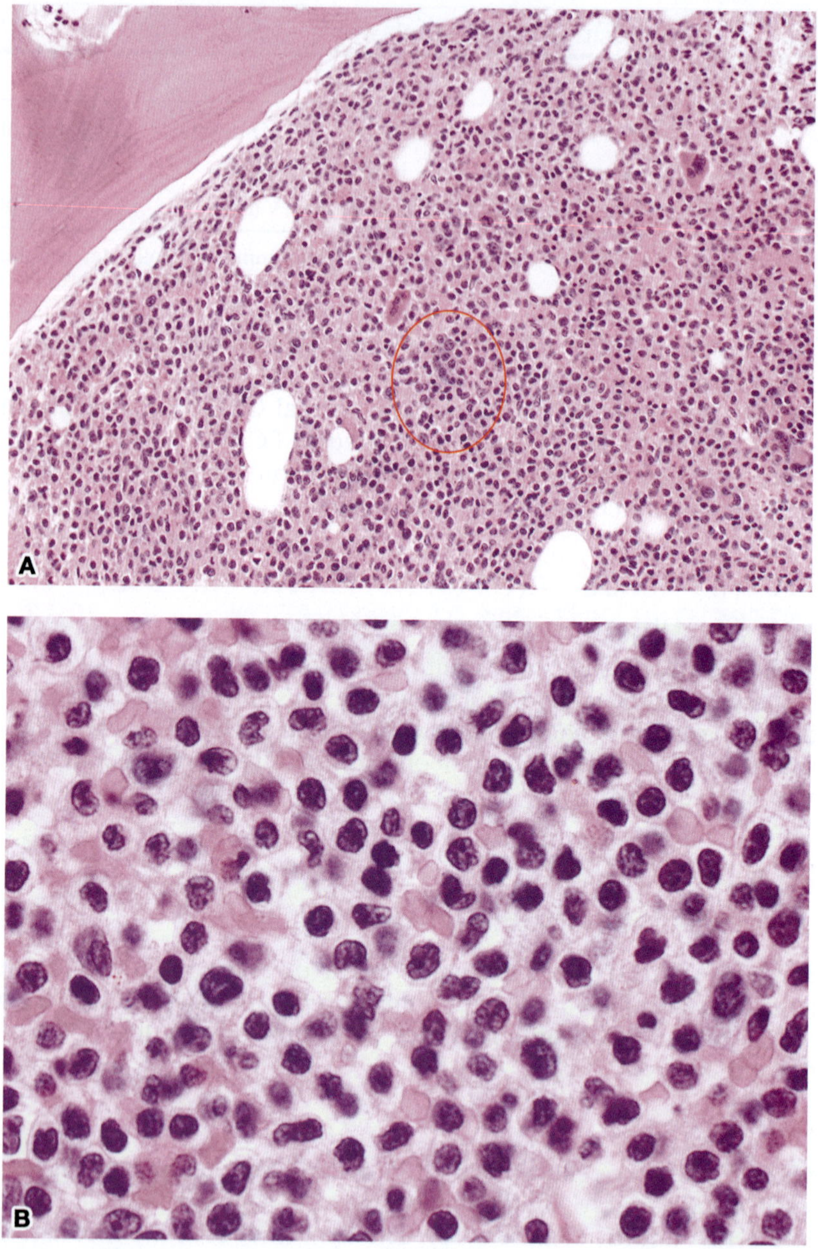

FIGURE 8.13 **Hairy cell leukemia (HCL) in the bone marrow.** A, In some cases, HCL can appear as a variably subtle interstitial and septal lymphoid infiltrate. B, An immunohistochemical stain for BRAF is positive on the hairy cells, confirming the diagnosis. Other immunohistochemical markers useful for diagnosis, albeit not specific, include DBA44, CD123, cyclin D1, and Annexin A1.

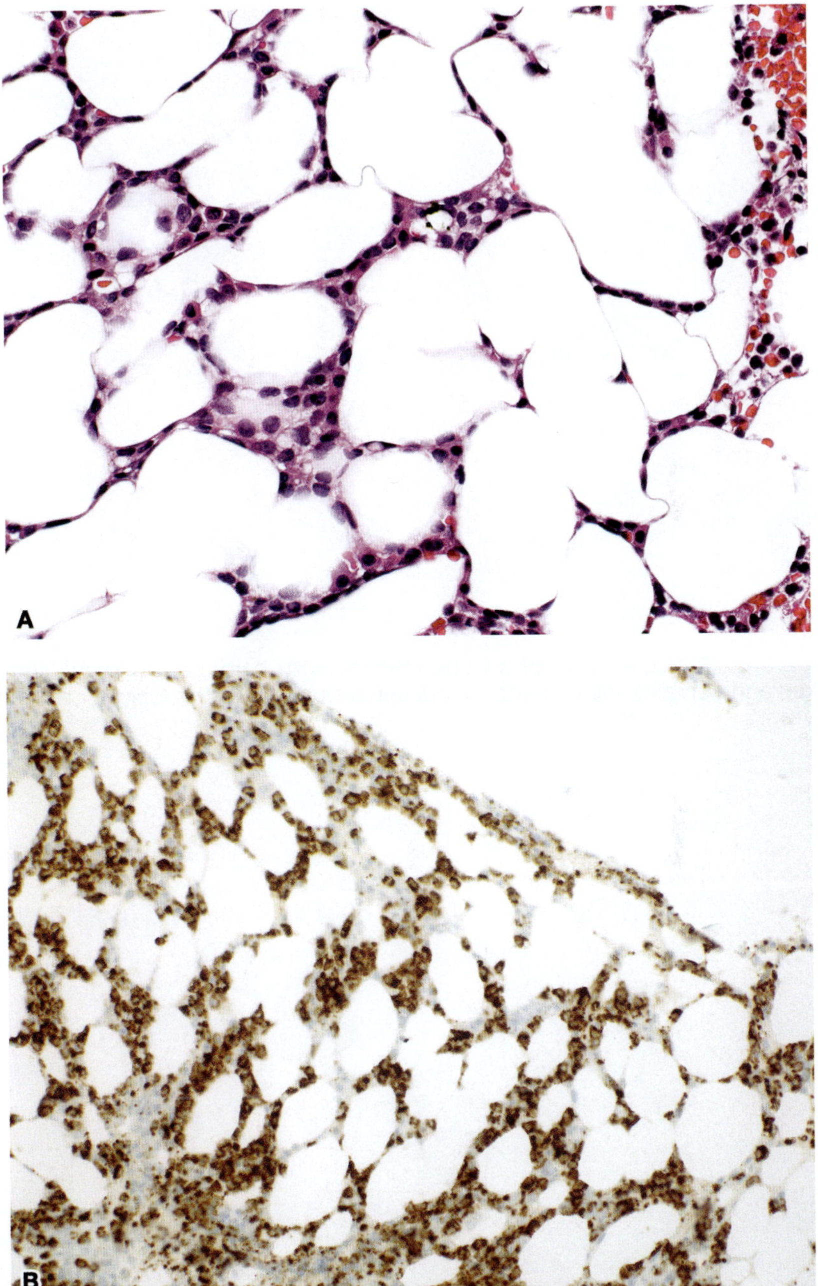

FIGURE 8.14 **Hairy cell leukemia (HCL) in the bone marrow.** A, At low power, the abnormal cells are medium sized and have abundant cytoplasm, giving them a "fried egg" appearance on hematoxylin and eosin. Compare to residual erythroid cells in the circle. B, At very high power, cells can have irregular nuclei but nucleoli are absent or very small, and the abundant cytoplasm clearly separates the cells.

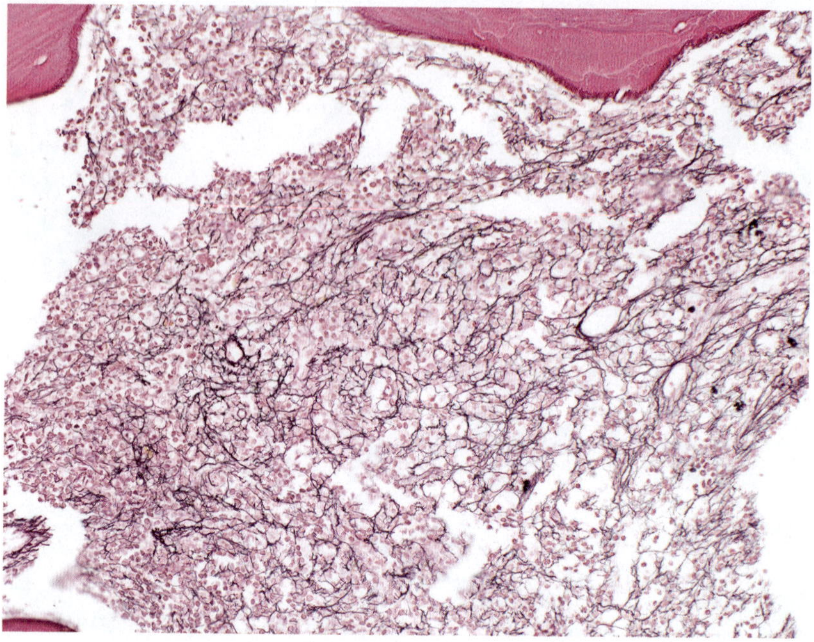

FIGURE 8.15 **Reticulin stain of a bone marrow with hairy cell leukemia shows a marked and complex investment of reticulin around cells.** This typically can result in a "dry tap."

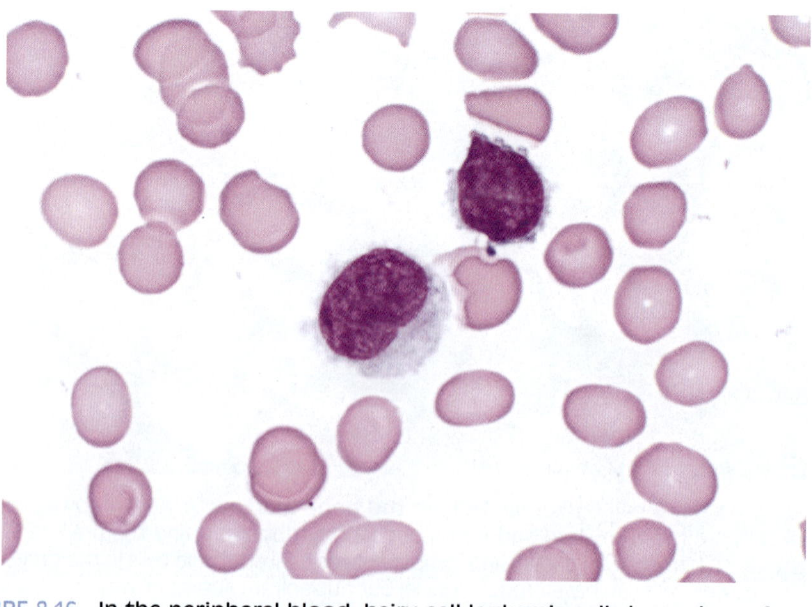

FIGURE 8.16 **In the peripheral blood, hairy cell leukemia cells have circumferential cytoplasmic projections, giving the cells a "hairy" appearance.**

The spleen may be involved and shows atypical cells in the red pulp forming "blood lakes."

Immunophenotype

FC shows that the cells are positive for bright CD20 and CD11c, in addition to CD103 and CD25 (Figure 8.17; eFigure 8.13). By IHC and/or special stains, the cells are positive for Cyclin D1, CD123, DB44, Annexin A1, Trap, and BRAF. The differential diagnosis includes variant HCL, which is indistinguishable from typical HCL by FC, except for negativity for CD25, and SMZL, which has a very different overall phenotype (see later).

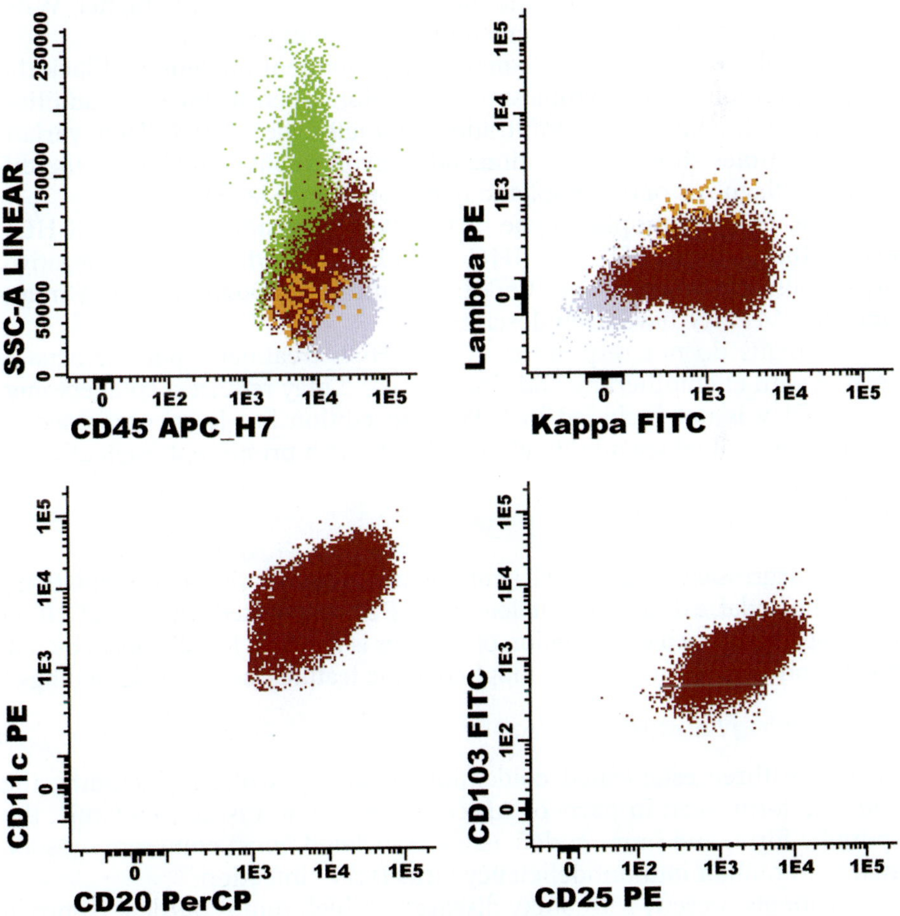

FIGURE 8.17 **Flow cytometry of hairy cell leukemia.** Note that there are very few monocytes (highlighted in orange in CD45/side scatter [SCC] plot top left) and that the leukemic cells (brown) occupy the same general area on this plot that monocytes would be found. Leukemic cells have low light chain restriction (top right), bright CD20 (bottom left), and coexpress bright CD11c, CD25, and CD103 (bottom left).

Genetics

Mutations in *BRAF* V600E are characteristic of HCL and are not found in other B cell lymphomas. Although chromosomal abnormalities have been detected, none are specific.

Prognosis

Despite the remissions achieved with purine analog treatment, up to half of all patients will relapse. Other treatment opportunities include anti-CD22 and BRAF inhibitors.

Hairy Cell Leukemia Variant

Hairy cell leukemia variant (HCL-v) is a much less common disease than even the rare classic HCL. Patients tend to present with higher WBC counts and typically have preserved monocyte counts.

Morphologically, the cells may have prominent nucleoli and lack the typical circumferential cytoplasmic projections seen in HCL. In addition to the interstitial pattern of infiltration characteristic of HCL, HCL variant may sometimes show distinct sinusoidal involvement, bringing up the differential diagnosis of other splenic lymphomas (see later).

The FC immunophenotype of HCL-v is very similar to that of HCL except that it lacks CD25; by IHC, Annexin A1 and BRAF are negative. HCL-v also lacks the *BRAF-V600E* mutation, although recurrent mutations in *MAP2K1* have been described.

Patients do not respond to typical HCL treatment, but are usually treated with chemotherapy and rituximab and may require a splenectomy.

HCL-v is not included in WHO 5th edition but is encompassed in what is now called splenic B cell lymphoma with prominent nucleoli.

BURKITT LYMPHOMA/LEUKEMIA

BL is an aggressive mature B cell lymphoma that has a variety of presentations, including nodal, extranodal, and leukemic. BL is associated with a *MYC*::IGH rearrangement, but a combination of findings is required for diagnosis, including morphologic features, immunophenotypic features, and genetic findings.

Epidemiology and Presentation

There are three established epidemiology subtypes of BL, including the endemic form, seen in parts of Africa where malaria is also endemic, the sporadic form, and immunodeficiency associated, most commonly associated with human immunodeficiency virus (HIV) infection.

Patients present with bulky disease and high tumor burden. Approximately 30% of patients present with stage I/II and 70% present with stage III/IV. Patients with bulky disease may show a leukemic phase, but exclusive involvement of the BM or PB is rare. In addition, BM involvement is not always associated with leukemic (PB) involvement.

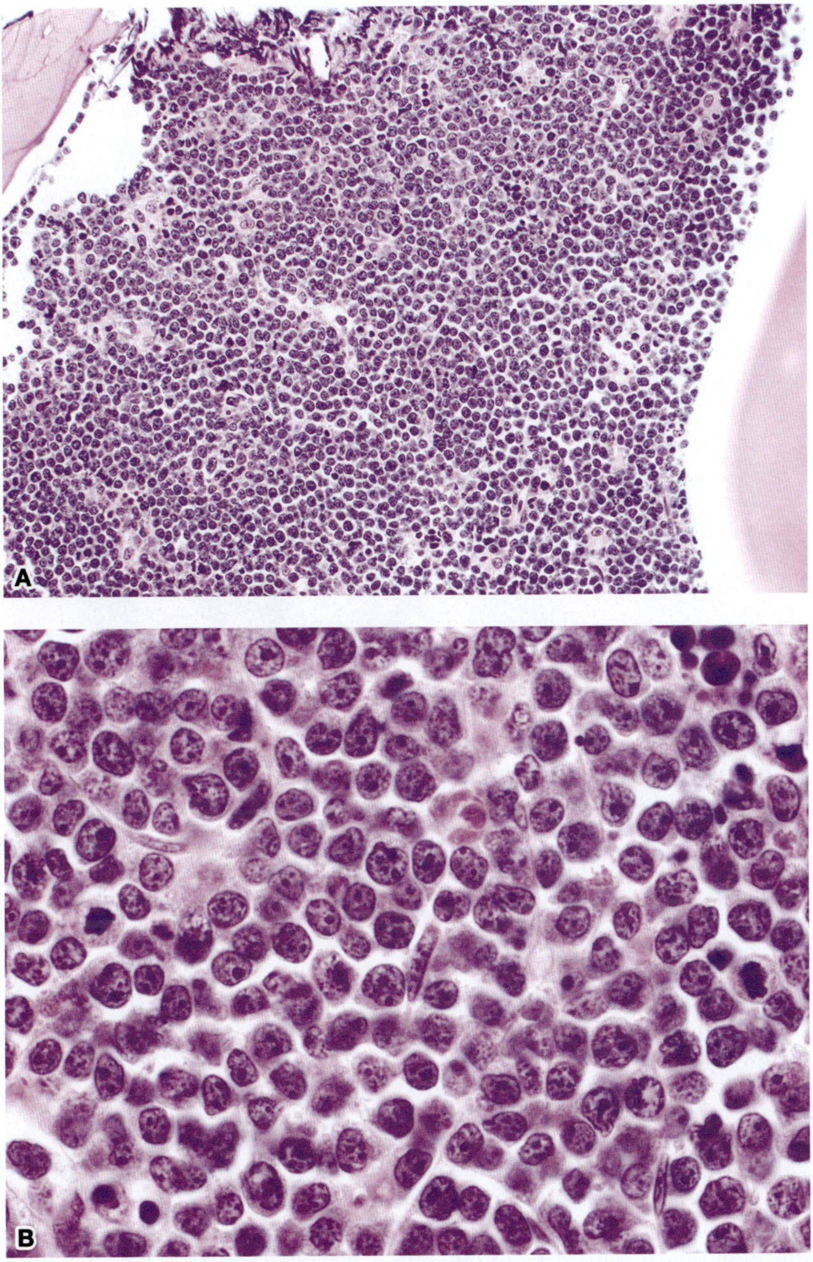

FIGURE 8.18 **Burkitt lymphoma (BL) in the bone marrow.** A, BL appears as a diffuse infiltrate of monotonous medium-sized cells. B, At higher power, BL cells have generally round nuclei and a small amount of cytoplasm with multiple nucleoli on a background of stippled chromatin. C, The bone marrow aspirate of a patient with BL shows medium-sized cells with small nucleoli, dark blue cytoplasm, and cytoplasmic vacuoles.

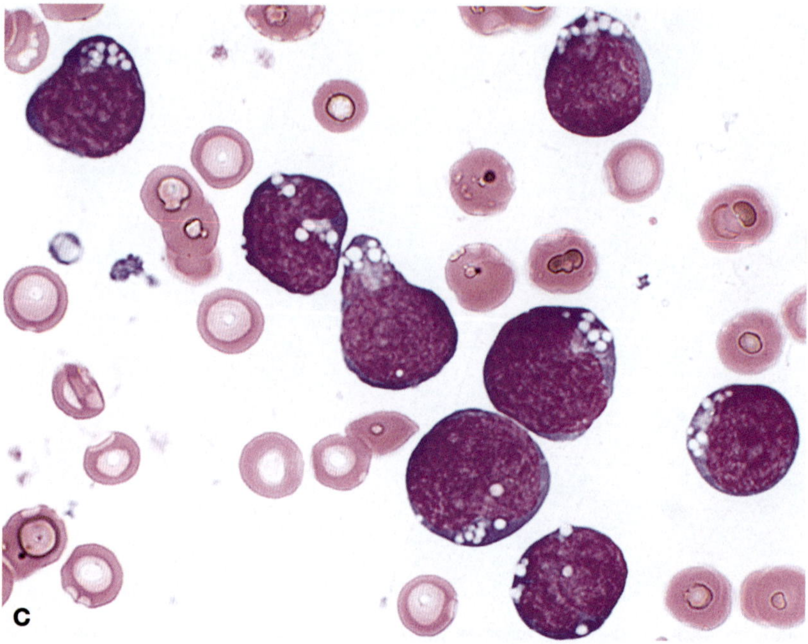

FIGURE 8.18 (continued)

Morphology

In BM biopsy sections, BL appears as a diffuse infiltration resembling acute leukemia (Figure 8.18A and B; eFigure 8.14).[12] Cells are monotonous, medium in size, and have a few small nucleoli. The "starry sky" appearance seen on LN biopsies may be subtle or difficult to detect in the BM, but there are increased mitosis and very few background T cells. The BM may be so packed that an aspirate results in a dry tap. In those cases that can be aspirated, the cells are medium sized with dark blue cytoplasm and cytoplasmic vacuoles (Figure 8.18C; eFigure 8.15). Some cases of BL may have plasmacytoid appearance (especially in cases associated with underlying immunodeficiency).

Immunophenotype

BL expresses mature B cell markers including CD19, CD20, and surface kappa or lambda, in addition to CD10. By FC, CD38, CD10, and light chains are usually bright, and CD20 may be dim (Figure 8.19). By IHC, BCL2 is usually negative (or weak), which helps differentiate this lymphoma from FL. Strong BCL2 expression in a tumor with high grade morphology effectively excludes BL and raises the suspicion of a high-grade B cell lymphoma (HGBCL) with translocations of *MYC* and *BCL2*, so-called "double-hit lymphoma." BL in HIV-positive patients may show extremely dim CD20 expression by FC and may be confused with B-ALL. Approximately 2% of pediatric cases with classic BL morphology and t(8;14) have an abnormal phenotype more consistent with a pre-B cell, positive for Tdt, CD34, and lacking CD20.

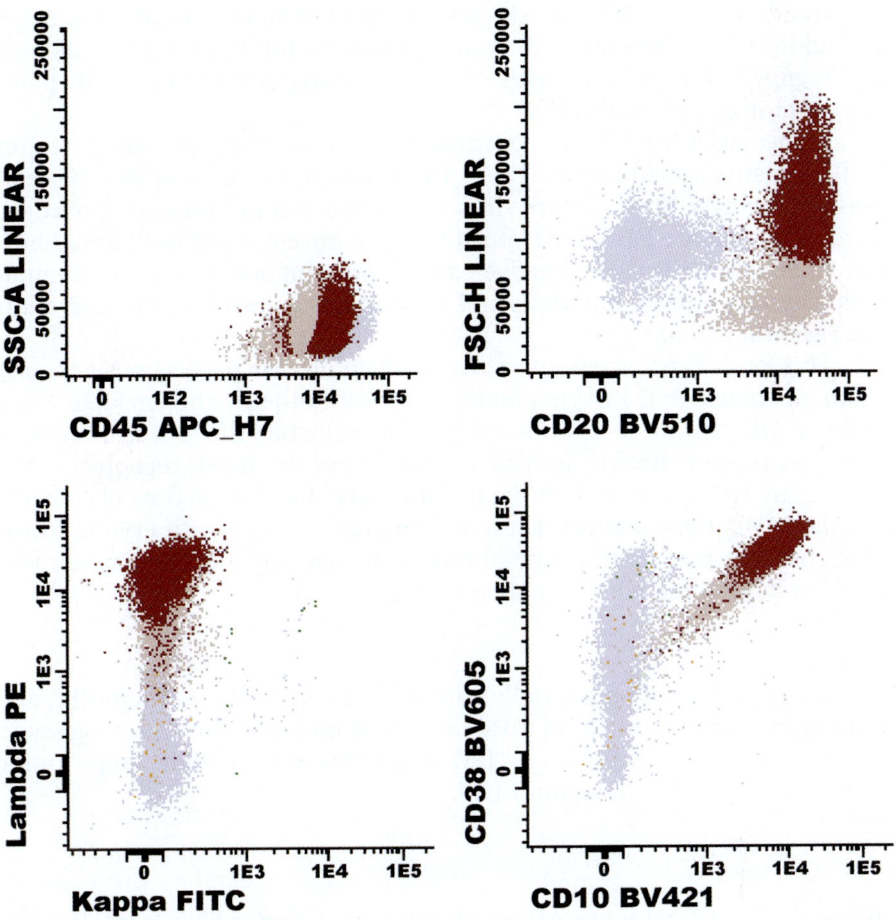

FIGURE 8.19 **Flow cytometry of Burkitt lymphoma.** Tumor cells (brown) have dimmer CD45 and higher forward scatter (FSC) than background lymphocytes (gray top panels). They show bright CD20 (top right panel), as well as bright clonal expression of light chains (bottom left panel) and CD10 and CD38 (bottom right panel). Burkitt lymphoma cells are fragile and often show degenerative changes (pale tan) with decreased light scatter and coordinated loss of antigen expression. SSC, side scatter.

Genetics

BL is characterized by *MYC::*IGH, which transposes the *MYC* oncogene on 8q24 and IGH on 14q32. *MYC* may have other translocation partners, including IGK on 2p12 or IGL on 22q11. For this reason, both breakapart and dual-color dual-fusion FISH probes should be utilized to evaluate *MYC* rearrangements. *MYC* breakpoints vary because of aberrant somatic hypermutation mediated by activation-induced cytidine deaminase (AID). Additional chromosomal abnormalities may also be present.

In addition to *MYC* translocations, up to 70% of sporadic BL cases have additional mutations in the transcription factor *TCF3/E2A* or its negative regulator *ID3*, which engage B cell signaling through the PI3K pathway, promoting cell survival.

Many cases of BL are positive for Epstein-Barr encoding region (EBER)-in situ hybridization (ISH). Interestingly, there is an inverse relationship between Epstein-Barr virus (EBV) status and mutational burden: those cases that are EBER-ISH positive often have a lower mutational burden, whereas EBER-ISH–negative cases have a higher frequency of mutations. Therefore, both mutations and EBV appear to result in the activation of B receptor signaling.

This lends credence to the polymicrobial disease pathogenesis theory, which postulates that EBV in combination with other pathogens like *Plasmodium falciparum* is responsible for the endemic BL found in central Africa because of chronic antigen stimulation of the B cell receptor.

Up to 10% of cases that would otherwise be classified as classic BL lack the *MYC* translocation. These may represent cases with cryptic translocations because of variant breakpoints or may represent the much less common lymphoma with 11q aberrations.

Prognosis

BL is an aggressive but potentially curable disease. Intensive chemotherapy leads to long-term survival in 70% to 90% of patients. Adverse prognostic factors include advanced stage, BM and CNS involvement, large tumor size (>10 cm), and high serum LDH.

DIFFUSE LARGE B CELL LYMPHOMA

This is a diverse category of neoplasms characterized by large B cells. Although the marrow may be completely replaced, even when there is only focal involvement. The term DLBCL is used to reflect the underlying pattern in tissue. DLBCL may involve the BM secondarily or, rarely, may represent primary, *de novo* disease, typically associated with lytic bone lesions.[13]

Epidemiology

This represents about 25% to 35% of NHLs and usually affects elderly people (median age in the seventh decade), but may be seen in younger patients. The exact etiology of the disease is unknown, although immunodeficiency has been identified as a factor.

Presentation

DLBCL can present as nodal (60%) or extranodal (40%) disease. B symptoms may be present; other symptoms depend on the site of involvement. Over half are advanced stage (III/IV) at diagnosis, but involvement of the BM is relatively uncommon and PB involvement is rare.

Morphology

The cells are large, with irregular nuclei, vesicular chromatin, and variably prominent nucleoli (Figure 8.20A and B). Because DLBCL cells may resemble immature marrow precursors, diagnosis requires immunophenotypic confirmation.

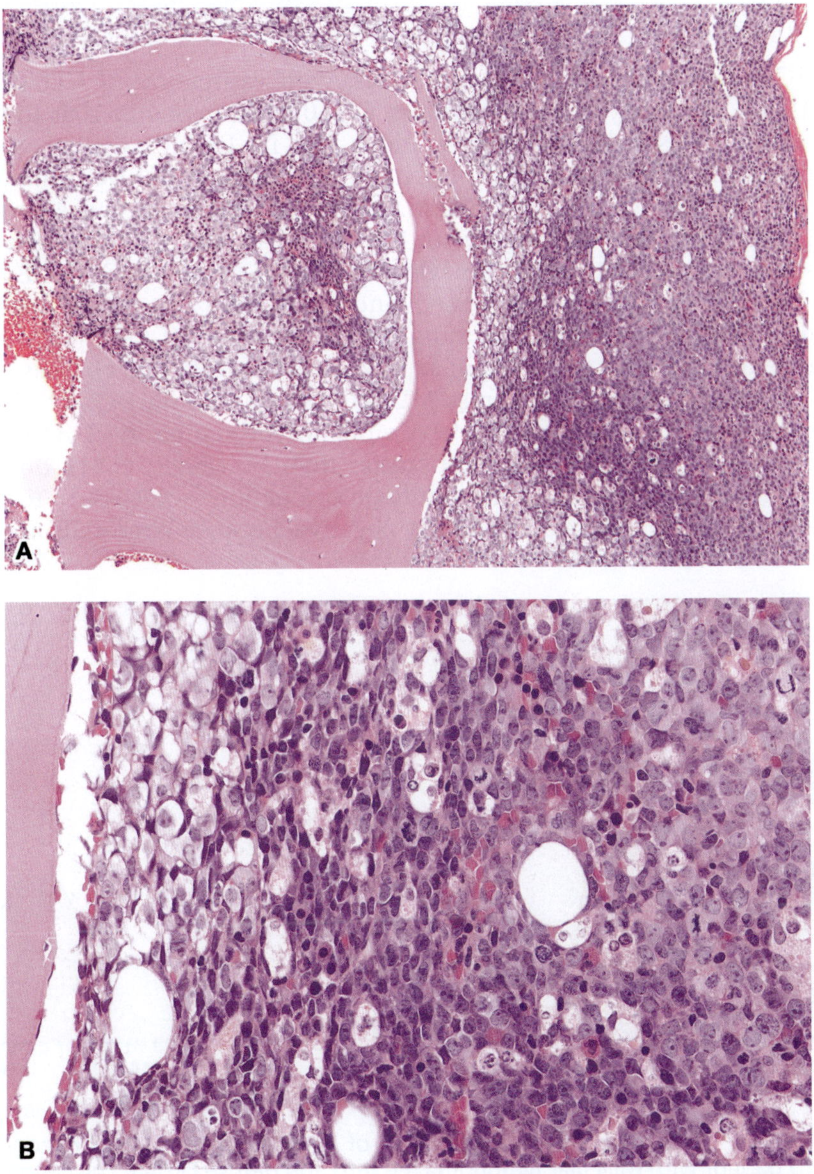

FIGURE 8.20 **Diffuse large B cell lymphoma in a patient with human immunodeficiency virus infection.** A, A low-power view of a bone marrow extensively replaced by sheets of large cells. B, High-power view of the same case showing large cells with abundant, sometimes vacuolated cytoplasm and prominent nucleoli.

Patients with DLBCL in tissues may have discordant or concordant BM histology: Low-grade lymphoma in the BM represents discordant morphology, and DLBCL in the BM represents concordant histology. Routine BM staging is often not performed in patients diagnosed with DLBCL, especially if fluorodeoxyglucose (FDG)-positron emission tomography (PET) imaging does not show evidence of marrow involvement.

Immunophenotype

DLBCLs are mature B cell lymphomas, with expression of CD20 and CD19, and a variety of other markers. CD30 is expressed in 10% to 20% of cases and has therapeutic implications. ISH for EBER is often positive, especially in cases with underlying immunodeficiency. DLBCLs may express CD5 (5%-10% of cases). These tend to be *de novo* and have a worse prognosis. They may express Cyclin D1, but these lack the *CCND1* translocations and SOX11 expression. Other markers, including CD10, BCL6, and MUM1, are variably expressed, and are the most common markers used as a surrogate for determining the cell of origin (COO) (see later). In general, cells with a GC origin express CD10 and BCL6, whereas post-GC cases lack CD10 and express MUM1 with or without BCL6.[14] Those cases with a GC origin typically have a phenotype similar to FL. DLBCLs tend to have higher forward light scatter than FL (Figure 8.21), but this is not always the case, and morphologic evaluation is necessary to confirm the diagnosis. FC may be falsely negative, because large cells are not recovered well.

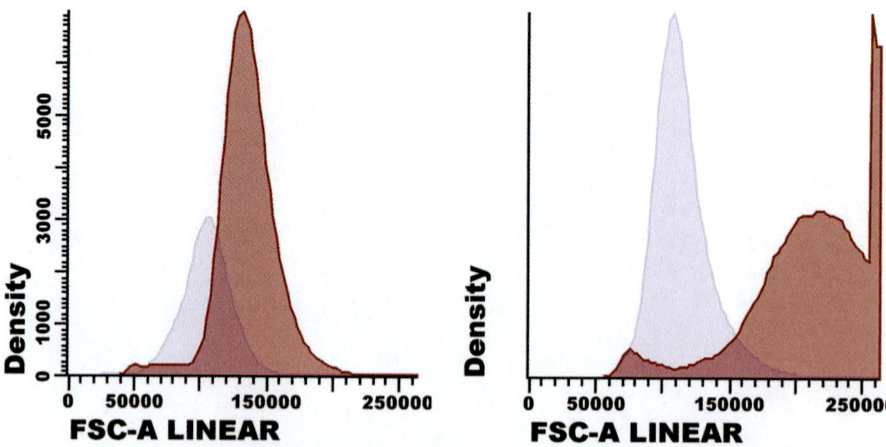

FIGURE 8.21 **Flow cytometric comparison of forward scatter (FSC) histograms from a patient with follicular lymphoma (FL, left) and diffuse large B cell lymphoma (DLBCL, right).** The FSC of the tumor is shown in brown and that of background T cells in blue. Germinal center–type DLBCL and FL can have the same flow immunophenotype, but FSC size can sometimes help distinguish them.

Genetics

GEP studies have uncovered two main molecular subtypes of DLBCL that reflect their COO: the GCB subtype and the Activated B cell (ABC) subtype; there is a third unclassifiable subtype, representing 10% to 15% of all DLBCL cases.[15] The GCB subtype is more common than the ABC subtype overall (60% of cases vs 40% of cases), but proportions differ in different patient populations. Historically, the ABC type has been considered to have a worse prognosis than GCB, although as therapy improves this may no longer hold.

The most common rearrangement involves *BCL6* at 3q27, and this is most often seen in the ABC subtype. Approximately 20% to 30% of cases have t(14;18) involving IGH::*BCL2*, typically in the GCB subtype. *MYC* translocations are detected in 8% to 14% of cases, seen in both subtypes, and these are associated with decreased survival. Cases of with the morphologic features of large B cell lymphoma with rearrangements of *MYC* and *BCL2* ("double-hit" lymphomas) are considered a separate diagnostic entity with worse prognosis; co-occurrence of *MYC* and *BCL6* translocations are no longer considered a separate entity in the most current classifications, because their prognosis does not seem as poor.

Mutations in DLBCL also vary based on the COO subtype. GCB DLBCLs have mutations in *EZH2* and *GNA13*, whereas ABC DLBCLs have mutations in *CARD11*, *MYD88*, and *CD79B*.

Prognosis

Patients treated with a CHOP regimen plus rituximab have a 5-year progression-free survival (PFS) of 60% and OS of 65%. With conventional therapy the ABC type had a worse prognosis than GCB, although as therapy improves this may no longer hold. The addition of bortezomib, lenalidomide, and ibrutinib to R-CHOP is beneficial to ABC subtypes. Clinically important prognostic factors include patient age and stage of disease, and to a lesser extent the tumor size, the sex of the patient, vitamin D deficiency, body mass index (BMI), the presence or absence of serum light chains and IgM paraprotein, lymphocyte and monocyte counts, and histology (concordant vs discordant). BM involvement by DLBCL predicts an increased risk of CNS relapse and is used in some institutions as a threshold to begin CNS prophylaxis.

Intravascular DLBCL is a rare systemic lymphoma that is detectable in the BM vessels (Figure 8.22A-C). Other subtypes of DLBCL may also be seen in the BM, albeit in low frequencies.

REVIEW OF INTERSTITIAL OR DIFFUSE B CELL INFILTRATES

- B cell neoplasms with a diffuse pattern include HCL, BL, and DLBCL. HCL additionally involves the spleen, whereas BL and DLBCL can involve any site.

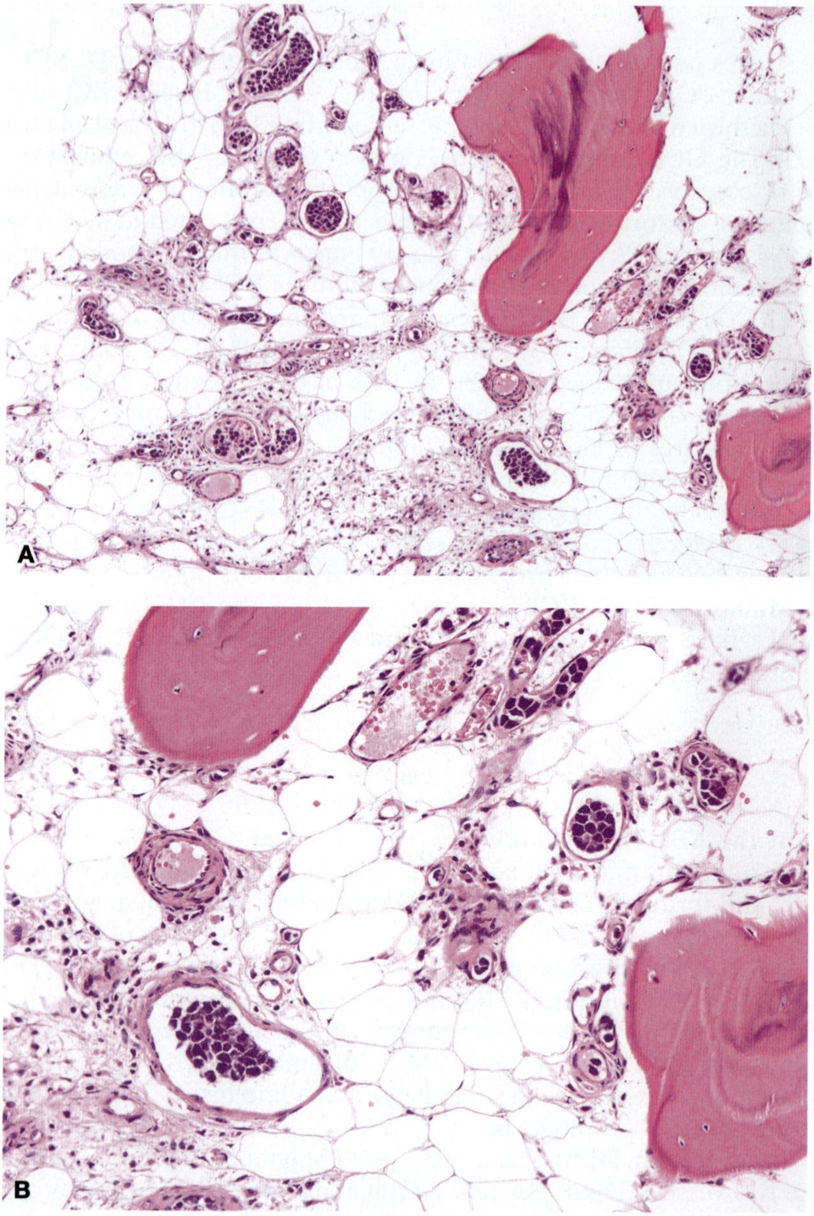

FIGURE 8.22 **A bone marrow involved by intravascular diffuse large B cell lymphoma.** A, Low-power view shows the distinct clusters of abnormal cells confined to vascular spaces. B, The same case at higher power shows the large cells with hyperchromatic irregular nuclei and a small amount of cytoplasm; these can appear loosely cohesive. C, An immunohistochemical stain for CD20 identifies these as B cells.

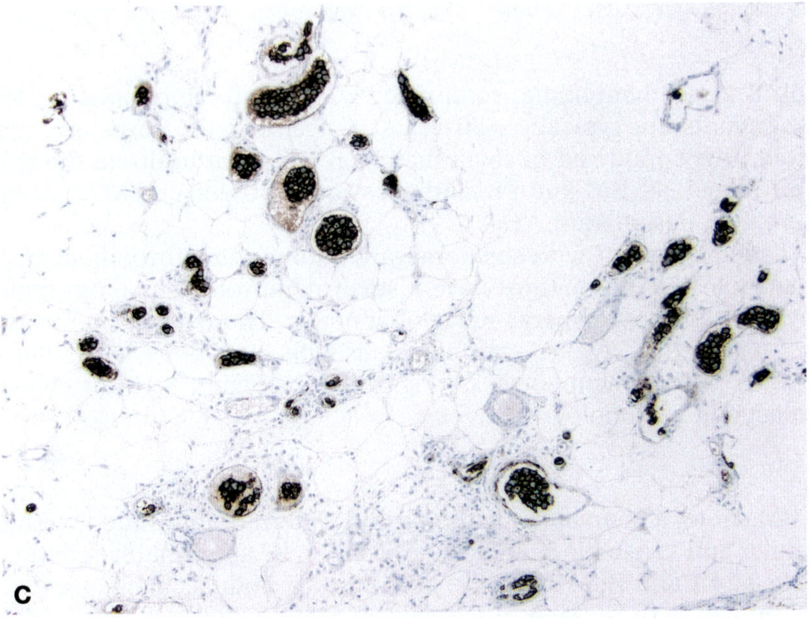

FIGURE 8.22 *(continued)*

- HCL and BL have characteristic phenotypic findings.
- By FC, HCL typically expresses bright CD20 and CD11c, as well as CD103, CD25, and CD200. By IHC, useful markers include Annexin, Cyclin D1, CD123, and BRAF. BL expresses CD10 and c-MYC and lacks BCL2.
- DLBCLs have a variety of immunophenotypes. FC plays a limited role in diagnosis because large cells may be lost, although forward scatter assessment may be helpful if cells are present.

B CELL LYMPHOMAS WITH MIXED OR OTHER PATTERNS OF INFILTRATION

Many lymphomas can show combined patterns of infiltration including a mixture of nodular and diffuse or interstitial involvement. CLL/SLL in particular may show this mixed pattern. Some lymphomas also show a distinctive sinusoidal pattern. In this pattern, abnormal cells are interspersed in sinusoids, often in linear aggregates of single-file cells. This may be subtle, and IHC is needed to help identify the abnormal population on tissue sections. The sinusoidal pattern may be predominant or even exclusive, or admixed with a nodular pattern.

SPLENIC MARGINAL ZONE LYMPHOMA

Epidemiology and Presentation

SMZL is a rare lymphoma, comprising <2% of all lymphomatous leukemias. Patients are typically >50 years of age, and the sexes are equally affected. It is comprised of small mature B cells that infiltrate the spleen, splenic hilar LNs, BM and PB, and occasionally the liver. SMZL does not present with peripheral LAD.[16]

Patients present with splenomegaly, autoimmune thrombocytopenia, and anemia. Up to one-third have a small paraproteinemia, but typically no hyperviscosity or hypergammaglobulinemia. There may be a lymphocytosis comprised of atypical lymphoid cells with short polar or bipolar villi, known as "villous lymphocytes" (Figure 8.23; eFigure 8.16) or cells with plasmacytoid morphology.

Morphology

The BM shows a characteristic dimorphic pattern of infiltration, with both a nodular and single-file sinusoidal infiltration by abnormal lymphoid cells (Figure 8.24A and B; eFigure8. 17). Within the nodules, there are two cell types similar to those seen in the spleen: Small lymphoid cells and large, marginal zone-like lymphoid cells. This infiltrate may be subtle, and IHC is very helpful in the diagnosis (Figure 8.25; eFigure 8.18).

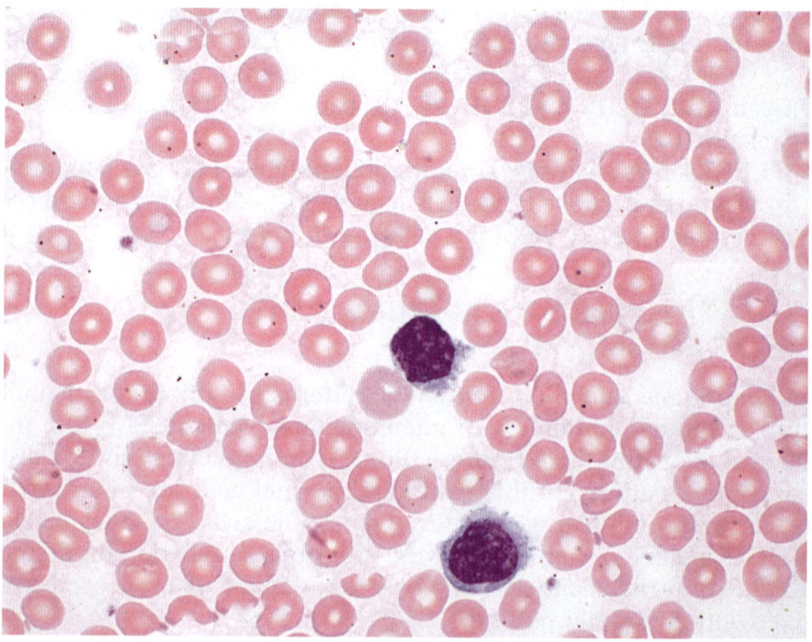

FIGURE 8.23 **Peripheral blood in a patient with splenic marginal zone lymphoma.** This lesion was originally described as "splenic lymphoma with villous lymphocytes" because the atypical cells have short polar villi or projections.

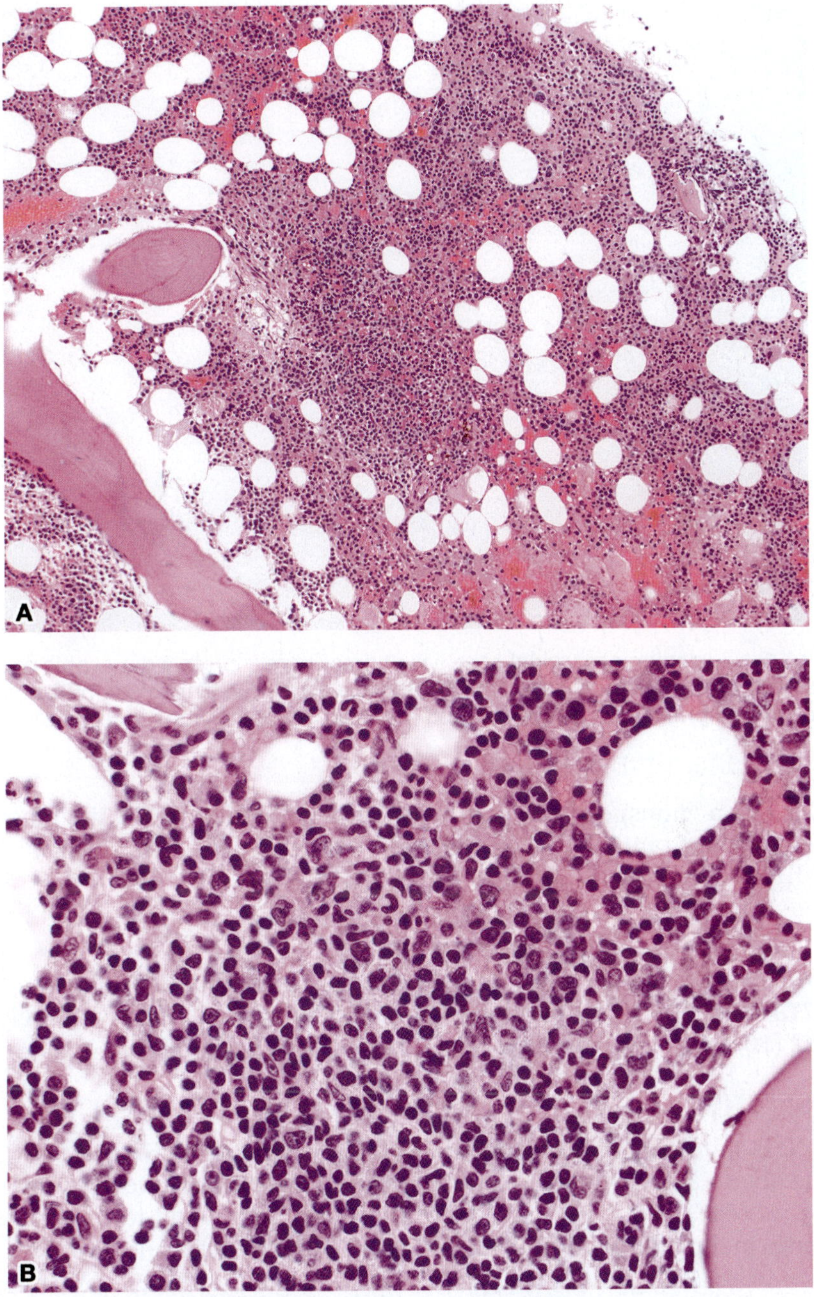

FIGURE 8.24 **Splenic marginal zone lymphoma (SMZL) in the bone marrow.** A, Low-power view showing a somewhat vague nonparatrabecular lymphoid aggregate. B, High-power view showing mostly small mature atypical lymphoid cells with round to irregular nuclei and rare larger lymphoid cells.

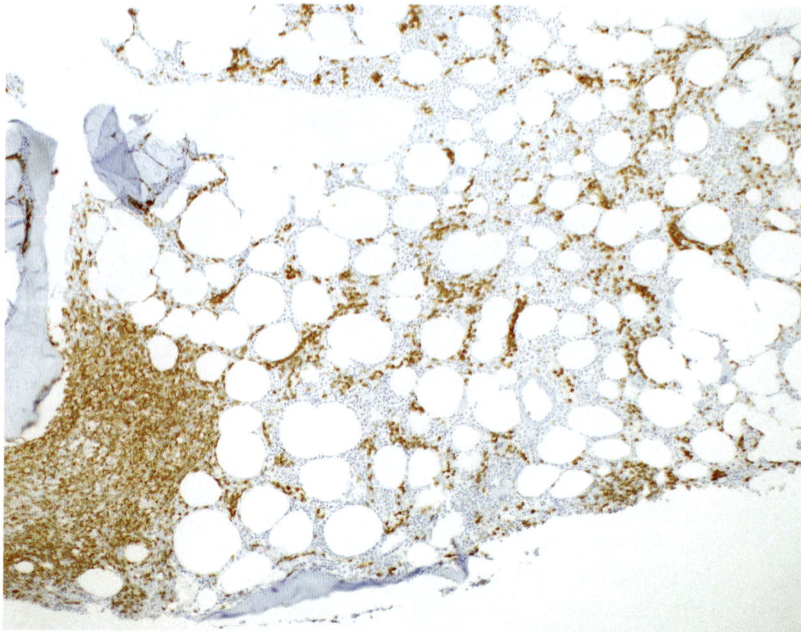

FIGURE 8.25 In splenic marginal zone lymphoma there is often a dimorphic pattern of infiltration, comprising both a nodular and a single-file sinusoidal infiltration of abnormal lymphoid cells, as highlighted here by CD20 immunohistochemical stain.

Immunophenotype

SMZL has a “nonspecific” phenotype, with expression of CD20 and other B cell markers, and a lack of CD5, CD10, CD200, CD103, Annexin A1, and BRAF.

Genetics

Approximately 30% have heterogeneous deletion chromosome 7q. *NOTCH2* is most often mutated (10%-25% of cases) followed closely by *KLF2* (10%-40%). Both mutations are associated with del(7q).

Prognosis

SMZL is indolent, with a 10-year survival probability of 67% to 95%. Patients obtain a hematologic response with rituximab treatment or splenectomy. About 10% to 15% will transform to a high-grade lesion. Adverse findings include large tumors and *NOTCH2* expression, among others.

Splenic diffuse red pulp small B cell lymphoma (SDRPL)

Splenic diffuse red pulp small B cell lymphoma (SDRPL) is a less common neoplasm that has a similar pattern of BM involvement as SMZL. It cannot be definitively distinguished from SMZL without splenic histology, although there may be differences in the mutational profile. As noted earlier, HCL-v can also be histologically similar in the BM although its FC immunophenotype is different.

LYMPHOPLASMACYTIC LYMPHOMA (LPL)

Lymphoplasmacytic lymphoma (LPL) is a mature B cell neoplasm comprised of a mixture of small B cells, B cells with plasmacytic differentiation, and plasma cells. LPL infiltrates the BM and PB and may or may not involve the spleen and peripheral LNs.[17]

Waldenström macroglobulinemia (WM) is LPL with BM involvement and an IgM monoclonal gammopathy or IgM paraprotein of any concentration. Although many patients with LPL meet the criteria for WM, these terms are not synonymous, although they may occasionally be used interchangeably.[18] Some patients with LPL lack paraproteins or have a non-IgM paraprotein; minor subsets have both IgM and IgG paraproteins. Likewise, the presence of a lymphoma with IgM gammopathy is not diagnostic of LPL, as it occurs in other lymphoid neoplasms like marginal zone lymphomas and CLL/SLL.

The diagnosis of LPL requires the exclusion of all other small B cell lymphomas with specific features, but it may be difficult to differentiate LPL from other lymphomas, so that some cases can only be diagnosed as "small B cell lymphoma with plasmacytic features," especially when molecular information is not available.

Epidemiology and Presentation

LPL is diagnosed most commonly in elderly patients and has a male predominance. In some reports, LPL has been associated with hepatitis C and Type II cryoglobulinemia. Immune stimulation leading to increased lymphoplasmacytic proliferations may increase the risk of LPL. However, the lymphoplasmacytic proliferation, even if clonal, may not be progressive and can regress after antiviral treatment.

Presentation

Patients present with weakness, fatigue, and anemia caused by BM infiltration.

Approximately 30% of patients have symptoms of PB hyperviscosity, which may arise for a number of reasons. The IgM paraprotein may act as an autoantibody, leading to autoimmune phenomenon and sequela, or may act as a cryoglobulin, causing cryoglobulinemia in up to 20% of patients. Coagulopathies may result from the IgM-binding clotting factors interacting with platelets and fibrin.

The IgM paraprotein interacts with antigens on the myelin sheath surrounding nerves and patients may present with peripheral neuropathies. Rarely, LPL involves the CNS, a phenomenon known as "Bing-Neel syndrome."

LPL often involves the PB, but the WBC count is usually lower than in CLL/SLL. A clonal cytotoxic T cell population can also sometimes be detected in the PB.

Morphology

Morphologic features of LPL in the BM include a nodular and interstitial infiltrate (Figure 8.26A; eFigure 8.19). Occasionally, the infiltrate may

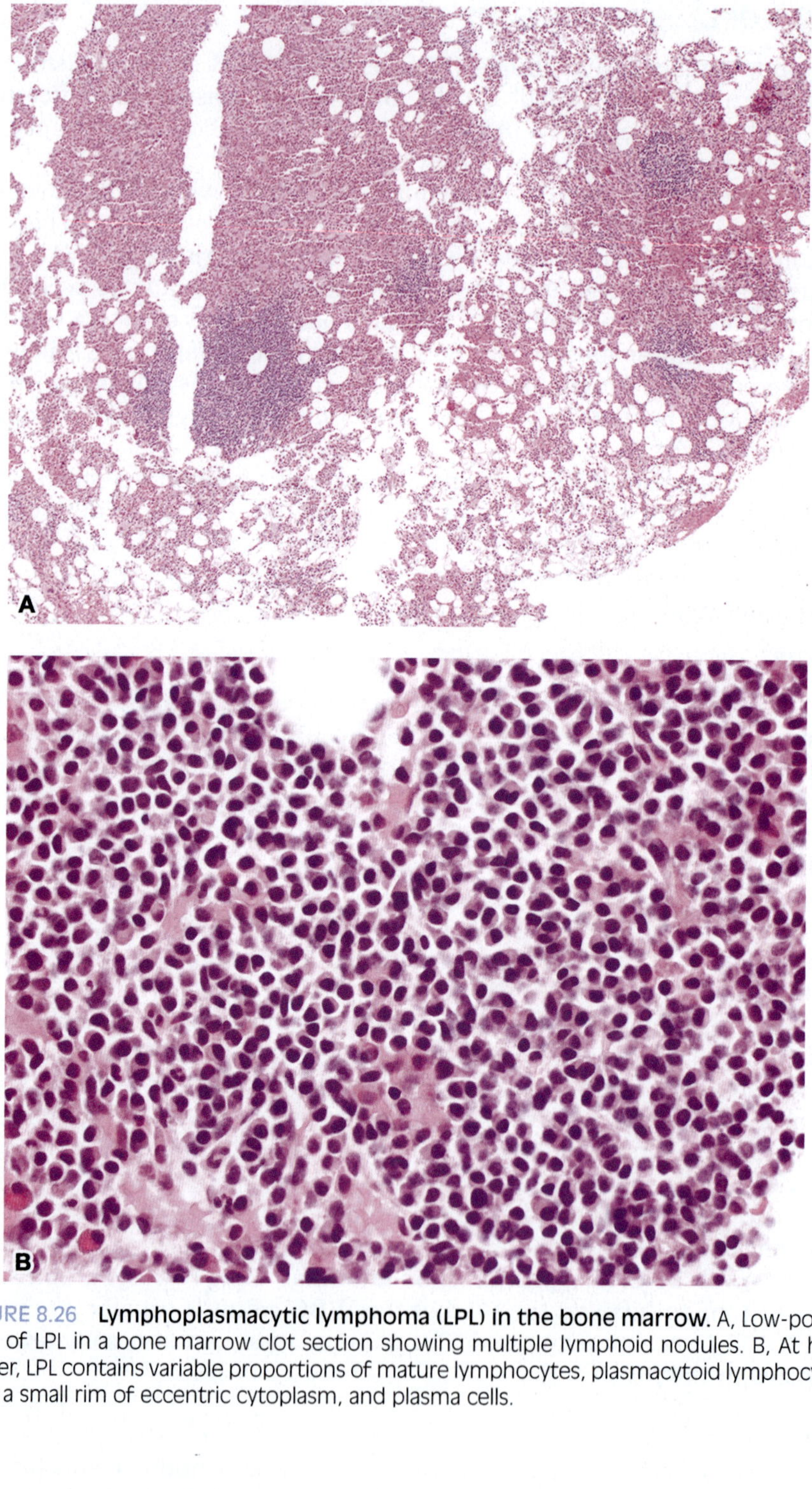

FIGURE 8.26 **Lymphoplasmacytic lymphoma (LPL) in the bone marrow.** A, Low-power view of LPL in a bone marrow clot section showing multiple lymphoid nodules. B, At high power, LPL contains variable proportions of mature lymphocytes, plasmacytoid lymphocytes with a small rim of eccentric cytoplasm, and plasma cells.

be paratrabecular, which raises FL in the differential diagnosis. The infiltrate is comprised of lymphoid cells with admixed plasmacytoid cells and plasma cells (Figure 8.26B). Mast cells may also be increased (eFigure 20). Plasma cells, which may be numerous, can cluster away from the other lymphoid cells and may be confused with a plasma cell neoplasm (PCN). Interestingly, this may be the only population remaining after treatment.

Immunophenotype

The abnormal B cells are positive for CD20 and CD38 and variable CD23. A minority may express CD5 or CD10, but this is uncommon (eFigure 8.21). In addition to the abnormal lymphoid population, an accompanying monoclonal plasma cell population with the same light chain restriction as the lymphoid population is detectable in LPL (Figure 8.27A-C). The plasma cells in LPL are positive for CD38, CD19, and CD45; the latter two are often negative in PCM. CD138 is typically positive but may be lost. Compared with normal plasma cells, or the plasma cells seen in MZL with plasmacytic differentiation they are more likely to be MUM1-negative and PAX5-positive.

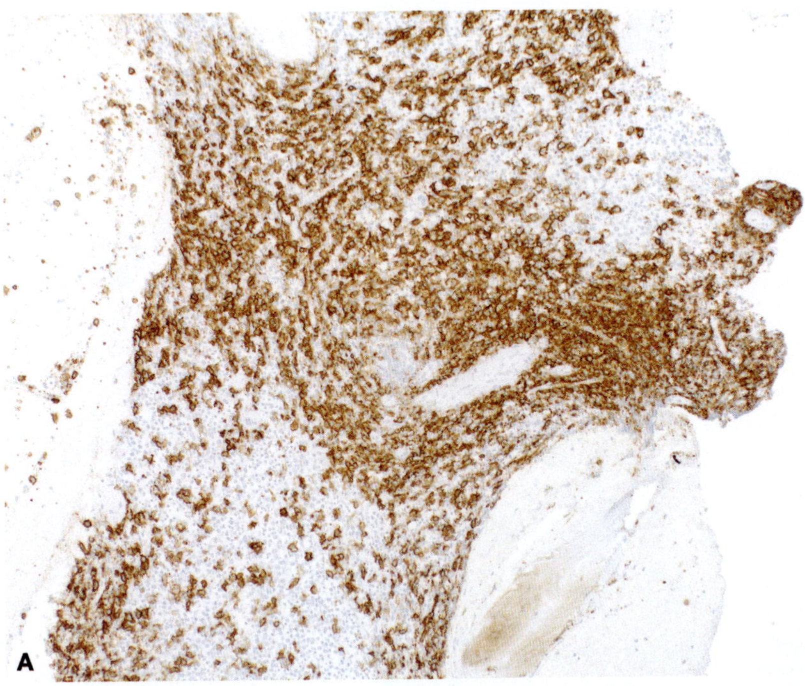

FIGURE 8.27 **Immunohistochemical stains of lymphoplasmacytic lymphoma.** A, CD20 stains B cells in the aggregate and extending into marrow space. B, CD138 stains smaller numbers of admixed plasma cells. C, The plasma cells are positive for IgM.

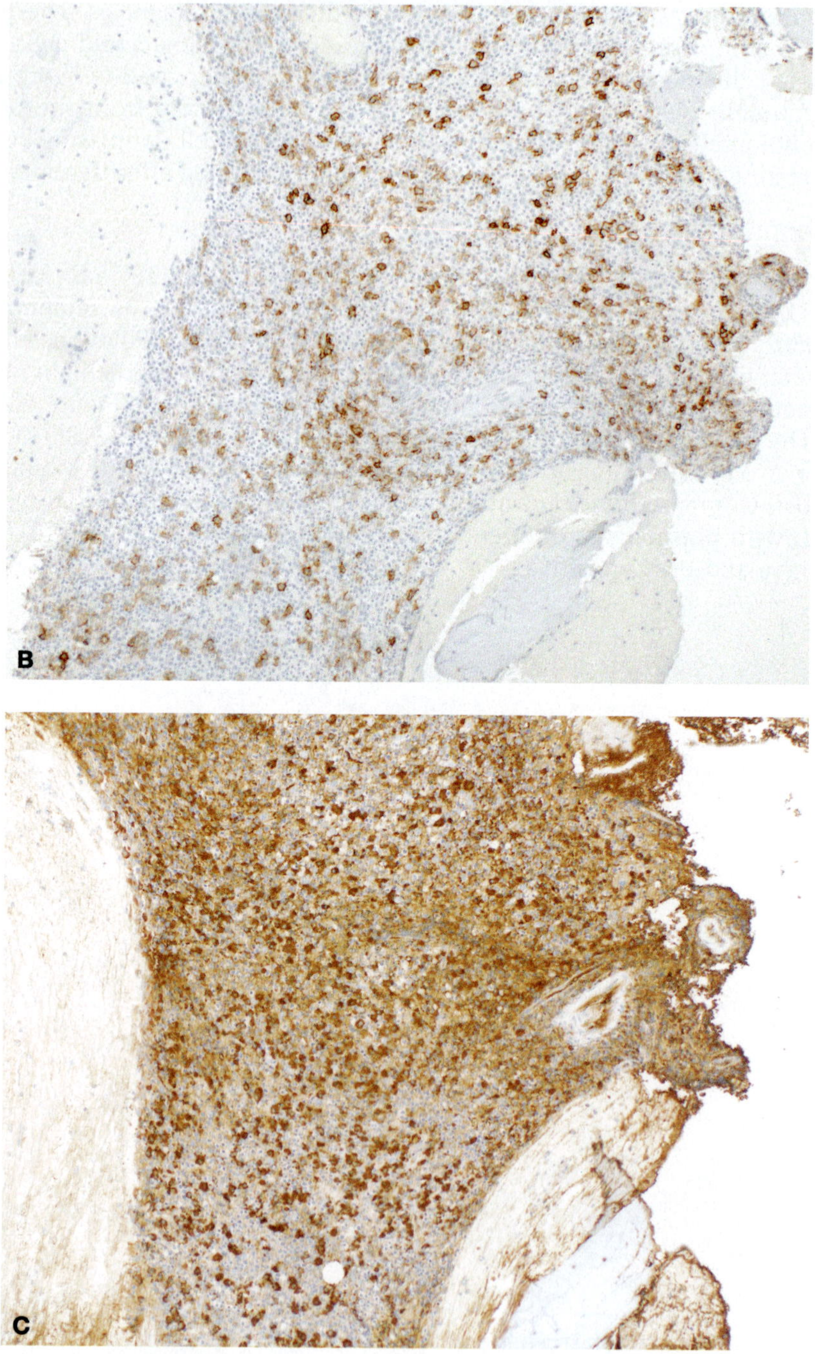

FIGURE 8.27 (*continued*)

Genetics

More than 90% of LPL cases have *MYD88* mutations. However, *MYD88* mutations can also be seen in other lymphomas, including other small B cell lymphomas, non-GCB DLBCL, primary cutaneous DLBCL leg type, primary CNS DLBCL, and testicular DLBCL. Up to 30% of LPLs also have truncating *CXCR4* mutations. Mutations in other genes including *ARIDIA*, *TP53*, *MT2D*, and *CD79a* lead to decreased NF-κB signaling. Although there are no specific chromosomal abnormalities, trisomy 4 and del(6q) are found in 20% and 50% of cases, respectively.

Prognosis

LPL is generally indolent with a 5- to 10-year survival. Adverse features include advanced age, cytopenias, poor performance status, and increased serum β2 microglobulinemia. The International Scoring System also includes increased serum paraprotein (>70 g/dL) as a risk factor.

MYD88 mutation–negative cases have a worse prognosis than typical LPL and a lower response to ibrutinib. Transformation to a large cell lymphoma can occur and portends a poor prognosis.

REVIEW OF MIXED OR OTHER INFILTRATION PATTERNS

- Many of these, with the exception of CLL/SLL, have nonspecific phenotypes (CD5−, CD10−).
- HCL-v, SDRPL, and SMZL can show an intrasinusoidal pattern. SMZL also typically shows nodules scattered throughout the marrow, although definitive distinction among these cannot be done by BM histology alone. HCL-v is similar to HCL in many ways but has a different phenotype and lacks *BRAF* mutations (Table 8.4).
- Lymphomas with plasmacytic differentiation include LPL, PCNs, and MZL.
- LPL does not have a definitively diagnostic phenotype, although it can be suspected if clonal IgM plasma cells are present in addition to B cells; molecular testing for the *MYD88* mutation in a histologically compatible case can be considered diagnostic.

TABLE 8.4 Other CD5-Negative, CD10-Negative B Cell Malignancies

Neoplasm	Size	CD20	CD25	CD103	CD11c	Annexin	BRAF
HCL	Small-medium	+ bright	+	+	+	+	+
HCL-v	Small-medium	+ bright	−	+	+	−	−
SMZL	Small-medium	+	+	−	+	−	−

HCL, hairy cell leukemia; HCL-v, HCL variant; SMZL, splenic marginal zone lymphoma.

SINGLE CELL B CELL INFILTRATION IN AN INFLAMMATORY BACKGROUND

This pattern is most often seen in lymphomas with large cells, including T cell/histiocyte-rich large B cell lymphoma (TCHRLBL) and CHL. Rare scattered large cells are present in the interstitium, usually within a background of histiocytes or inflammatory cells, forming a recognizable lesion, often associated with fibrosis. DLBCL can also rarely present with isolated or small groups of large cells.

FC has a limited role in this category of neoplasms because neoplastic cells are so rare, and often fragile.

T CELL HISTIOCYTE-RICH LARGE B CELL LYMPHOMA

Epidemiology and Presentation

This is a rare subtype of lymphoma, representing <10% of all large B cell lymphomas, primarily affecting middle-aged patients.[19] Fever, malaise, and HSM are common symptoms. Patients may also present with cytopenias, which suggests BM involvement.

TCHRLBCL may arise *de novo* or from nodular lymphocyte–predominant (NLP) Hodgkin lymphoma. Unlike NLP, which is usually localized, TCHRLBCL is systemic, involving multiple LNs as well as the BM and other tissues. There is a much higher frequency of BM involvement in TCHRLBCL than other types of DLBCL.

Morphology

Tissue evaluation shows very few abnormal large B cells in a background of histiocytes and T cells (Figure 8.28A and B; eFigure 8.22). Unlike NLP there is no significant small B cell component in the background, and the large cells may be difficult to identify without the aid of IHC.

Immunophenotype

The large B cells express CD20 and often CD10 and BCL6 (Figure 8.29A-C; eFigure 8.23). These cells are so few that they are not identified by FC, but rather require morphologic evaluation for diagnosis. The background T cells and histiocytes have unremarkable phenotypes.

Genetics

These neoplasms have clonally rearranged Ig genes and show abundant somatic hypermutation. There are no known recurrent karyotypic abnormalities.

Prognosis

This is an aggressive disease. Half of all cases are advanced at diagnosis and have an intermediate IPI score. Patients with a diagnosis of TCHRLBL should get a staging BM biopsy.

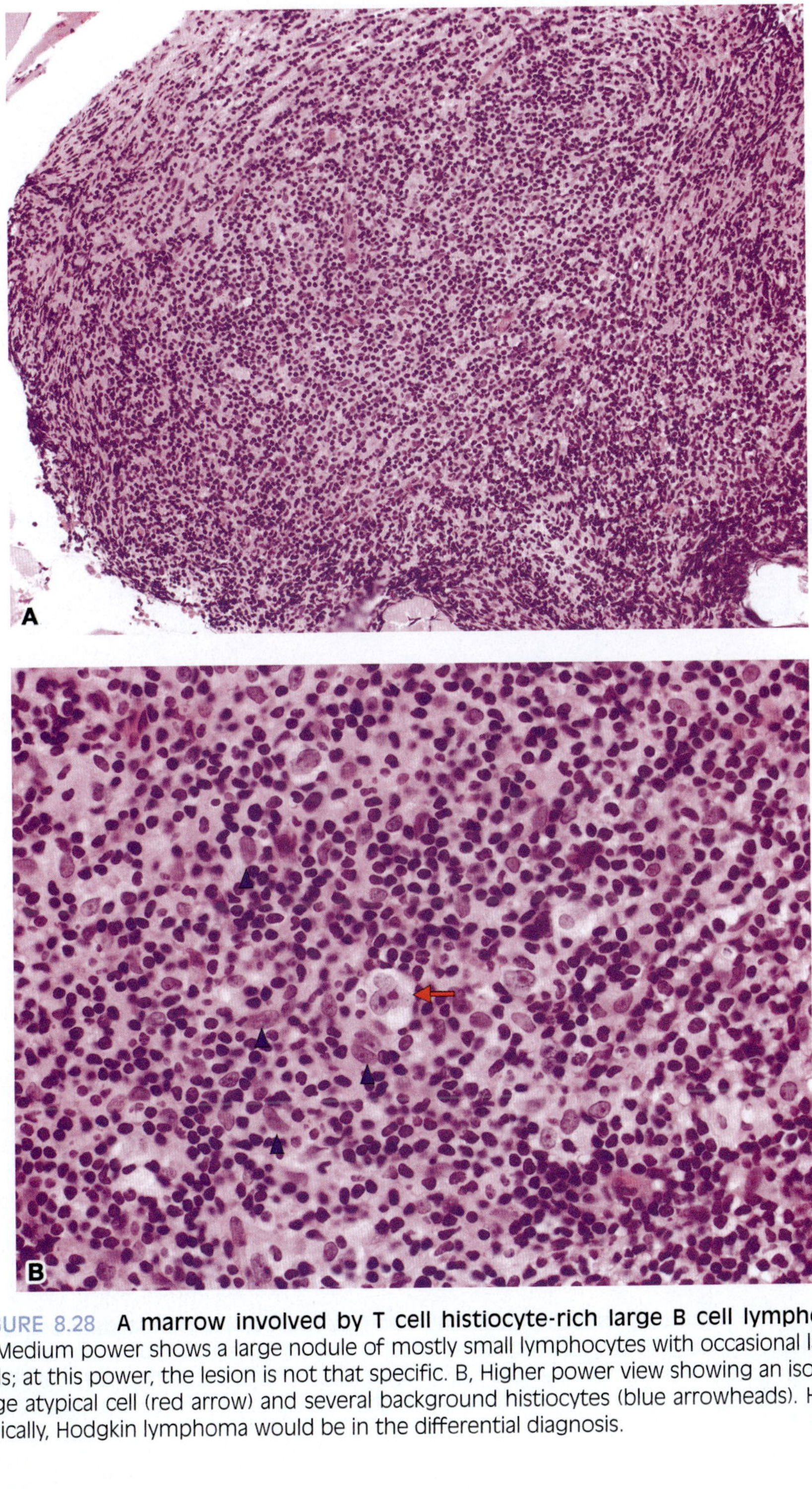

FIGURE 8.28 **A marrow involved by T cell histiocyte-rich large B cell lymphoma.** A, Medium power shows a large nodule of mostly small lymphocytes with occasional larger cells; at this power, the lesion is not that specific. B, Higher power view showing an isolated large atypical cell (red arrow) and several background histiocytes (blue arrowheads). Histologically, Hodgkin lymphoma would be in the differential diagnosis.

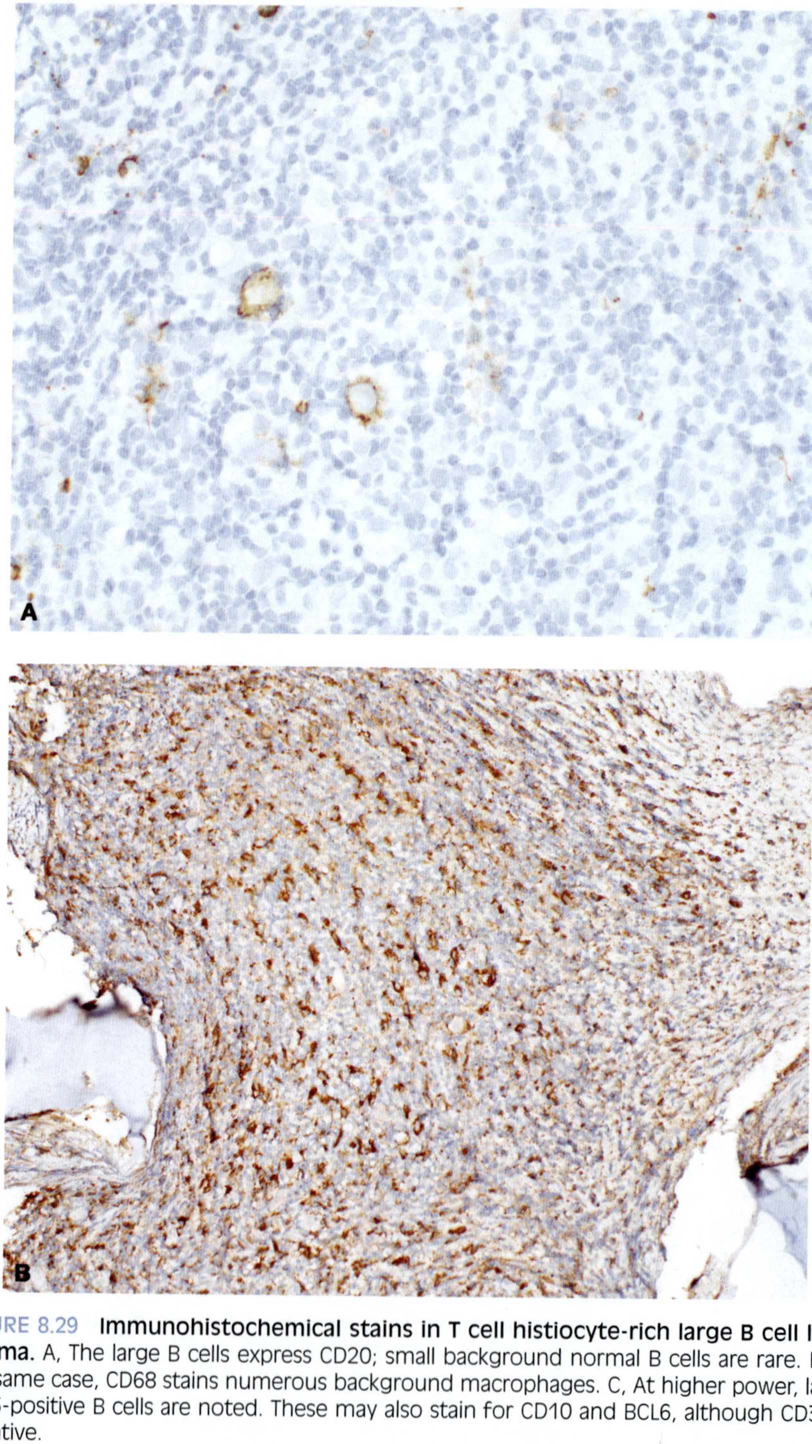

FIGURE 8.29 **Immunohistochemical stains in T cell histiocyte-rich large B cell lymphoma.** A, The large B cells express CD20; small background normal B cells are rare. B, In the same case, CD68 stains numerous background macrophages. C, At higher power, large PAX5-positive B cells are noted. These may also stain for CD10 and BCL6, although CD30 is negative.

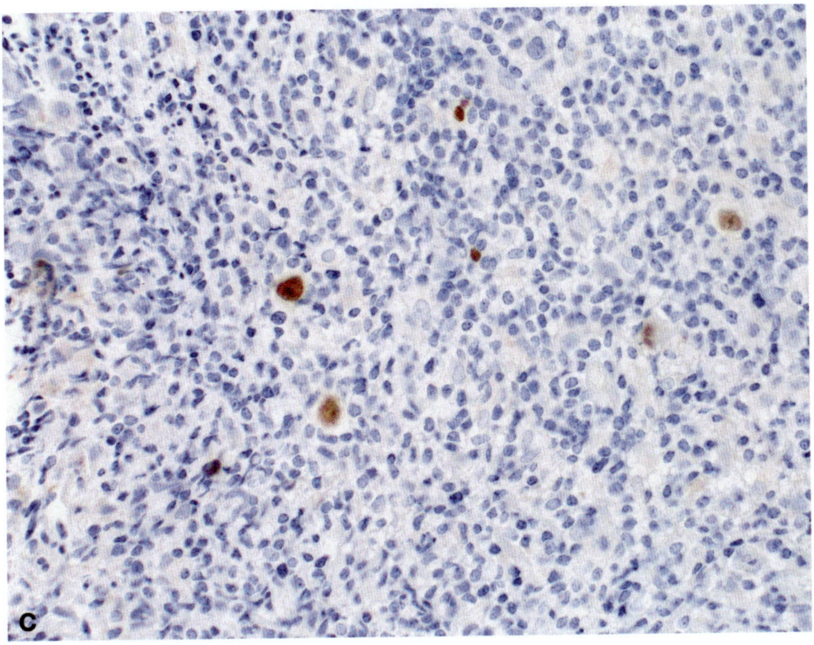

FIGURE 8.29 (*continued*)

CLASSIC HODGKIN LYMPHOMA

Hodgkin lymphomas are a unique set of diseases that typically affect LNs with a contiguous pattern of dissemination. They are also histologically unique in their cellular composition, with very few malignant Hodgkin Reed-Sternberg (HRS) cells in an inflammatory background (Figure 8.30A). Hodgkin lymphomas comprise CHL and NLP; in this chapter, we focus on CHL, as NLP is exceedingly rare in the BM.

Epidemiology and Presentation

Most patients with CHL present with nodal disease, especially cervical, mediastinal, axillary, and para-aortic. BM involvement is rare (5%).[20] The most common subtype of CHL is nodular sclerosis (NS), followed by mixed cellularity (MC), lymphocyte rich (LR), and lymphocyte depleted (LD). Each of these has varying degrees of association with EBV, as well as propensity for BM involvement. MC has the highest association with EBV (75% of cases), especially in patients with HIV, and shows BM involvement in 10% of cases. LD, the rarest subtype of CHL, is often found in retroperitoneal LNs, abdominal organs, and BM.

Morphology

The malignant cell in CHL is the Hodgkin or Reed-Sternberg cell. Hodgkin cells are large cells with a single nucleus and macronucleoli, and

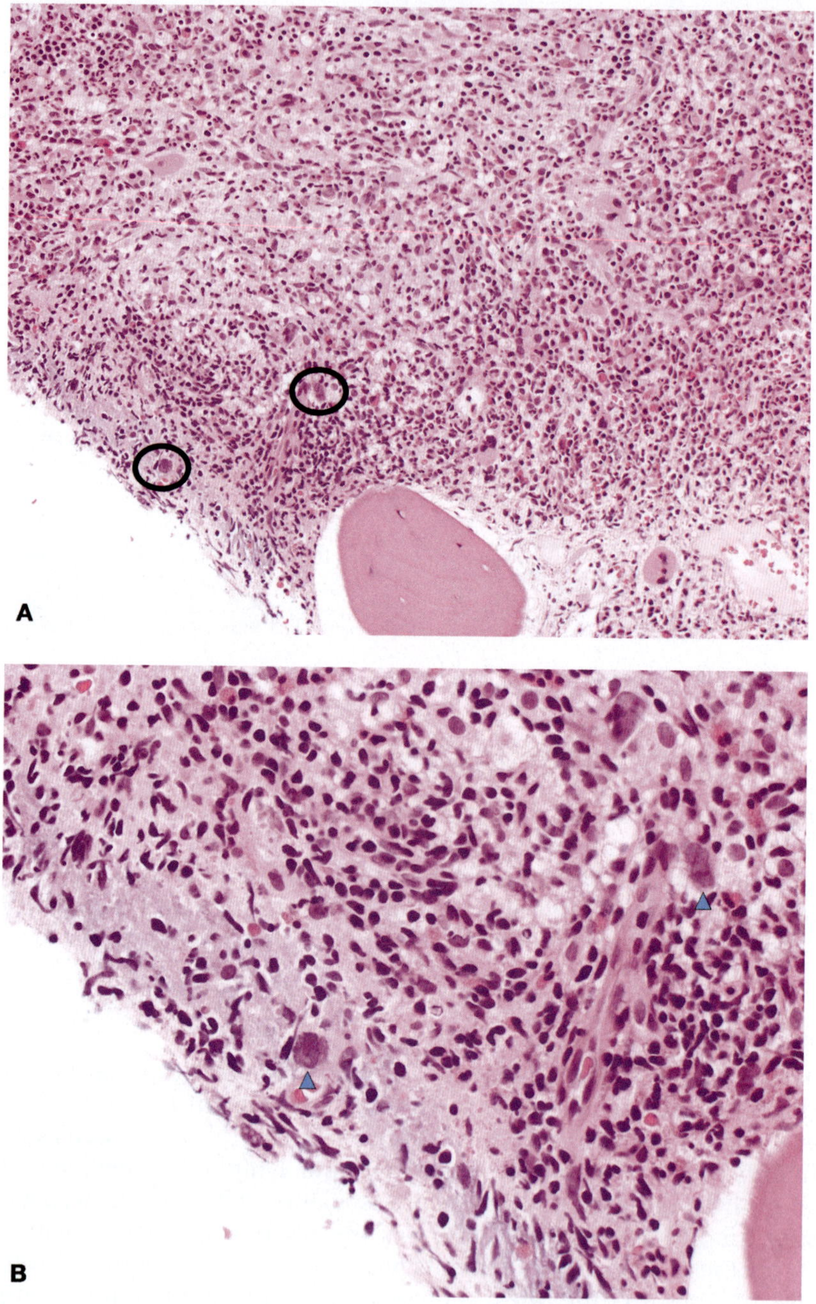

FIGURE 8.30 **Bone marrow involved by classic Hodgkin lymphoma (CHL).** A, On hematoxylin and eosin, the lesion is loosely fibrotic and consists of a mixture of small lymphocytes, eosinophils, plasma cells, and histiocytes, with occasional Hodgkin cells (circled). B, At higher power, the large atypical Hodgkin cells can be seen (blue arrowheads).

Reed-Sternberg cells are large, multinucleated cells with multiple large nucleoli (Figure 8.30B; eFigure 8.24). As they commonly are found together, they are often referred to as HRS cells. The HRS cells are scattered, usually singly or in small clusters, within an inflammatory infiltrate, comprised of lymphocytes, plasma cells, histiocytes, and eosinophils (eFigure 8.25). In the BM, HRS cells may be difficult to identify by H&E alone. Occasionally, granulomas may be seen in conjunction with CHL, and this may be a useful diagnostic clue, although granulomas by themselves are not diagnostic of marrow involvement in patients with known CHL.

Immunophenotype

The HRS cells are positive for CD30, MUM1, and dim PAX5 and are variably positive for CD15 (Figure 8.31; eFigure 26). They lack typical B cell markers, CD20 and CD79a. In tissue sections, they are typically ringed by T cells. As noted earlier, FC is not useful in BM staging of CHL.

Genetics

HRS cells have clonal Ig rearrangements in most cases, but genetic information is not generally utilized for the diagnosis of CHL.

Prognosis

Typical CHL has a relatively good prognosis. Treatment with standardized chemotherapy regimens has led to a >85% cure rate. Treatments are tailored to stage (using Ann Arbor system); BM involvement is considered advanced (stage IV) disease. Other clinical findings, such as tumor size, the presence

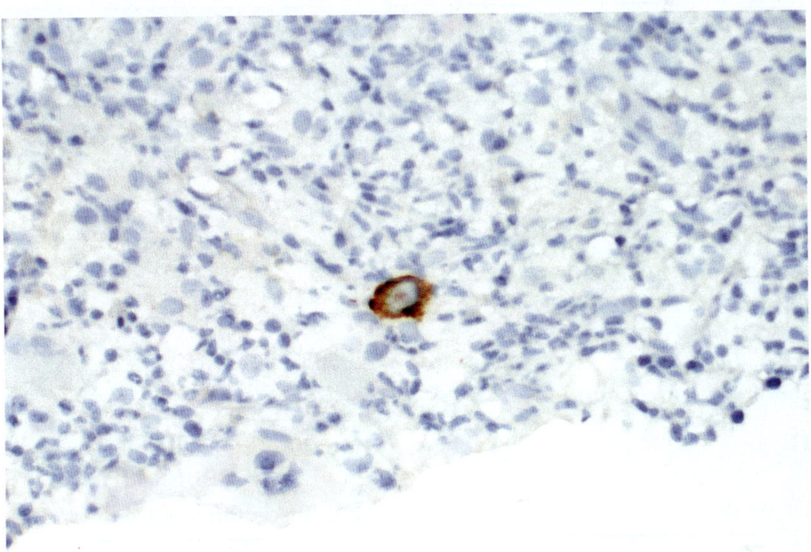

FIGURE 8.31 An immunohistochemical stain for CD30 is positive on Hodgkin cells.

or absence of extranodal disease, erythrocyte sedimentation rate (ESR), and involvement of multiple nodes may affect prognosis. Advanced stage patients are prognosticated using the IPI. FDG-PET scans after initial therapy can identify poor risk patients who require additional therapy. Novel treatments with anti-CD30 and anti-PD1 agents have shown some success.

REVIEW OF SINGLE CELL INFILTRATIONS

- TCHRLBL and CHL are not detectable by FC and require morphologic evaluation. They can be histologically similar but IHC can distinguish them.

MATURE T cell LYMPHOMAS/LEUKEMIAS

Mature T cell leukemias/lymphomas are designated "peripheral," because, unlike lymphoblasts of T cell ALL (T-ALL), they do not arise from the central thymic compartment. These neoplasms are much rarer than mature B cell neoplasms and tend to be more aggressive, with a few exceptions.

Classification of T cell Neoplasms

There are >30 different types of mature T cell neoplasms, only a subset of which involve the BM. Among those that do, many cannot be classified based only on marrow findings. This chapter focuses on six T cell malignancies that involve the BM (Table 8.5), some of which always or nearly always involve the bone, although PB and other sites are often involved. For the remaining types, marrow involvement is secondary, usually from nodal disease.

TABLE 8.5 **T cell Leukemia/Lymphoma Bone Marrow Involvement**

Bone marrow involvement	Pattern of infiltration	Phenotype
Primary involvement		
T-PLL	Diffuse	CD4+/CD8− (60%); CD4+/CD8+ (25%)
HSTCL	Sinusoidal	Cytotoxic γδ
Often Primary involvement		
ATLL	Diffuse	CD4+,CD7−,+/− CD25
T-LGL	Sinusoidal + Nodules	Cytotoxic αβ
Secondary involvement		
AITL	Focal clusters or diffuse	Follicular T helper; EBER-ISH
PTCL-NOS	Focal clusters or diffuse	Often CD4, αβ

AITL, angioimmunoblastic T cell lymphoma; ATLL, adult T cell leukemia/lymphoma; EBER, Epstein-Barr encoding region; HSTCL, hepatosplenic T cell lymphoma; ISH, in situ hybridization; LGL, large granular lymphocytic leukemia; PTCL-NOS, peripheral T cell lymphoma, not otherwise specified; T-PLL, T-prolymphocytic leukemia.

Immunophenotype

As mentioned earlier, it is rarely possible to differentiate B cell and T cell malignancies by morphology alone, especially in the marrow. FC or IHC is instrumental in determining the cellular lineage and detecting antigen aberrancy.

Unlike B cells, which can be easily assessed for light chain restriction, T cells are more complex, and assessment of clonality is less straightforward (see Chapter 3). Most often, pathologists rely on other features, including aberrant phenotypic patterns.

Nonetheless, FC is helpful in differentiating T cells from NK cells, subtyping T cells based on receptor expression, and subclassifying T cell neoplasms.

T cells express surface CD3 and pan T cell antigens at predictable levels of intensity with some normal variation in CD7 expression. CD3 is associated with a surface T cell receptor (TCR), which is either an alpha-beta (TCRαβ) or gamma-delta (TCRγδ) type. TCRαβ T cells are more prevalent than their counterpart and express either CD4 or CD8, with the former predominating in normal marrows. CD4-positive T cells are categorized as "helper" or "regulatory" T cells, whereas CD8-positive T cells are known as "cytotoxic" T cells that express cytotoxic markers like TIA1, granzyme B, and perforin. TCRγδ T cells express bright CD3, variable CD5, and lack CD4 and CD8. Intensity of expression of most markers (other than CD8) is relatively tightly regulated on T cells, so that abnormal levels of expression of a T cell antigen raises the suspicion of a T cell neoplasm. A highly skewed CD4:CD8 ratio can also be helpfu

NK cells are unique cells with innate killing abilities. Present in all lymphoid organs as well as in the GI tract and LNs, NK cells are especially abundant in the PB, comprising 10% to 20% of the total lymphocyte count. Morphologically, NK cells are large granular lymphocytes (LGLs). NK cells express bright CD7 by FC and lack surface CD3 expression, but because they express the epsilon subunit of the TCR, they are generally positive for cytoplasmic CD3 by IHC, with subsets positive by FC. NK cells also express CD56, CD16, and CD2, as well as cytotoxic markers (TIA1, granzyme B, and perforin), but are usually negative for CD5 and lack TCRαβ or TCRγδ.

Like NK cells, immature T cells express cytoplasmic, but not surface, CD3 and have characteristic phenotypes and patterns of normal maturation.

Immature NK cells have brighter CD56 expression than mature NK cells by FC. However, CD56 is an activation marker, which is not specific to NK cells.

T Cell/NK Cell clonality

Unlike B cells, T cells have a more complex pattern of TCR gene rearrangements, discussed at length in Chapter 3. In brief, FC can establish clonality by detecting restricted TCR Vβ family usage.[21] In addition, αβ T cells will express either T cell receptor beta constant (TRBC) 1 or 2, so that in analogy to surface Ig light chain, TRBC restriction can be used as a clonality metric, although to date only antibodies against TRBC1 have been produced.[22] Normal T cell populations have a variety of Vβ repertoires and a mixed population of TRBC1-positive and -negative cells.

NK cells lack a TCR, but they do express surface killer cell Ig-like receptors (KIRS), which are recognized by major histocompatibility complex (MHC) Class I receptors. There are 30 KIRS subtypes, normally heterogeneously expressed on NK cells, but only a few are routinely assessed by FC.

T cell LYMPHOMAS WITH INVARIABLE OR HIGH-FREQUENCY BM INVOLVEMENT

T cell Prolymphocytic Leukemia

Epidemiology and Presentation

This rare clonal neoplasm results in the proliferation of abnormal mature T cells in the PB and BM.[23] Patients present with very high WBC counts (>100 × 10^9 K/L), diffuse LAD, and tissue involvement at the time of diagnosis, including involvement of the PB, BM, LNs, liver, and spleen. Skin involvement is common (20%), and patients often present with cytopenias because of BM infiltration.

Morphology

The PB shows small abnormal lymphoid cells with nongranular basophilic cytoplasm, irregular nuclei, visible nucleoli, and cytoplasmic blebs (Figure 8.32). The BM shows diffuse infiltration by abnormal cells, although diagnosis cannot be made based on histology alone.

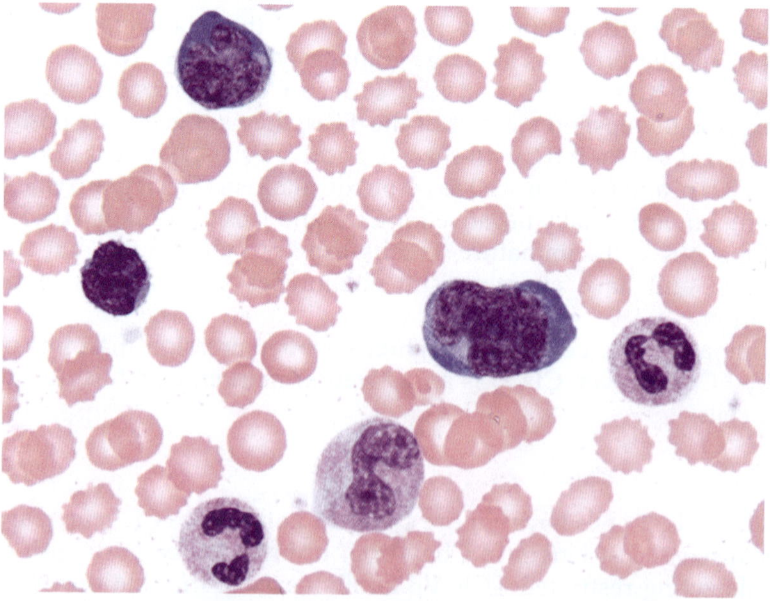

FIGURE 8.32 **The peripheral blood in a patient with T-prolymphocytic leukemia (T-PLL) showing highly atypical large lymphocytes with complex nuclear shapes and ropy chromatin.** Nucleoli are inconspicuous here but can be more prominent.

IMMUNOPHENOTYPE

The abnormal T cells express T cell markers, including CD3, CD5, and CD2. CD7 is bright, and surface CD3 may be dim or even absent in some cases (Figure 8.33). In more than half of cases, the abnormal cells express both CD4 and CD8, a phenomenon that raises a differential diagnosis of an immature T cell neoplasm. However, T-PLL lacks immature markers including Tdt and CD1a. Increased expression of CD52 is detected and may be used as a target of therapy. Cells may also overexpress the oncoprotein TCL1, which can be identified by FC or IHC.

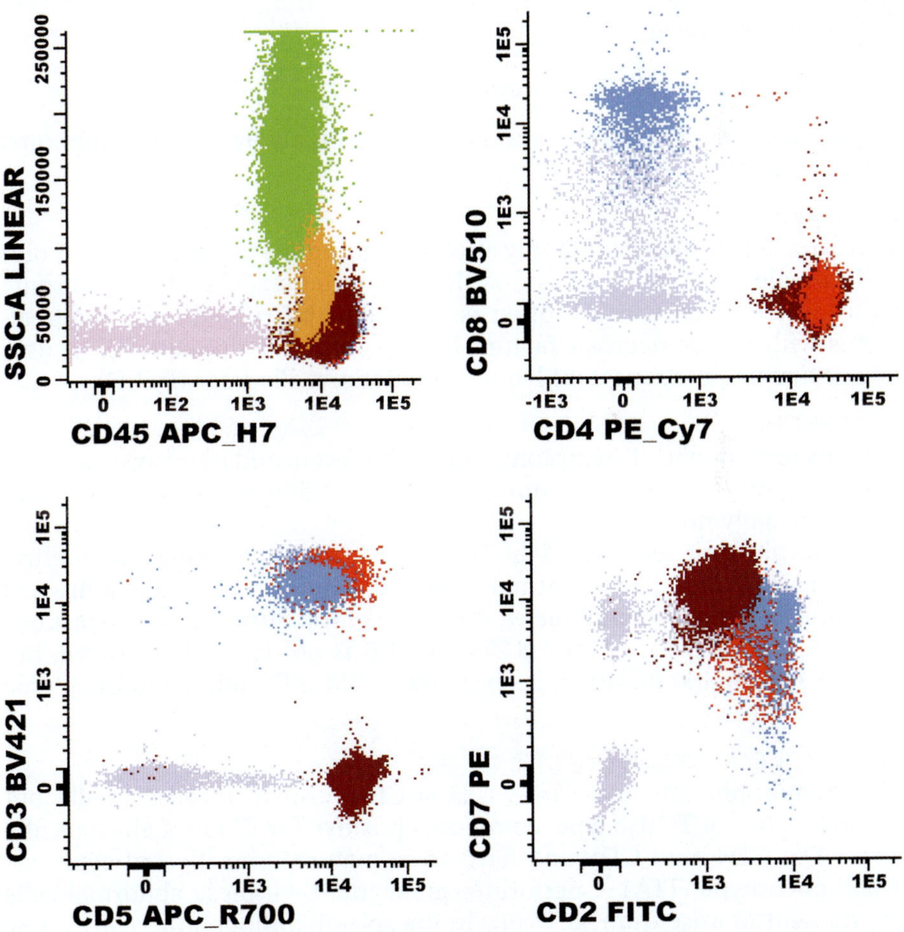

FIGURE 8.33 **Flow cytometry of T-prolymphocytic leukemia (T-PLL).** On CD45 vs side scatter (SSC; top left panel) abnormal cells (brown) have bright CD45 (myeloid cells: green, monocyte: orange; nucleated red blood cells: pink). They also have bright CD7 and CD5 and dimmer than normal CD2 (bottom panels). In this case, they lack surface CD3, although that is not typical. T-PLL can be CD4+ and CD8− as in this case (top right panel) or coexpress CD4 and CD8. (Normal CD4 and CD8 T cells: red and blue, respectively; other lymphocytes: gray.)

Genetics
This lymphoma is characterized by abnormalities involving chromosome 14. Up to 80% of cases have inv(14)(q11q32), which juxtaposes *TRA* at 14q11 and the oncogene *TCL1A/TCL1B* at 14q32, leading to overactivation. A further 10% of cases have t(14;14), and some have t(14;X), involving the *CMTCP* gene at Xq28, analogous to *TCL1A/TCL1B*. These translocations are considered initiating events but are not sufficient for leukemogenesis. An additional 70% to 80% of cases have abnormalities of chromosome 8, including trisomy 8 or t(8;8).

Prognosis
This is an aggressive disease with a 1- to 2-year survival. Rare reports of a chronic or indolent T-PLL have been reported. Treatment with anti-CD52 may improve survival.

Hepatosplenic T cell Lymphoma

Hepatosplenic T cell lymphoma (HSTL) is a highly aggressive lymphoma with a poor prognosis.[24]

Epidemiology
This rare disease most commonly affects young adults (average 35 years old) with a male predominance and is thought to be associated with chronic antigenic stimulation, as it is often associated with Crohn disease and treatments with tumor necrosis factor (TNF)-α inhibitor (infliximab), or as a late occurring posttransplant lymphoproliferative disorder (PTLD).

Presentation
Patients present with B symptoms, including fevers and night sweats. HSM and sometimes massive splenomegaly (1,000-3,500 g) are common, but there is usually no LAD.

Morphologic features of the BM include a unique sinusoidal infiltration (Figure 8.34). The abnormal cells are monomorphic, medium-sized lymphoid cells with round nuclei, dispersed chromatin, and inconspicuous nucleoli (Figure 8.35; eFigure 8.27). The PB is not typically involved, but there may be marked cytopenias because of BM infiltration and/or splenic sequestration.

Immunophenotype (eFigure 8.28)
The immunophenotype of HSTCL is of CD3-positive T cells, usually, but not invariably, of TCRγδ type, commonly positive for CD56. Cells typically lack CD5, CD4, and CD8 and have an immature/nonactivated cytotoxic T cell phenotype (TIA1+, perforin−, granzyme B−); these abnormal cells are thought to arise from γδ T cells in the spleen, although there are a few reports of cases with a αβ phenotype. Both subtypes are similar in morphology, cytogenetics, and gene expression.

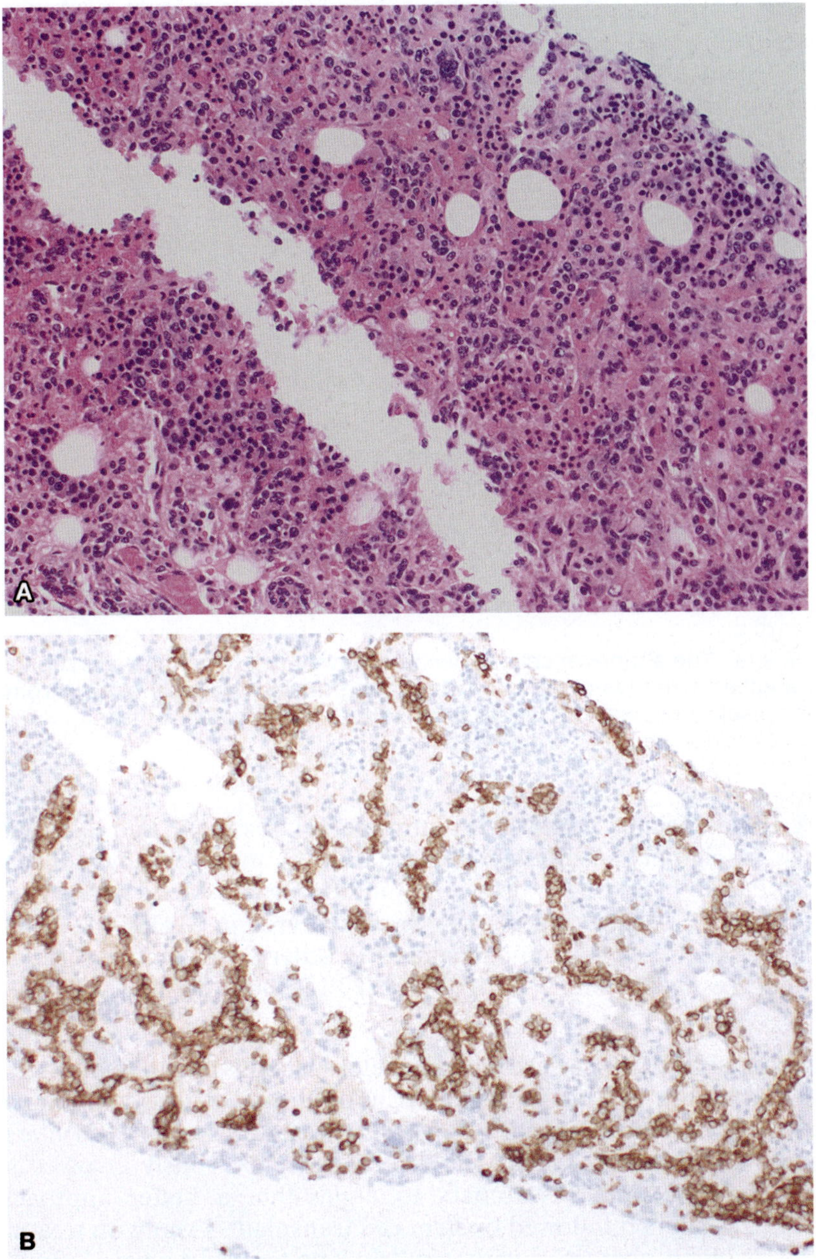

FIGURE 8.34 The Bone marrow in a case of hepatosplenic T cell lymphoma shows a very subtle pattern of sinusoidal infiltration that can be difficult to see on hematoxylin and eosin (A), but is readily revealed on an immunohistochemical stain for CD3 (B).

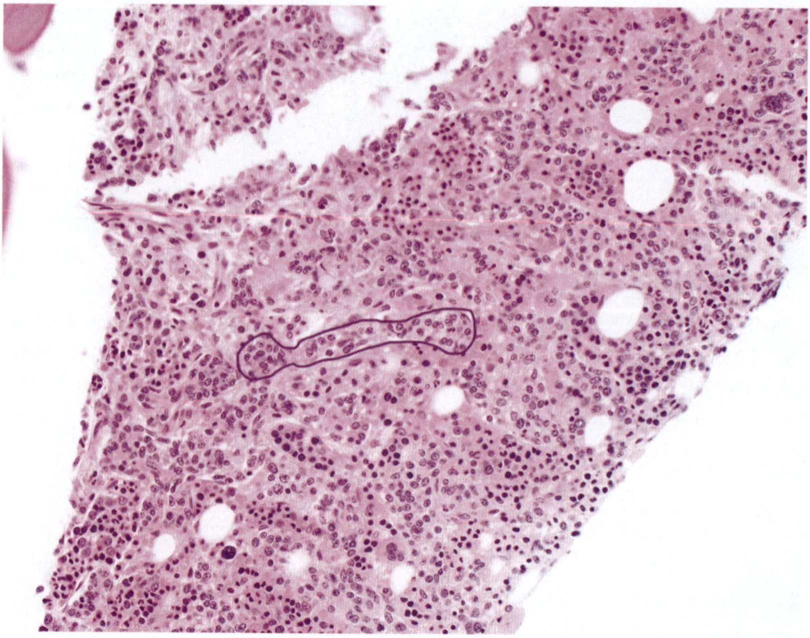

FIGURE 8.35 **The abnormal cells in hepatosplenic T cell lymphoma are monomorphic, medium-sized lymphoid cells with round nuclei, relatively open chromatin, and inconspicuous nucleoli.** The abnormal cells, circled in this bone marrow biopsy section, typically infiltrate in a sinusoidal pattern.

Genetics

HSTCL is associated with isochromosome 7q, trisomy 8, and loss of Y, although the significance of these abnormalities is not fully known. It is associated with an increased expression of multidrug resistance gene, *ABCB1*.

Recently, *STAT5B* mutations were discovered in γδ HSTCL. The very same mutation was also found in subsets of other T cell lymphomas including an aggressive form of T-LGL (2%),[25] T-PLL (36%),[26] and T-ALL (8%).

Prognosis

The treatment for this disease is highly heterogeneous and includes steroids, alkylating agents, CHOP-like regimens, and purine analogs. Approximately 60% to 70% of patients respond to first-line treatment with CHOP-like regimen, but they also experience early relapses at previously involved sites, which has led some researchers to argue that a better approach is non-CHOP regimen followed by stem cell transplant. Even with treatment, HSTCL is highly aggressive with very few long-term survivors.

Adult T cell Leukemia/Lymphoma

Epidemiology

This clonal T cell neoplasm is associated with human T cell lymphotropic virus 1 (HTLV1) infection and is endemic in those parts of the world with a high prevalence of HTLV1, including southwest Japan, parts of the

Caribbean, and central Africa. It is a disease of adults (average age 50-60 years), occurring after a long latency period. Many patients with adult T cell leukemia/lymphoma (ATLL) suffer from immunodeficiency and have concurrent infections with other opportunistic organisms.[27]

Presentation

The disease is widely disseminated at diagnosis, including widespread LAD, skin involvement (50% of patients), and PB involvement. The presence of PB involvement does not correlate with the extent of BM involvement, which suggests that other sites, like the skin, may seed the PB.

There are several clinical variants, or phases of disease, from smoldering to chronic to lymphomatous to acute. Acute is the most common and involves the PB and occasionally the BM. Patients in this phase often have hypercalcemia, with or without lytic bone lesions.

Morphology

Pleomorphic lymphoid cells with lobular nuclei, known as "flower cells," are identified in the PB (Figure 8.36; eFigure 8.29). These cells are also identified in the BM, often forming focal sheets (Figure 8.37; eFigure 8.30). Osteoclastic activity is increased, leading to hypercalcemia, even in BMs without overt lymphomatous involvement.

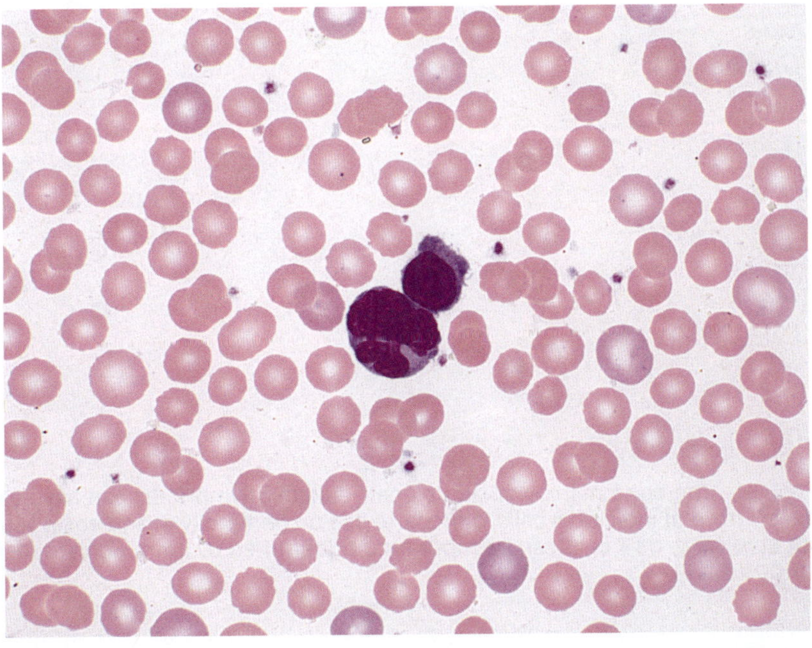

FIGURE 8.36 The peripheral blood of a patient with adult T cell leukemia/lymphoma containing pleomorphic lymphoid cells with lobular nuclei, known as "flower cells."

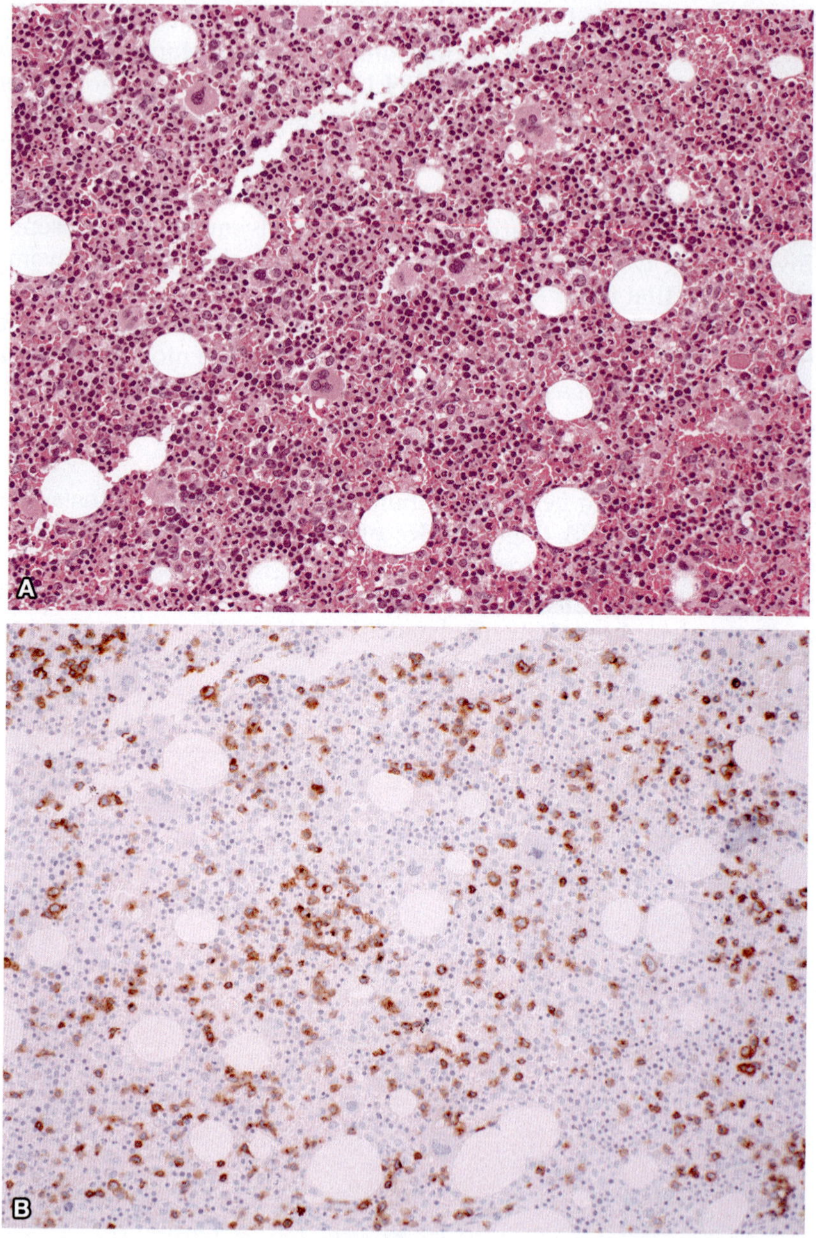

FIGURE 8.37 The bone marrow in adult T cell leukemia/lymphoma can have a very subtle infiltrate of individual cells, difficult to see on hematoxylin and eosin section (A) but atypical large T cells can be more readily identified by immunohistochemistry for CD3 (B).

Immunophenotype

Abnormal cells express T cell markers, including CD3 and CD4, often express CD25, an activation marker, and lack CD7. They may express CD30 but lack cytotoxic markers.

Genetics

The integration of HTLV1 and production of viral proteins activate cellular genes to promote leukemogenesis. However, HTLV1 infection alone is not sufficient to cause the disease. *HBZ*, a gene that is responsible for many signal pathways, differentiation, and growth, is expressed in all cases of ATLL and may be crucial for its development. Other genetic mutations have been shown, including *CCR4* mutations.

Prognosis

Prognostic factors include the subtype, the patient age, performance status, and serum calcium and LDH levels. Survival is generally poor but can range from weeks to years. Death usually results as a consequence of other opportunistic infections.

LGL Leukemia

This chronic, indolent disorder results in a proliferation of clonal cytotoxic T cells or NK cells (known as LGLs) in the PB.[28] Diagnosis requires identification of clonal proliferation of LGLs of T cell lineage (2000/μL or greater) in the PB, persisting for 6 months or more. Distinguishing LGL leukemia from a reactive disorder may be difficult without a complete clinical history.

Epidemiology

Patients with myasthenia gravis and certain autoimmune disorders, such as rheumatoid arthritis (RA), have a higher chance of being afflicted with this cytotoxic proliferation. Patients who have undergone stem cell transplants also appear to have a higher chance of presenting with a clonal LGL population of cells.

LGL most commonly affects middle-aged and elderly adults (50-60 years of age), with a similar sex distribution (M=F). Approximately two-thirds of patients are symptomatic at presentation, often showing signs and symptoms of cytopenias, especially significant neutropenia and infections. Patients may also have anemia, but usually not pancytopenia.

Presentation

The CBC reveals leukocytosis, with a high lymphocyte count, most characteristically with neutropenia and anemia. Some patients may present with pure red cell aplasia. The PB smear characteristically shows LGLs, which are medium-to-large cells with slightly eccentric oval nuclei, ample blue-gray cytoplasm, and small azurophilic granules (Figure 8.38A and B; eFigure 8.31). LGLs are normal PB cells and may be increased in reactive disorders, or as a sequela of viral infections, and even reactive proliferations may sometimes be clonal, further complicating diagnosis.

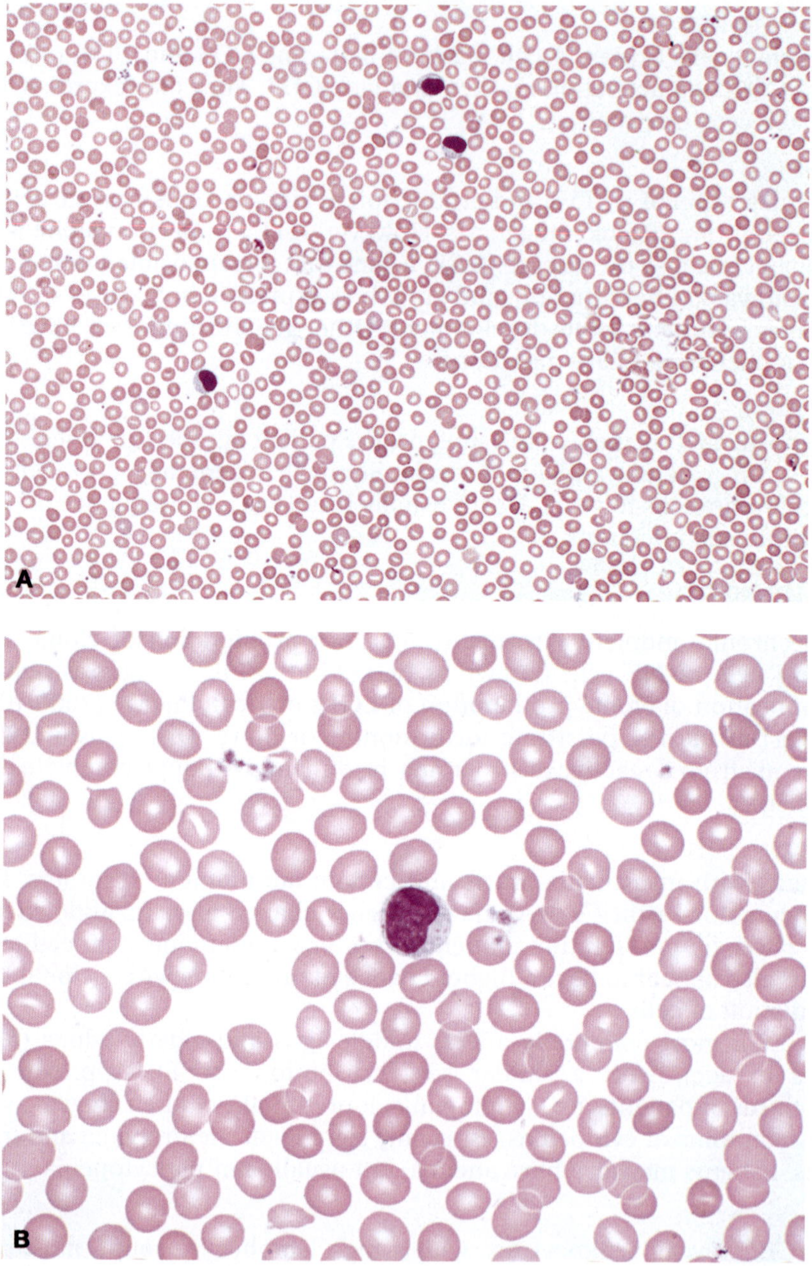

FIGURE 8.38 **Figure A shows a peripheral blood smear at low power with scattered large granular lymphocytes (LGLs).** At higher power (B), LGLs are medium-to-large cells with slightly eccentric oval nuclei, ample blue-gray cytoplasm, and small azurophilic granules.

MORPHOLOGY

The morphologic features of the BM include a subtle interstitial infiltrate (Figure 8.39; eFigure 8.32) by CD8-positive cytotoxic T cells, often in sinusoidal single-file lines (Figure 8.40A and B). There are also scattered small lymphoid aggregates, often composed of mostly CD4-positive T cells.

IMMUNOPHENOTYPE

The LGLs are most prevalent in the PB, and this is the best specimen to evaluate via FC. They are CD8-positive T cells with relatively dim CD5, CD56, and often CD57 with loss of CD27 and/or CD28. CD11c may be expressed on some, and these have been associated with a more aggressive course. Unlike many other cytotoxic T cell disorders, LGLs are TCRαβ. Rarely, LGLs may be CD4-positive. The most characteristic findings in the PB flow include lymphocytosis with relative neutropenia, an inverted CD4:CD8 ratio, and a population of atypical LGLs. If these findings are present, molecular studies of the PB are recommended.

GENETICS

TCR gene rearrangements are recommended in patients with the characteristic findings described above.

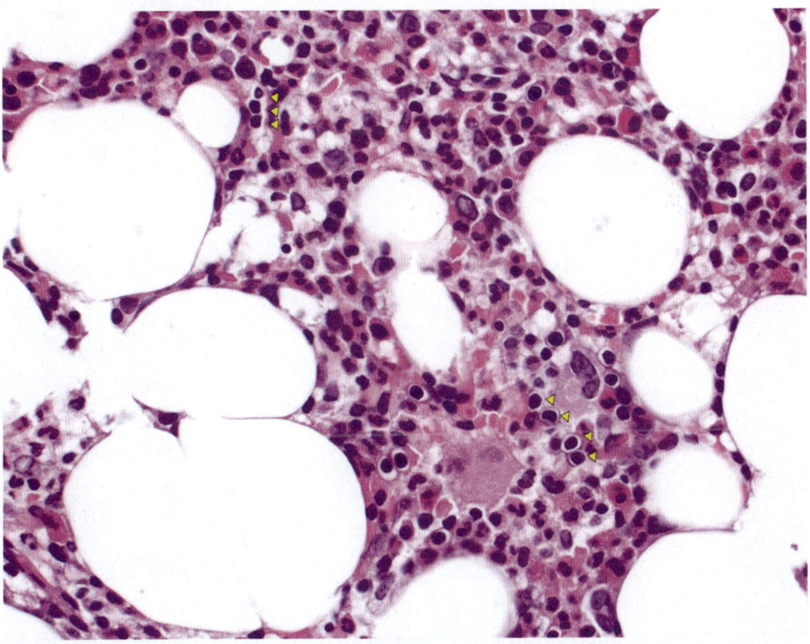

FIGURE 8.39 **A bone marrow involved by large granular lymphocytic leukemia.** There is a subtle interstitial infiltrate by atypical lymphoid cells with a distinct rim of cytoplasm (upper left; yellow arrowheads).

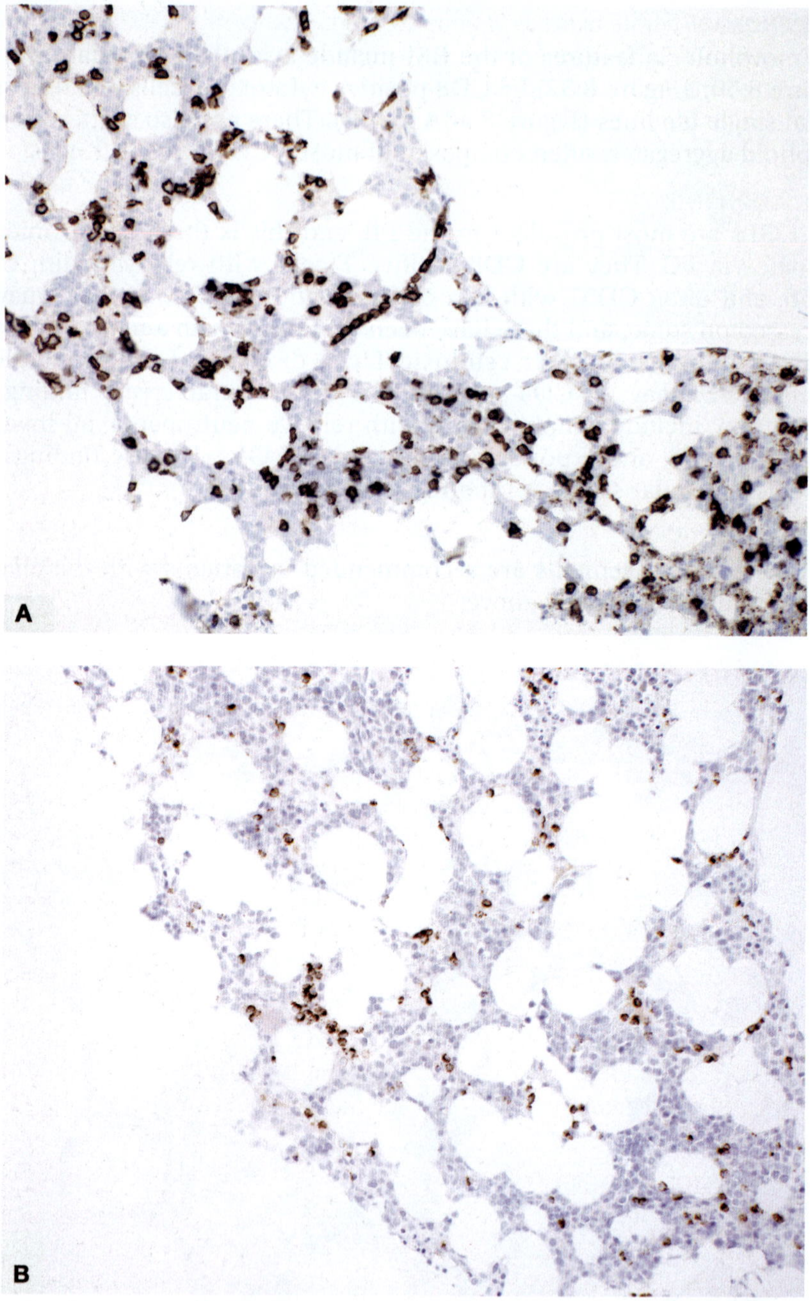

FIGURE 8.40 **Immunohistochemical stains in large granular lymphocytic leukemia.** A, CD8-positive T cells are seen in the interstitium and in sinusoids, often in single-file lines. B, The abnormal cells are positive for the cytotoxic marker, perforin.

Recently, whole-exome sequencing studies detected *STAT3* mutations in up to 40% of T-LGL cases,[29] especially in patients with neutropenia and RA. The mutations increase STAT3 dimerization, which results in greater transcriptional activity than the wild type, leading to increased phosphorylation and nuclear localization. *STAT3* mutation is associated with a good prognosis.

Somatic *STAT5B* mutations were subsequently detected in 2% of T-LGL. This mutation leads to increased transcriptional activity, and the clinical course is aggressive, unlike normal T-LGL.

Treatment

The decision to treat depends on the severity of the cytopenias. Usually, methotrexate or cyclophosphamide or corticosteroids are used and occasionally anti-CD52.

Aggressive NK cell Leukemia

Aggressive NK cell leukemia (ANKL) is a rare, aggressive neoplasm of mature NK cells (eFigure 8.33). It most often affects patients in eastern Asia and has an association with EBV infection. The prognosis of ANKL is poor, with an average life expectancy of <1 year.[30]

PERIPHERAL T CELL LYMPHOMAS WITH SECONDARY BM INVOLVEMENT

Angioimmunoblastic T cell Lymphoma

Angioimmunoblastic T cell lymphoma (AITL) is one of the most common subtypes of peripheral T cell lymphoma, not otherwise specified (PTCL-NOS) and is recognizable by its growth pattern and T follicular helper (TFH) phenotype. It is a systemic disease, involving multiple LNs, the spleen, liver, skin, and BM.

Epidemiology and Presentation

AITL most commonly affects middle-aged to elderly patients. Patients are typically very sick and present with advanced stage disease, with diffuse adenopathy, polyclonal hypergammaglobulinemia, skin rashes, pleural effusions, and arthralgias.

Morphology

The abnormal infiltrate is highly polymorphous and may comprise single or multiple loose nodular infiltrates (Figure 8.41A; eFigure 8.34).[31] Many of the abnormal T cells show relatively abundant clear cytoplasm and irregular nuclei with condensed chromatin. Like in the LN, there may be increased small vessels, abundant immunoblasts, and scattered EBER-ISH–positive B cells.

Immunophenotype

AITL expresses pan T cell markers (Figure 8.41B), often with decreased surface CD3 by FC and decreased CD7 by FC and IHC. These express the TFH phenotype, with expression of CD4, CD10, variable BCL6, PD1, and ICOS.

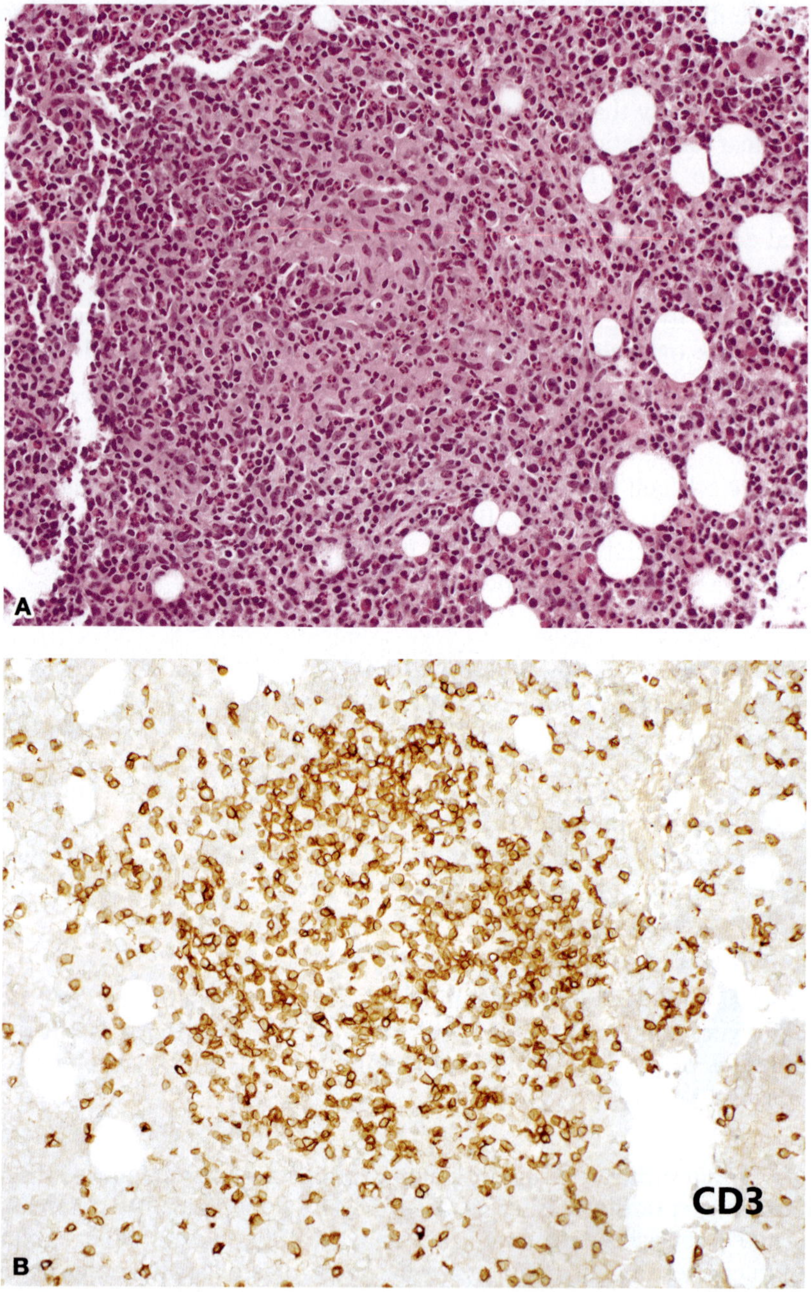

FIGURE 8.41 **Bone marrow involved by angioimmunoblastic T cell lymphoma.** A, High power shows a focal lesion in the bone marrow comprised of a mixture of small lymphocytes, histiocytes, eosinophils, plasma cells, and immunoblasts. B, An immunohistochemical stain for CD3 highlights the abnormal lymphoid cells.

Genetics

Most have clonal TCRs (75%-90%), and a significant portion also has clonal B cells (25%-30%) due to the EBV-positive B cell expansion. Chromosomal abnormalities are detected in up to 90%. Mutations in *IDH2*, *TET2*, *DNMT3a*, and *RHOA* are also commonly found.

Prognosis

These have a variable course, with a relatively poor prognosis (<3 years). Some factors that affect patient survival include patient sex, the presence or absence of mediastinal LAD, and the presence or absence of anemia.

Peripheral T Cell Lymphoma, Not Otherwise Specified

PTCL-NOS is considered a diagnosis of exclusion, once other more specific peripheral T cell leukemias/lymphomas have been ruled out. This category is thought to represent a heterogeneous group of mature T cell malignancies, although significant work is being done to help categorize these neoplasms based on molecular mutations and GEPs.

Epidemiology and Presentation

Commonly, patients present at advanced stage, with involvement of multiple LNs, BM, liver, spleen, and extranodal sites.[3] The PB may be involved, but pure leukemic presentation is rare. Patients often have B symptoms and may have eosinophilia and pruritus.

Morphology

Morphologically, the abnormal T cells are medium-to-large with variable pleomorphism (eFigure 35).

Immunophenotype

PCTL-NOS shows an aberrant T cell phenotype in most cases. Most are TCRαβ, and there is usually decreased expression of one or more of the pan T cell markers, often CD5 and CD7. They may express CD30, usually to a lesser extent than anaplastic large cell lymphoma (ALCL), ALK1 positive or negative. The Ki67 proliferative index is usually high.

Genetics

Complex karyotypes are expected, with recurrent gains and losses. Mutations involving the transcription factors *TBX21* (T-BET) and *GATA3*, which are master regulators of Th1 and/or Th2 differentiation, have been detected and may help further subclassify PTCL-NOS.

Prognosis

This is an aggressive disease with poor response to therapy and frequent relapses. The IPI and stage of disease are associated with prognosis, although BM involvement and the Ki67 proliferative index may also be associated with prognosis. Treatment includes autologous BM stem cell transplant.

OTHER T cell LYMPHOMAS

Among other well-characterized T cell lymphomas, only a few can be found in the BM and those are uncommon. Mycosis fungoides, particularly when it disseminates as Sézary syndrome, can involve marrow, typically in an interstitial pattern. Similarly, ALCL can involve marrow, either focally or as a subtle infiltrate of large atypical cells.

REVIEW OF MATURE T cell LEUKEMIA/LYMPHOMA BM INVOLVEMENT

- T cell leukemias/lymphomas are less common than B cell leukemias/ lymphomas and are often aggressive.
- T cell malignancies often show aberrant immunophenotypes by FC, with aberrant levels of expression of one or more T cell antigens.
- ATLL is associated with HTLV1 and is endemic in parts of the world with a high seroprevalence of the virus.
- LGL leukemia is more prevalent in patients with autoimmune disorders, with indolent behavior, and is associated with a good prognosis, except if it has mutations in *STAT5*.
- Many, but not all types of T cell lymphomas that present with nodal or extranodal tissue disease can secondarily involve the marrow.

REFERENCES

1. Clark P, Normansell DE, Innes DJ, Hess CE. Lymphocyte subsets in normal bone marrow. *Blood*. 1986;67(6):1600-1606.
2. Arber DA, George TI. Bone marrow biopsy involvement by non-Hodgkin's lymphoma: frequency of lymphoma types, patterns, blood involvement, and discordance with other sites in 450 specimens. *Am J Surg Pathol*. 2005;29(12):1549-1557.
3. Viswanatha D, Foucar K. Hodgkin and non-Hodgkin lymphoma involving bone marrow. *Semin Diagn Pathol*. 2003;20(3):196-210.
4. Kipps TJ, Stevenson FK, Wu CJ, et al. Chronic lymphocytic leukaemia. *Nat Rev Dis Primers*. 2017;3:16096.
5. Hallek M, Cheson BD, Catovsky D, et al. iwCLL guidelines for diagnosis, indications for treatment, response assessment, and supportive management of CLL. *Blood*. 2018;131(25):2745-2760.
6. Arber DA, Orazi A, Hasserjian R, et al. The 2016 revision to the World Health Organization classification of myeloid neoplasms and acute leukemia. *Blood*. 2016;127(20):2391-2405.
7. Sander B, Quintanilla-Martinez L, Ott G, et al. Mantle cell lymphoma—a spectrum from indolent to aggressive disease. *Virchows Arch*. 2016;468(3):245-257.
8. Campo E, Jaffe ES, Cook JR, et al. The international consensus classification of mature lymphoid neoplasms: a report from the clinical advisory committee. *Blood*. 2022;140: 1229-1253.
9. Freedman A, Jacobsen E. Follicular lymphoma: 2020 update on diagnosis and management. *Am J Hematol*. 2020;95(3):316-327.
10. Kussick SJ, Kalnoski M, Braziel RM, Wood BL. Prominent clonal B-cell populations identified by flow cytometry in histologically reactive lymphoid proliferations. *Am J Clin Pathol*. 2004;121(4):464-472.

11. Maitre E, Cornet E, Troussard X. Hairy cell leukemia: 2020 update on diagnosis, risk stratification, and treatment. *Am J Hematol.* 2019;94(12):1413-1422.
12. Zamò A, Johnston P, Attygalle AD, Laurent C, Arber DA, Fend F. Aggressive B-cell lymphomas with a primary bone marrow presentation. *Histopathology.* 2020;77(3):369-379.
13. Chang H, Hung YS, Lin TL, et al. Primary bone marrow diffuse large B-cell lymphoma: a case series and review. *Ann Hematol.* 2011;90(7):791-796.
14. Hans CP, Weisenburger DD, Greiner TC, et al. Confirmation of the molecular classification of diffuse large B-cell lymphoma by immunohistochemistry using a tissue microarray. *Blood.* 2004;103(1):275-282.
15. Alizadeh AA, Eisen MB, Davis RE, et al. Distinct types of diffuse large B-cell lymphoma identified by gene expression profiling. *Nature.* 2000;403(6769):503-511.
16. Piris MA, Onaindía A, Mollejo M. Splenic marginal zone lymphoma. *Best Pract Res Clin Haematol.* 2017;30(1-2):56-64.
17. Juárez-Salcedo LM, Castillo JJ. Lymphoplasmacytic lymphoma and marginal zone lymphoma. *Hematol Oncol Clin North Am.* 2019;33(4):639-656.
18. Wang W, Lin P. Lymphoplasmacytic lymphoma and Waldenström macroglobulinaemia: clinicopathological features and differential diagnosis. *Pathology.* 2020;52(1):6-14.
19. Tousseyn T, De Wolf-Peeters C. T-cell/histiocyte-rich large B-cell lymphoma: an update on its biology and classification. *Virchows Arch.* 2011;459(6):557-563.
20. Laurent C, Arber DA, Johnston P, Fend F, Zamò A, Attygalle AD. Diagnosis of classic Hodgkin lymphoma on bone marrow biopsy. *Histopathology.* 2020;76(7):934941.
21. van den Beemd R, Boor PPC, van Lochem EG, et al. Flow cytometric analysis of the Vβ repertoire in healthy controls. *Cytometry.* 2000;40(4):336-345.
22. Horna P, Shi M, Olteanu H, Johansson U. Emerging role of T-cell receptor constant β chain-1 (TRBC1) expression in the flow cytometric diagnosis of T-cell malignancies. *Int J Mol Sci.* 2021;22(4):1817.
23. Staber PB, Herling M, Bellido M, et al. Consensus criteria for diagnosis, staging, and treatment response assessment of T-cell prolymphocytic leukemia. *Blood.* 2019;134(14): 1132-1143.
24. Yabe M, Miranda RN, Medeiros LJ. Hepatosplenic T-cell lymphoma: a review of clinicopathologic features, pathogenesis, and prognostic factors. *Hum Pathol.* 2018;74:5-16.
25. Rajala HL, Eldfors S, Kuusanmäki H, et al. Discovery of somatic STAT5b mutations in large granular lymphocytic leukemia. *Blood.* 2013;121(22):4541-4550.
26. Kiel MJ, Velusamy T, Rolland D, et al. Integrated genomic sequencing reveals mutational landscape of T-cell prolymphocytic leukemia. *Blood.* 2014;124(9):1460-1472.
27. Vadillo E, Dorantes-Acosta E, Pelayo R, Schnoor M. T-cell acute lymphoblastic leukemia (T-ALL): new insights into the cellular origins and infiltration mechanisms common and unique among hematologic malignancies. *Blood Rev.* 2018;32(1):36-51.
28. Lamy T, Moignet A, Loughran TP, Jr. LGL leukemia: from pathogenesis to treatment. *Blood.* 2017;129(9):1082-1094.
29. Koskela HL, Eldfors S, Ellonen P, et al. Somatic STAT3 mutations in large granular lymphocytic leukemia. *N Engl J Med.* 2012;366(20):1905-1913.
30. Ishida F. Aggressive NK-cell leukemia. *Front Pediatr.* 2018;6:292.
31. Xie Y, Jaffe ES. How I diagnose angioimmunoblastic T-cell lymphoma. *Am J Clin Pathol.* 2021;156(1):1-14.

9

PLASMA CELL DISORDERS

Plasma cells (PCs) are terminally differentiated B cells that secrete cytoplasmic immunoglobulin (Ig) in their critical role as defenders in the adaptive immune response. PCs travel throughout the body and are present mainly in the bone marrow (BM), lymph nodes (LNs), and other tissues. In this chapter, we focus on PCs in the BM.

PCs may be increased in the BM in both reactive and neoplastic conditions, and therefore, additional data, including patient history, PC phenotype, and/or clonality studies, are critical in differentiating between benign reactive conditions and neoplastic or malignant conditions.[1]

Reactive plasmacytosis: Reactive PC proliferations are detectable in patients with certain infections, particularly viral infections. Patients with HIV may have BM biopsies that show a pronounced polytypic plasmacytosis. Other causes of reactive plasmacytosis are listed in Table 9.1.

Neoplastic plasmacytosis: Plasma cell neoplasms (PCNs) evolve over time from expansions of clonal PCs. They are clinically recognized because of the mass effect of the PCs, the interaction of PCs with the BM microenvironment, and/or the damage done by their Ig.

TABLE 9.1 Causes of Reactive Plasmacytosis
Infection
Malignancy
Inflammation
Castleman disease
Iron deficiency
Megaloblastic anemia
Hemolytic anemia
Diabetes mellitus
Cirrhosis
Streptokinase treatment

PLASMA CELL NEOPLASMS

Epidemiology and Presentation

There are several subtypes of PCNs (Table 9.2) that are categorized based on: (a) the number of clonal PCs in the BM; (b) the amount of Ig in the serum, and (c) the accompanying clinical symptoms.[2]

TABLE 9.2 Plasma Cell Neoplasm Subtypes

Plasma cell neoplasm subtypes	Defining features	Symptomatic?
MGUS	<3 g/dL <10% clonal PC in BM	NO
Myeloma		
• Smoldering myeloma	10%-60% clonal PC in BM	NO
• Overt multiple myeloma	>60% clonal PC in BM or any % PC with symptoms	YES
• Nonsecretory myeloma		YES
• Plasma cell leukemia	PC >20% of total WBC or absolute count >2000/μL	YES
Plasmacytoma		
• Solitary	PC lesion in bone <10% PC in uninvolved BM	YES or NO
• Extramedullary	PC lesion in extramedullary site	YES or NO
Associated with paraneoplastic process		
• POEMS	Polyneuropathy, organomegaly, endocrinopathy, monoclonal gammopathy, and skin changes	YES
• TEMPI	Telangiectasias, erythropoietin, monoclonal gammopathy, perinephric fluid, and intrapulmonary shunting	YES
Monoclonal Ig deposition disease		
• Amyloidosis	Deposition of monoclonal Igs that form B-pleated sheets (amyloid) and cause organ damage	YES
• Systemic light and heavy chain	Deposition of monoclonal Igs (light or heavy chains) that do NOT form B-pleated sheets (amyloid), but still cause organ damage	YES

BM, bone marrow; Ig, immunoglobulin; MGUS, monoclonal gammopathy of undetermined significance; MM, multiple myeloma; PC, plasma cells; WBC, white blood cell.

Clonal PCs: These are detected by morphologic evaluation of the BM biopsy and with the aid of ancillary studies, namely immunohistochemistry (IHC), in situ hybridization (ISH), or flow cytometry (FC). The quantity of clonal PCs helps subclassify PCNs, as discussed in the following:

1. **Increased serum/urine monoclonal Ig:** Depending on the PCN subtype, patients present with varying levels of homogeneous Ig secreted by PCs in the serum (paraproteinemia, also known as monoclonal protein, or "M-protein") or urine, indicating a clonal PC population. Patients with suspected PCNs should be assessed for paraproteinemia either by serum protein electrophoresis (SPEP) or urine protein electrophoresis (UPEP), followed by immunofixation electrophoresis (IFE) or similar studies (Table 9.3).

   In addition to SPEP/UPEP and IFE, screening for elevated serum free light chains (SFLCs) at diagnosis is recommended.[3] This

TABLE 9.3 Clinical and Laboratory Tests for PCNs

Name	Test	Description
SPEP	Patient serum is added to an agarose gel followed by electrophoresis, leading to the separation of serum proteins into five distinct zones: albumin, α1, α2, β, and γ.	Paraproteins display as a discreet band, known as a monoclonal protein ("M-protein" or "M-spike") in the γ region, and occasionally in the α or β regions.
UPEP	Similar to SPEP, but using patient urine.	Excessive serum protein overwhelms the kidney and escapes filtration into the urine. These monoclonal light chains in the urine, known as "Bence-Jones proteins," cause damage to the renal tubules, and ultimately damage the kidneys.
IFE	To characterize the monoclonal band on the SPEP or UPEP, patient serum or urine is placed in separate wells of an agarose gel. Following electrophoresis, antiserum is applied to the gel (anti-IgG, anti-IgA, anti-IgD, κ and λ), and the gel is stained.	Distinct bands representing the heavy and light chains of the paraprotein are visualized.
FLC	Automated immunoassays quantitate the FLCs in serum or urine.	These are prognostic and recommended to assess "nonsecretory" PCNs.

FLC, free light chain; IFE, immunofixation electrophoresis; PCNs, plasma cell neoplasms; SPEP, serum protein electrophoresis; UPEP, urine protein electrophoresis.

assay measures the amount of Ig free light chains in the serum, which is useful for those patients with PCNs that are nonsecretory or oligosecretory or in patients with amyloid or light chain deposition disorder, as the traditional methods of measuring monoclonal Ig (SPEP) may result in a false negative. SFLC assays are prognostic and are used to monitor patients for response. However, treatment-related suppression of the uninvolved light chain might make this test unreliable.

The presence of M-proteins is not specific to PCN; other B cell malignancies can secrete paraproteins, most notably chronic lymphocytic leukemia/small lymphocytic lymphoma (CLL/SLL), marginal zone lymphoma, and lymphoplasmacytic lymphoma (LPL).

Up to 30% of patients with PCNs have reduction in the other Igs, or hypogammaglobulinemia, which predispose these patients to infections. Hypogammaglobulinemia, without an M-protein, may also be seen in patients who secrete light chains only, rather than the complete Ig molecule. In those instances, SPEP/IFE studies are often necessary.

2. **Clinical symptoms:** Patients may or may not present with clinical symptoms, often referred to as "CRAB" symptoms: Hyper**c**alcemia, **R**enal abnormalities, **A**nemia, and **B**one lesions (Table 9.4).

The PCNs comprise monoclonal gammopathy of undetermined significance (MGUS, non-IgM type), plasma cell myeloma (PCM; including smoldering myeloma [SM] and overt multiple myeloma [MM]), and plasmacytoma. Other rare tissue disorders, including heavy chain disease and heavy and light chain deposition disease, are beyond the scope of this chapter.

Morphology

Normal PCs are slightly larger than lymphocytes and have eccentric nuclei with blocky chromatin, resembling a "clock face" (eFigure 9.1). The cytoplasm is abundant, and because of the excessive protein production, there is prominent endoplasmic reticulum, which is visible as a perinuclear space, or "hof" (Figure 9.1A and B).

TABLE 9.4 Symptoms of Plasma Cell Neoplasms

	Symptom	Caused by
C	Hypercalcemia	Osteoclast activity leads to increased calcium.
R	Renal	Bence-Jones proteins lead to renal tubular damage.
A	Anemia	Plasma cells infiltrate the bone marrow, decreasing normal hematopoiesis.
B	Bone lesions	Osteoblast activity leads to bone resorption.

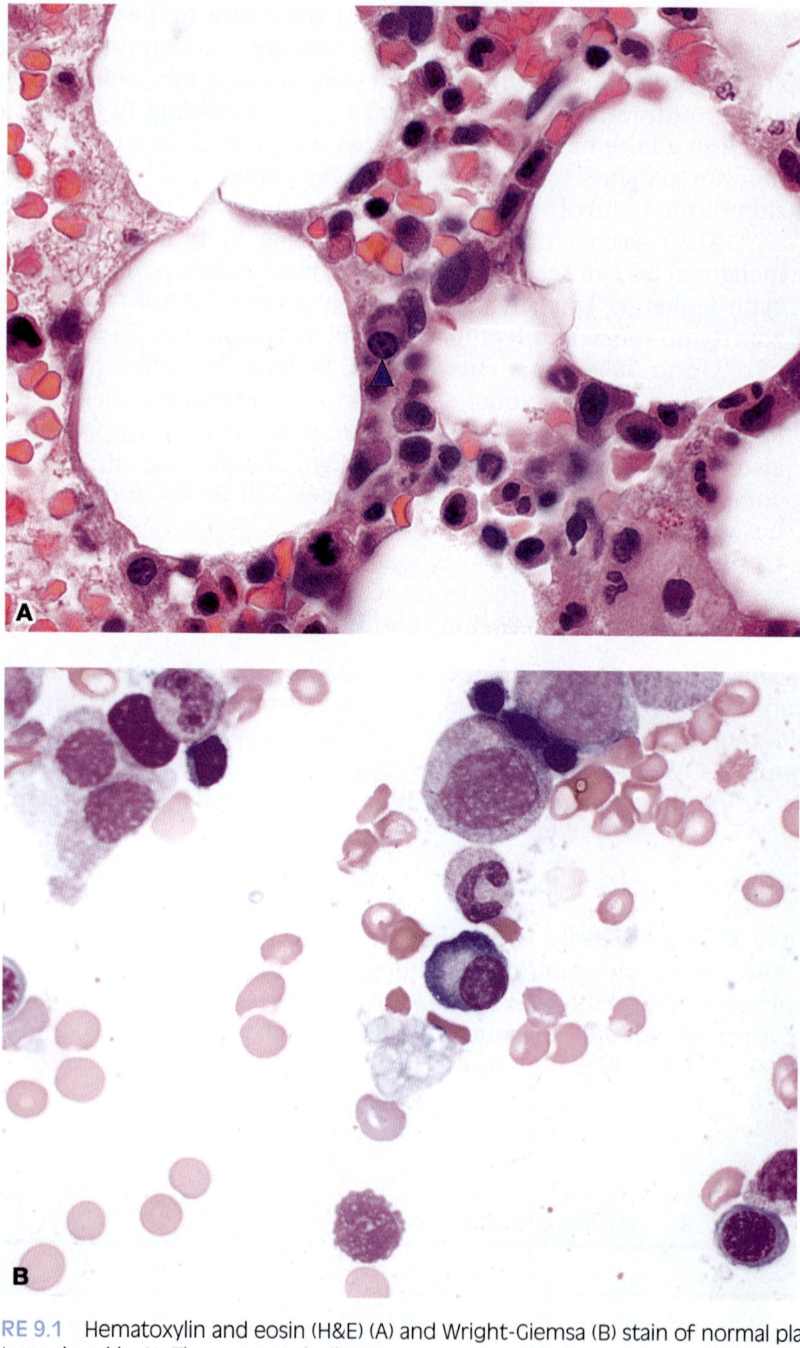

FIGURE 9.1 Hematoxylin and eosin (H&E) (A) and Wright-Giemsa (B) stain of normal plasma cells (arrowhead in A). These are typically scattered throughout marrow and have eccentric nuclei and have prominent endoplasmic reticulum, which is visible as a perinuclear space, or hof.

PCs may have different morphologies: They may be binucleate or trinucleate (Figures 9.2A and B), may or may not have nucleoli, and may vary in size. The cytoplasm may have a characteristic cytoplasmic appearance due to Ig, as seen in “flame cells” (Figure 9.3; eFigure 9.2). They can have

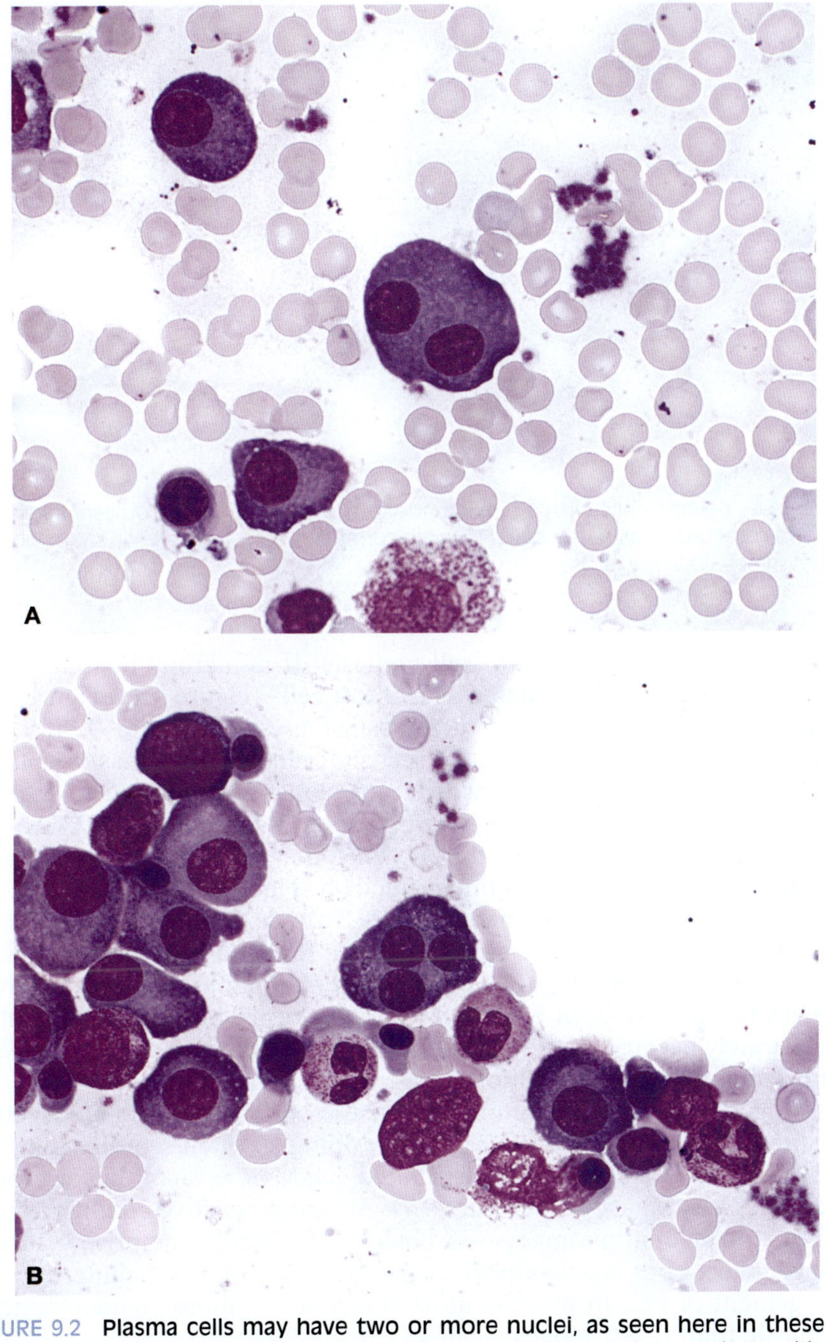

FIGURE 9.2 **Plasma cells may have two or more nuclei, as seen here in these WG stained aspirate smears (A and B).** Although these images are from patients with myeloma, these may be seen in reactive conditions as well.

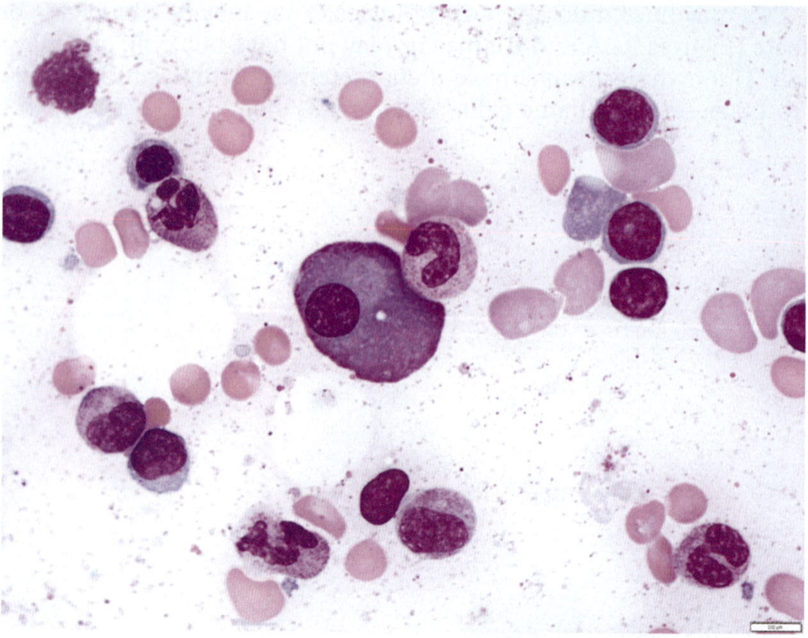

FIGURE 9.3 **Plasma cells with a pinkish hue at the edge of the cytoplasm as shown here are referred to as flame cells.** They are commonly associated with immunoglobulin A. Photograph courtesy of Dr. Rena Xian.

cytoplasmic Ig inclusions ("Russell bodies"). If numerous Russell bodies are present, the PC is designated as a "Mott cell" (Figure 9.4; eFigure 9.3). Plasma cells can also contain cytoplasmic crystals (Figure 9.5). These abnormal appearing forms may be seen in reactive as well as neoplastic conditions, so that definitive evidence of clonality is needed to make a diagnosis of a PCN. However, the presence of Dutcher bodies (Figure 9.6; eFigure 9.4), inclusion bodies that obscure the nucleus, or plasmablasts, immature large PCs with prominent nucleoli (Figure 9.7; eFigure 9.5), are more reliable indicators of a neoplastic PC.[4]

PCs may be difficult to aspirate from a BM and are variably present in BM aspirate smears (Figure 9.8; eFigure 9.6). Quantitation for classification has historically been based on aspirate counts, but this is difficult to do accurately because of the patchy involvement of myeloma in marrow, so that it requires counting multiple areas on numerous coverslips.

In general, it is often simpler to use the core biopsy or a clot section to estimate the number of PCs, although doing so often requires the help of IHC stains. PCs are usually distributed singly or as small linear groups around vessels (Figure 9.9; eFigure 9.7). Although reactive conditions may lead to a polyclonal plasmacytosis, benign PCs usually comprise <20% of total cellularity, but may comprise as much as 50% of total cellularity.[5] The arrangement of PCs in prominent islands is much more characteristic of neoplastic than reactive plasmacytosis (Figure 9.10).

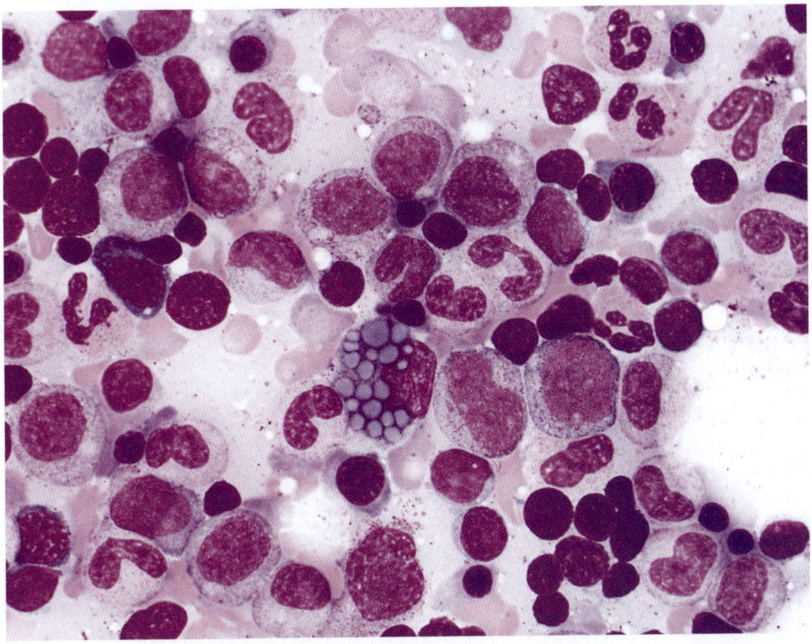

FIGURE 9.4 **Russell bodies are spherical globules of immunoglobulin.** When they accumulate in the cytoplasm of plasma cells as shown here, the cells are referred to as Mott cells after the surgeon who first identified them.

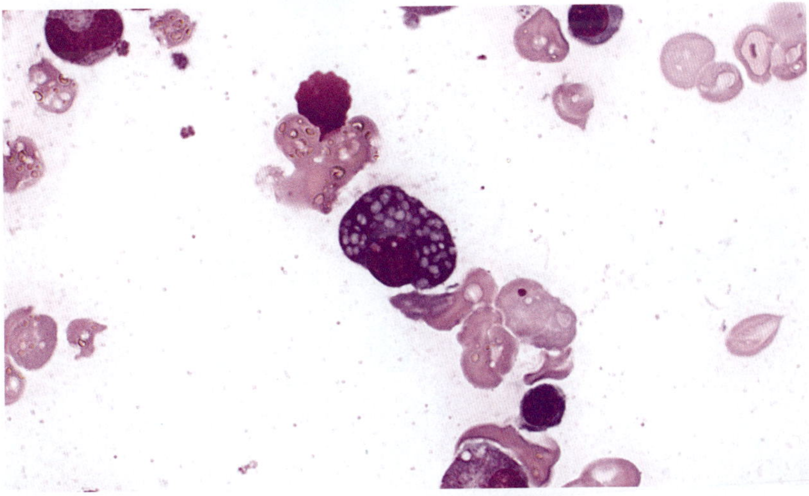

FIGURE 9.5 **In some plasma cell disorders, plasma cells may have cytoplasmic crystals and can have a variety of shapes including needle-like, or more oblong or rounded, as shown here.**

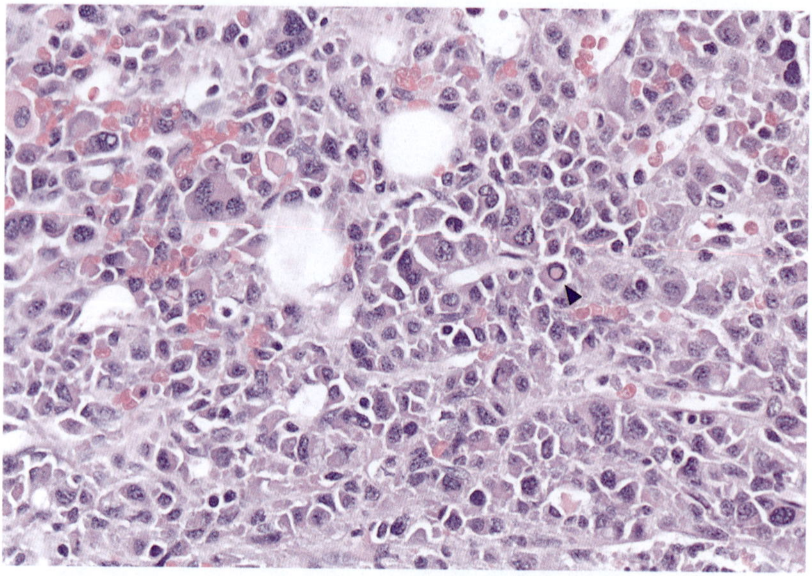

FIGURE 9.6 Dutcher bodies, or nuclear pseudo-inclusions (such as the one shown at the arrowhead) are thought to be specific for plasma cell dyscrasias.

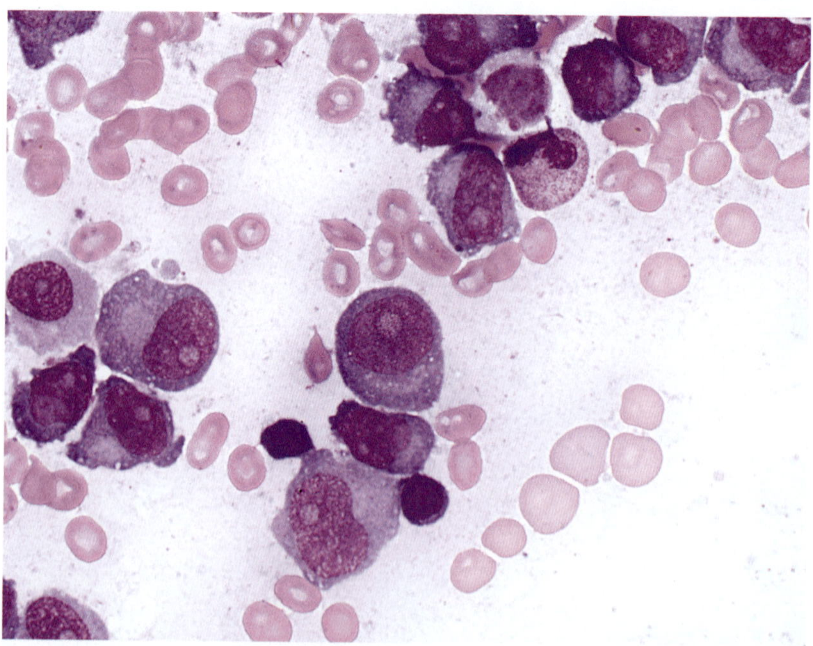

FIGURE 9.7 Plasmablasts are immature large plasma cells with prominent nucleoli. As shown here on the aspirate smear, they typically maintain eccentrically placed nuclei and a cytoplasmic hof.

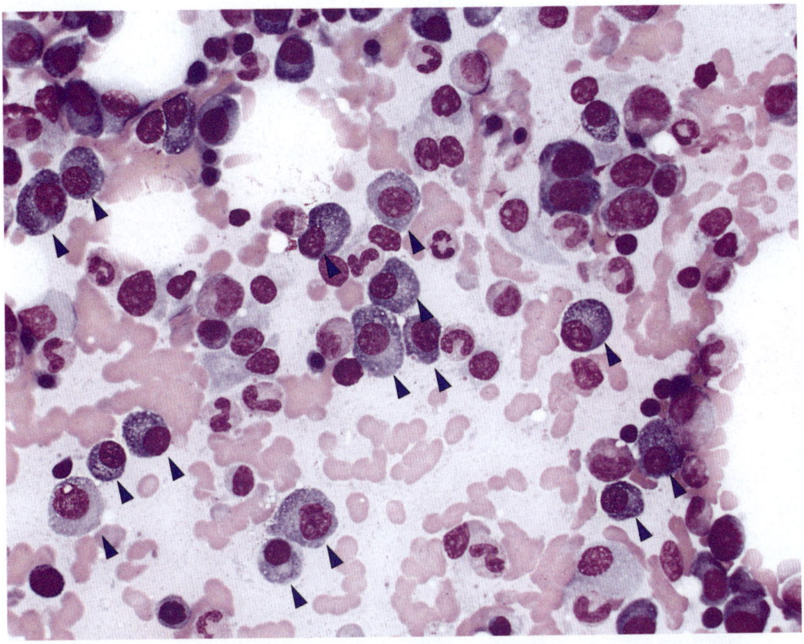

FIGURE 9.8 Plasma cells (arrowheads) are typically abundant on an aspirate in cases of plasma cell myeloma, although they may vary in number from field to field.

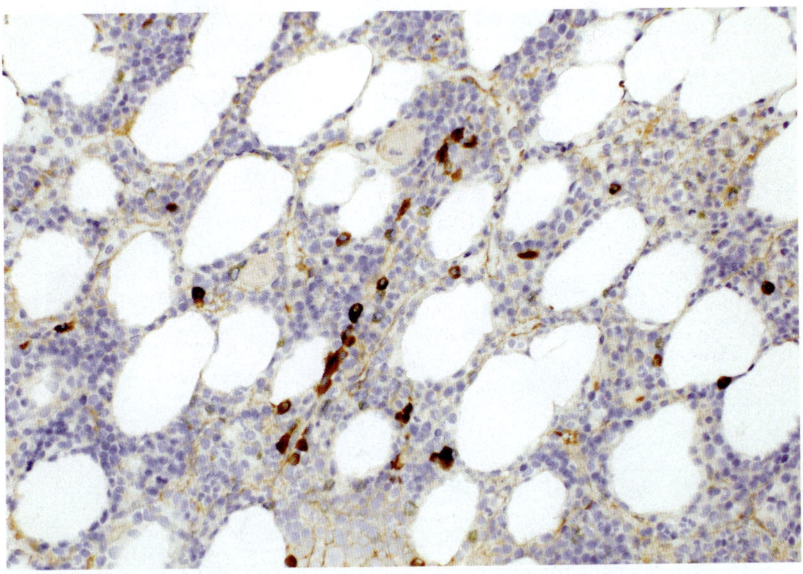

FIGURE 9.9 Plasma cells, highlighted here by an immunohistochemical stain for CD138, often cluster along vessels in normal bone marrow core biopsies.

Although normally there is no significant PC population in the peripheral blood (PB), a few circulating PCs may be seen in certain conditions, including infections (Figure 9.11; eFigure 9.8).

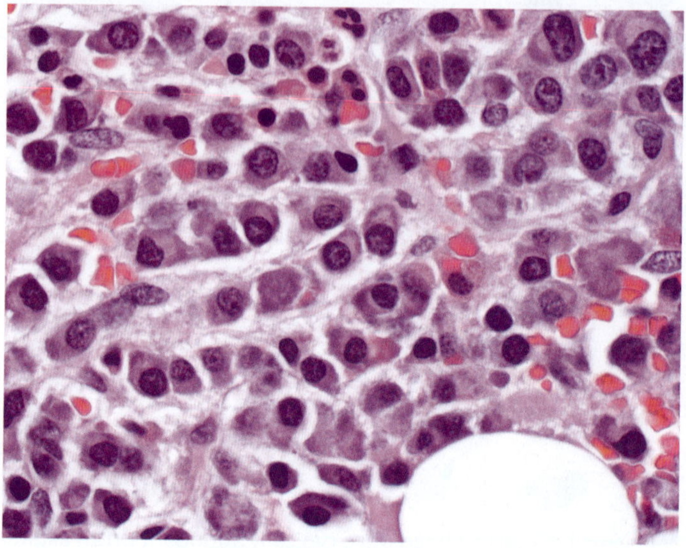

FIGURE 9.10 Although marrow plasma cells can be increased in many reactive conditions, when they are found in sheets as shown here, they almost always indicate a neoplastic process.

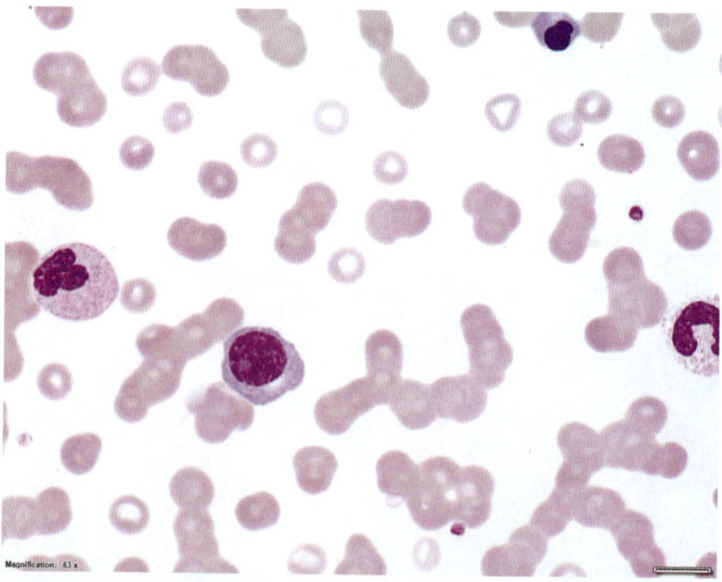

FIGURE 9.11 Plasma cells may be seen circulating in the blood of some individuals with nonneoplastic process, including autoimmune diseases or chronic infections. This case, however, was from a patient with plasma cell myeloma. A plasma cell is seen in the peripheral blood, in a background of RBCs with Rouleaux. Photograph courtesy of Dr. Xiaojun Wu.

Immunophenotype

In addition to IHC and ISH, FC plays an important diagnostic role in PCNs, although FC often underestimates the number of PCs in a sample and should not be relied upon for quantitation (eFigure 9.9).[6] After treatment, when PCs are significantly decreased, detecting residual clones by IHC can be difficult, so that FC is preferable when evaluating a BM for low-level residual disease. However, IHC has value to demonstrate abnormal plasma cells with CD56 or cyclin D1, or to demonstrate clonality when there is a small clonal cluster in a background of polyclonal PCs.

Normal PCs express B cell markers CD19, CD79a, and CD38, but lack CD20 and PAX5. They express CD138 and MUM1 and are polytypic for κ and λ light chains. FC is useful to help distinguish normal from abnormal PCs (Figure 9.12).

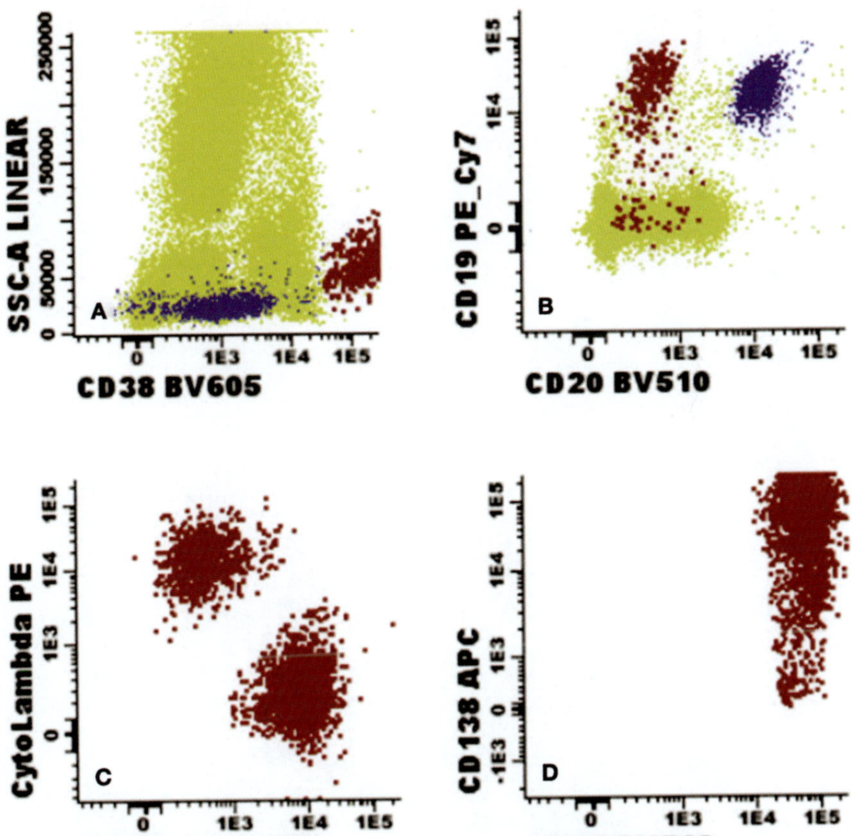

FIGURE 9.12 By flow cytometry, normal plasma cells (brown) are brightly positive for CD38 (A), but in contrast to normal B cells (blue, B), they lack CD20. Most express CD19 at levels similar to that of normal B cells, but a small subset is CD19 negative. They are polytypic for cytoplasmic κ and λ (C). CD138 is expressed (D) but often will have the broad distribution shown here because CD138 can be shed from plasma cells over time when in suspension. SSC, side scatter.

Abnormal PCs: Using IHC, abnormal PCs may lack CD19 and may aberrantly express CD20, CD56, and/or cyclin D1 (Figure 9.13A-C) and are light chain restricted (Figure 9.14). By FC, CD56, CD117, and CD200 are often upregulated in myeloma, whereas CD19, CD27, CD81, and CD45 are

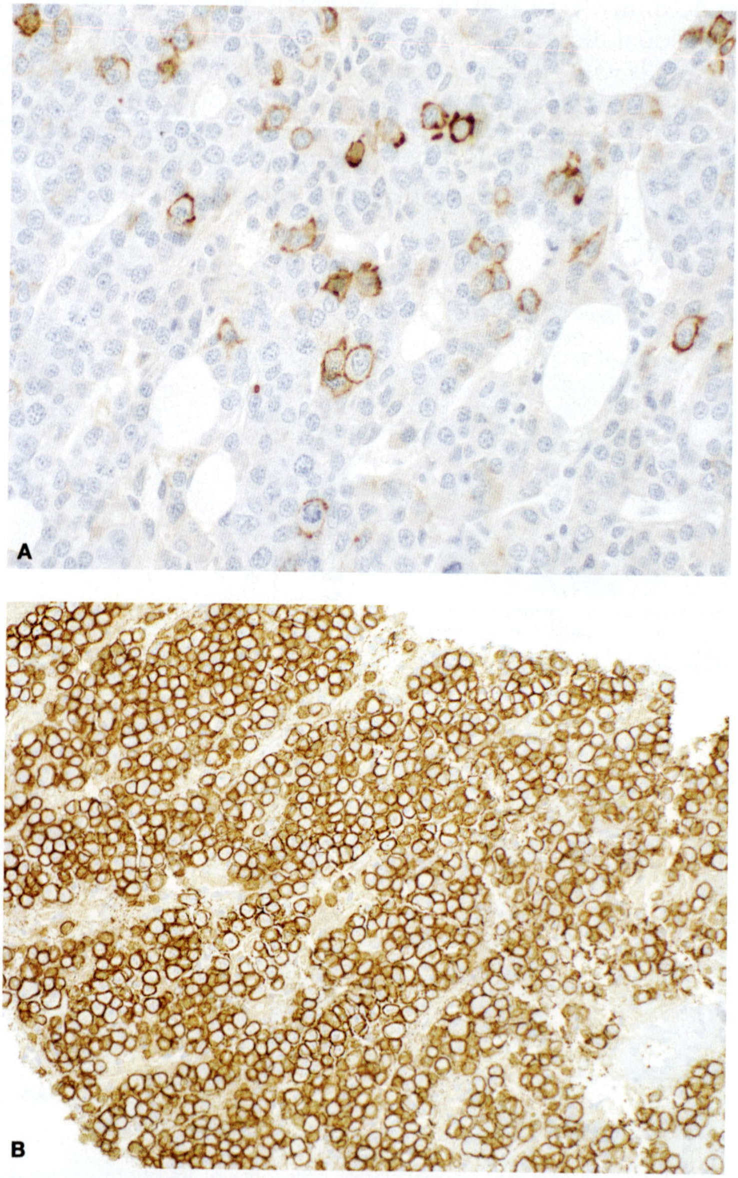

FIGURE 9.13 **Immunohistochemical stains can often demonstrate abnormal immunophenotypes of plasma cells (PCs) in PC neoplasms.** Although most cases of multiple myeloma (MM) will lack CD20, focal expression, as shown here, is not uncommon (A). A small subset of normal PCs express CD56, but uniform CD56 expression on PCs is always aberrant (B).

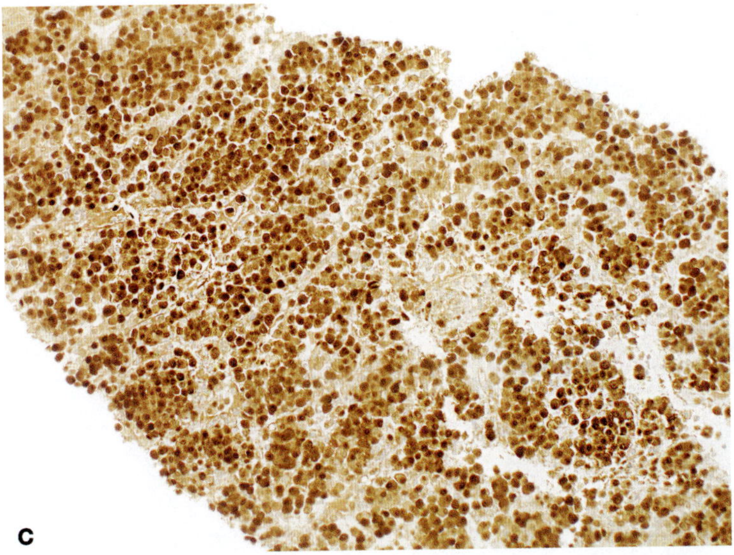

FIGURE 9.13 ***(continued)*** Cyclin D1 expression is seen in cases of MM associated with the t(11;14) translocation (C).

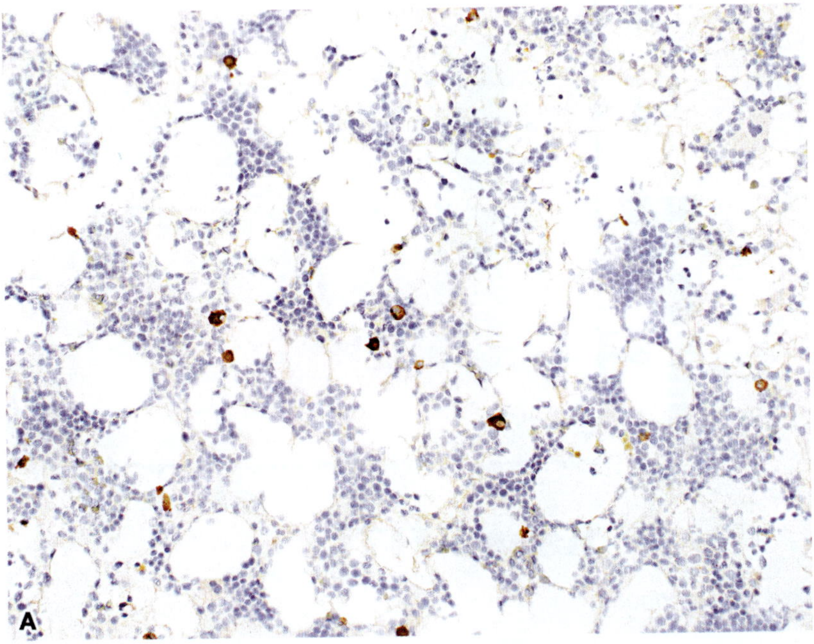

FIGURE 9.14 Clonal plasma cells (PCs) are monotypic for κ or λ by immunohistochemistry. In Figure A, kappa stains only rare plasma cells, while in Figure B, lambda stains numerous lambda-restricted plasma cells. By flow cytometry, the abnormal PCs are monotypic for cytoplasmic κ and λ but are negative for surface κ and λ (C).

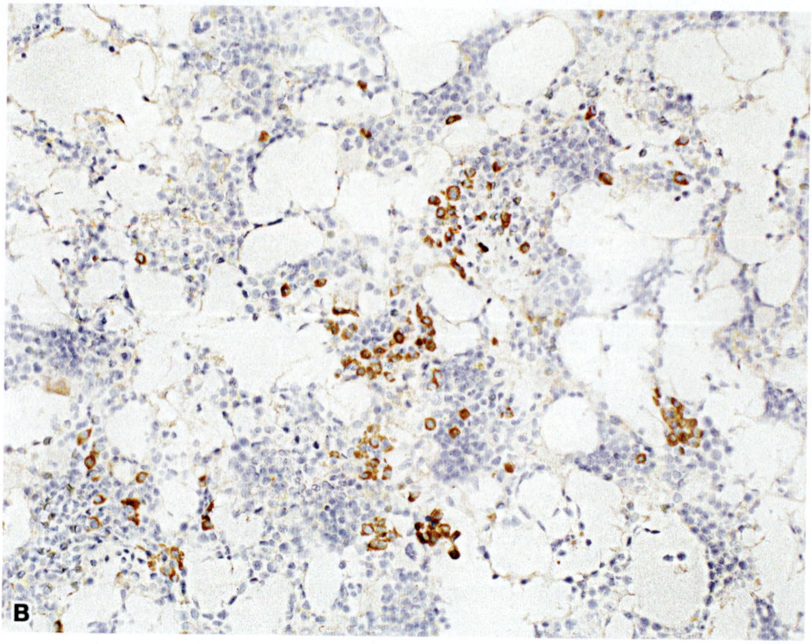

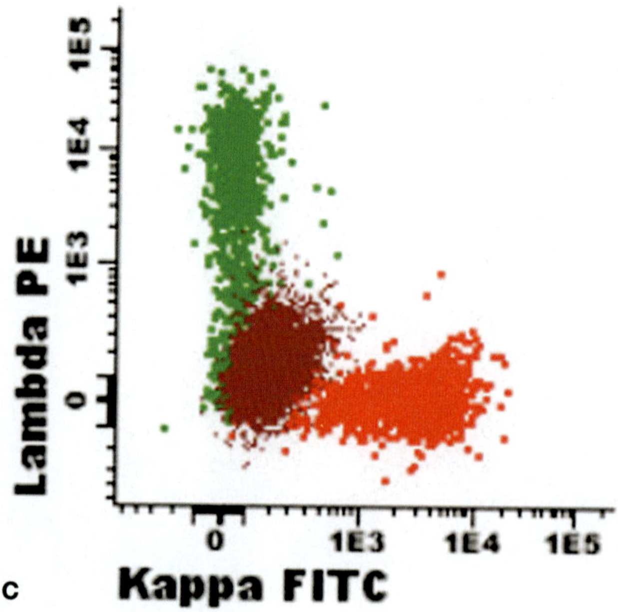

FIGURE 9.14 (*continued*)

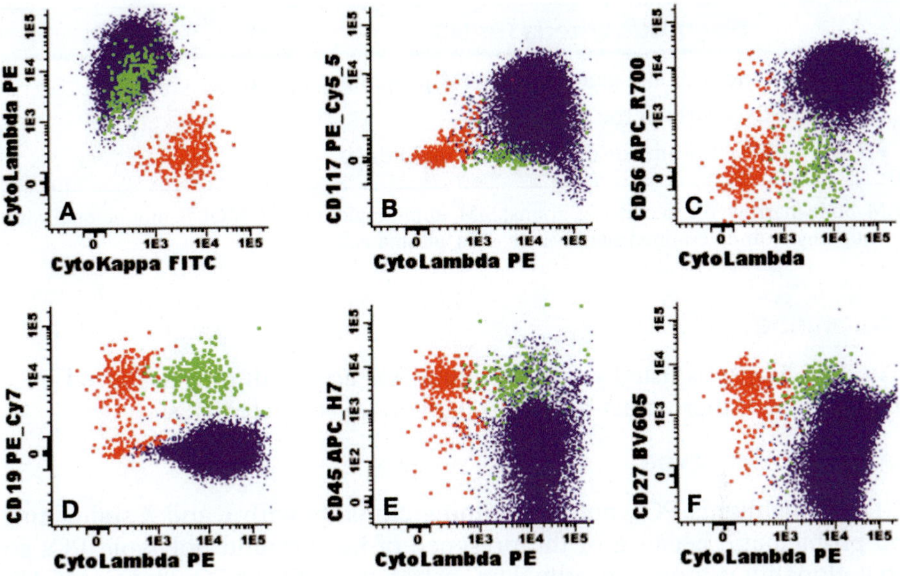

FIGURE 9.15 **Abnormal plasma cells (PCs) in a plasma cell neoplasm (PCN).** PCs show monotypic expression of cytoplasmic light chain (λ in this case; dark blue population) compared to the polytypic expression of the few background normal PCs (red and green populations) (A). In PCNs, CD117 and CD56 are often up-regulated (B and C, respectively), whereas CD19 is almost always negative (D) and CD45 and CD27 are characteristically down-regulated (E and F, respectively).

characteristically downregulated or negative (Figure 9.15). It should be noted, however, that there are small numbers of normal CD19-negative and/or CD56-positive PCs. The small cell/lymphoplasmacytic variant of PCM can express CD20 and cyclin D1. These variants have translocations involving *CCND1*.

MONOCLONAL GAMMOPATHY OF UNDETERMINED SIGNIFICANCE

MGUS is an asymptomatic clonal expansion of PCs, usually detected by SPEP. It can be separated into two distinct categories based on the secreted Ig subtype. In this chapter, we will focus on non-IgM MGUS, because IgM MGUS is more typically associated with lymphoproliferative disorders and considered a different entity.

Epidemiology and Presentation

Patients are usually elderly, and the risk increases with age. Over 5% of people over the age of 70 have MGUS. There is a male predominance, and it is more common in Black populations compared with White populations.

The diagnosis of MGUS requires evidence of a non-IgM monoclonal gammopathy (M-protein) <3 g/dL, clonal PCs <10% in the BM, and no CRAB symptoms or evidence of amyloidosis (Table 9.5).

TABLE 9.5 Diagnostic Criteria for MGUS
• Non-IgM monoclonal gammopathy (M-protein) <3 g/dL
• Clonal PCs <10% in the BM
• No CRAB symptoms or evidence of amyloidosis

BM, bone marrow; dL, deciliter; g, grams; IgM, immunoglobulin M; MGUS, monoclonal gammopathy of undetermined significance; PCs, plasma cells.

Morphology

The BM biopsy is usually normocellular for age, with only scattered PCs. By definition, there must be <10% light chain restricted PCs.

Immunophenotype

CD138 highlights PCs, but determining clonality with κ and λ stains may be problematic because of the presence of background polytypic PCs so that clonality is more typically demonstrated by IFE or FC. By FC, MGUS can show the same phenotypic abnormalities seen with myeloma, but typically has more background polyclonal PCs.

Genetics

Most patients with MGUS have a normal karyotype, but abnormalities are often detected by fluorescence in situ hybridization (FISH) studies. The most common abnormalities are the same as those seen in overt MM and include rearrangements of *IGH* at 14q32 and *CCND1* at 11q13, hyperdiploidy (40% of cases), and deletion of 13q (30%-40% of cases).

Prognosis

Some factors that affect prognosis include the size and type of the M-protein. For example, patients with >25 g/dL monoclonal gammopathy have a significantly higher rate of progression to MM in comparison with patients with <5 g/dL.

It is important to recognize and subcategorize these neoplasms because they have different rates of progression to overt MM and different clinical implications (Table 9.6).[7]

In general, patients with non-IgM MGUS progress to MM at a rate of approximately 1% per year. The proportion of abnormal PCs by FC has been suggested as predictive of progression of MGUS to myeloma.[8]

PLASMA CELL MYELOMA

PCM, defined as >10% clonal PCs in the BM or >3 g/dL M-protein, may arise either *de novo*, from progression of a preceding MGUS, or in a

TABLE 9.6 Rate of Progression to Overt MM

Subtype	Rate of progression to overt MM
MGUS	1%/year
Smoldering myeloma	10%/year for 5 years; 3%/year for next 5 years; 1.5% for every year thereafter

MGUS, monoclonal gammopathy of undetermined significance; MM, multiple myeloma.

TABLE 9.7 Diagnostic Criteria for Multiple Myeloma/PCM

Smoldering myeloma: asymptomatic PCM

- Clonal PCs comprise >10%, but <60% of total cellularity in the BM
- And/or M-protein >3 g/dL
- No CRAB symptoms or evidence of amyloidosis

Multiple myeloma: symptomatic PCM

- Presence of CRAB symptoms
- Or the presence of >60% clonal PCs in BM

BM, bone marrow; CRAB, hypercalcemia, renal abnormalities, anemia, bone lesions; PC, plasma cell; PCM, plasma cell myeloma.

patient with a prior solitary plasmacytoma. PCM can be subdivided into SM or overt MM based on the presence or absence of "CRAB" symptoms (Table 9.7).

Epidemiology and Presentation

Although a rare malignancy overall, comprising only 1% of all malignancies, it is one of the more common hematopoietic malignancies, comprising 10% to 15% of hematolymphoid neoplasms. Most cases occur in elderly patients, and it is exceedingly rare in young patients. Chronic infections, radiation exposure, and other toxic exposures are some of the risk factors that are theorized to cause PCM.

Patients present with CRAB symptoms and may additionally have abnormal laboratory studies including hypercalcemia, hyperuricemia, hypoalbuminemia, and high creatinine. Bone abnormalities, including lytic lesions, compression fractures, or osteoporosis, are detected on imaging in up to 70% of patients.

Almost all patients have M-proteins in their serum or urine, with a distribution similar to that seen in MGUS: 50% are IgG, 20% are IgA, 20% are light chain only, and <10% are IgD, IgE, or biclonal. Other manifestations of PCM include neurologic abnormalities and bleeding. Patients typically present with generalized or multifocal disease in the BM, especially in areas of active hematopoiesis.

Morphology

BM biopsy of the iliac crest is helpful to identify PCM, which presents as interstitial, focal clusters or sheets of PCs (eFigure 9.10). SM presents with 10% to 60% PCs (Figure 9.16), and overt MM presents with >60% PCs (Figure 9.17A and B). PCs, especially in the SM subtype, are admixed within a background of normal hematopoiesis. Bone trabecula may be thinned or show evidence of prominent remodeling, and in many cases, biopsies may be fragmented because of the poor quality of bone trabeculae. Osteoclasts, multinucleated bone-remodeling cells, may also be seen (Figure 9.18; eFigures 9.11 and 9.12).

The BM aspirate shows either scattered PCs or sheets of PCs, depending on both the number and the nature of the abnormal PCs in the specimen. As noted above, abnormal PCs are cytologically highly variable. PCs are present in the PB in up to 15% of cases of PCM.

Patients with PCM have renal abnormalities because of excretion of abundant urine protein (Bence-Jones protein), which damages renal tubules during reabsorption. Microscopic eosinophilic material can be seen in renal tubules, representing Bence-Jones proteins. Renal disease can also be caused by concurrent amyloidosis, or rarely by infiltration by PCs.

Extramedullary involvement can occur in almost any organ and typically indicates advanced disease, although isolated plasmacytomas can occur and have a better prognosis. Patients with plasmacytomas should have BM examined to look for evidence of systemic disease.

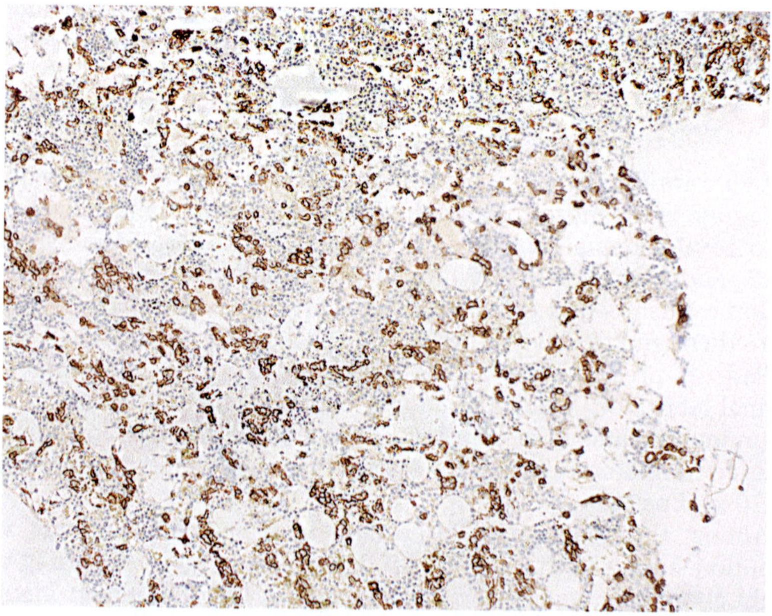

FIGURE 9.16 **Plasma cells (PCs) in marrow sections are readily highlighted by a CD138 immunostain that makes estimation of PC numbers easier.** This case of smoldering myeloma has >10% but <60% PCs.

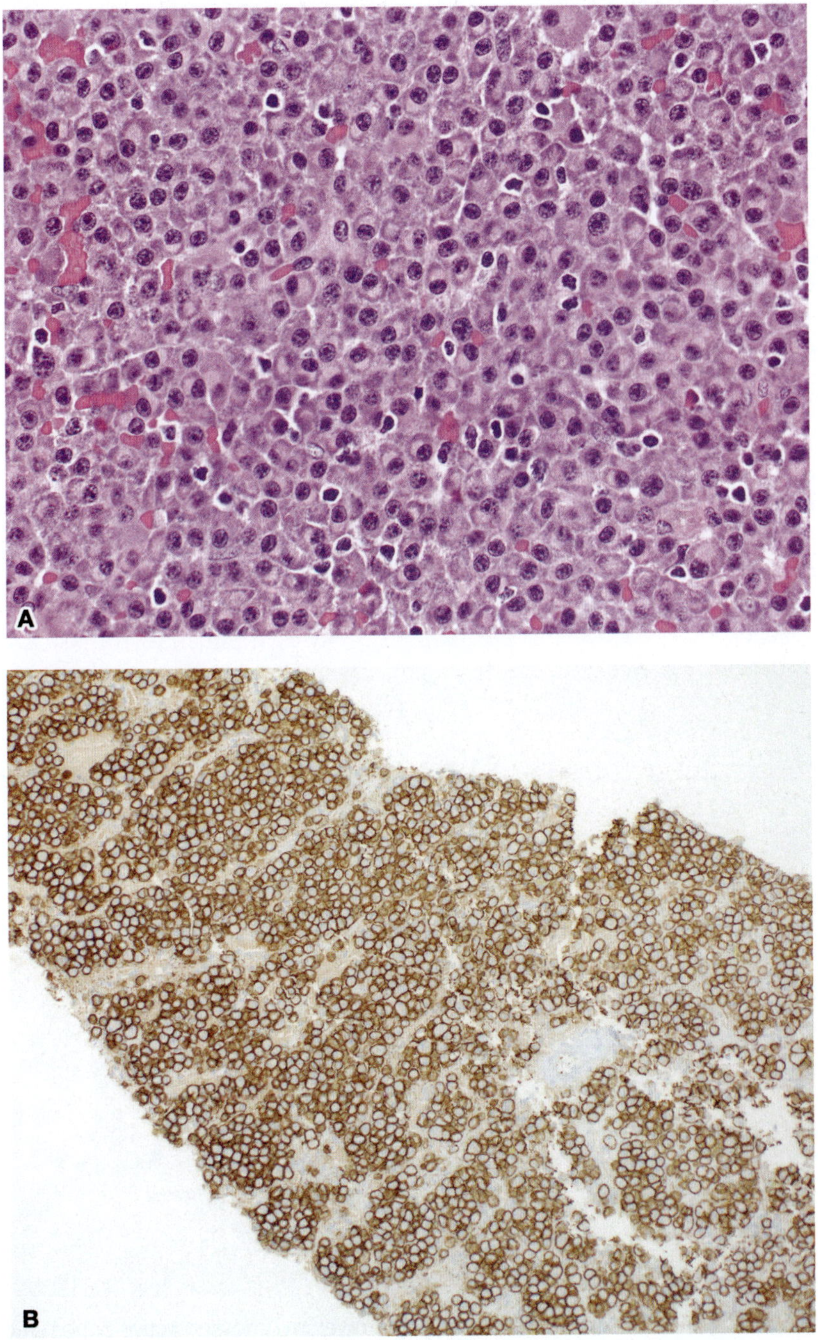

FIGURE 9.17 Hematoxylin and eosin (H&E) (A) and CD138 immunostain (B) in a case of overt multiple myeloma (MM) showing the typical sheeting out of plasma cells (PCs). When PCs account for >60% of cells, patients are considered to have active MM irrespective of the presence of any symptoms.

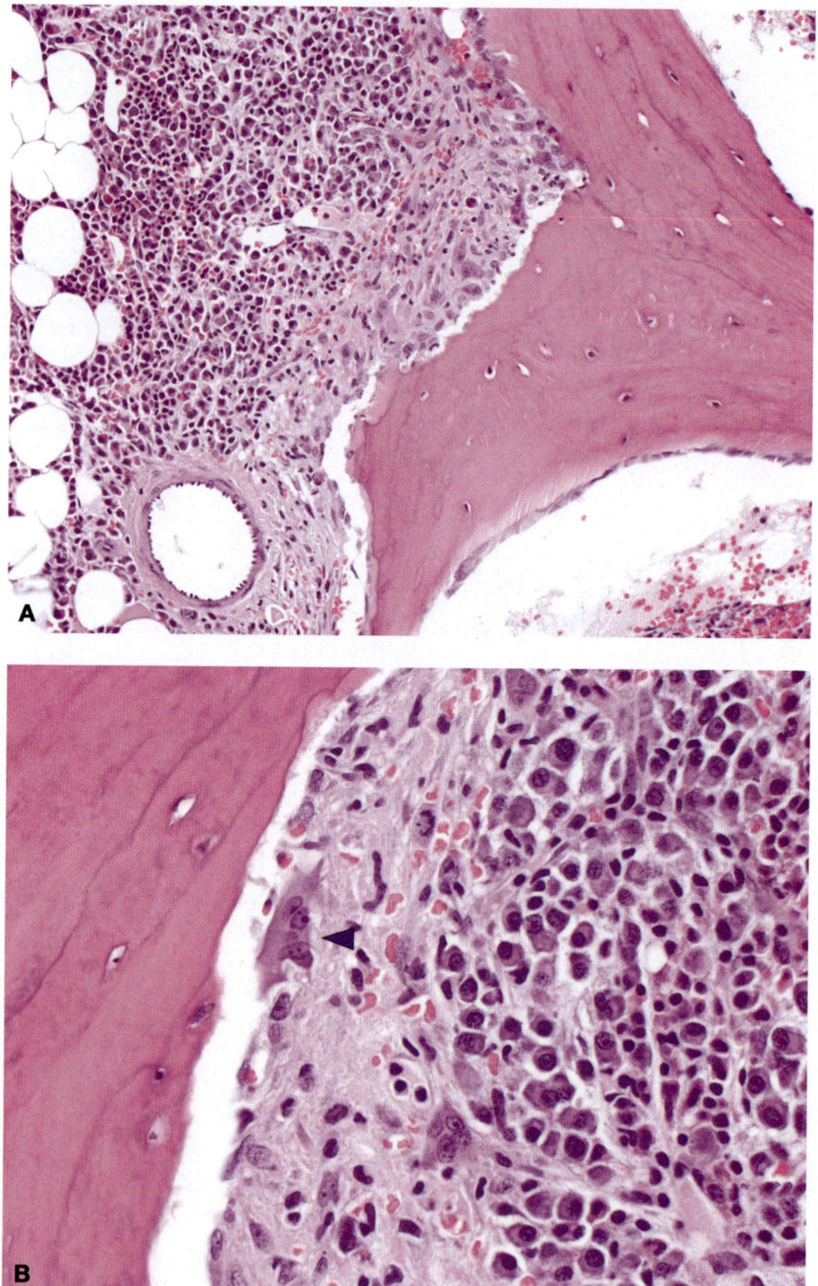

FIGURE 9.18 Bone marrow in a case of multiple myeloma showing active bone remodeling with numerous osteoclasts and osteoblasts and paratrabecular fibrosis (A). High power highlighting a multinucleated osteoclast (B, arrowhead).

Immunophenotype

The phenotype of PCMs is similar to that described in abnormal PCs and MGUS above.The phenotype of PCMs is similar to that described in abnormal PCs and MGUS above.

Genetics

Up to one-third of patients have abnormalities detected by karyotype, and up to 90% have abnormalities detected by FISH. About 40% of cases or PCM are hyperdiploid and seven recurring translocations are found in another 40% (Table 9.8).[9,10] The ICC recognizes hyperdiploid myeloma, and 3 families of translocations with IGH as distinct entities: *CCND1* (t(11;14)); *MAF* (t(14;16) and t(14;20)); and *NSD2* (MMSET, t(4;14)). Virtually all myeloma will show clonal rearrangement of Ig heavy chain genes, a feature especially useful for monitoring (see later).

Prognosis

PCM shows a spectrum of clinical courses, from asymptomatic to aggressive, and survival varies widely, from <6 months to >10 years. Patients with comorbidities and advanced age (>70) have poorer prognosis.

The International Staging System (ISS) for PCM considers clinical information, including serum β_2 microglobulin and albumin levels, as strong predictors of survival.[11] The Revised ISS (R-ISS) includes cytogenetic abnormalities and categorizes patients into standard, intermediate, and high-risk categories. Other prognostic factors include lactate dehydrogenase (LDH), creatinine, hypergammaglobulinemia, Ki-67 proliferative

TABLE 9.8 Genetics of Plasma Cell Neoplasms

Primary genetic events–MGUS	Secondary events–SMM/overt MM
Hyperdiploidy	**Mutations**
• Trisomies 3, 5, 7, 9, 11, 15, 19, 21	• *NRAS, KRAS, BRAF, FAM46C, EGR1, CYL, FGFR3, DIS3, PRKD2, PRDM1, CCND1, IRF4, MAF/MAFB*
Monosomy	**Gains/Del**
• Chromosome 13/del(13q)	• Del(17p)[a]; *TP53* • Del(12p) • Gain 1q
***IGH* translocations**	**Other translocations**
• t(4;14)[a], t(14;16)[a], t(11;14), t(6;14), t(14;20)	• *MYC*

MGUS, monoclonal gammopathy of undetermined significance; MM, multiple myeloma; SMM, smoldering multiple myeloma.

[a]Considered high-risk cytogenetics.

TABLE 9.9 International Staging System

ISS stage	Description
I	Serum β_2-microglobulin <3.5 mg/L, serum albumin ≥3.5 g/dL
II	Not ISS stage I or III
III	Serum β_2-microglobulin ≥5.5 mg/L

ISS, International Staging System.

TABLE 9.10 Revised International Staging System

R-ISS stage	Definition
I	ISS stage I and standard-risk CA[a] by iFISH[a] and normal LDH
II	Not R-ISS stage I or III
III	ISS stage III and either high-risk CA[b] by iFISH or high LDH

CA, cytogenetic analysis; iFISH, interphase florescence in situ hybridization; ISS, International Staging System; LDH, lactate dehydrogenase; R-ISS, revised International Staging System.
[a]Standard-risk CA = no high-risk CA.
[b]High-risk CA = presence of del(17p) and/or translocation t(4;14) and/or translocation t(14;16).

index, extent of BM infiltration, plasmablastic morphology, and serum soluble receptor for interleukin (IL)-6 (Tables 9.9 and 9.10).

Monitoring of PCM: Patients with PCM are routinely followed for response using routine laboratory parameters including SPEP and free light chain analysis. With more effective treatments, including new chemotherapeutic agents, targeted immunotherapy, and BM transplantation, there is increasing use of highly sensitive techniques to detect minimal residual disease (MRD), as the goal of these treatments is to achieve MRD negativity.

MRD can be detected either by FC, based on finding small populations of PCs with aberrant immunophenotypes as described earlier, or by next-generation sequencing (NGS) methods to look for unique clonal sequences present in the pretreatment sample.[12] Sensitivity of the latter is generally considered greater and can detect $1/10^6$ clonal sequences or fewer, although these require a pretreatment sample to define the clone; FC assays typically achieve sensitivities about a log less. Additionally, FC methods may be made more difficult because of the widespread use of anti-CD38 immunotherapy; alternative markers such as CD229, CD319, and CD269 (BCMA) have been proposed, for disease monitoring[13] although newer agents targeting these are also being used in trials.

RARE PCM SUBTYPES

Nonsecretory PCM

This rare subtype comprises only 1% of all PCM, and these patients present with CRAB symptoms and evidence of marrow involvement but have an absence of M-protein on SPEP. Most nonsecretors (85%) produce abnormal Ig, as seen by IHC/ISH on BM sections, but have impaired secretion of the Ig.

Plasma Cell Leukemia

Although patients with PCNs may have rare circulating PCs, a diagnosis of plasma cell leukemia (PCL) requires >20% circulating PCs.[14] Often, there is total BM replacement and other organs are involved. PCL is the primary presentation in 2% to 4% of overt MM. PCL may be secondary, representing transformation, in 1% of MM. PCL often expresses CD20 and lacks CD56 (80%). This disease is considered aggressive, and patients typically have poor survival.

REFERENCES

1. Gorden L, Smith C, Graber SE. Marked plasmacytosis and immunoglobulin abnormalities following infusion of streptokinase. *Am J Med Sci.* 1991;301(3):186-189.
2. Rajkumar SV. Multiple myeloma: 2022 update on diagnosis, risk stratification, and management. *Am J Hematol.* 2022;97(8):1086-1107.
3. Dispenzieri A, Kyle R, Merlini G, et al. International Myeloma Working Group guidelines for serum-free light chain analysis in multiple myeloma and related disorders. *Leukemia.* 2009;23(2):215-224.
4. Fujino M. The histopathology of myeloma in the bone marrow. *J Clin Exp Hematopathol.* 2018;58(2):61-67.
5. Wei A, Juneja S. Bone marrow immunohistology of plasma cell neoplasms. *J Clin Pathol.* 2003;56(6):406-411.
6. Tembhare PR, Yuan CM, Venzon D, et al. Flow cytometric differentiation of abnormal and normal plasma cells in the bone marrow in patients with multiple myeloma and its precursor diseases. *Leuk Res.* 2014;38(3):371-376.
7. Kyle RA, Larson DR, Therneau TM, et al. Long-term follow-up of monoclonal gammopathy of undetermined significance. *N Engl J Med.* 2018;378(3):241-249.
8. Pérez-Persona E, Mateo G, García-Sanz R, et al. Risk of progression in smouldering myeloma and monoclonal gammopathies of unknown significance: comparative analysis of the evolution of monoclonal component and multiparameter flow cytometry of bone marrow plasma cells. *Br J Haematol.* 2010;148(1):110-114.
9. Cardona-Benavides IJ, de Ramón C, Gutiérrez NC. Genetic abnormalities in multiple myeloma: prognostic and therapeutic implications. *Cells.* 2021;10(2):336.
10. Gutiérrez NC, García-Sanz R, San Miguel JF. Molecular biology of myeloma. *Clin Transl Oncol.* 2007;9(10):618-624.
11. Palumbo A, Avet-Loiseau H, Oliva S, et al. Revised International Staging System for multiple myeloma: a report from international myeloma working group. *J Clin Oncol.* 2015;33(26):2863-2869.
12. Holstein SA, Bahlis N, Bergsagel PL, et al. The 2020 BMT CTN myeloma intergroup workshop on immune profiling and minimal residual disease testing in multiple myeloma. *Transplant Cell Ther.* 2021;27(10):807-816.
13. Soh KT, Tario JD, Jr, Hahn T, Hillengass J, McCarthy PL, Wallace PK. CD319 (SLAMF7) an alternative marker for detecting plasma cells in the presence of daratumumab or elotuzumab. *Cytometry B Clin Cytom.* 2021;100(4):497-508.
14. Gundesen MT, Lund T, Moeller HEH, Abildgaard N. Plasma cell leukemia: definition, presentation, and treatment. *Curr Oncol Rep.* 2019;21(1):8.

10

ABNORMALITIES OF BONE AND STROMA, INFECTIONS, AND OTHER NONHEMATOLYMPHOID DISORDERS

A bone marrow (BM) biopsy examination is not complete without an assessment of the non-hematopoietic constituents. Evaluation of the other BM components provides useful information about patient health and can indicate abnormalities that may otherwise go undiagnosed. This chapter reviews some of the findings one may encounter when examining BM specimens.

ABNORMALITIES OF BONE

Morphologic evaluation of the bony structures in the biopsy may provide clues to an underlying physiologic or pathologic process. In a normal state, bone is constantly undergoing a process of tightly regulated remodeling via osteoblast-mediated bone deposition and osteoclast-mediated bone absorption.[1] The balance between these two processes helps maintain normal bony structures and calcium homeostasis.

Disorders characterized by excess bone resorption appear as a thinning of the bony trabeculae, as in osteoporosis (Figure 10.1; eFigure 10.1), typically seen in elderly or postmenopausal patients.

In addition, certain disease states associated with resorption have characteristic histologic findings:

1. **Plasma cell neoplasms** may secrete or express potent cytokines that lead to increased osteoclastic bone resorption, resulting in hypercalcemia. This process leads to the characteristic radiographic "punched-out" bone lesions in myeloma. Bony remodeling (Figure 10.2; eFigure 10.2) is frequently evident in marrow biopsies as both osteoclastic and osteoblastic activity.
2. **Chronic renal disease** leads to mineral and bone disorders, known as renal osteodystrophy. Damaged kidneys are unable to convert vitamin D into calcitriol, creating a calcium imbalance, which leads

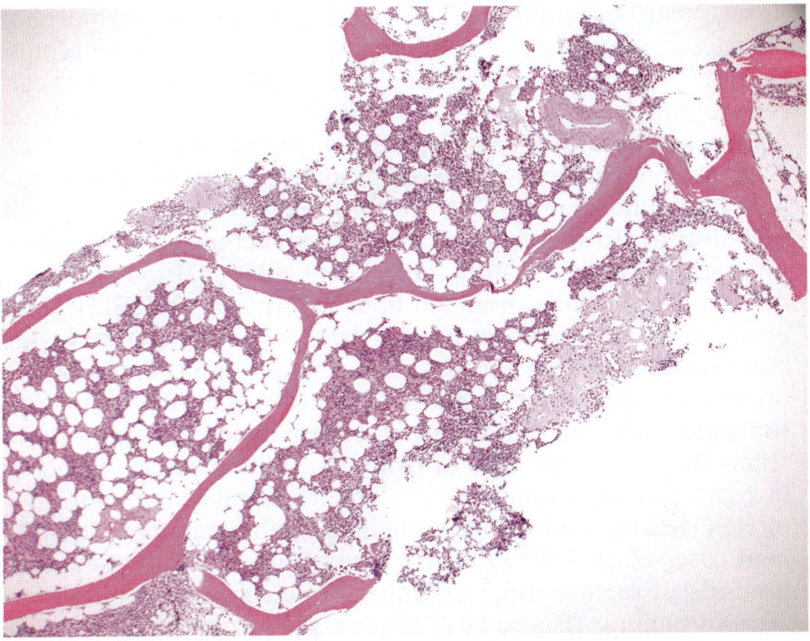

FIGURE 10.1 Osteopenia occurs as a result of excess bone resorption over deposition and appears as a thinning of the bony trabeculae.

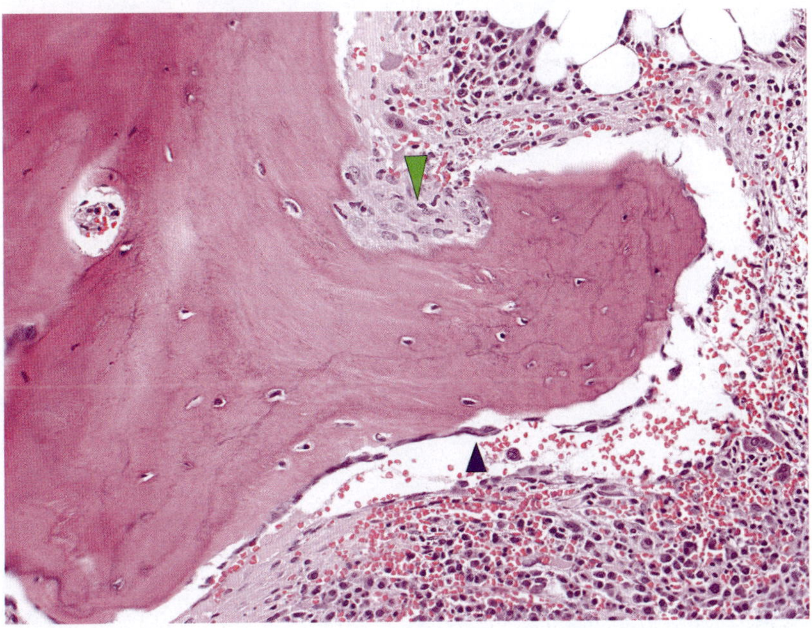

FIGURE 10.2 Increased osteoclastic activity associated with plasma cell myeloma. Osteoclastic resorption results in a scalloped appearance of bone (green arrowhead); bone deposition (blue arrowhead) also occurs as evidenced by osteoblast proliferation.

to secondary hyperparathyroidism (HPTH) and similar morphologic changes (see later). Additionally, damaged kidneys cannot remove excess phosphorus from the blood, which triggers additional calcium release from bones.

3. **Hyperparathyroidism** may cause osteitis fibrosa cystica (OFC), a skeletal abnormality that develops through the overproduction of parathyroid hormone (PTH). PTH normally acts to maintain calcium homeostasis. In the event of decreased calcium or increased phosphorus, PTH acts to restore the calcium balance through the activity of osteoclasts, which results in bone resorption. In HPTH, the overproduction of PTH activates osteoclasts, which in turn cause cortical bone destruction and fibrous cyst formation. In OFC, the BM shows osteoclastic and osteoblastic activity with hemosiderin-laden macrophages and osteoclast-lined cyst formation, with intratrabecular "tunneling," or focal areas of demineralization similar to those seen in renal osteodystrophy. In OFC, which is more common in cases of HPTH associated with parathyroid carcinoma compared with benign cases of HPTH,[2] osteoclast-like giant cells and vascularized fibrous tissue replace BM, resulting in non-neoplastic lesions known as "Brown tumors" (Figure 10.3; eFigure 10.3).

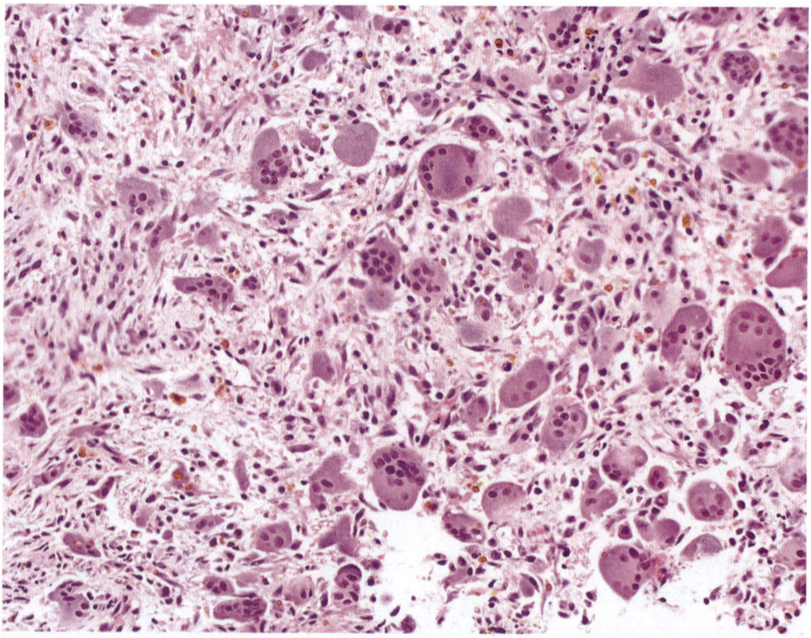

FIGURE 10.3 **In osteitis fibrosa cystica, the excessive osteoclastic activity can produce Brown tumors characterized as proliferations of giant cells in a fibrous background with numerous hemosiderin-laden macrophages.** Photo courtesy of Dr. John Gross.

Osteosclerosis, or thickened bone (eFigure 10.4), is always pathologic:

1. **Paget disease** (osteitis deformans) is the second most common bone remodeling disease after osteoporosis, affecting 1% to 2% of elderly white patients. The disease, which may involve a single bone (monostotic) or multiple bones (polyostotic), is associated with increased RANKL, which stimulates osteoclastic differentiation.[3] Morphologically, osteoclasts are increased and have multiple nuclei with inclusion bodies resembling viral particles. Viral infection has been proposed as the underlying etiology, although this theory is controversial. Even in the absence of active remodeling, Paget disease can be recognized as a disorganized array of osteoid deposition (Figure 10.4), accompanied by increased vascularity. The abnormal bony deposition is not as strong as normal bone, and patients are at increased risk of fracture or deformity.
2. **Myeloproliferative neoplasms (MPNs)**: These neoplasms, especially primary myelofibrosis (PMF) or polycythemia vera, commonly show thickened trabecular bone in late stages, often accompanied by extensive marrow fibrosis. Underlying cellular changes of MPN may or may not be present.
3. **Other tumors**: Metastatic tumors are frequently associated with osteolytic changes in BM biopsies but can sometimes produce osteosclerosis (Figure 10.5).

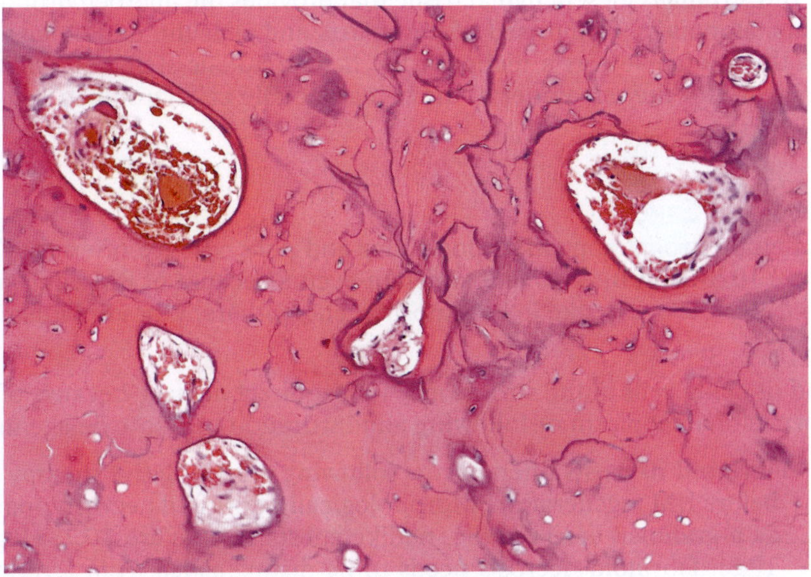

FIGURE 10.4 **Paget disease results in a disorganized array of osteoid deposition.** Photo courtesy of Dr. John Gross.

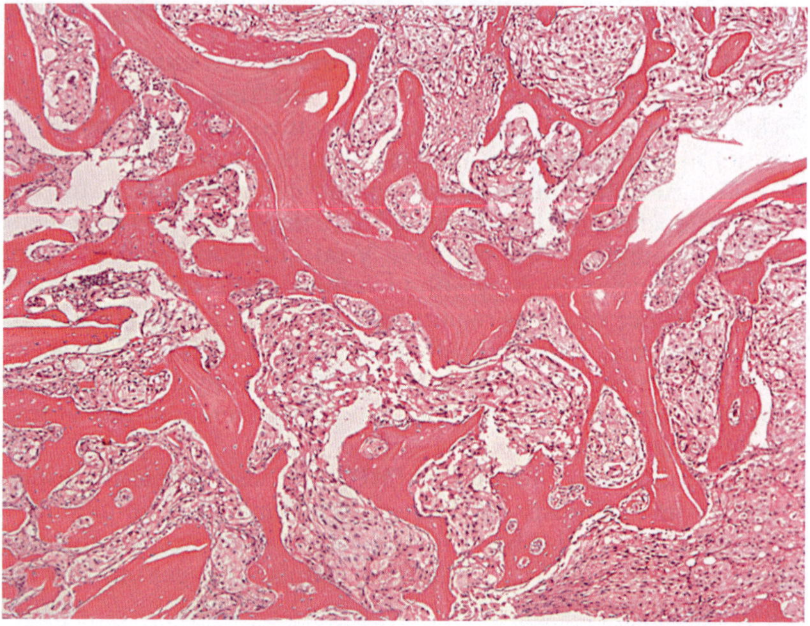

FIGURE 10.5 **Although most metastatic tumors produce osteolytic lesions, prostatic carcinoma in particular is associated with prominent osteosclerosis, visible here as thickened bony trabeculae.**

STROMA

The BM stroma is mesenchymal tissue that provides the microenvironment for hematopoiesis. Comprised of fibroblasts and reticulin and collagen fibers, the stroma acts as a niche for the hematopoietic stem cell and as a framework for the remainder of the hematopoietic cellular milieu.

Stromal Abnormalities

Edematous Stroma

Edematous stroma appears hypocellular and pale because of excess fluid (Figure 10.6A and B). This phenomenon occurs because of BM damage after a traumatic event, like toxin exposure, chemotherapy, or viral infection.

Necrotic Stroma

Dead or dying cells in the stroma may reflect direct damage because of the presence of a neoplasm or following administration of cytotoxic agents.

Fibrinoid necrosis often occurs following myeloablative therapy and before BM regeneration. Morphologically, fibrinoid necrosis appears as a granular, eosinophilic, netlike substance (Figure 10.7; eFigure 10.5). Fibrinoid necrosis needs to be distinguished from aspiration artifact, gelatinous transformation (serous fat atrophy), and amyloid deposition.

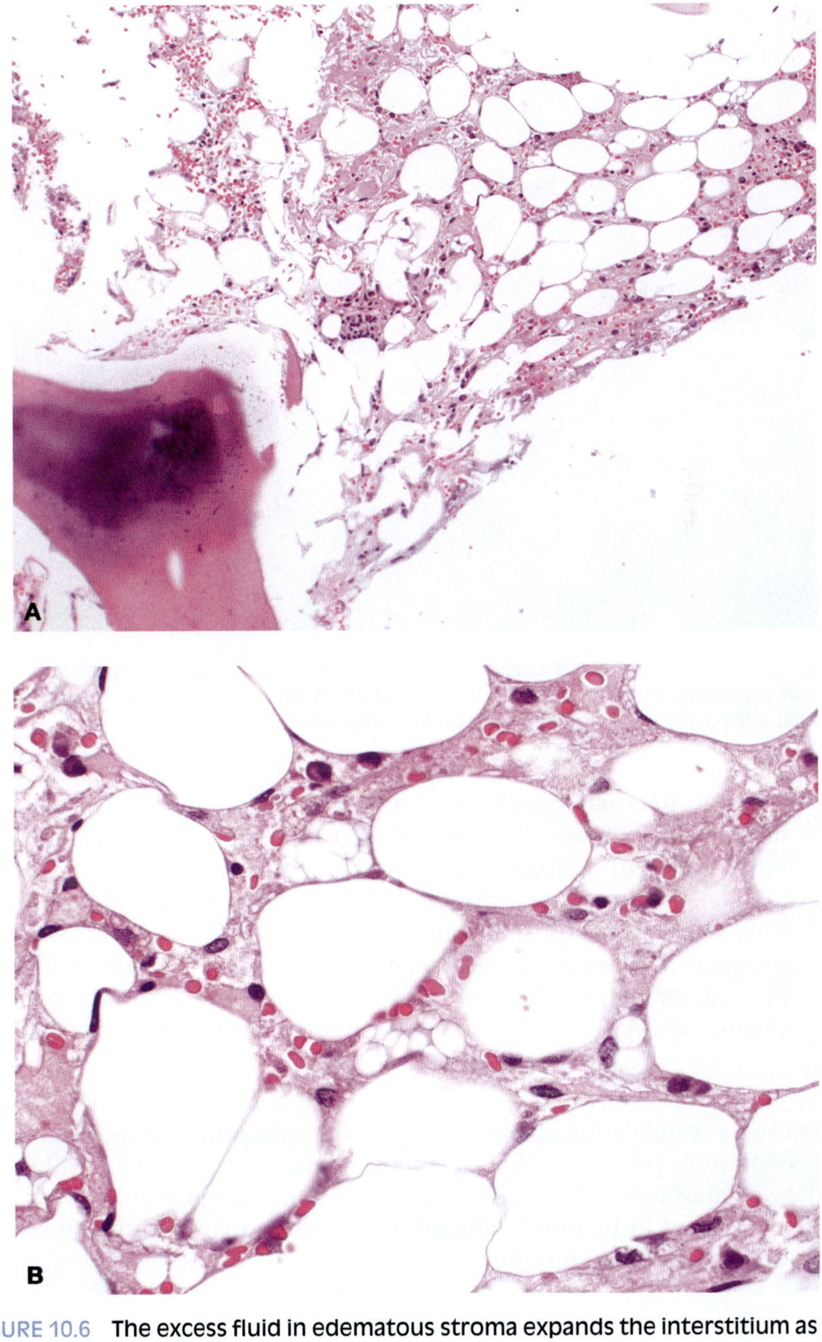

FIGURE 10.6 The excess fluid in edematous stroma expands the interstitium as pale pink, often granular material, as seen here in this bone marrow biopsy at low power (A) and high power (B).

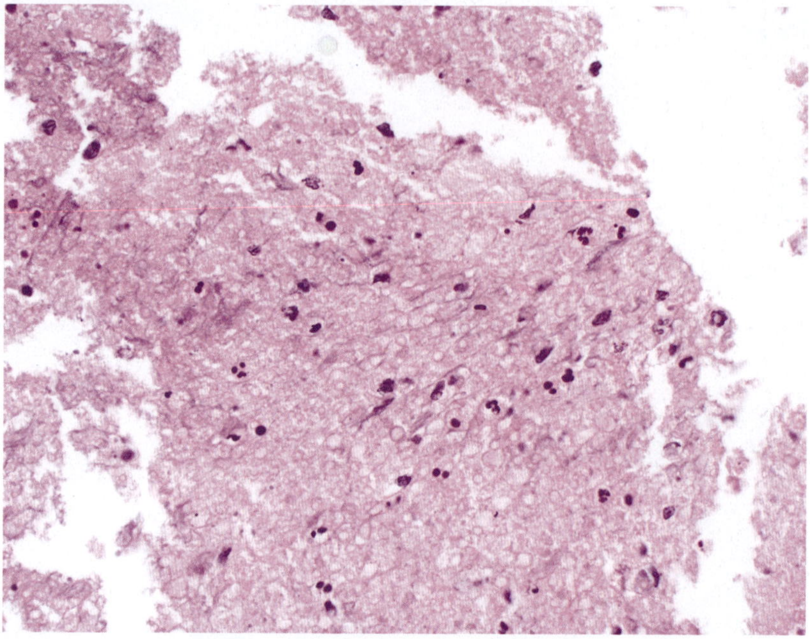

FIGURE 10.7 Marrow necrosis as a result of bone marrow damaging events such as toxin exposure, chemotherapy, or viral infection typically appears as amorphous material with admixed degenerating cellular elements.

Ischemic necrosis results from a lack of blood supply. It is uncommon, seen in fewer than 5% of BM biopsies, although it may be more frequent in particular disorders, including rapidly growing neoplasms like acute lymphoblastic leukemia (ALL). Patients with sickle cell disease in particular are prone to fat embolisms, which produce BM necrosis that can manifest as acute chest syndrome. Finding cellular outlines of dead cells, sometimes called ghost cells (Figure 10.8A and B), supports the diagnosis of ischemic necrosis.[4]

Gelatinous Transformation/Serous Fat Atrophy

This process results in fat atrophy and partial replacement of adipose tissue by eosinophilic, gelatinous, homogeneous, agranular material (hyaluronic acid) associated with BM hypoplasia (Figure 10.9; eFigure 10.6). This phenomenon occurs in metabolic disorders including extreme nutritional deprivation, cachexia, or starvation.[5,6]

Fibrosis

Fibroblasts produce increased amounts of collagen in response to various stimuli (eFigure 10.7). Fibrosis is typically associated with MPNs like PMF, and occasionally myelodysplastic syndrome (MDS) and/or acute myeloid leukemia (AML). Other neoplastic entities associated with BM fibrosis

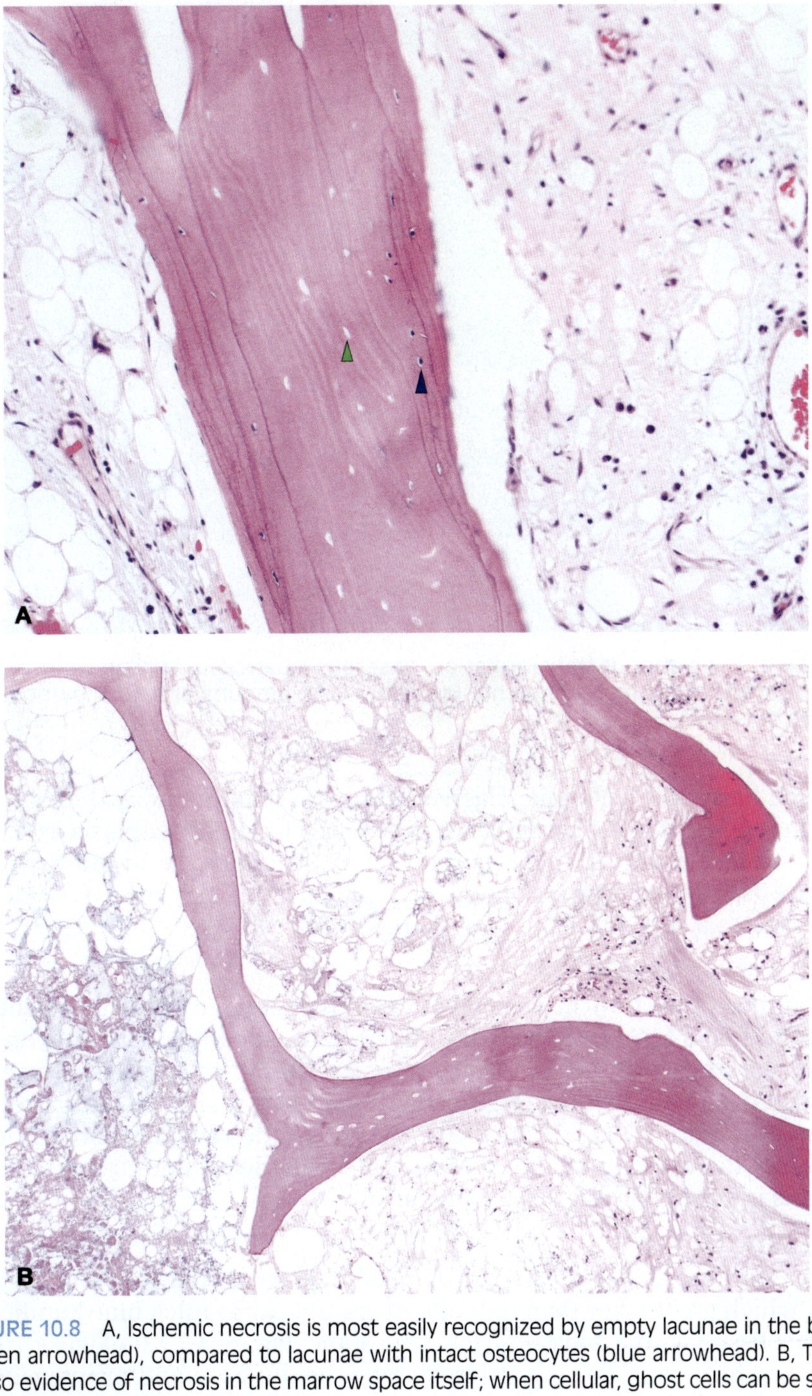

FIGURE 10.8 A, Ischemic necrosis is most easily recognized by empty lacunae in the bone (green arrowhead), compared to lacunae with intact osteocytes (blue arrowhead). B, There is also evidence of necrosis in the marrow space itself; when cellular, ghost cells can be seen. Photos courtesy of Dr. John Gross.

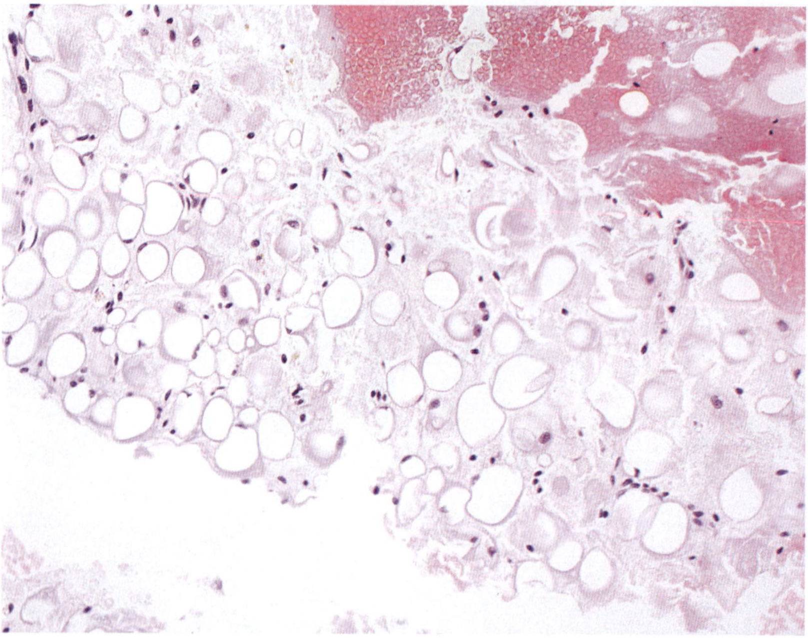

FIGURE 10.9 Gelatinous transformation, or serous fat atrophy, appears as increased pink proteinaceous material within fat cells as the amount of lipid they hold becomes depleted.

include hairy cell leukemia, classical Hodgkin lymphoma, and metastatic carcinoma. However, fibrosis is not necessarily a sign of neoplasia as it may be a sequela of infections, especially viral infections, or in autoimmune disease (see later). The detection of significant fibrosis on a BM biopsy necessitates a search for the underlying cause.

Reticulin Fibrosis

The primary reaction in stromal fibrosis is increased reticulin. Delicate reticulin fibers form a spiderweb of fibers, occasionally identifiable on hematoxylin and eosin (H&E) stain as a "streaming" effect caused by cells trapped in the meshworks (Figure 10.10) and best identified with a reticulin stain (Figure 10.11; eFigure 10.8). Grading the reticulin fibrosis helps establish the severity of the fibrosis and helps determine progression of fibrosis in future biopsies (see Chapter 6).[7]

Collagen Fibrosis

Increased fibrosis occurs after prolonged damage to the BM. Collagen fibers, which are thicker than reticulin fibers, appear as thick blue bundles of fibrous tissue with a Masson trichrome stain (Figure 10.12; eFigure 10.9). Collagen fibrosis is also graded, reflecting the duration and/or intensity of the insult.

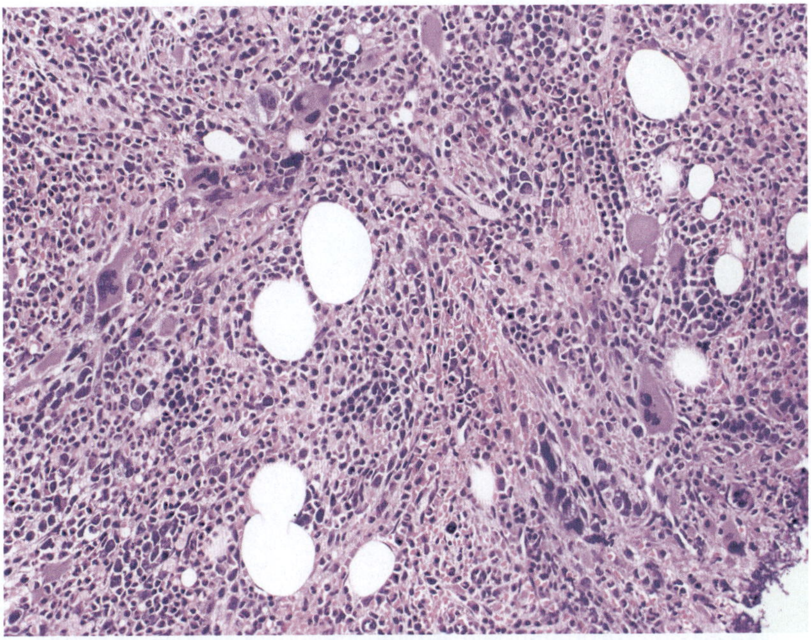

FIGURE 10.10 Fibrosis on hematoxylin and eosin appears as a "streaming" effect that entraps and distorts cells within the fibrotic meshwork.

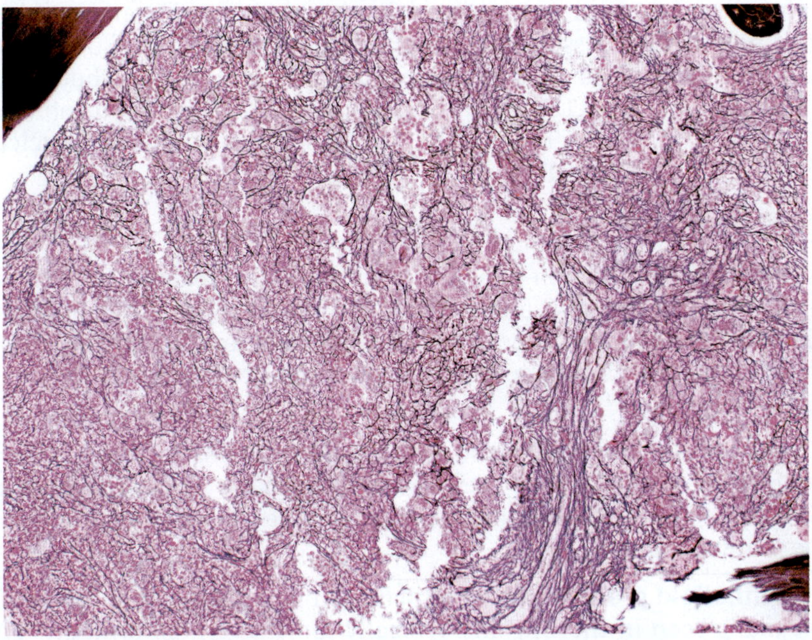

FIGURE 10.11 In a fibrotic marrow, reticulin deposition is the first process to occur. Delicate reticulin fibers form a spiderweb of fibers, best identified with a silver stain.

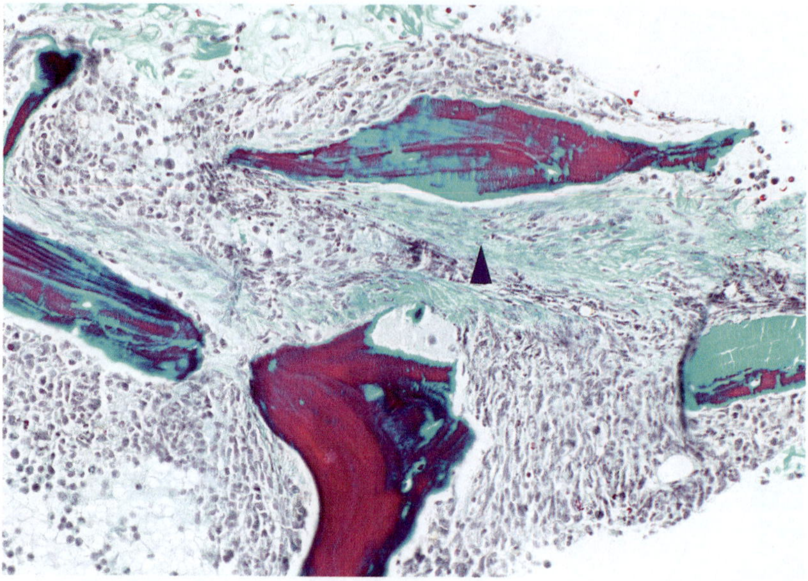

FIGURE 10.12 Collagen fibers, which are thicker than reticulin fibers, are identified using a Masson trichrome stain as blue-green thick bundles of fibrous tissue (arrowhead).

Fibrosis often results in an aspiculate BM aspirate ("dry tap"), a hemodiluted sample inadequate for evaluation. In these instances, a touch prep is helpful to assess cellular morphology. The fibers cause a physical distortion of red blood cells (RBCs) into teardrop shapes as they exit the BM sinuses (Figure 10.13). Fibrosis can also lead to leukoerythroblastosis (LEB) in the peripheral blood (PB), manifesting as circulating nucleated RBCs, giant platelets, and a myeloid left shift.

Histiocytosis

Most histiocytoses are non-neoplastic and represent reactive or accumulation disorders, although clonal histiocytic disorders and rare malignant histiocytic neoplasms may be seen. Histiocytoses may be diffuse or focal, with clusters of distinctive cells. Some examples are listed below.

Granulomas

Granulomas are non-neoplastic focal clusters of histiocytes. There are several types of granulomas seen in the BM, many of which are due to systemic infections, whether or not organisms can be demonstrated in the tissue section.[8]

Epithelioid granulomas, of which there are many types, are not normally seen in the BM and typically indicate an abnormality. These may be associated with systemic infections, autoimmune or neoplastic conditions, like lymphoma (particularly Hodgkin lymphoma),

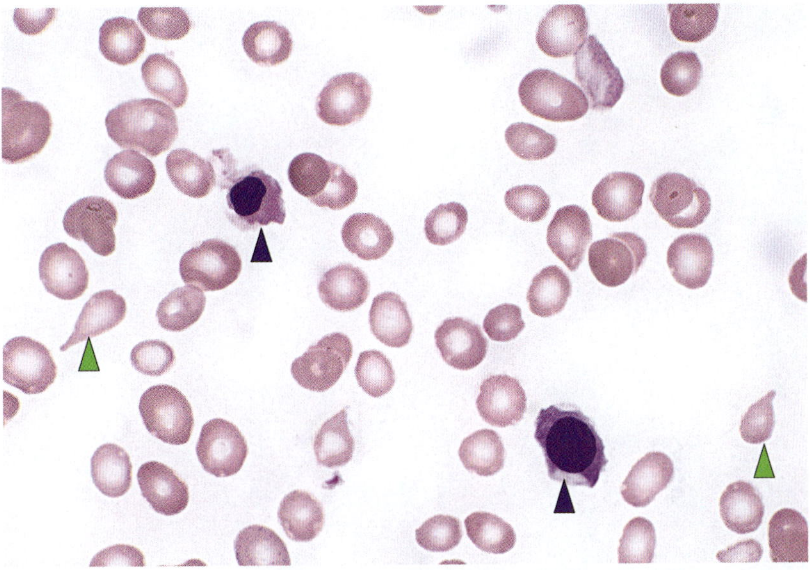

FIGURE 10.13 Marrow fibrosis produces physical distortion of peripheral red blood cells into teardrop shapes (green arrowheads); nucleated red cells (blue arrowheads) are also common in the peripheral blood of patients with marrow fibrosis.

or sarcoidosis (eFigure 10.10). These granulomas are composed of histiocytes forming a cluster (Figure 10.14; eFigure 10.11) and thus mimicking epithelium, with no associated necrosis (as opposed to caseating granulomas). Immunosuppressed patients, particularly those with untreated HIV, are unlikely to have well-formed granulomas and may only show a poorly cohesive collection of histiocytes.

Caseating granulomas are clusters of histiocytes with central necrosis. These are usually associated with infectious organisms, especially *Mycobacterium* species. Mycobacteria and other infectious organisms (fungi, yeast) can sometimes be seen with special stains, like acid-fast bacilli (AFB), Grocott methenamine silver (GMS), or Schiff fungus (Figure 10.15; eFigure 10.12).

Ring granulomas are identified on tissue sections as a ring of histiocytes surrounding a central empty space. These granulomas are identified in infectious processes, most notably Q fever, discussed later.

Multinucleated giant cells are histiocytes with multiple nuclei, which do not cluster, but are usually seen associated with other histiocytes in epithelioid granulomas. These are nonspecific and may be seen in a variety of conditions.

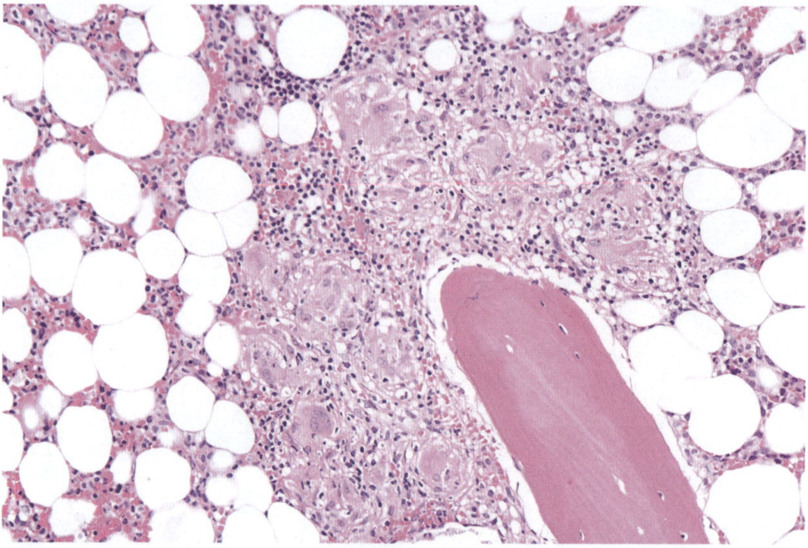

FIGURE 10.14 **Granulomatous inflammation in a marrow in a patient with sarcoidosis.** These epithelioid granulomas are comprised of large pink histiocytes in clusters with admixed small lymphocytes. Giant cells may or may not be present.

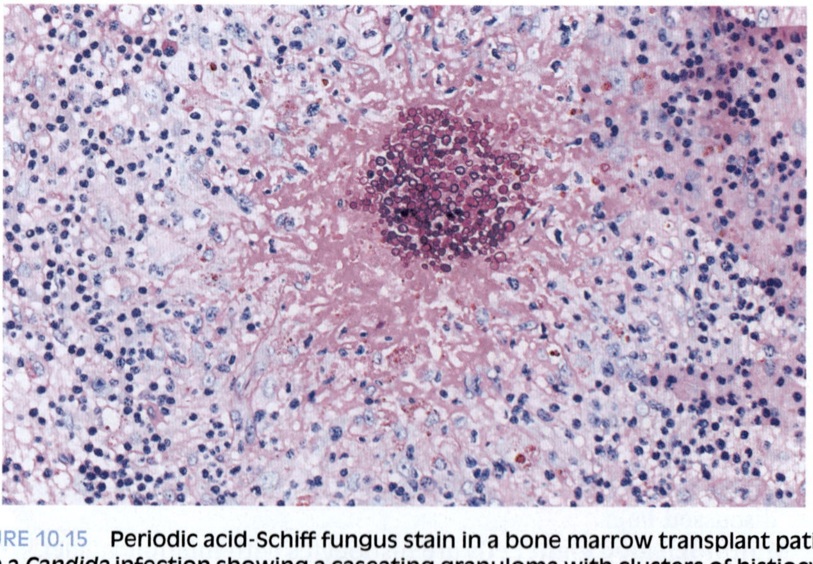

FIGURE 10.15 **Periodic acid-Schiff fungus stain in a bone marrow transplant patient with a *Candida* infection showing a caseating granuloma with clusters of histiocytes with organisms seen in the area of central necrosis.** Caseating granulomas are almost always associated with infectious organisms even if organisms cannot be demonstrated by special stains.

Lipogranulomas are normally seen in a subset of BM specimens (Figure 10.16). These are small focal collections of histiocytes with varying amounts of pink cytoplasm that become vacuolated as they absorb adipose tissue, often surrounded by a rim of lymphocytes.

As opposed to granulomas, **diffuse histiocytosis** is rare in the BM and is more likely to suggest a significant abnormality. Diffuse, non-neoplastic histiocytic lesions include hemophagocytic lymphohistiocytosis (HLH), storage diseases, and other rare reactive conditions.

Other nonspecific increases in histiocytes may be seen with myeloablative therapy, fat necrosis, and with certain lymphomas and also may occur after BM transplantation.

Hemophagocytic lymphohistiocytosis is a clinical syndrome that describes a pathologic systemic activation of histiocytes/macrophages, occasionally referred to as macrophage activation syndrome (MAS). HLH may be either primary or secondary:

Primary: Primary HLH is an autosomal recessive disorder with loss-of-function mutations in genes encoding perforin or other proteins that are primarily responsible for destroying activated immune cells. Patients are usually diagnosed at an early age. The treatment is BM transplant.

Secondary: Secondary HLH usually arises because of an infection, autoimmune disorder, or malignancy, which causes widespread activation of the innate immune system. This usually occurs in immunocompromised patients and is often triggered by a viral infection.

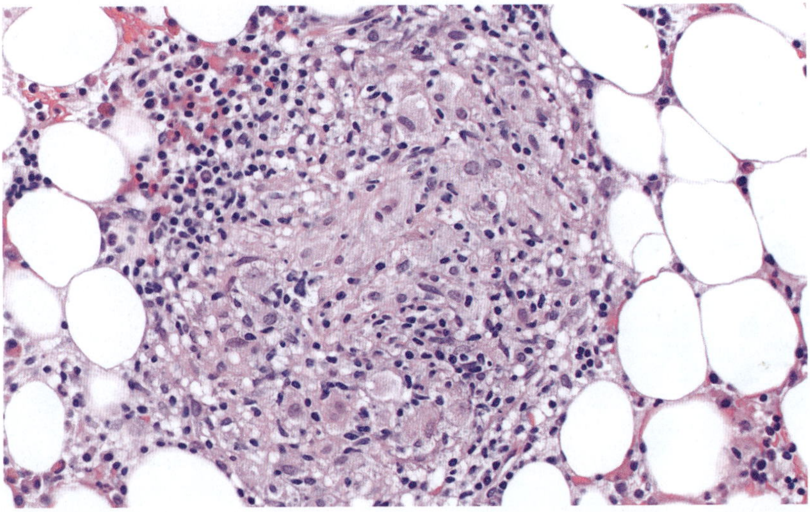

FIGURE 10.16 **Lipogranulomas are common in bone marrow and do not represent evidence of a systemic illness.** They can be recognized as clusters of histiocytes and admixed lymphocytes with variable amounts of lipid in vacuoles.

Cytokines activate macrophages and promote phagocytosis by upregulating adhesion molecules and major histocompatibility complex (MHC) molecules. Treatment not only requires managing the cytokine storm but also depends on the removal of the underlying cause.

In both primary and secondary HLH, patients present with high fever, hepatosplenomegaly, and variable lymphadenopathy. Other manifestations include abnormalities of liver function tests, coagulopathies, and cytopenias.[9]

Morphologic findings include phagocytic histiocytes in the BM aspirate or other tissues (Figure 10.17; eFigure 10.13). The histiocytes are bland-appearing with unremarkable nuclei and increased intracellular phagocytic debris.

Hemophagocytosis is not always identified in HLH and is not necessary for the diagnosis. Additionally, phagocytosis may be seen in patients without HLH, so this diagnosis is not based on morphology alone. Only florid hemophagocytosis should be reported as morphologic evidence of HLH. Diagnostic criteria include finding several of a list of abnormalities (Table 10.1), only one of which is the presence of hemophagocytosis.

Liposomal storage disorders are rare genetic disorders causing specific lysosomal enzyme defects and the subsequent accumulation of substrate proteins within histiocytes. There are many subtypes, but the most common include Gaucher disease and Niemann-Pick (NP) disease.

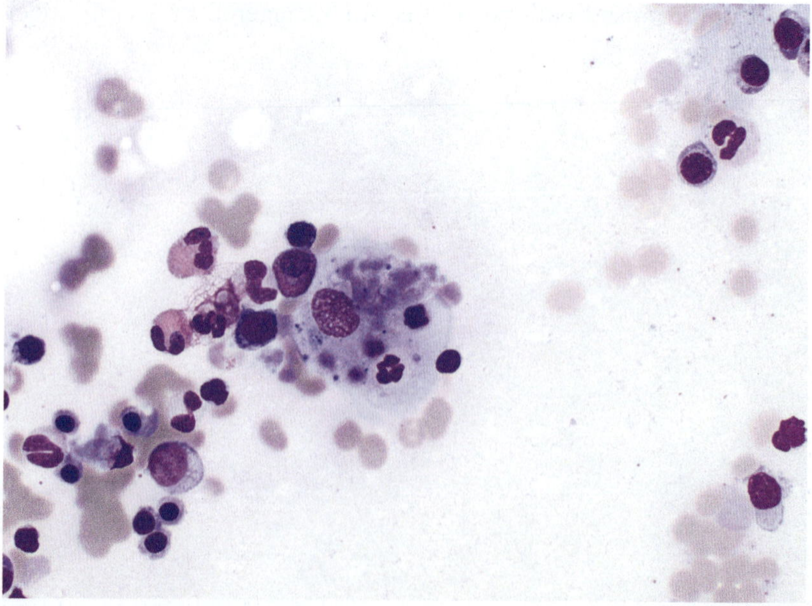

FIGURE 10.17 **A phagocytic macrophage in a patient with hemophagocytic lymphohistiocytosis (HLH).** Although this finding is not specific for HLH, and not all patients with HLH will display phagocytosis, it is considered one criterion in the clinical diagnosis.

TABLE 10.1 Clinical and Laboratory Findings in HLH

Finding	Value	Because of
Fever	>38.5°C	• Increased Interleukins
Cytopenias	ANC <1000/µL	• Increased INFγ
	Hgb <9 g/dL	• Increased TNFα
	Plt <100 000/µL	• Hemophagocytosis
Hypertriglyceridemia	Fasting TG (triglycerides) >265 mg/dL	• Decreased LPL because of TNFα
Low fibrinogen	<150 mg/dL	• Increased fibrinogen cleavage because of increased plasminogen activator secretion from macrophages
High ferritin	>500 ng/dL	• Secreted from activated macrophages
High soluble CD25 (IL-2 receptor)	>2400 U/mL	• Secreted from activated lymphocytes
Splenomegaly	Clinical exam	• Infiltration by T cells and NK cells
Hemophagocytosis	BM; Spleen bx	• Activated macrophages

ANC, absolute neutrophil count; BM, bone marrow; bx, biopsy; Hgb, hemoglobin; HLH, hemophagocytic lymphohistiocytosis; IL, interleukin; INFγ, interferon gamma; LPL, lipoprotein lipase; NK, natural killer; Plt, platelets; TNFα, tumor necrosis factor alpha.

The histiocytes in Gaucher disease have a low nuclear-to-cytoplasmic ratio and an amphophilic, striated "tissue paper"-like appearance of the cytoplasm (Figure 10.18A and B; eFigure 10.14). NP histiocytes are vacuolated, foamy macrophages. Sea-blue histiocyte syndrome is a subtype of NP, characterized by large histiocytes with blue cytoplasm, but the morphology is not specific; these as well as Gaucher-like or "pseudo-Gaucher histiocytes" are also seen in other conditions including those with increased cell turnover, particularly chronic myeloid leukemia (Figure 10.19) and hyperlipidemia.

Clonal histiocytoses include Rosai-Dorfman disease (RDD), Langerhans cell histiocytosis (LCH), and other rare non-LCH entities. Although many of these other histiocytoses may involve bone, they are only very rarely detected on routine marrow biopsies.

Rosai-Dorfman disease or sinus histiocytosis with massive lymphadenopathy (SHML) can occur anywhere in the body, even the bone, although it is rare in the BM.[10] The cells are large, with unique nuclear features. The cells display emperipolesis, which is characterized by cells passing through the ample histiocytic cytoplasm (Figure 10.20A and B; eFigure 10.15). The cells are positive for S100 and histiocytic markers, CD68 and CD163. At least a subset of cases are clonal and many have *RAS/MAPK* mutations.[11]

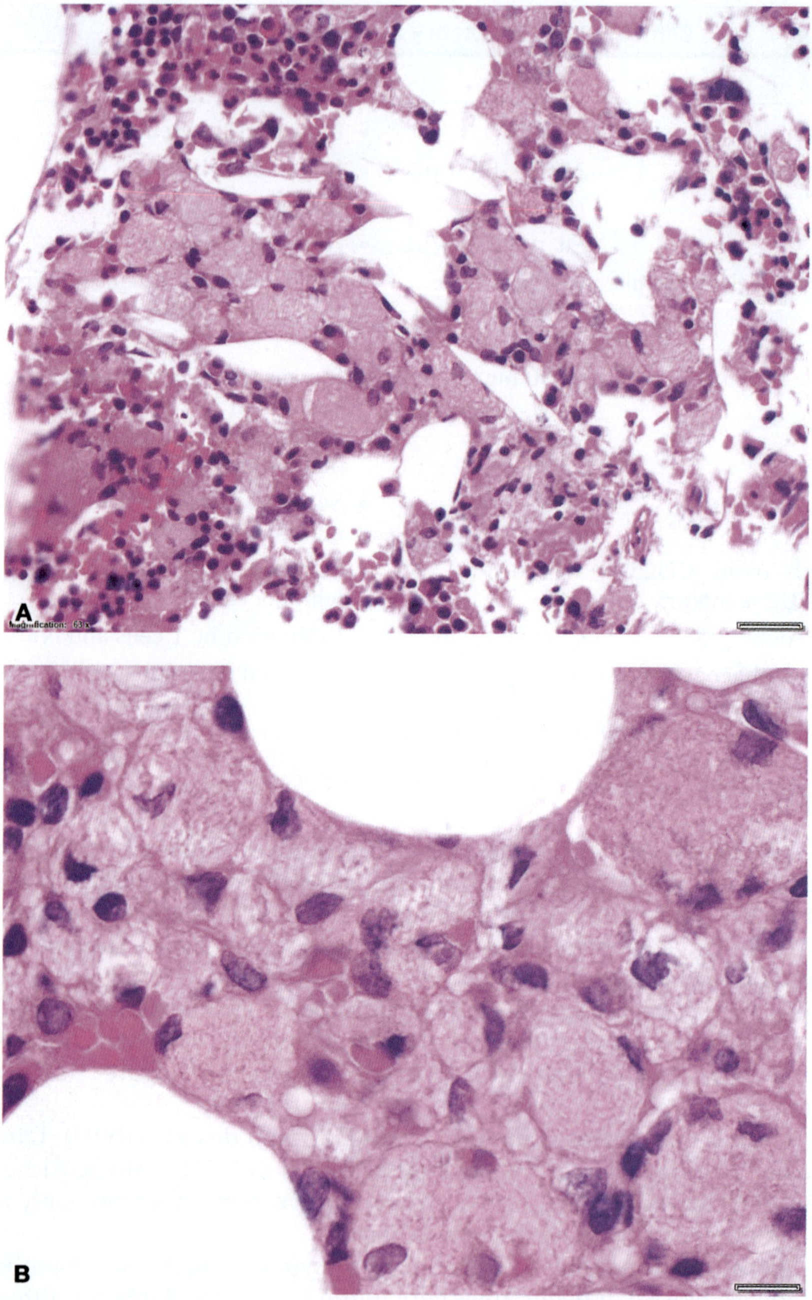

FIGURE 10.18 **Macrophages in a patient with Gaucher disease displaying so-called "wrinkled tissue paper" cytoplasm (A low power; B high power).** Photos courtesy of Dr. Xiaojun Wu.

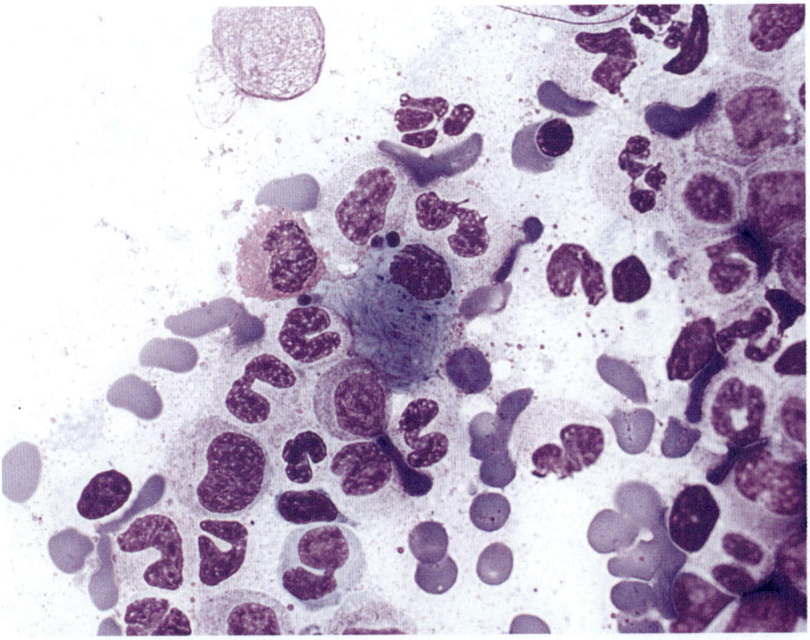

FIGURE 10.19 **Gaucher-like or pseudo-Gaucher cell in the bone marrow of a patient with chronic myelogenous leukemia (CML).** These sea-blue histiocytes are common in CML and may also be seen in other hematologic diseases with high cell turnover.

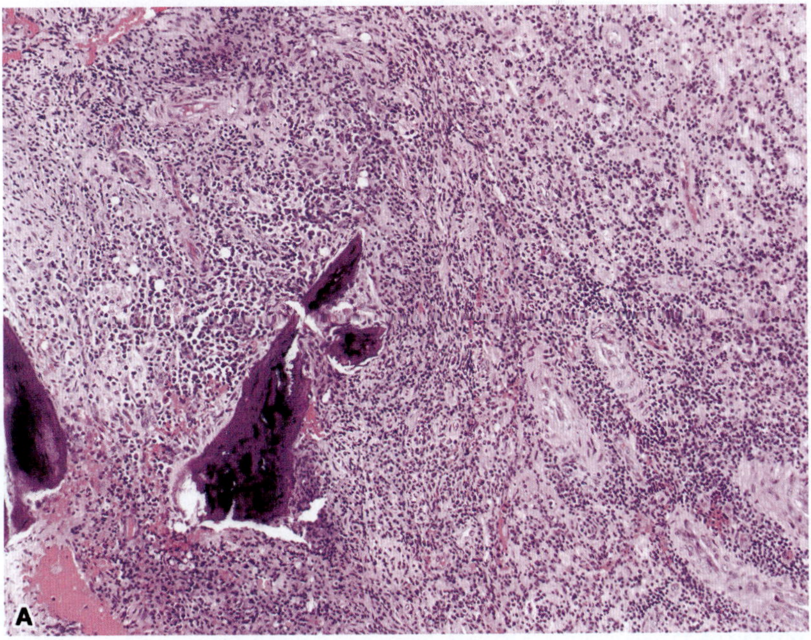

FIGURE 10.20 Rosai-Dorfman disease is relatively uncommon in bone marrow, but appears as a space-occupying lesion with a mixed inflammatory infiltrate with abundant plasma cells and variable numbers of characteristic macrophages in the background (A).

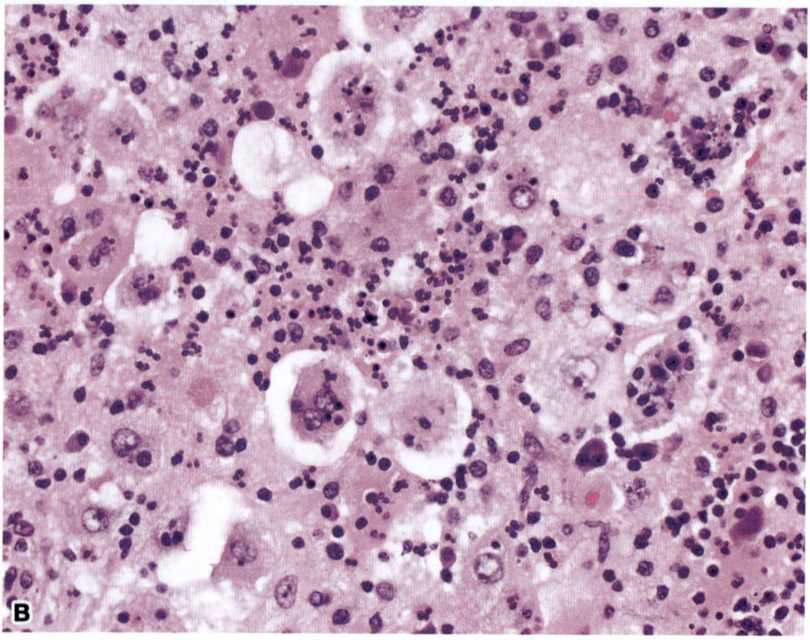

FIGURE 10.20 (*continued*) At high power (B), the macrophages have large round nuclei and display emperipolesis. Photos courtesy of Dr. John Gross.

Langerhans Cell Histiocytosis: Langerhans cells (LCs) usually reside in the skin and function as antigen-presenting cells in the lymph nodes (LNs). They are also found normally in small numbers in the BM. LCH is associated with *BRAF* V600E mutations, which cause a gain of function of the MAPK pathway, leading to LC proliferation, most often in LNs and skin, but occasionally in the BM.

Up to 20% of multisystem LCH have BM involvement, which appears as a diffuse histiocytosis on the core biopsy.[12,13] The cells have bland nucleoli and ample pink cytoplasm. LCs are positive for Langerin and BRAF immunohistochemistry (IHC), in addition to S100 and CD1a (Figure 10.21A-C; eFigure 10.16).

Erdheim-Chester disease (ECD) is a rare non-LC disorder of foamy histiocytes that involves the bone and extranodal tissue and has classic clinical and radiologic findings, including long bone osteosclerosis at the metadiaphysis.[14] Like LCH, patients with ECD may have activating mutations in the MAPK pathway. The cell of origin is uncertain, but is postulated to be a myeloid progenitor cell, as a subset of these patients have concurrent myeloid neoplasms, including chronic myelomonocytic leukemia (CMML).[15]

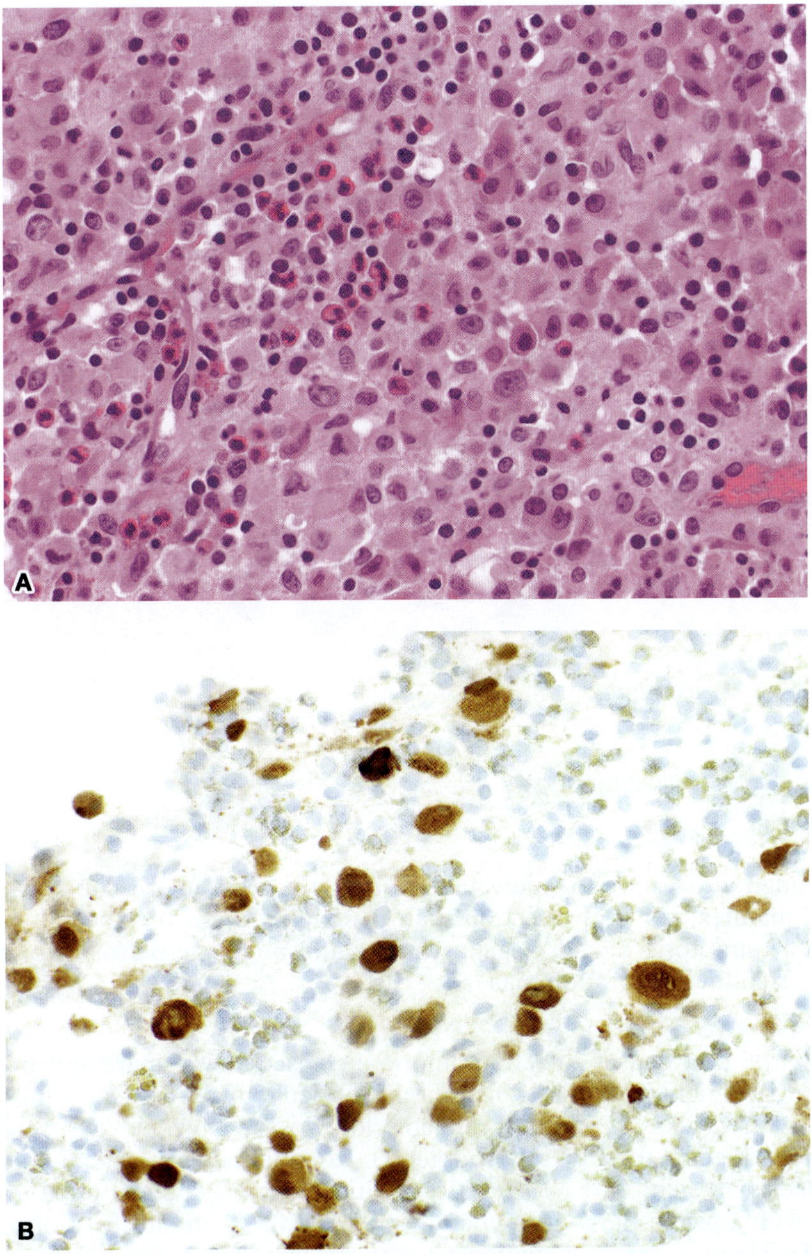

FIGURE 10.21 **Langerhans cell histiocytosis.** Hematoxylin and eosin section showing relatively small histiocytes with eccentric nuclei with a prominent admixture of eosinophils (A). Immunohistochemical stains are positive for S100 (B) and CD1a (C). Photos courtesy of Dr. John Gross.

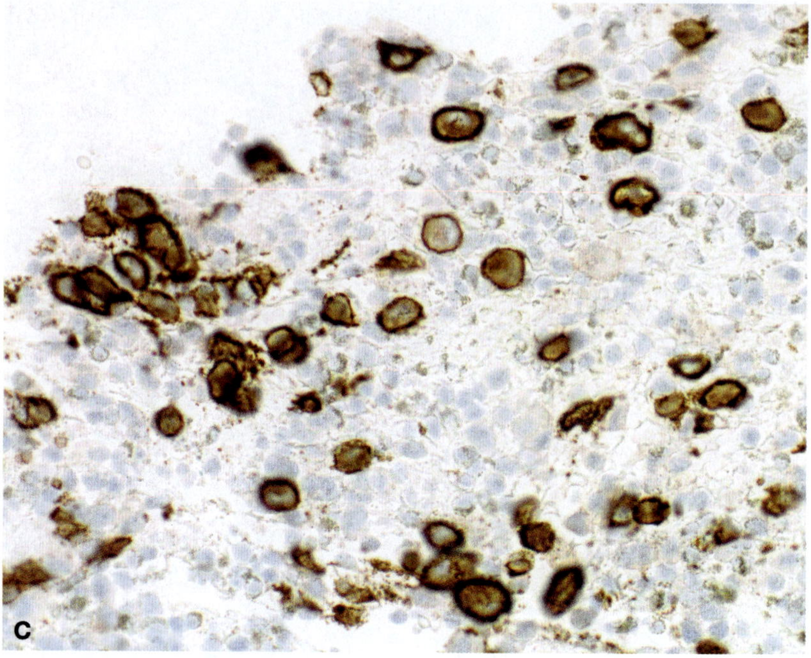

FIGURE 10.21 *(continued)*

INFECTIOUS ORGANISMS

Viral Infections

Although viruses are not detectable through routine microscopic evaluation, manifestations of infection may, depending upon the specific virus, include apoptotic/naked megakaryocytes and polytypic plasmacytosis, as well as epithelioid granulomas.[4]

Epstein-Barr Virus

The virus that causes infectious mononucleosis shows characteristic PB findings, which may mimic lymphoma or leukemia. Atypical lymphoid cells with variably prominent nucleoli, known as "Downey cells," are often identified in the PB (see Chapter 1). In patients with systemic mononucleosis, Epstein-Barr virus (EBV)–positive cells may be identified in the BM with Epstein-Barr virus–encoded RNA (EBER) in situ hybridization (ISH). There is rarely a significant marrow lymphocytosis, which, along with immunophenotyping, may help distinguish mononucleosis from lymphoid neoplasms. Often, in addition, there are small histiocytic clusters or epithelioid granulomas.

Human Immunodeficiency Virus

This RNA virus infects and destroys the host's CD4-positive T cells, which leads to CD4 lymphopenia that is the hallmark of the disease. In the BM, there may be atypical small naked megakaryocytes and dysplastic myeloid cells in addition to a marked polytypic plasmacytosis. Similar to infection with EBV, HIV may show increased epithelioid granulomas, even in those patients without opportunistic infections. Although no longer common in the era of effective antiviral therapy, patients with HIV used to have infections with *Mycobacterium avium* complex, which manifest as poorly formed granulomas with abundant organisms detected with AFB stains. Patients with HIV are at an increased risk of not only infections, but are also prone to develop lymphomas that may also involve the marrow.

Parvovirus B19

This virus, which replicates only in erythroid progenitors, causes an acquired anemia characterized by near absence of mature RBCs in the BM. Abnormal proerythroblasts are present, with characteristic prominent nuclear inclusions (Figure 10.22; eFigure 10.17), but there is essentially always a maturation arrest. Immunocompromised patients, like those following BM transplant, may be at a higher risk. Parvovirus infection is common in patients with sickle cell anemia and is responsible for the so-called aplastic crisis.

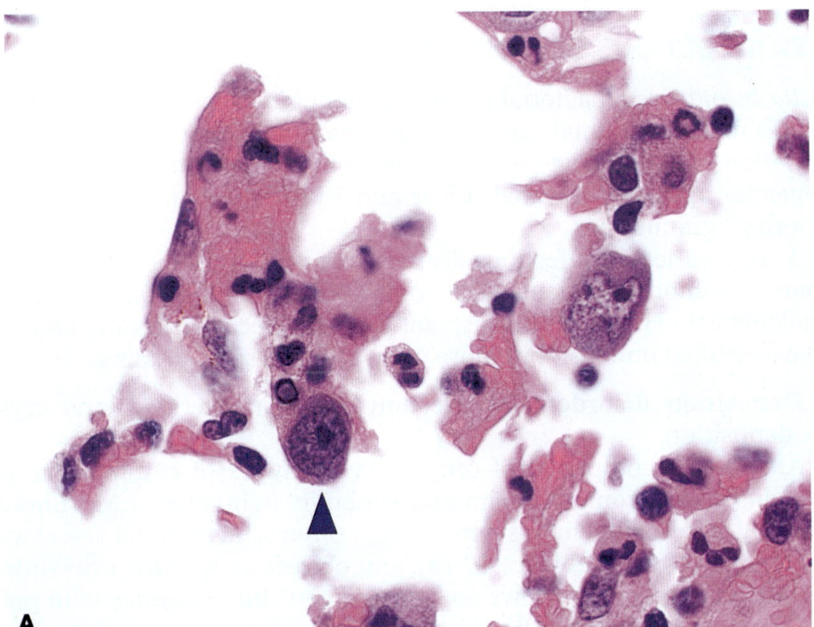

FIGURE 10.22 Parvovirus infection showing the characteristic giant pronormoblasts with prominent nuclear inclusions in a hematoxylin and eosin section (A) and on the aspirate smear (B) (arrowheads). Maturing erythroid elements are essentially absent.

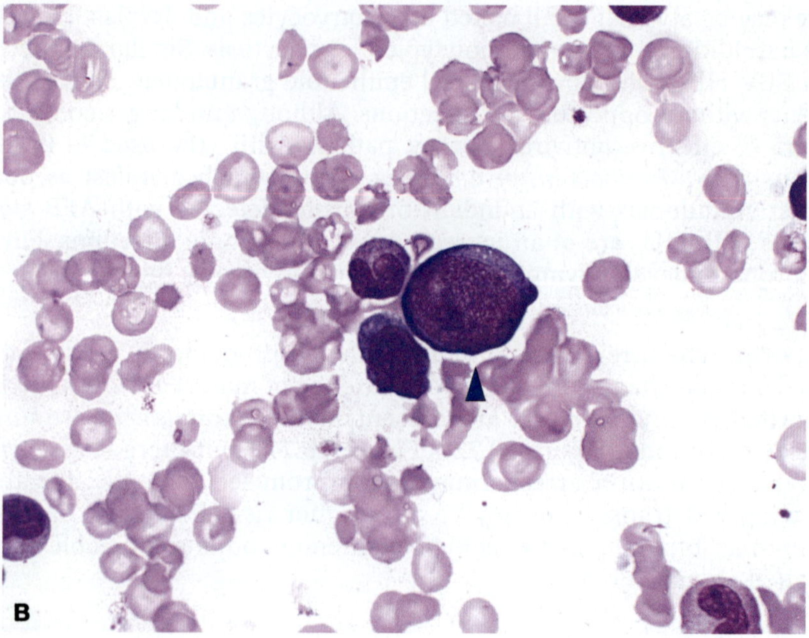

FIGURE 10.22 (*continued*)

OTHER INFECTIOUS ORGANISMS

Coxiella burnetii is a bacterial organism that causes acute Q fever. The organism is found in animals and is an occupational hazard for farmers and veterinarians. Thrombocytopenia is present in 25% of patients, and hepatic enzymes are typically elevated. Liver and BM biopsies may show classic "fibrin-ring" granulomas.

A wide variety of infectious diseases can be seen in the BM, but these are most common in patients with compromised immune systems, including patients with HIV or posttransplant patients. Occasionally, the organism may be identified on H&E but more often requires special stains.

Deposition disorders include amyloid, iron overload, and crystal deposition.

Amyloid is comprised of one of several types of extracellular proteins, most commonly immunoglobulin light chain. Morphologically, it is homogeneous and smudgy, often seen in blood vessel walls (Figure 10.23A; eFigure 10.18), and occasionally in the interstitium. A Congo red stain shows an "apple green" birefringence with polarization (Figure 10.23B; eFigure 10.19). Ultrastructural features include twisted β-pleated sheets of fibrils of varying lengths.

Iron overload may be seen in hereditary hemochromatosis, chronic liver disease, and diseases with chronic red cell destruction, although

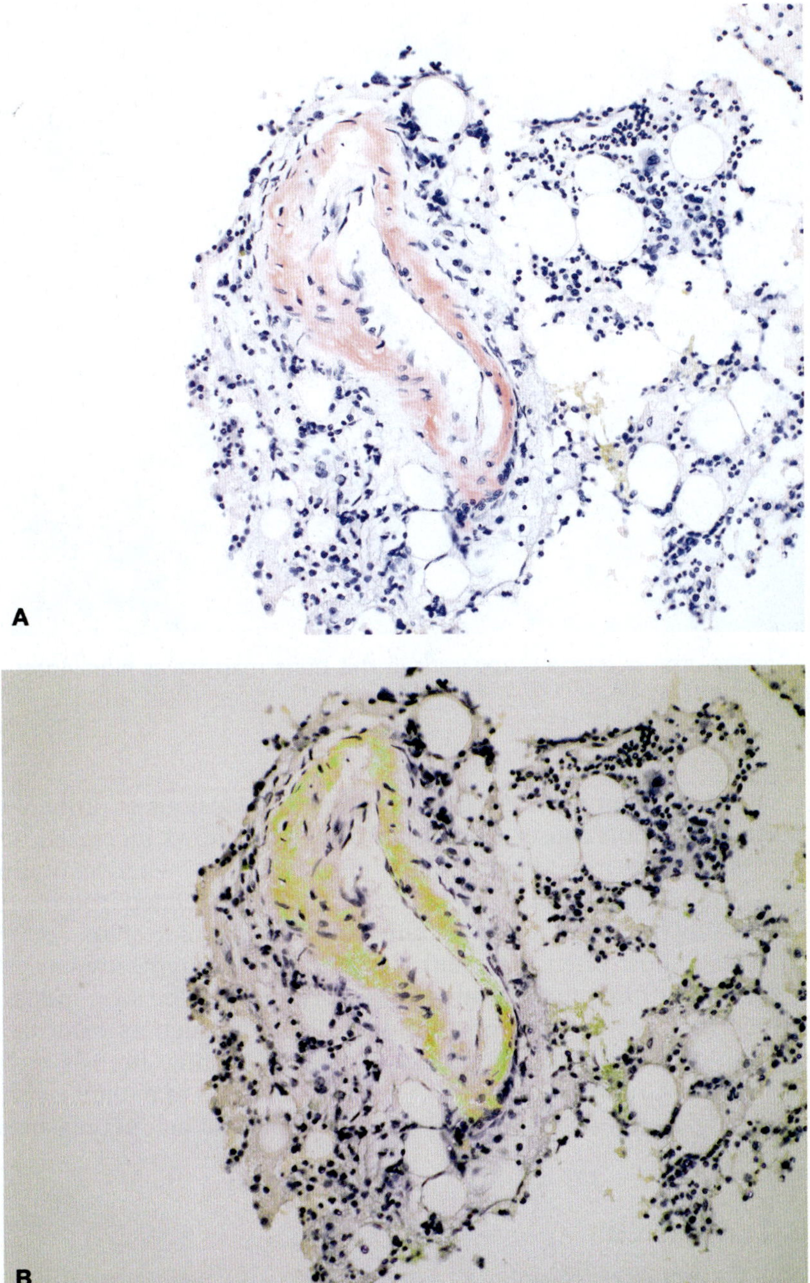

FIGURE 10.23 **In a bone marrow section, amyloid deposition is most evident in vessels.** Congo red (A) highlights amyloid that appears orangeophilic on hematoxylin and eosin stain and shows "apple green" birefringence under polarized light (B).

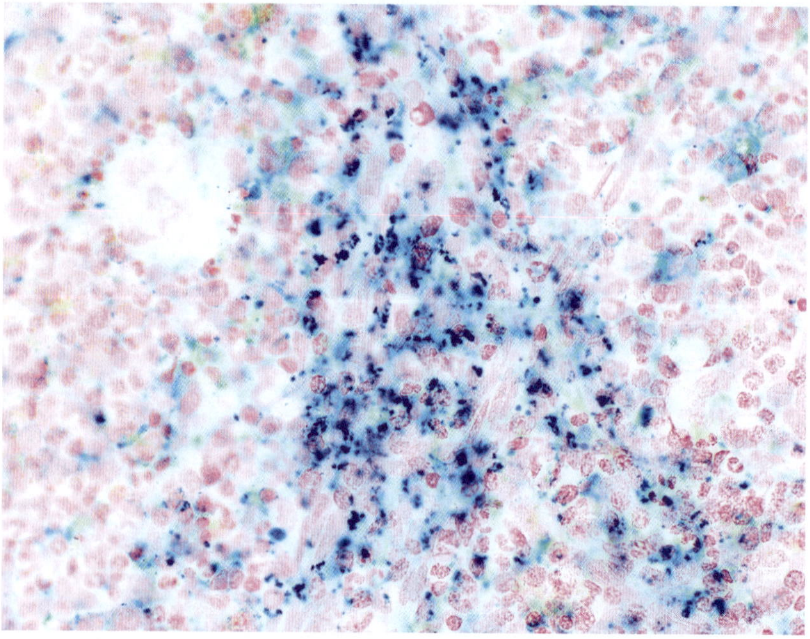

FIGURE 10.24 Iron overload is apparent in this bone marrow, as highlighted by a Prussian blue stain.

iatrogenic iron overload from multiple transfusions is probably the most common cause. A Prussian blue stain shows increased histiocytic storage iron (Figure 10.24; eFigure 10.20), whereas erythroid iron may or may not be increased. Transfusion-related iron overload typically has a beaded appearance on Prussian blue stain.

Crystals most often represent a fixation artifact typically caused by formalin or mercurial fixatives. True crystals may be seen in marrow macrophages in rare constitutional disorders such as oxalosis and cystinosis, and the background marrow may show fibrosis or bony changes. Crystals can also be seen in histiocytes in patients with immunoglobulin deposition disorders and plasma cell neoplasms (see Chapter 9).[16]

OTHER DISORDERS

Systemic lupus erythematosus (SLE) is an idiopathic immunologic disorder that may present with a myriad of systemic manifestations, including cytopenias. Although BM examination is not usually indicated, patients with severe, unexpected cytopenias may require one.

The BM is variably cellular in SLE: SLE patients with increased large granular lymphocyte (LGL) populations or those taking certain medications may have hypocellular marrows, whereas patients with autoantibodies or hemolytic anemias may present with hypercellular marrows. Lymphocytes and plasma cells are also often increased in BM biopsies of patients with SLE. In comparison with the general population, patients with SLE are at increased risk of osteoporosis, osteonecrosis, and osteomyelitis.[17]

Autoimmune myelofibrosis: Some patients with SLE or other autoimmune disorders who have a BM examined for cytopenia may rarely have a fibrotic marrow that morphologically resembles an MPN. Most often, the BM is hypercellular with erythroid hyperplasia, intrasinusoidal hematopoiesis, and scattered small lymphoid aggregates.[18]

METASTATIC CARCINOMA

Patients with newly diagnosed malignancies typically undergo BM biopsies to assess the stage of disease. Additionally, detecting cytopenias in a patient with a known malignancy should prompt a BM biopsy. Metastatic disease should be especially considered in older patients with unexplained cytopenias.

The type of metastatic carcinoma most often identified in the BM depends on the demographic of the patient and the proclivity of the tumor to home to the BM (Table 10.2).[19]

PEDIATRIC PATIENTS

Small round blue cell tumors (SRBCTs), more commonly seen in the pediatric population, resemble lymphoid or erythroid cells on a core biopsy, and minimal involvement may be very difficult to detect with the naked eye. Special stains are warranted for staging BMs in patients with these malignancies (Figure 10.25A and B; eFigure 10.21).

TABLE 10.2 The Most Common Bone Marrow Metastases Seen in Pediatric Patients Versus Adults

Pediatric patient	Adult patient
Neuroblastoma	Breast
Retinoblastoma	Prostate
Ewing sarcoma	Gastrointestinal
Rhabdomyosarcoma	Lung
Medulloblastoma	Kidney

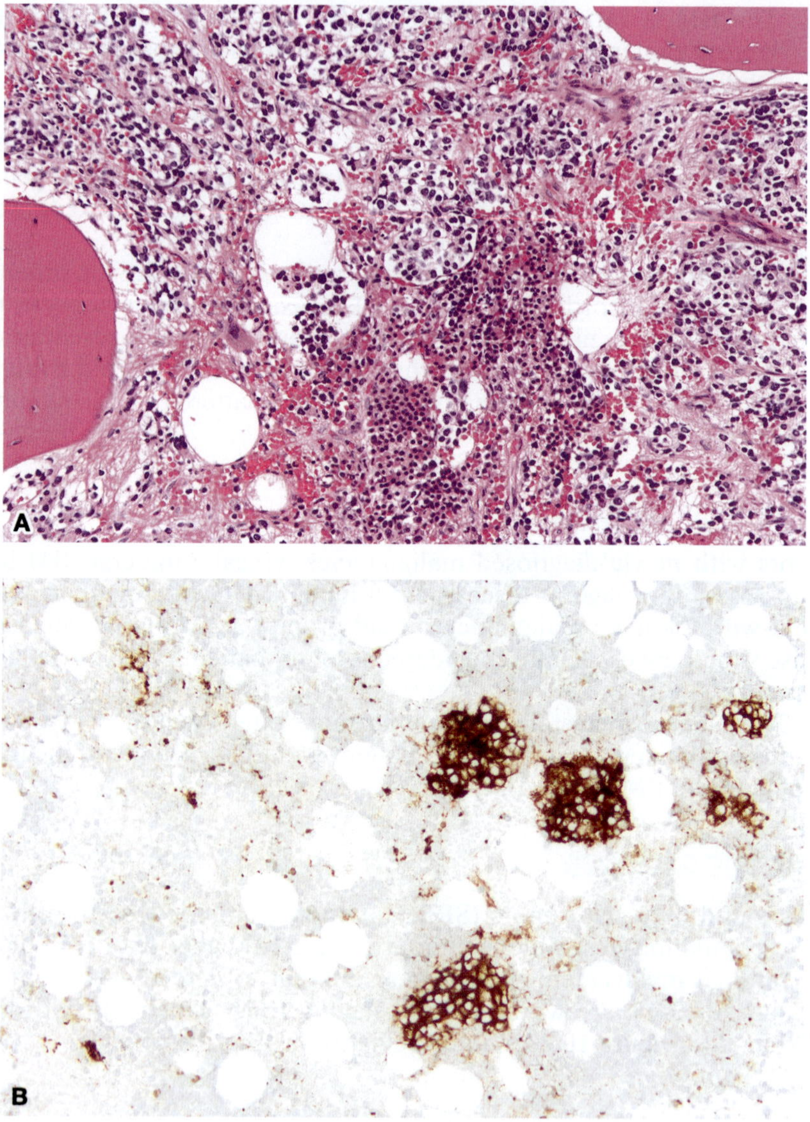

FIGURE 10.25 Small round blue cell tumors in pediatric patients may resemble erythroid or lymphoid cells, although when abundant, as in this case of neuroblastoma, form distinct nests (A). Immunohistochemistry, in this case for synaptophysin (B), is often necessary to identify these metastases, especially if only very small deposits are present.

Additionally, SRBCTs may mimic ALL, as both these disorders are comprised of small cells with scant cytoplasm. In such instances, a panel of IHC stains may be necessary for a diagnosis.

ADULT PATIENTS

The adult population is more often affected by metastatic epithelial carcinomas, including breast cancer (eFigure 10.22), prostate cancer (eFigure 10.23), gastrointestinal (GI) cancer, and lung cancer. These subtypes are more prone to travel to the BM. Metastatic lesions may cause osteolytic lesions, osteoblastic (or sclerotic) lesions, or both.[20]

Lobular breast carcinoma has a unique, single-cell pattern of infiltration, which may be difficult to detect on H&E and may require IHC stains (Figure 10.26A and B). Some cancers are associated with such extensive fibrosis that it obscures tumor cells, so that IHC for epithelial markers may be needed to identify the metastasis. Other metastatic tumors are bland-appearing and may be mistaken for histiocytic cells or other cells, but are easily recognized by IHC (Figure 10.27A and B).

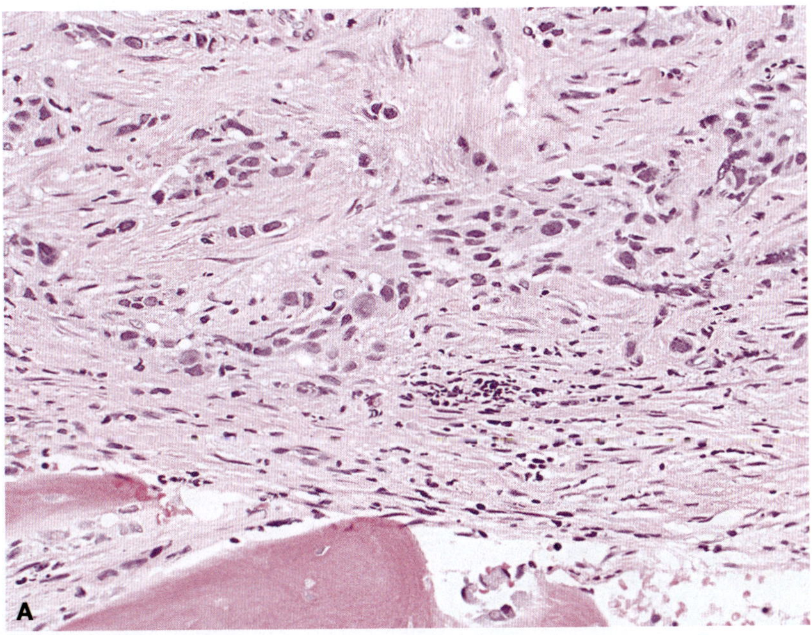

FIGURE 10.26 Metastatic breast carcinoma can appear as small nests of cells, or even individual cells trapped in a fibrous stroma (A) and can be highlighted by immunohistochemical stains for cytokeratin (B).

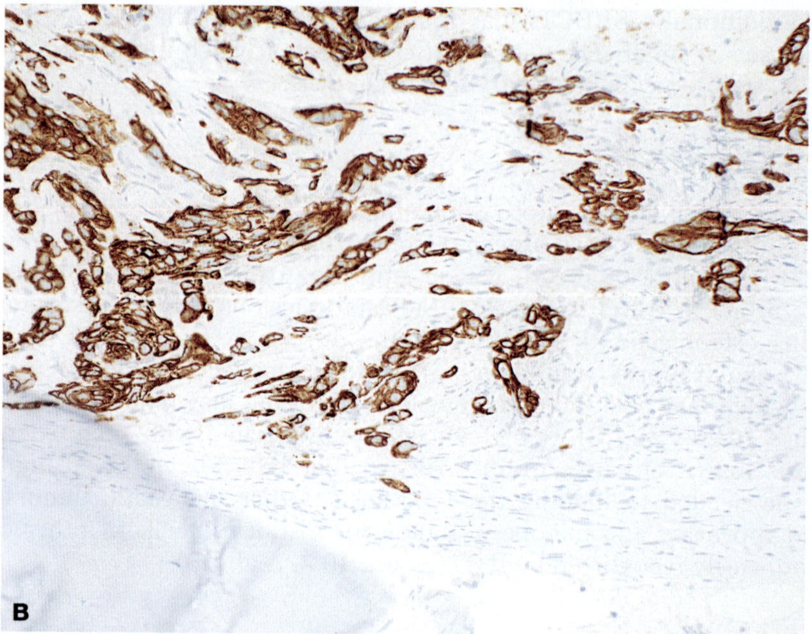

FIGURE 10.26 (*continued*)

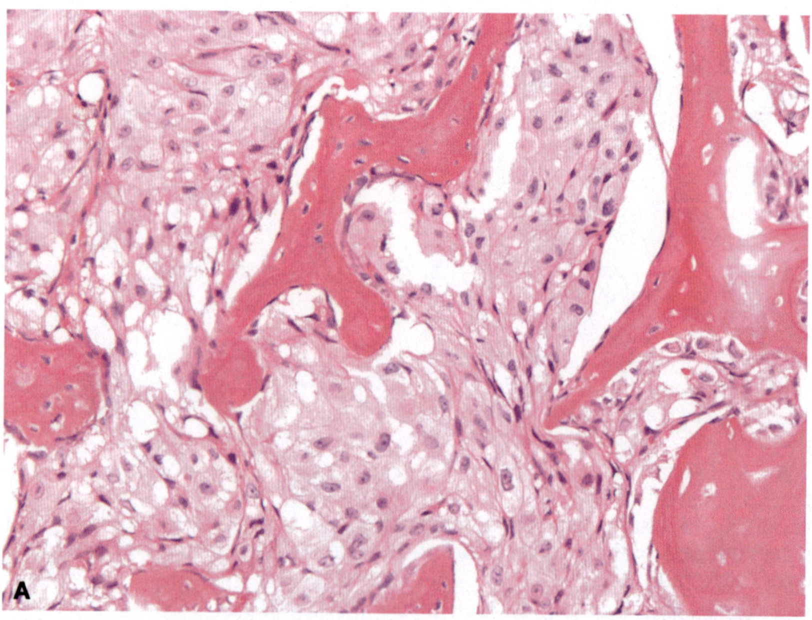

FIGURE 10.27 At high power (A), prostatic tumor cells can be very bland and resemble histiocytes, but can be identified with immunohistochemical stains for NKX 3.1 (B).

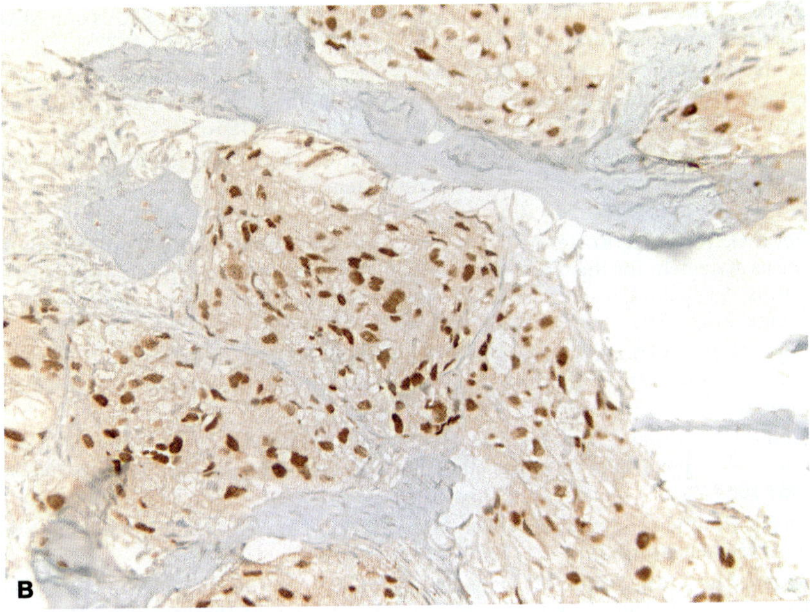

FIGURE 10.27 (*continued*)

REFERENCES

1. Høilund-Carlsen PF, Hess S, Werner TJ, Alavi A. Cancer metastasizes to the bone marrow and not to the bone: time for a paradigm shift! *Eur J Nucl Med Mol Imaging*. 2018;45(6):893-897.
2. Silverberg SJ, Shane E, de la Cruz L, et al. Skeletal disease in primary hyperparathyroidism. *J Bone Miner Res*. 1989;4(3):283-291.
3. Shaker JL. Paget's disease of bone: a review of epidemiology, pathophysiology and management. *Ther Adv Musculoskelet Dis*. 2009;1(2):107-125.
4. Diebold J, Molina T, Camilleri-Broët S, Le Tourneau A, Audouin J. Bone marrow manifestations of infections and systemic diseases observed in bone marrow trephine biopsy review. *Histopathology*. 2000;37(3):199-211.
5. Böhm J. Gelatinous transformation of the bone marrow: the spectrum of underlying diseases. *Am J Surg Pathol*. 2000;24(1):56-65.
6. Naeim F, Nagesh Rao P, Song SX, Phan RT. Morphology of abnormal bone marrow and extramedullary hematopoiesis. In: Naeim F, Nagesh Rao P, Song SX, Phan RT, eds. *Atlas of Hematopathology*. 2nd ed. Academic Press; 2018:89-104.
7. Bauermeister DE. Quantitation of bone marrow reticulin–a normal range. *Am J Clin Pathol*. 1971;56(1):24-31.
8. James DG. A clinicopathological classification of granulomatous disorders. *Postgrad Med J*. 2000;76(898):457-465.
9. Rosado FGN, Kim AS. Hemophagocytic lymphohistiocytosis: an update on diagnosis and pathogenesis. *Am J Clin Pathol*. 2013;139(6):713-727.
10. Huang Q, Chang KL, Weiss LM. Extranodal Rosai-Dorfman disease involving the bone marrow: a case report. *Am J Surg Pathol*. 2006;30(9):1189-1192.

11. Garces S, Medeiros LJ, Patel KP, et al. Mutually exclusive recurrent KRAS and MAP2K1 mutations in Rosai-Dorfman disease. *Mod Pathol.* 2017;30(10):1367-1377.

12. Kumar M, Updesh Singh Sachdeva M, Naseem S, et al. Bone marrow infiltration in Langerhan's cell histiocytosis – an unusual but important determinant for staging and treatment. *Int J Hematol-Oncol Stem Cell Res.* 2015;9(4):193-197.

13. Galluzzo ML, Braier J, Rosenzweig SD, Garcia de Dávila MT, Rosso D. Bone marrow findings at diagnosis in patients with multisystem Langerhans cell histiocytosis. *Pediatr Dev Pathol.* 2010;13(2):101-106.

14. Goyal G, Young JR, Koster MJ, et al. The Mayo clinic histiocytosis working group consensus statement for the diagnosis and evaluation of adult patients with histiocytic neoplasms: Erdheim-Chester disease, Langerhans cell histiocytosis, and Rosai-Dorfman disease. *Mayo Clin Proc.* 2019;94(10):2054-2071.

15. Goyal G, Ravindran A, Liu Y, et al. Bone marrow findings in Erdheim-Chester disease: increased prevalence of chronic myeloid neoplasms. *Haematologica.* 2020;105(2): e84-e86.

16. Brodie C, Agrawal S, Rahemtulla A, O'Shea D, Lampert I, Naresh KN. Multiple myeloma with bone marrow extracellular crystal deposition. *J Clin Pathol.* 2007;60(9): 1064-1065.

17. Rella V, Rotondo C, Altomare A, Cantatore FP, Corrado A. Bone involvement in systemic lupus erythematosus. *Int J Mol Sci.* 2022;23(10):5804.

18. Vergara-Lluri ME, Piatek CI, Pullarkat V, et al. Autoimmune myelofibrosis: an update on morphologic features in 29 cases and review of the literature. *Hum Pathol.* 2014;45(11):2183-2191.

19. Kucukzeybek BB, Calli AO, Kucukzeybek Y, et al. The prognostic significance of bone marrow metastases: evaluation of 58 cases. *Indian J Pathol Microbiol.* 2014;57(3): 396-399.

20. Macedo F, Ladeira K, Pinho F, et al. Bone metastases: an overview. *Oncol Rev.* 2017;11(1):321.

INDEX

Note: Page numbers followed by *f* and *t* indicates figures and tables respectively.

B